Adam C⟨...⟩

Dept of

Royal London Hospital

Whitechapel London E1.

Mechanical Circulatory Support

Edited by ————————————————————

Terence Lewis FRCS

Department of Cardiothoracic Surgery,
The Royal London Hospital, London, UK

Timothy R Graham MD FRCS MBES

The Cardiothoracic Surgical Unit,
The Queen Elizabeth Hospital, Birmingham, UK
Formerly Department of Cardiothoracic Surgery, The Royal London Hospital

Co-editors ————————————————————

O HOWARD FRAZIER MD
Department of Cardiac Transplantation,
Texas Heart Institute, Houston, Texas, USA

J DONALD HILL MD
Department of Cardiac Surgery, California Pacific
Medical Center, San Francisco, California, USA

D GLENN PENNINGTON MD
Department of Surgery, St Louis University School
of Medicine, St Louis, Missouri, USA

STANLEY SALMONS BSc PhD ARCS DIC MBES FZS
British Heart Foundation Skeletal Muscle Assist
Research Group, Department of Human Anatomy
and Cell Biology, University of Liverpool, Liverpool, UK

Edward Arnold

A member of the Hodder Headline Group
LONDON BOSTON SYDNEY AUCKLAND

Distributed in the Americas by
Little, Brown and Company, 34 Beacon Street, Boston, MA 02108
First published in Great Britain 1995 by
Edward Arnold, a division of Hodder Headline PLC,
338 Euston Road, London NW1 3BH

Whilst the advice and information in this book is believed to be true
and accurate at the date of going to press, neither the authors nor the publisher
can accept any legal responsibility or liability for any errors or omissions
that may be made. In particular (but without limiting the generality of the
preceding disclaimer) every effort has been made to check drug dosages;
however it is still possible that errors have been missed. Furthermore,
dosage schedules are constantly being revised and new side-effects
recognized. For these reasons the reader is strongly urged to consult the
drug companies' printed instructions before administering any of the drugs
recommended in this book.

British Library Cataloguing in Publication Data
A catalogue record for this book is available from the British Library

ISBN 0 340 57602 2

1 2 3 4 5   95 96 97 98 99

Typeset in 10/11 pt Baskerville by
Wearset, Boldon, Tyne and Wear.
Printed and bound in Great Britain by
The Bath Press, Avon

Contents

SECTION VIII   General Issues

List of contributors

JR Anderson, Department of Cardiac Surgery, St George's Hospital, London, UK

DL Bader, Interdisciplinary Research Centre in Biomedical Materials, Queen Mary and Westfield College, University of London, London, UK

CT Bowles, Harefield Hospital, Harefield, Middlesex, UK

M Buxton, Health Economics Research Group, Brunel University, Uxbridge, UK

C Cabrol, Department of Thoracic and Cardiovascular Surgery, La Pitie Hospital, Paris, France

AF Carpentier, Division of Cardiothoracic Surgery, Broussais Hospital, Paris, France

J-C Chachques, Division of Cardiothoracic Surgery, Broussais Hospital, Paris, France

JM Chen, Division of Circulatory Physiology, Columbia Presbyterian Medical Center, New York, NY, USA

MR Cleavinger, University of Arizona Heart Center, Tucson, Arizona, USA

S Cockroft, Anaesthetic Department, Salisbury District Hospital, Salisbury, UK

JG Copeland, University of Arizona Heart Center, Tucson, Arizona, USA

A Coumbe, Department of Morbid Anatomy, The Royal London Hospital, UK

KA Dasse, Department of Research and Development, Thermo Cardiosystems Inc, Woburn, Massachusetts, USA

PH Deleuze, Centre de Recherches Chirurgicales, CHU Henri Mondor, Creteil, France

JJ Dunning, Transplant Unit, Papworth Hospital, Papworth Everard, Cambridge, UK

Sir Terence English, Papworth Hospital, Papworth Everard, Cambridge, UK

DJ Farrar, Department of Cardiac Surgery, California Pacific Medical Center, San Francisco, California, USA

RK Firmin, Heart Link ECMO Centre, The Glenfield Hospital, Leicester, UK

J Fisher, Harefield Hospital, Harefield, Middlesex, UK

OH Frazier, Department of Cardiac Transplantation, Texas Heart Institute, Houston, Texas, USA

J Gandjbakhch, Department of Thoracic and Cardiovascular Surgery, La Pitie Hospital, Paris, France

SL Gigg, Interdisciplinary Research Centre in Biomedical Materials, Queen Mary and Westfield College, University of London, London, UK

LAR Golding, Department of Biomedical Engineering, Cleveland Clinic Foundation, Cleveland, Ohio, USA

TR Graham, Department of Cardiothoracic Surgery, Queen Elizabeth Hospital, Birmingham, UK; (formerly The Royal London Hospital, UK)

PA Grandjean, Division of Cardiothoracic Surgery, Broussais Hospital, Paris, France

JD Hill, Department of Cardiac Surgery, California Pacific Medical Center, San Francisco, California, USA

TL Hooper, Department of Cardiothoracic Surgery, Wythenshawe Hospital, Manchester, UK

JS Jassawalla, Baxter Healthcare Corporation, Novacor Division, Oakland, California, USA

J Kuo, Department of Cardiothoracic Surgery, University Hospital Wales, Cardiff, UK

M Leat, University of Arizona Heart Center, Tucson, Arizona, USA

P Lebesnerais, Centre de Recherches Chirurgicales, CHU Henri Mondor, Creteil, France

Ph Leger, Department of Thoracic and Cardiovascular Surgery, La Pitie Hospital, Paris, France

H Lennartz, Klinikum der Philipps-Universitaet Marburg, Interdisziplinaeres Medizinisches Zentrum, Marburg, Germany

H Levin, Division of Circulatory Physiology, Columbia Presbyterian Medical Center, New York, NY, USA

T Lewis   Department of Cardiothoracic Surgery, The Royal London Hospital, London, UK

SJ Ley, Department of Cardiac Surgery, California Pacific Medical Center, San Francisco, California, USA

S Lick, University of Arizona Heart Centre, Tucson, Arizona, USA

DY Loisance, Centre de Recherches Chirurgicales, CHU Henri Mondor, Creteil, France

MP Macris, Cullen Cardiovascular Research Laboratories, Texas Heart Institute, Houston, Texas, USA

JP Mazzucotelli, Centre de Recherches Chirurgicales, CHU Henri Mondor, Creteil, France

T McCarthy, 10 Brierville, Durham City DH1 4QE, UK

R Millner, Department of Cardiothoracic Surgery, St George's Hospital, London, UK

PE Oyer, Department of Cardiothoracic Surgery, Stanford University School of Medicine, Stanford, California, USA

GM Pantalos, Departments of Surgery and Bioengineering, and Artificial Heart Research Laboratory, University of Utah, Salt Lake City, Utah, USA

DJ Parker, Department of Cardiac Surgery, St George's Hospital, London, UK

A Pavie, Department of Thoracic and Cardiovascular Surgery, La Pitie Hospital, Paris, France

GA Pearson, Department of Child Health, Leicester University, UK

DG Pennington, Department of Surgery, St Louis University Medical Center, St Louis, Missouri, USA

JR Pepper, Royal Brompton Hospital, London, UK

VL Poirier, Thermo Cardiosystems Inc, Woburn, Massachusetts, USA

PM Portner, Baxter Healthcare Corporation, Novacor Division, Oakland, California, USA

G Rabago, Department of Thoracic and Cardiovascular Surgery, La Pitie Hospital, Paris, France

S Salmons, Department of Human Anatomy and Cell Biology, University of Liverpool, Liverpool, UK

RG Smith, University of Arizona Heart Center, Tucson, Arizona, USA

LW Stephenson, Division of Cardiothoracic Surgery, Wayne State University, Detroit, Michigan, USA

MT Swartz, Department of Surgery, St Louis University Medical Center, St Louis, Missouri, USA

J Szefner, University of Arizona Heart Center, Tucson, Arizona, USA

KM Taylor, Cardiothoracic Surgical Unit, Royal Postgraduate Medical School, Hammersmith Hospital, London, UK

G Tedy, Department of Thoracic and Cardiovascular Surgery, La Pitie Hospital, Paris, France

MJ Underwood, Department of Cardiothoracic Surgery, Bristol Royal Infirmary, Bristol, UK

J Waggoner, Heart Link ECMO Centre, The Glenfield Hospital, Leicester, UK

J Wallwork, Transplant Unit, Papworth Hospital, Papworth Everard, Cambridge, UK

RK Wampler, Johnson & Johnson Interventional Systems, Rancho Cordova, California, USA

D Wheeldon, Transplant Unit, Papworth Hospital, Papworth Everard, Cambridge, UK

PS Withington, The Royal London Hospital, London, UK

Sir Magdi Yacoub, Department of Cardiothoracic Surgery, Harefield Hospital, Middlesex, UK

Preface

The support of a failing heart by mechanical means is a rapidly growing field of medicine. Widely differing concepts are employed which harness many technologies. When considered at first the whole subject seems confusing and disjointed.

The aim of this book is to bring together the science of the subject with clinical reality and to show not only what is possible, or soon to be possible, but also what is clinically indicated and ethical.

All the contributors are at the very forefront of the various technologies discussed. They deal with the trials as well as the tribulations of their work, and their accumulated experience will help those entering the subject to avoid the known pitfalls and to marry the appropriate technology to the right clinical problem.

This book was developed from two highly successful specialized meetings held at the Royal London Hospital in 1990 and 1993, when it became quite clear that a written forum was urgently needed to present the experience already gained across the whole field of mechanical circulatory support.

We are extremely grateful to all the contributors who covered their fields so comprehensively and objectively, and especially to the section editors who collated their chapters so carefully.

It is an honour to have a foreword from Denton Cooley MD—not only a cardiac surgical giant of our time, but also one of the very earliest workers to venture into this difficult but rewarding field.

We hope that this book will enhance the understanding of the whole subject of mechanical circulatory support.

Terence Lewis
Timothy Graham

Foreword

Denton A Cooley

The advent of mechanical circulatory assist devices is one of the twentieth century's greatest surgical technological triumphs. Because these devices are now so widely used, we tend to forget that, only 50 years ago, many experts viewed the heart as largely off-limits. This attitude began to change during the Second World War, when battlefield trauma forced surgeons to make new inroads into the heart. With the clinical introduction of cardiopulmonary bypass in 1953, the stage was set for a dazzling array of open-heart procedures, ranging from correction of intracardiac defects to bypassing of diseased arteries. These breakthroughs culminated in the world's first human heart transplant, performed by Christiaan Barnard in 1967. Surgeons all over the world soon duplicated this feat. In 1968, I performed the first successful cardiac transplant operation in the United States. Although the initial results were promising, we and others were rapidly disillusioned as the patients succumbed to tissue rejection. Because of this dismal turn of events, heart transplantation was abandoned in many centres until the early 1980s.

Meanwhile, researchers intensified their efforts to create a workable circulatory assist device. These efforts were directed toward two main goals: (1) producing a total artificial heart that could either temporarily support or permanently replace the natural heart, and (2) devising a ventricular assist device that could sustain the natural heart until it recovered or was replaced.

The history of mechanical circulatory assistance parallels that of cardiac transplantation. Although devices to support the failing heart were envisioned as early as the 1930s, research remained intermittent for decades. A major breakthrough occurred in 1961, when Moulopoulos and associates developed the intra-aortic balloon pump. Six years later, this device was introduced clinically by Kantrowitz's group. Since then, it has proved extremely valuable for patients with potentially reversible left ventricular impairment. The concept is remarkably simple: when inserted into the thoracic aorta, the inflatable balloon augments the cardiac output by as much as 25%. Even today, this approach remains the most common form of circulatory assistance, serving as a bridge to heart transplantation in some cases.

In the early 1960s, Tetsuzo Akutsu and Willem Kolff undertook a series of animal experiments involving a total artificial heart. During the ensuing decade, these researchers gradually attained survivals with the artificial heart of more than a week. Meanwhile, in 1969, spurred on by the apparent success of clinical heart transplantation, we implanted the Liotta total artificial heart in a 47-year-old man who could not be weaned from bypass following ventriculoplasty for repair of diffuse left ventricular fibrosis. This was the first implantation of a total artificial heart in a human being. The heart supported our patient for 64 hours, until he could undergo a heart transplant. By confirming that a mechanical device could serve as a bridge to transplantation, this success paved the way for two-staged replacement of the human heart.

Not until July 1981 was a second total artificial heart implanted, again by our team. The recipient was a 36-year-old man whose heart had failed immediately after a coronary artery bypass operation. The artificial heart had also been created by Akutsu, who was then working in our laboratories. The Akutsu heart kept the patient alive for 39 hours until we found a suitable allograft for transplant. After his heart transplant, the patient lived for slightly more than a week before succumbing to infection and multiple organ failure.

In late 1982, the total artificial heart again captured public attention when William DeVries' team, at the University of Utah, implanted a Jarvik-7 prosthesis into Barney Clark, who survived for 112 days. This prosthesis, which was designed by Willem Kolff and Robert Jarvik, closely resembled the Akutsu pump that our team had implanted the previous year. In contrast, however, the Jarvik-7 prosthesis was envisioned as a permanent heart substitute.

In 1984 and 1985, four additional patients received a Jarvik-7 heart, including one patient who lived for a history-making 620 days. None of the patients, however, escaped the blood-clotting and thromboembolic complications that have so far plagued artificial hearts used clinically. By 1987, implantations of the total artificial heart for the purpose of permanent cardiac replacement had ceased. In fact, the US Food and Drug Administration declared a moratorium on this practice. The Hershey and CardioWest total artificial hearts have, however, recently been approved by the FDA for use as a bridge to transplantation in the USA. These and other types of artificial hearts are being used elsewhere in the world as well.

In the early 1980s, the advent of new methods for diagnosing and controlling tissue rejection led to a revival of interest in cardiac transplantation. Now that its time had come, this technique quickly became an accepted therapeutic option. Since 1980, thousands of adults and children have received heart transplants worldwide. A continuing challenge, however, remains: the great discrepancy between the number of transplant candidates and the number of available donors. Without some type of circulatory assistance, up to 40% of these desperately ill patients die before a donor organ can be located.[1] For this reason, the total artificial heart is sometimes used as a bridge to transplantation. More commonly, however, bridging is provided by temporary ventricular assistance.

In the early 1970s, the National Heart, Lung, and Blood Institute initiated research on development of implantable left ventricular assist devices (LVADs) that would be lightweight enough for clinical use. Unlike the artificial heart, assist devices function in series with the patient's own heart. By receiving blood from the atrium or ventricle and directing it into the great vessels, these devices can support both the systemic and pulmonary circulations.

The world's first staged cardiac transplantation involving an LVAD was performed by our Texas Heart Institute team in 1978. The patient was a 21-year-old man in whom ischaemic contracture of the ventricle ('stone heart' syndrome) had developed immediately after double-valve replacement. Upon being implanted in the patient's abdomen, the single-chambered, externally powered, pneumatic blood pump maintained the patient's entire circulation for five days. After a suitable heart donor was located, transplantation was performed. Unfortunately, the patient died of infectious complications ten days later.

During the 1980s, progress in materials and designs yielded a new generation of cardiac assist devices that have proved highly effective as either short- or long-term bridges to cardiac transplantation. These devices include piston (pusher-plate) and sac-type pumps that provide pulsatile blood flow, as well as axial pumps that provide continuous, nonpulsatile flow by means of high-speed rotors. Depending upon the system, the pump may be external or internally implanted. Moreover, it may be driven by pneumatic or electrical power.

As a bridge to transplant, we currently use the HeartMate (Thermo Cardiosystems Inc., Woburn, Massachusetts), a pulsatile, abdominally positioned pump, which is driven either pneumatically or electrically. The HeartMate has served as a major focus for our research efforts during the past decade. We are currently using the electrical version of the HeartMate in selected patients as a bridge to transplant. This device has supported one of our patients for 505 days. Other internal electrical pumps are being used in other centres. The Abiomed BVS-5000, an external device, is also approved by the FDA as a bridge to transplant and is being used successfully by many centres for short-term support.

Today's circulatory assist systems are safe enough that they should be implanted early, before end-stage organ failure occurs. In the USA alone, mechanical circulatory support might benefit as many as 16 000 to 66 000 patients per year,[2] including numerous cardiac transplant candidates. Support may be continued for prolonged periods, with a low risk of sudden death. When appropriate mechanical assistance is begun before transplantation, the patient can be expected to have a good outcome. By reducing time in the intensive care unit and returning the patient to self care, costs are also reduced.

Successful as they are, short-term mechanical circulatory support systems cannot make up for the shortage of donor hearts. Therefore, as we approach the next century, finding a suitable alternative to transplantation has become a primary research goal. Although the total artificial heart shows great promise, versions under development still must undergo many years of testing before they can be reconsidered for permanent implantation. In particular, researchers must find a way to minimize the risks of haemorrhage, thromboembolism, infection or stroke associated with this device.

Within the next few years, an implantable left ventricular assist system with an internal power supply and control mechanism will almost certainly become available. This device might be satisfactory for long-term use in some patients *in lieu* of heart transplantation. Our early evidence lends some hope that prolonged rest may also allow eventual recovery of native heart function, which might ultimately permit removal of the device. Already, initial clinical trials of the battery-operated HeartMate LVAD as a bridge to transplant at the Texas Heart Institute have shown the effectiveness of this device for long-term support. With this externally rechargeable device, heart transplant candidates are able to move around freely and even leave the hospital. Our patient who was supported for 505 days went to movies, ate in restaurants, and was even able to work.

The entire spectrum of assisted circulation and total heart replacement is addressed fully in this volume. My brief summary is intended merely to whet the reader's appetite. In saluting the contributors to this book, I applaud not only the world-renowned authorities whose names figure prominently in these pages but also the patients who have contributed significantly to the development of these devices. May the insights presented here be a stimulus for further breakthroughs in the evolution of mechanical cardiac support systems.

Houston, Texas

References

1. Levinson MM, Copeland JG. The artificial heart and mechanical assistance prior to heart transplantation. In: Cerilli CJ (ed), *Organ Transplantation and Replacement*. Philadelphia: JB Lippincott, 1987: 661–679.
2. Poirier V. The quest for the permanent LVAD: we must continue, we must push forward. *ASAIO Trans* 1990; **36**, 787–788.

Section I _____

Introduction

1

A selective history of mechanical circulatory support

George M Pantalos

Diseases desperate grown
By desperate appliance are reliev'd,
Or not at all.

William Shakespeare: *Hamlet*, act 4, scene 3

The goal of the mechanical circulatory support community is to develop devices and techniques which restore cardiac and circulatory function so that patients may be rehabilitated to the point where they once again become productive members of society. From the vantage point of a relative apprentice in the 'guild of mechanical circulatory supporters', I would offer that we have emerged from our infancy and progressed through childhood with our adolescent stage of development approaching on the horizon. To paraphrase the words of Shakespeare's Hamlet, we are no longer a 'desperate appliance guild', rather we are becoming a 'dependable appliance guild' as a consequence of years of dedicated effort by the master craftsmen and all the associates of the guild. Revisiting selected words and events of the heritage on which we are building will provide insights and revitalize our spirits as we work towards future advances in the field of mechanical circulatory support.

> . . . For it is the heart by whose virtue and pulse the blood is moved, perfected, made apt to nourish and is preserved from corruption and coagulation. . . . It is indeed the fountain of life, the sources of all action.
>
> William Harvey, *Exercitatio Anatomica de Motu Cordis et Sanguinis in Animalibus*, 1628[1]

With great respect and admiration for our British colleagues who have organized this treatise on mechanical circulatory support, it is only appropriate to begin this historical review by recognizing the work of British pioneers who laid the foundation for us to build on. William Harvey presented the foundational description of heart and circulatory function in 1628. Nearly a hundred years later in 1733, the Reverend Stephen Hales,[2] when not dealing with matters theological, explored the rheological and physiological nature of cardiovascular function by making the first direct measurement of arterial blood pressure—in a horse! Waterloo Bridge over the River Thames in London was the site for the initial attempts of flow measurement by Michael Faraday.[3] At this location in 1832, Faraday put the first electromagnetic flow probe around the 'aorta of England' to initiate a series of experiments that would eventually provide us with a mechanism for measuring blood flow when using mechanical circulatory support devices. Then, in the early part of this century, Ernest Starling[4] advanced our understanding of cardiac pump function—vital to the management of circulatory support patients—by relating the ventricular contractile force, oxygen consumption and work per beat in an isolated heart preparation to the ventricular diastolic size (as a part of his 'Law of the Heart').

The history of circulatory support is much more than a chronological recounting of dates and achievements. It is an amalgam of moments of serendipidous insight and observation interspersed between extended periods of methodical effort in the laboratory and, eventually, in the hospital. Driven by various motivations, here we find surgeon and nurse, engineer and inventor, patient and loved ones bound together in the uncanny juxtaposition of medical hubris to selfless compassion and dedication to healing the afflicted. For this review of circulatory support, we must consider principles, pumps, pioneers and their predicaments, places and policies, and always patients, whom we desire to help. Although this text is entitled *Mechanical Circulatory Support*, it is essential to recognize that biologically as well as mechanically powered pumps have been employed in many settings to restore cardiac and circulatory function. Indeed, biological pumps in the form of retrained muscles or donor hearts often demonstrated concepts of cardiac support or replacement in the clinical setting before having the opportunity to attempt the same interventions with mechanical devices.

> . . . if the place of the heart could be supplied by injection—and if for the regular continuance of this injection, there could be furnished a quantity of arterial blood, whether natural, or artificially formed, supposing such a formation possible—then life might be indefinitely maintained in any portion.
>
> JJC Le Gallois, *Experiences in the Principle of Life,* 1813[5]

> The success of work with isolated organs is closely related to success in designing devices that serve to maintain the blood circulation in the surviving organ.
>
> Sergei S Bryukhonenko, *An Apparatus for Artificial Blood Circulation,* 1928[6]

Le Gallois is credited with initial efforts at heart replacement, though this concept can be traced back to the third century BC in China.[7,8] According to a Chinese legend, the hearts of two men suffering from an 'imbalanced equilibrium of energies' were exchanged to achieve proper balance for both. As often occurs in fields of endeavour, independent and unrecognized projects in a similar period are undertaken only to be acknowledged at a later date. Such a situation is exemplified by the early investigations of organ and whole-body perfusion by Carrel and Lindbergh in the USA,[9] Gibbon in the USA[10] and Bryukhonenko in Russia.[6] In 1927 Bryukhonenko successfully demonstrated for the first time that

whole-body perfusion was feasible using a complex arrangement of pumps, tubes and valves he called his 'autojector'. However, it was another 26 years before Gibbon clinically performed the closure of an atrial septal defect with successful cardiopulmonary bypass using the heart–lung machine he had developed. Ironically, Lindbergh did not have the opportunity to witness the clinical application of the mechanical oxygenator until 1967.

> They're infiltrating every sphere,
> Except perhaps theology,
> And now we find the engineer
> Researching in biology.
>
> There on the operating floor
> If you should stop and peer . . .
> With surgeons ankle-deep in gore
> You'll see an engineer.
>
> Gibson, *The Biological Engineer?* 1964

The alliance between Lindbergh and Carrel is of particular note since it represents the advent of the engineer into the clinical domain. Because the training and mindset of the surgeon and physician is very different from that of the engineer, the collaborative integration of the professions is awkward at best and filled with tension at worst. However, given a common sense of purpose and cross-professional education, this tension has led to the creative synergy needed for advancements in mechanical circulatory support.

> The effective use of this pump in patients who require cardiac assistance does not have wide clinical application for a number of reasons: For one thing, the cost of using it clinically is almost prohibitive. For another, its clinical application necessitates a major operation with thoracotomy. . . . Mechanical assistance for long-term support or possible total replacement of the biologic heart therefore remains unachieved insofar as a satisfactory blood interface is concerned. The blood interface is perhaps the most critical problem yet to be solved in the development of an artificial heart.
>
> Michael DeBakey, 1971[11]

Although the challenge of 'how to do it' has always confronted investigators, ever present is the question of 'should we continue to do it?'. Following the first few clinical applications of cardiopulmonary bypass by Gibbon in 1953, and pulsatile, paracorporeal ventricular assistance by DeBakey in 1966, the answer to the second question was 'no'. With further insights and technological advancements, this answer was subsequently reversed over the years by the efforts of other colleagues in the field in many other countries.

> Although final evaluation must await more data, balloon pumping appears to be effective in cardiogenic shock.
>
> Adrian Kantrowitz, 1968[12]

Many approaches using continuous and pulsatile mechanical blood pumps for circulatory support have been investigated. In 1961, Dennis and colleagues[13] provided the first clinical application of left ventricular assistance using a roller pump with uptake cannulation insertion via an atrial trans-septal puncture and return cannulation through the femoral artery. A roller pump was successfully used by Spencer[14] in 1963 to provide continuous-flow ventricular assistance for a postcardiotomy, cardiogenic shock patient to achieve ventricular recovery followed by patient discharge and long-term survival. Several methods of providing counterpulsation by diastolic augmentation of aortic pressure were explored by Moulopoulos, Topaz, Kolff[15] and others, culminating in an intraaortic balloon pump clinical trial by Kantrowitz and colleagues in 1967 while working in New York City.[12] The dramatic reversal of cardiogenic shock by intra-aortic balloon pumping in this first series of patients stimulated a multicentre study and the eventual worldwide use of nearly 80 000 devices per year.[16] Continuing efforts by Kantrowitz and colleagues in Detroit led to a modified intra-aortic balloon pump called the 'dynamic aortic patch', which resulted in the first patient discharged with a mechanical circulatory support device in 1971.[17] By the mid-1970s, intracorporeal and paracorporeal pulsatile ventricular assist devices were being tested for both the 'bridge-to-transplant' and 'support-to-weaning' indications by Norman in Houston using a textured blood-contacting surface device[18] and by Pierce in Hershey using a smooth blood sac device.[19] The virtues and drawbacks of atrial and ventricular cannulation for assist device uptake along with patient selection, anticoagulation strategy and device control mode were among the issues to be resolved. Haemodynamic and other criteria for initiating ventricular assistance were delineated by these clinical trials. The clinical trial series in Houston presented the first opportunity to attempt to bridge a patient to cardiac transplantation with a ventricular assist device in 1978,[20] although successful bridge-to-transplantation with patient discharge and long-term follow-up was not achieved until 1984 by Hill and colleagues in San Francisco[21] and by Oyer and colleagues at Stanford University.[22]

Since 1988, a catheter-mounted, axial-flow assist pump developed by Wampler has provided nearly total support without the need of a thorocotomy.[23] An early concept by Anstadt[24] that has recently been re-evaluated clinically is direct mechanical ventricular actuation. Using this technique, a lateral thorocotomy is used to rapidly place the pneumatically actuated compression cup around the ventricles, providing synchronous, external compression of the heart. This device has been used successfully in patients at Duke University Medical Center both as a bridge-to-transplantation[25] and for a week of resuscitative support in a patient suffering cardiogenic shock secondary to an acute viral myocarditis. Muscle-powered cardiac assistance has been limited; nonetheless, building on the clinical efforts of Petrovsky[26] and other investigators, encouraging clinical trials were initiated in the 1980s by Carpentier in Paris[27] and by Magovern in Pittsburgh.[28] The optimal training regimen for stimulating the latissimus dorsi muscle remains a challenge.

The annual use of ventricular assist devices as reported by the American Society for Artificial Internal Organs and the International Society for Heart and Lung Transplantation is shown in Fig. 1.1. Since 1987, ventricular assist devices have been used in over 200 cases annually with the majority used in postcardiotomy cardiogenic shock situations.[29] The reduced number of ventricular assist cases in recent years may reflect a reduced number of voluntary reports as the use of these devices becomes more widespread, rather than indicating a true reduction in the number of cases. The majority of assist applications employed a roller pump or a centrifugal pump to provide 'depulsed' or 'continuous' flow with many different cannulation approaches requiring sternotomy or thorocotomy. Of the patients requiring ventricular assistance in the setting of postcardiotomy cardiogenic shock, half are usually weaned from the devices, but only about half of those patients are ultimately discharged, which is indicative of the difficulties these cases present to the health care team. The average duration of support for these patients regardless of the need for single or biventricular assistance has been 3 days.

> '*Christ, it's going to work!*'
> Christiaan Barnard[30] upon cardioverting the first
> cardiac allograft in 1967

Cardiac replacement efforts pursued many avenues, including work by Kolff and his associates at the Cleveland Clinic who sustained the circulation of a dog with a polyvinyl chloride artificial heart for 90 minutes in 1957,[31] only to find out

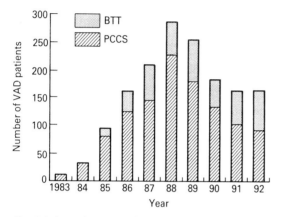

Fig. 1.1 Annual number of ventricular assist device applications for all cases (pulsatile and continuous flow pumps, single and bi-ventricular support) report to the ASAIO and ISHLT combined registry for the clinical use of mechanical ventricular assist pumps and total artificial hearts, as of March 1993. BTT = bridge-to-transplantation, PCCS = postcardiotomy cardiogenic shock.

years later than Demikhov had performed a similar experiment in 1937.[32] It was not until 1967 that allograft transplantation was clinically attempted in South Africa by Barnard in a 55-year-old man.[33,34] Within days, Kantrowitz, then working in New York City, performed the first paediatric cardiac transplantation in a 19-day-old boy.[35] Although long-term survival was not realized with either patient, these two attempts illustrate the desire to provide circulatory support and cardiac replacement for both the adult and paediatric patient populations. Following an initial flurry of cardiac transplantation activity (Fig. 1.2), clinical efforts subsided until the advent of cyclosporin A for control of donor organ rejection episodes in the early 1980s.[37] By 1986, the transplantation activity worldwide exceeded 2000 cases annually with a 5-year survival of nearly 70%,[38] with the limitation on the number of transplantations performed being the availability of suitable donor organs. Hence, the pressing desire for an acceptable alternative to donor allografts including the consideration of mechanical devices.

> We took a patient who probably would have been dead by midnight, took him to the operating room and removed his heart. . . . It was almost a spiritual experience for everyone in the room.
> William DeVries, following the first permanent
> artificial heart implantation, 1982[39]

Clinical utility of the total artificial heart for bridging to transplantation was first demonstrated in Houston by Cooley and Liotta in 1969,[40]

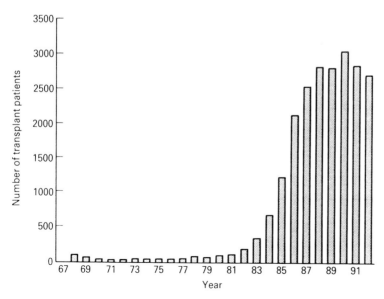

Fig. 1.2 Annual number of heart transplants worldwide, compiled from reports by the Stanford University international heart transplantation registry (for 1967–80) and the registry of the International Society for Heart and Lung Transplantation (for 1981–92).[36]

and again in 1981,[41,42] prior to the first permanent implantation of a total artificial heart in Salt Lake City by DeVries and Joyce in 1982.[43] Initial attempts to discharge TAH recipients were made in Louisville by DeVries[44] and in Stockholm by Semb in 1985 with the periodic use of a small, portable heart driver developed by Heimes in Aächen.[45,46] The long-term outcome with those patients was poor, causing a cessation of 'permanent' artificial heart implantations. However, the shorter term results of using artificial hearts for bridging-to-transplantation were encouraging, leading to widespread clinical trials of the approach initiated by the first successful total artificial heart bridge-to-transplantation by Copeland and Levinson in 1985 in Tucson.[47] To date, 11 different kinds of artificial hearts have been used in over 260 cases for the bridge-to-transplant application (Table 1.1). As with the early activity with cardiac transplantation, the number of artificial heart implantations grew rapidly (Fig. 1.3), only to decline due to device-related complications, the availability of alternative devices, the interruption in 1990 by the US Food and Drug Administration of the Jarvik-7-70 artificial heart clinical trial sponsored by Symbion Inc.,[48,49] and possibly the shortage of suitable donor organs.

> Up until the day they did the actual implant, I thought I was going to get better. They came to me that morning and told me that I wasn't going to get better and I probably wasn't going to make it through the week, so I said ok, let's do it. When

> I woke up, I felt better right away. It was amazing how much better I felt.
>
> Michael Templeton, while being supported by an implanted, portable LV assist system in January 1992

The use of implantable LV assist systems in the bridge-to-transplant application started again in 1984.[22,50,51] The extended period of time before donor heart acquisition and the ability to restore end-organ function and rehabilitate LV assist system patients[52] reactivated efforts to provide monitored patient discharge and improved quality of life by Kormos and Griffith in Pittsburgh in 1990,[53,54] and by Frazier in Houston in 1992.[51] Patients still needing to be tethered to control consoles have been able to live in modified dwellings with their families and take complete care of themselves, while patients with portable controllers have been able to enjoy periodic stays at home and travel about their locale.

The overall effectiveness of devices for bridging-to-transplantation from the major clinical trial series is presented in Table 1.2. Based on the percentage of patients surviving and the actuarial survival statistics for the bridge-to-transplant process,[55,56] there is a trend suggesting that patients bridged with ventricular assist devices have better outcomes than patients bridged with artificial hearts. It should be noted, however, that the diversity of patient entry criteria and clinical protocols used for the different devices, as well as the 'learning curve effect' and variability in the duration of support, preclude the judgement

Table 1.1 Device type, number of patients and patient outcome for total artificial hearts used as a bridge-to-transplantation, reported by the University of Utah Institute for Biomedical Engineering artificial heart registry as of January 1995.

Device	Patient numbers	Transplanted (Tx)	Alive at discharge	%Tx	%Tx alive at discharge
Liotta	1	1	0	100	0
Akutsu	1	1	0	100	0
Jarvik-7	41	26	15	63	58
Jarvik-7-70	147	109	74	74	68
Penn State	3	1	0	33	0
Phoenix	1	1	0	100	0
Berlin	7	2	1	29	50
BRNO (Czech)	6	3	0	50	0
Unger	4	2	1	50	50
Poisk	16	3	2	19	67
Vienna	2	1	0	50	0
CardioWest	36	23	22	68	96
All 12 devices	265	173	115	65%	66%

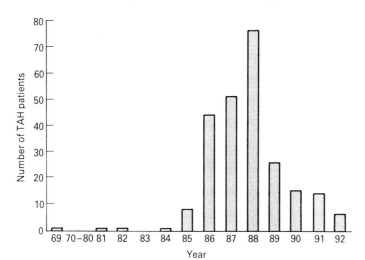

Fig. 1.3 Annual number of total artificial heart implantations for bridging-to-transplantation and permanent support reported by the artificial heart registry of the University of Utah Institute for Biomedical Engineering, as of March 1993.

Table 1.2 Device type, duration of support, number of patients and patient outcomes for the major clinical trials with ventricular assist devices and total artificial hearts used as a bridge-to-transplantation, as reported by the clinical trial sponsors at January 1995.

Device	Average duration (days)	Patients implanted	Patients transplanted†	Patient survival‡
Novacor (LVAS, all patients)	48 (1–370)	274 (18 waiting)	154 (60% IMPLTD) (3 in HTX recovery)	139 (92% HTX)* (55% IMPLTD)
Novacor (LVAS, wearable controller only)	64 (1–314)	95 (18 waiting)	46 (60% IMPLTD) (2 in HTX recovery)	42 (95% HTX)* (56% IMPLTD)
TCI§ (LVAS, pneumatic only)	67 (<1–343)	223 (2 waiting)	147 (67% IMPLTD)	131 (89% HTX)* (59% IMPLTD)
Thoratec (LVAD and BiVAD)	26 (<1–247)	326 (13 waiting)	199 (64% IMPLTD)	171 (86% HTX)* (55% IMPLTD)
Thoratec (LVAD only)	36 (<1–247)	113 (3 waiting)	75 (68% IMPLTD)	70 (93% HTX)* (64% IMPLTD)
Symbion (J7–100 and J7-70 TAH)‖	26 (1–603)	198	144 (73% IMPLTD)	85 (59% HTX)* (43% IMPLTD)
Symbion (LVAD AND BiVAD)¶	19 (1–164)	44	27 (61% IMPLTD)	22 (81% HTX)** (50% IMPLTD)
CardioWest (C-7-70)	32 (1–186)	36 (2 waiting)	23 (68% IMPLTD)	22 (96% HTX)* (65% IMPLTD)

* Reported by the sponsor as patient discharge.
** Reported by the sponsor as patients who were currently living at the time of the report or who had survived at least 30 days post-HTX.
§ TCI = Thermo Cardiosystems: Patient enrollment into TCI clinical trial closed upon FDA pre-market approval for the bridge-to-transplant application, September 1994.
‖ Clinical trial halted: Data as of October 1, 1992.
¶ Clinical trial halted: Data as of May 1, 1991.
† % IMPLTD = patients HTX/(patients implanted − patients waiting).
‡ % HTX = (Patients surviving − patients waiting − patients in recovery)/(patients transplanted − patients in recovery).
% IMPLTD = (patients surviving − patients waiting − patients in recovery)/(patients implanted − patients waiting − patients in recovery).

at this time that ventricular assist devices are clearly superior to total artificial hearts. Indeed, Kormos recently pointed out that patients entered into their clinical trial of the Jarvik-7 total artificial heart in Pittsburgh were in worse condition than the patients entered into their clinical trial of the Novacor LV assist system that was initiated a few years later.[57] It is encouraging to see reported that, despite the long period of support usually required prior to transplantation, for patients with some of the ventricular assist devices and total artificial hearts used for bridging, the actuarial survival outcome of the patients post-transplant has been equivalent or better than those cardiac transplant recipients who did not require mechanical circulatory support prior to transplantation.[55] However, for all the devices used, the lower percentage of patients implanted that go on to long-term, post-transplant survival reiterates the level of difficulty these cases present to the patient care team and the need for improved patient selection criteria and improved patient care protocols.

The current, extensive clinical trial experience with all these devices has demonstrated improving pump reliability and patient outcomes. However, there remains the need to overcome haemorrhagic, thrombotic and infectious complications with these devices. These issues are addressed throughout this book.

> In the past few years, the FDA has been severely criticized for its implementation of the amendments. A rethinking is now in order. The widening gap between Congress's expectation, as reflected in the specific statutory requirements, and the actual implementation of the law must be examined. The failure of the FDA to implement several major statutory provisions intended to ensure the safety and effectiveness of medical devices leads to one of two conclusions: either the safety and effectiveness of medical devices are not being ensured or the provisions are superfluous.
>
> David Kessler *et al.*[58] three years before he became FDA Commissioner

> The Food and Drug Administration has withdrawn its approval to continue three studies being conducted by Symbion Inc., the manufacturer of the Jarvik artificial heart. . . . The FDA believes that, on balance, the deficiencies in the Symbion studies were great enough that the risks to patients were outweighing the benefits. It is still possible that Symbion's studies could resume in the future if the problems are corrected. The

> agency has offered to work with the company in correcting the deficiencies, and it is willing to reconsider its decision if the company turns things around.
>
> FDA Press Office, January 1990[46]

> Ladies and gentlemen, I am here today to tell you that I place a high priority on enforcing the law. This is not the idle talk of a new commissioner. Today, the US Attorney's office in Minneapolis is filing on FDA's behalf a seizure action against. . . .
>
> David Kessler, four months after becoming FDA Commissioner in 1991[59]

> Hello. My name is Ron Parr of the FDA. I am here to help you.
>
> Ron Parr, FDA Division of Small Manufacturers Assistance, 1993

Any discussion of mechanical circulatory support devices is not complete without some consideration of the regulatory requirements currently imposed upon the use of these devices. The early clinical use of mechanical circulatory support devices was conducted prior to the perceived need for medical device regulation. Then, in 1976 the Medical Device Amendments to the Food, Drug and Cosmetics Act (Public Law 94–295) were enacted, followed later by the Safe Medical Devices Act of 1990.[60–62] These legislated actions were intended to create a regulatory process to oversee the clinical investigation and subsequent marketing of medical devices with the goal of approving devices that are safe and effective for patients. Though well-intended, the regulatory process has become cumbersome and stifling for clinical investigators, cost-prohibitive and adversarial for the clinical trial sponsors, and overwhelming for the reviewers at the US Food and Drug Administration. Despite this demonstrated bureaucratic morass, many federal health ministries around the world are initiating similar regulatory programmes. Indeed, we all desire to have safe and effective devices, and a realistic level of regulatory oversight with intolerance of misconduct is understandable; and yet a certain amount of clinical responsibility needs to be allowed to prevail. Perhaps it is time to heed the admonition of cardiac surgical pioneer Dwight Harken when he said 'Perfection may be the enemy of good'. We all wish to have the 'perfect' device, but the experience of our heritage has taught us that with every device there are developmental deficiencies that always need to be overcome. Somewhere between the prototype and the 'perfect' end-product there is a 'good' device that can 'do good' for many people while advancing techniques of circulatory support patient care and device development. A reality of life that must be kept in perspective is that medical devices are not absolutely risk-free, but then again, neither is life in general.

It is encouraging to recognize that despite the formidable regulatory challenges, ABIOMED® (Danvers, Massachusetts) received FDA market approval of their BVS 5000® temporary biventricular support system for postcardiotomy cardiogenic shock applications in November 1992 and Thermo Cardiosystems (Woburn, Massachusetts) received FDA market approval of their Heart-Mate® left ventricular assist system for bridging-to-transplantation in September of 1994.

Final thoughts

A final, historical observation by this apprentice of the mechanical circulatory support guild is that we not only strive to support the circulation, but we strive to support each other and the collective advancement of the field. Compared with other professional communities, our guild has always been impressive because of its lack of secrecy and intellectual assault and the abundance of genuine openness and cooperation. When one looks at the big picture, we are really on the fringe far from the mainstream of medical and surgical practice, though we are working our way in closer. Maybe it is this perspective that has supported the behaviour that it is better to preserve the species than to be preoccupied with the pecking order within.

One can suspect that this desire for openness and exchange comes from the very reason we are in this trade in the first place: to give people suffering from a life-threatening cardiac crisis the best possible chance of survival and rehabilitation. We have all spent sleepless nights in the operating room, intensive care unit and laboratory so that we learn how to provide better cardiopulmonary mechanical support. The reinforcement received from the openness and exchange with colleagues has nurtured that process time and again. Ultimately we are trying to do the best we can to provide hope for people in need of circulatory support and provide ourselves with the reassurance that we will continue to learn and improve from each other's experience and creativity.

Every time we commit to a procedure, be it total artificial heart or ventricular assist device, we are headed into murky waters with the final destination and precise course yet to be determined. But the waters, though murky, are not completely unknown; they are becoming better charted with research, development experience, and insight by the members of the guild. It is unlikely that we will ever have complete control over our course and final destination, but we do have control over how we attempt to improve our techniques. Openness and exchange should always be a part of that pursuit in the future.'

It is possible to detach oneself from the role of investigator in mechanical circulatory support and member of a care providing team to take an introspective glimpse at what we are doing. It often comes in the intensive care unit in the middle of the night, between hourly readings when things are stable for the moment. There we are, nurses, surgeons, engineers, cardiologists and technicians working together, trying to help someone in the process of restoring a vital existence. Recalling the words of RG Ingersoll: 'And in the night of death, hope sees a star, and listening love hears the rustle of a wing'. In this situation, we know that the rustling wing of the messenger will surely come. What we do not know is the destination of the messenger. Yet, what we do know is that we have a realistic hope for the desired outcome; a hope that is built on years of research, experience, openness and exchange. What else will serve us better? What else will sustain us as we pass from our past through the challenges facing the guild in the future? Our history has just ended; our future has just begun. Let us continue to pursue that future together.

Acknowledgements

Many 'members of the guild' generously provided resource material to augment the preparation of this historical review, including: Sergei Dzemeshkevich (Russian National Research Centre of Surgery, Moscow), Timothy Graham (Royal London Hospital), Jean Kantrowitz (L·VAD Technology Inc.), Harvey Borovetz (University of Pittsburgh), Steve Parnis (Texas Heart Institute), Richard Smith (University of Arizona Medical Center), Phil Miller (Novacor Inc.), Mark Anstadt (Duke University Medical Center), Cindy Miller (Pennsylvania State University), Susan Quaal (Department of Veterans Affairs Medical Center, Salt

Lake City), Kurt Dasse (Thermo Cardiosystems Inc.), David Farrar (Thoratec Inc.), and Steve Langford (CardioWest Technologies Inc.). Assistance in the preparation of this chapter was kindly given by Carol Rice, Scott Everett, Natalie Sparks and Brad Mortimer at the Artificial Heart Research Laboratory of the Institute for Biomedical Engineering at the University of Utah. To all of these people, I would like to express my grateful thanks and appreciation for their contributions.

References

1. Harvey W. *Exercitatio Anatomica de Motu Cordis et Sanguinis in Animalibus* (Anatomical Studies on the Motion of the Heart and Blood). English translation by CD Leake, 5th edn. Springfield, Ill: Charles C Thomas, 1970.
2. Hales S. *Statical Essays: Vol. 2, Containing Haemastaticks; or an Account of Some Hydraulic and Hydrostatical Experiments Made on the Blood and Blood-Vessels of Animals.* London: Innys and Manby, 1733.
3. Faraday M. Experimental researches in electricity. *Phil Trans Roy Soc* 1832; **122**, 287–288.
4. Starling EH. *The Linacre Lecture on the Law of the Heart Given at Cambridge, 1915.* London: Longmans, Green, 1918.
5. LeGallois CJJ. *Experiences on the Principle of Life.* Philadelphia: Thomas, 1813. Translation of: LeGallois CJJ, *Experiences sur le Principe de la Vie,* Paris, 1812.
6. Bryukhonenko SS. An apparatus for artificial blood circulation (in warm-blooded animals). Bulletin, 1928.
7. Wong KC. China's contribution to the science of medicine. *China Med J* 1929; **43**, 1193–1209.
8. Wong KC, Lien-Teh W. *History of Chinese Medicine.* Shanghai: National Quarantine Service, 1936.
9. Lindbergh CA. An apparatus for the culture of whole organs. *J Exp Med* 1935; **62**, 409.
10. Gibbon JH. Application of a mechanical heart and lung apparatus to cardiac surgery. *Minn Med* 1954; **37**, 171–180.
11. DeBakey ME. Left ventricular bypass pump for cardiac assistance. *Am J Cardiol* 1971; **27**, 3–11.
12. Kantrowitz A, Tjonneland S, Freed PS, Phillips SJ, Butner AN, Sherman JL. Initial clinical experience with intraaortic balloon pumping in cardiogenic shock. *JAMA* 1968; **203**, 113–118.
13. Dennis C, Hall DP, Moreno JR, Senning A. Left atrial cannulation without thoracotomy for total left heart bypass. *Acta Chir Scand* 1962; **156**, 190.
14. Spencer FC, Eiseman B, Trinkle JK, Rossi NP. Assisted circulation for cardiac failure following intracardiac surgery with cardiopulmonary bypass. *J Thoracic & Cardiovas Surg* 1965; **49**(1): 56–73.
15. Moulopoulos SD, Topaz SR, Kolff WJ. Extracorporeal assistance to the circulation and intraaortic balloon pumping. *ASAIO Trans* 1962; **8**, 86–88.
16. Alan R. *Cardiac Assist Devices: An Emerging Life-Saving Technology.* Kidder Peabody Equity Research Industry Report, 18 October 1988: 12.
17. Kantrowitz A, Krakauer J, Rubenfire M, *et al.* Initial clinical experience with a new permanent mechanical auxiliary ventricle: the dynamic aortic patch. *ASAIO Trans* 1972; **18**, 159–167.
18. Norman JC, Duncan JM, Frazier OH, Hallman GL, Ott DA, Reul GJ, Cooley DA. Intracorporeal (abdominal) left ventricular assist devices or partial artificial hearts. *Arch Surg* 1981; **116**, 1441–1445.
19. Pierce WS, Parr GVS, Myers JL, Pae WE, Bull AP, Waldhausen JA. Ventricular-assist pumping in patients with cardiogenic shock after cardiac operations. *New Engl J Med* 1981; **305**, 1606–1610.
20. Norman JC, Brook MI, Cooley DA, *et al.* Total support of the circulation of a patient with postcardiotomy stone-heart syndrome by a partial artificial heart (ALVAD) for 5 days followed by heart and kidney transplantation. *Lancet* 1978; **1**, 1125.
21. Hill JD, Farrar DJ, Hershon JJ, Compton PG, Avery GJ, Levin BS, Brent BN. Use of a prosthetic ventricle as a bridge to cardiac transplantation for postinfarction cardiogenic shock. *New Engl J Med* 1986; **314**, 626–628.
22. Portner PM, Oyer PE, McGregor CGA, *et al.* First human use of an electrically powered implantable ventricular assist system. *Artif Organs* 1985; **9**(A), 36.
23. Frazier OH, Wampler RK, Duncan JM, Dear WE, Macris MP, Parnis SM, Fuqua JM. First human use of the hemopump, a catheter-mounted ventricular assist device. *Ann Thorac Surg* 1990; **49**, 299–304.
24. Anstadt MP, Anstadt GL, Lowe JE. Direct mechanical ventricular actuation: a review. *Resuscitation* 1991; **21**, 7–23.
25. Lowe JE, Anstadt MP, Trigt PV, Smith PK, Hendry PJ, Plunket MD, Anstadt GL. First successful bridge to cardiac transplantation using direct mechanical ventricular actuation. *Ann Thorac Surg* 1991; **52**, 1237–1245.
26. Petrovsky BV. Surgical treatment of cardiac aneurysms. *J Cardiovasc Surg (Torino)* 1966; **7**, 87.
27. Carpentier A, Chachques JC. Myocardial substitution with a stimulated skeletal muscle: first successful clinical case (Letter). *Lancet* 1985; **1**, 1267.
28. Magovern GJ, Park SB, Magovern GJ, Bencart DH, Tullis G, Rozar E, Kayo R, Christlieb I. Latissimus dorsi as a functioning synchronously paced muscle component in the repair of a left ventrical aneurysm (Letter). *Ann Thorac Surg* 1986; **41**, 116.
29. Miller CA, Pae WE, Pierce WS. Combined registry for the clinical use of mechanical ventricular assist

devices: postcardiotomy shock. *ASAIO Trans* 1990; **36**, 43–46.

30. The ultimate operation. *Time* 1967, 15 December, 64–72.

31. Akutsu T, Kolff WJ. Permanent substitutes for valves and hearts. *ASAIO Trans* 1958; **4**, 230.

32. Demikhov VP. Chapter 5 in: Haigh B (ed), Experimental transplantation of vital organs. Moscow Translation. Medquiz, 1960: 212–213.

33. Barnard CN. A human cardiac transplant: an interim report of a successful operation performed at Groote Schuur Hospital, Capetown. *S Afr Med J* 1967; **41**, 1271.

34. Barnard CN. Human cardiac transplantation. *Am J Cardiol* 1968; **22**, 584.

35. Kantrowitz A, Haller JD, Joos H, Cerruti MM, Carstensen HE. Transplantation of the heart in an infant and an adult. *Am J Cardiol* 1968; **22**, 782.

36. Kaye MP. The registry of the International Society of Heart and Lung Transplantation: tenth official report, 1993. *J Heart Lung Transpl* 1993; **12**, 541–548.

37. Schroeder JS, Hunt S. Cardiac transplantation update, 1987. *JAMA* 1987; **258**, 3142–3145.

38. Frangomeni LS, Kaye MP. Registry: International Society for Heart Transplantation, 1988. *Clin Transplant* 1988; **2**, 150–151.

39. Clark M, Copeland JB, Shapiro D, Abramson P, Hagar M, Sandza R. An incredible affair of the heart. *Newsweek* 1982; 13 December, 70–79.

40. Cooley DA, Liotta D, Hallman GL, Bloodwell RD, Leachman RD, Milam JD. Orthotopic cardiac prosthesis for two-staged cardiac replacement. *Am J Cardiol* 1969; **24**, 723–730.

41. Cooley DA, Akutsu T, Norman JC, Serrato MA, Frazier OH. Total artificial heart in two-staged cardiac transplantation. *Bull Texas Heart Inst* 1981; **8/3**, 305–319.

42. Cooley DA. Staged cardiac transplantation: report of three cases. *J Heart Transplant* 1982; **1**, 145.

43. DeVries WC, Anderson JL, Joyce LD, Anderson FL, Hammond EH, Jarvik RK, Kolff WJ. Clinical use of the total artificial heart. *New Engl J Med* 1984, **310**, 273–278.

44. DeVries WC. The permanent artificial heart: four case reports. *JAMA* 1988; **259**, 849.

45. Heimes HP, Klasen F. Completely integrated wearable TAH-drive unit. *Int J Artif Organs* 1982; **5**, 157–159.

46. Heimes HP. Wearable drive systems. In: Unger F (ed), *Assisted Circulation Vol 2*. Berlin: Springer-Verlag, 1984: 367.

47. Copeland JG, Levinson MM, Smith R, *et al.* The total artificial heart as a bridge to transplantation: a report of two cases. *JAMA* 1986; **256**, 2991–2996.

48. 'Statement on Jarvik Artificial Heart'. FDA Press Office, Rockville, MD, 11 January 1990.

49. Olsen DB. The FDA and the artificial heart. *Artif Organs* 1990; **14**, 173.

50. Dasse KA, Chipman SD, Sherman CN, Levine AH, Frazier OH. Clinical experience with textured blood contacting surfaces in ventricular assist devices. *ASAIO Trans* 1987; **33**, 418–425.

51. Frazier OH, Rose EA, Macmanus Q, Burton NA, Lefrak EA, Poirier VL, Dasse KA. Multicenter clinical evaluation of the heartmate 1000 IP left ventricular assist device. *Ann Thorac Surg* 1992; **53**, 1080–1090.

52. Dasse KA, Frazier OH, Lesniak JM, Myers T, Burnett CM, Poirier VL. Clinical responses to ventricular assistance versus transplantation in a series of bridge to transplant patients. *ASAIO Trans* 1992; **38**, M622–626.

53. Dew MA, Kormos RL, Roth LH, Armatige JM, Pristas JM, Harris RC, Capretta C, Griffith BP. Life quality in the era of bridging to cardiac transplantation: bridge patients in an outpatient setting. *ASAIO Trans* 1993; **39**, 145–152.

54. Kormos RL, Borovetz HS, Pristas JM, *et al.* Out of hospital facility for the Novacor bridge to transplant: the Pittsburgh family house experience. *ASAIO Abst* 1991; **20**, 13.

55. Johnson KE, Liska MB, Joyce LD, Emery RW. Use of total artificial hearts: summary of world experience, 1969–91. *ASAIO Trans* 1992; **38**, M486–492.

56. Rasamamy N, Portner PM. Novacor LVAS: results with bridge to transplant and chronic support. In: Ott RA, Gutfinger DE, Gazzaniga AB (eds), *Cardiac Surgery and Mechanical Cardiac Assist*. Philadelphia: Hanley & Belfus Inc., 1993: 363–376.

57. Kormos RL, Armitage JM, Capretta CJ, Pristas JM, Winowich S, Griffith BP. Infection in Novacor bridge to transplant patients. *J Heart Lung Transplant* 1992; **11**, 197.

58. Kessler DA, Pape SM, Sundwall DN. The Federal regulation of medical devices. *New Engl J Med* 1987; **317**, 357.

59. The Man with the Plan. *Time* 1991; 15 July: 59.

60. Acharya A, Lemperle B. Role of FDA in a ventricular assist device program. In: Quaal SJ (ed), *Cardiac Mechanical Assistance Beyond Balloon Pumping*. St Louis: Mosby Yearbook Inc., 1992: 244–255.

61. Holstein HM. The Safe Medical Devices Act of 1990. *Regulatory Affairs* 1991; **3**, 91.

62. Kahan JS, Holstein H, Munsey R. The implications of the Safe Medical Devices Act of 1990. *Med Dev Diag Ind*, February 1991.

2

The physiology of left ventricular assistance

Kurt A Dasse, Howard Levin, O Howard Frazier and Timothy R Graham

Introduction

Irrespective of the aetiological basis for the disease, the clinical objectives in utilizing ventricular assist technology are to restore adequate blood flow and to preserve end-organ function. Whether the patient is in cardiogenic shock resulting from acute left ventricular failure or in chronic congestive heart failure, the indication to implant an LVAD is low-output syndrome. More often than not, because initiation of ventricular assistance has been delayed, peripheral end-organ dysfunction must also be treated.

The haemodynamic principles in utilizing an LVAD for acute or chronic LV failure are essentially the same. However, appropriate selection of a device, the specific physiological challenges to be overcome, and the individual management of the acute versus chronically debilitated patient may differ based on the physiological status of the individual at the time of LVAD implantation. The purpose of this chapter is to discuss basic haemodynamic considerations in the use of an LVAD, the physiological considerations of the host, as well as current thoughts regarding optimal operation of an assisting device.

An LVAD, like a normal healthy ventricle, will produce a stroke volume proportional to the preload. Factors that limit the preload or filling of the device, such as elevated pulmonary vascular resistance or right ventricular dysfunction, will limit the output of the device. Each pump has a specific fill sensitivity, that dictates the maximal flows that can be achieved as well as its responsiveness to the demand for flow. A properly designed LVAD will maintain left atrial pressure within a constant range. As long as the left atrial pressure remains within this range the LVAD may be considered to be functioning properly; however, this does not ensure that adequate flows will be achieved despite proper performance. Low pulmonary venous return, independent of the cause, will result in low pump output. In other words, like a healthy ventricle, the device will simply pump whatever volume of blood it gets, and if treatment of the patient fails to optimize filling, the clinical objectives will not be met.

The target population

Pathophysiology of cardiac failure

The typical LVAD candidate is in cardiac failure resulting from a reduction in myocardial contractility secondary to ischaemic or myopathic heart disease. The cardiac output and oxygen delivery are reduced, a condition that usually results in compensatory vasoconstriction and an increase in systemic vascular resistance. While systemic arterial pressure is at least transiently preserved, this generally causes impedance to left ventricular ejection and an increase in left ventricular filling pressure. The elevated systemic pressure triggers a vicious cycle whereby the compromised cardiac contractility coupled with the increased vascular impedance contribute to the low-output condition.

In acute heart failure, the cardiac index is generally reduced to $2.0–2.4 \, l/min/m^2$ with an $S\text{v}_{O_2} \leqslant 55\%$.[1] Left ventricular filling pressure generally exceeds 15 mmHg, and the systemic vascular resistance increases to $\geqslant 1600$ dynes cm^{-5}. If the cardiac index is reduced to less than $2.0 \, l/min/m^2$, or if the compensatory increase in vascular resistance fails to occur, hypotension will further complicate the clinical picture. The emerging haemodynamic state is often one of rapid deterioration that requires immediate pharmacological support. If the condition becomes refractory to drugs, and if intra-aortic balloon pumping proves incapable of stabilizing the patient, left ventricular assistance may be the only avenue available for supporting the patient.

Classic haemodynamic indications for LVAD use

The specific indications for left ventricular assistance were originally developed in the mid-1970s to guide selection of postcardiotomy candidates. Although the patient population presently contains a mix of acute and chronic LV failure patients, most if not all of the clinical groups continue to select patients based on similar criteria. The LVAD candidate typically has a pulmonary capillary wedge pressure (LAP) $\geqslant 20$ mmHg, with either a systolic blood pressure $\leqslant 80$ mmHg or a cardiac index $\leqslant 2.0 \, l/min/m^2$. A variety of exclusion criteria also exist that are intended to restrict the use of such devices in patients unlikely to benefit from univentricular support. Ongoing studies continue to delineate optimal patient selection criteria.

Exclusion criteria

There is considerable debate regarding which factors should be used to exclude a patient from left ventricular assistance; however, specific factors have been identified that appear to meet with universal agreement. For example, while it is possible to successfully treat a patient with mild to moderate right ventricular dysfunction, severe right ventricular failure characterized by a low RV ejection fraction, coupled with elevated pulmonary vascular resistance or an increased transpulmonary pressure gradient, has proven to be associated with a poor outcome. Likewise, irreversible hepatic dysfunction, based on elevated serum enzymes and positive biopsy findings prior to LVAD implantation, has been associated with a poor prognosis.

Less clear is whether renal failure should be regarded as a contraindication. Historically, renal failure has been cited as being highly predictive of mortality in patients suffering from acute cardiogenic shock who were treated with an LVAD.[2] More recently, others have reported that renal failure does not necessarily prevent successfully bridging a patient to transplantation.[3,4] A possible difference between these studies is related to the nature and/or rate of onset of the cardiac disorder.

Severe blood dyscrasia is also a serious contraindication. Uncontrollable bleeding due to a heparin sensitivity, low platelet count, or factors contributing to prolonged PT and/or PTT values can prevent successful use of the device. Other factors that are often used as exclusion criteria include: age, size, severe pulmonary disease, intractable arrhythmias, cerebral vascular disease, and active systemic infection.

Haematological consequences of ventricular assistance

Two measurements have been made routinely to document the haemodynamic effectiveness of ventricular assistance during circulatory support. TCI routinely obtains a measurement of the cardiac index for each patient within 24 hours prior to LVAD implantation. The value for each patient is then compared against the average 'pump index' value (pump flow/BSA). The average pump index for a cohort of 79 TCI patients was $2.6 \, l/min/m^2$, which represented a 37% increase over the baseline cardiac index which averaged $1.9 \, l/min/m^2$ (Table 2.1). Similar results were presented by Frazier *et al.*[5]

A concern in utilizing ventricular assist devices is damage to the cellular elements of the blood due to the effects of shear forces within the blood pump. Routine measurements of the haematocrit, haemoglobin, plasma free haemoglobin and platelet counts are typically made throughout support to assess the affect of pumping on the blood. A decrease in the haematocrit, haemoglobin or platelet count, or an increase in the plasma free haemoglobin values, signal possible damage

Table 2.1 Haemodynamic effectiveness of the HeartMate® 1000 IP LVAD.

Parameter	Mean value (l/min/m²) (n = 79)	Standard deviation	Increase over baseline
Average baseline CI*	1.9	0.6	NA
Average PI** throughout implant	2.6	0.51	37%

*CI = cardiac index (cardiac output/BSA)
**PI = pump index (pump flow/BSA)

Table 2.2 Haematological response to ventricular assistance.

Parameter (average values)	Mean (n = 79)	SD
Haematocrit (%)	33	4
Haemoglobin (g/dl)	11	1.3
Plasma free haemoglobin (mg/dl)	7.9	10.7
Platelet count (×10⁶/ml)	255	98

to the cellular elements. Minimal damage has been reported with the use of implantable pusher-plate type LVADs (Table 2.2).[5]

Considerations in treating acute *versus* chronic LV failure patients

Patients in acute LV failure may have distinctly different physiological challenges facing left ventricular support than patients in chronic LV failure. If the rate of onset of LV failure has been sudden, such as following a myocardial infarction, the right ventricle may not have had sufficient time to adjust to the retrograde challenges posed by the failing left ventricle. In contrast, a cardiomyopathy patient with a long history of cardiac disease may have an RV that has had an opportunity to accommodate to chronically elevated pulmonary pressures. A sudden elevation in the PVR (or transpulmonary pressure gradient) during the perioperative period may pose a greater threat to the unaccommodated, acutely stunned right ventricle compared with the accommodated right ventricle associated with chronic congestive heart failure. Accommodated or not, if the extent of myocardial damage is so severe that too little functional tissue remains, the RV will be incapable of actively delivering blood through the lungs to the left ventricle. Passive flow through the right ventricle may be possible provided the pulmonary

vascular resistance does not obstruct forward flow.

Biological recovery in the LVAD candidate

Recovery in the native heart

Scheinen *et al.*[6] recently cited evidence for recovery of the ventricular myocardium based on morphological comparisons of samples removed before and after prolonged ventricular assistance. Apical samples from the left ventricle of eight cardiomyopathy patients were electively removed at the time of LVAD implantation, and the histological appearance compared with samples obtained following ventricular assistance at the time of transplantation. Marked improvement in the histological properties of the myocardium was observed following an average of 79 days of ventricular assistance. Samples examined following ventricular assistance exhibited a marked decrease in myocyte attenuation compared with samples removed prior to circulatory support. These findings were supported by radiographic evidence indicating that the ventricular dimensions decreased substantially as a result of ventricular assistance.

Additional studies are presently in progress to assess changes in contractility of the natural heart during ventricular assistance, using transoesophageal echocardiography (TEE). Preliminary observations indicate that right and left ventricular ejection fractions significantly increase following initiation of left ventricular assistance. These findings, coupled with the observation that patients exhibit improved tolerance to brief 'pump off' tests over time, further support the conclusion that cardiac function improves as a result of ventricular assistance.

Hepatic, renal and pulmonary recovery

Bridge-to-transplant candidates with a history of progressive cardiac failure often exhibit significant multiorgan dysfunction shortly before or after LVAD implantation. The condition of the end organs appears to deteriorate due to poor perfusion. Restoration of an adequate driving pressure and flow to the peripheral organs has been shown to result in progressive improvement in the renal, hepatic and pulmonary status of the patient.[3,4,7] However, it has also been shown to

Table 2.3 Hepatic and renal responses to ventricular assistance.

Parameter	Baseline value before LVAD implant (n = 27)	At 30 days	Last value before transplant
Hepatic			
Total bilirubin (mg/dl)	2.3 ± 1.9	1.1 ± 1.1	0.7 ± 0.4
SGOT (U/l)	73 ± 71	74 ± 96	35 ± 19
Renal			
Creatinine (mg/dl)	1.7 ± 0.9	10 ± 0.6	1.2 ± 0.5
BUN (mg/dl)	37 ± 19	19 ± 19	19 ± 12

take up to six weeks for normal hepatic function to be restored following use of the device. In still other patients, the end organs continue to deteriorate despite improved flows for reasons that remain largely elusive.

Hepatic recovery

Marked improvement in hepatic function, based on changes in total bilirubin and serum enzyme values, has been observed for the majority of patients treated with the HeartMate® 1000 IP LVAD (Table 2.3). In a recent study, total bilirubin and SGOT values were each compared within 24 hours before LVAD implant, and just before transplant, for 27 patients who were successfully bridged for an average of 102 days.[3] The average final values just before transplant (total bilirubin = 0.7 mg/dl; SGOT = 35 U/l) were significantly reduced compared with the average baseline values (total bilirubin = 2.3 mg/dl; SGOT = 73 U/l); however, approximately six weeks' of support was required for the serum enzymes to be returned to normal values.

Renal recovery

In the same study described above, creatinine and BUN values were monitored at weekly intervals throughout support to assess renal function. Both parameters were found to be significantly reduced as a result of ventricular assistance. The final values just before transplant (creatinine = 1.2 mg/dl; BUN = 19 mg/dl) were significantly reduced compared with the baseline values just before LVAD implant (creatinine = 1.7 mg/dl; BUN = 37 mg/dl).

Pulmonary recovery

The rate of improvement of pulmonary function during ventricular assistance has been evaluated in a cohort of 12 patients treated with the Heart-Mate 1000 IP LVAD for periods greater than 30 days.[7] The mean cardiac index and pulmonary capillary wedge pressure returned to normal in all patients within 3 days on the LVAD. The mean pulmonary arterial pressure and pulmonary vascular resistance decreased, but not to normal. The mean CVP remained elevated throughout the first month and then eventually decreased to normal. Peak airway pressures improved allowing 10 of the 12 patients to be extubated by the fifth postoperative day. Preoperative evidence of pulmonary oedema was present on X-ray in 8 patients, and pulmonary hilar prominence was present in the remaining four. The pulmonary oedema resolved, but persisted for approximately a week after surgery in the majority of patients. Optimal recovery of pulmonary function required several weeks.

Loisance[8] reported recovery of pulmonary function following initiation of ventricular assistance, based on reductions in pulmonary capillary wedge pressure and clearing of third-space fluid in the lungs, within the initial days of mechanical circulatory support. In fact, the lungs were reported to be one of the first organs to respond to restoration of perfusion.

Exercise tolerance in the LVAD patient

If left ventricular assist devices are ultimately to serve as an alternative to transplantation, patients supported with this technology must respond physiologically to the cardiovascular demands of daily activities. Studies are in progress to assess the ability of LVAD patients to respond to circulatory demands during moderate exercise.[9] Within one month following the LVAD implant, patients are tested on stationary bicycles and upright treadmills with the work load ranging from 50 to 150 W power output. Haemodynamic and oxygen consumption measurements are performed before, during and after exercise with the LVAD operated in the asynchronous 'pump on full' mode. During exercise, the LVAD typically increases in beat rate with little change in stroke volume. The output of the device rises significantly in parallel with oxygen consumption. Fifteen to thirty minutes of exercise is generally well tolerated. Patients treated with the HeartMate LVAD, as well as the Novacor device, have been shown to adapt to the demands of normal daily activities without difficulty.

Synchronous and asynchronous pump operations

Pulsatile LVADs are generally operated in either synchronous or asynchronous control modes. When operated synchronously, the blood pump is set to eject at a predetermined point during the cardiac cycle. During asynchronous pumping, the device is timed to eject independently of the cardiac cycle.

Synchronous copulsation *versus* counterpulsation

There are two basic forms of synchronous pumping: co- and counterpulsation. Simultaneous ejection of the pump during biologic systole is termed synchronous copulsation. During copulsation, both the natural heart and LVAD fill simultaneously during biologic diastole, and empty during systole. Consequently, the left ventricle is volume (but not pressure) unloaded.

Alternatively, the device may be set to eject during biologic diastole, an option referred to as synchronous counterpulsation. In this mode, the left ventricle either passively or actively empties into the pump, pressure unloading (but not volume unloading) the left ventricle.

'Fixed rate' *versus* 'pump on full' asynchronous modes

A pulsatile blood pump may also be ejected at regular intervals independent of the cardiac cycle. Two options frequently used include 'fixed rate' and 'pump on full' modes. In the 'fixed rate' mode, the pump is set to eject at a rate that optimizes output. The rate may or may not be equivalent to the natural heart. In the 'pump on full' mode, the beat rate of the pump is varied to eject when full. As with the 'fixed rate' mode, the timing of ejection is independent of the cardiac cycle.

The eject time in any asynchronous mode wanders through the cardiac cycle. At times, the device is copulsing and at other times it is counterpulsing. The closer the rates are matched between the pump and the natural heart, the

longer it takes to wander through the cardiac cycle.

Although the HeartMate 1000 IP LVAD may be operated in both synchronous and asynchronous modes, the 107 patients treated to date were supported using only asynchronous pumping in either the 'fixed rate' or 'pump on full' control options. Asynchronous operation greatly simplifies management of the patient by eliminating the need to synchronize the device with the cardiac cycle. It is also practical in the presence of confounding arrhythmias.

At present there does not appear to be any physiological advantage of operating in the synchronous rather than the asynchronous mode. In a recent study by Pantalos *et al.*,[10] the effect of synchronous versus asynchronous operation of a pulsatile LVAD was investigated. The primary focus of the investigation was on determining the change in regional organ blood flow distribution and LV myocardial oxygen consumption (LV MVo_2) in response to each mode. Pulsatile LV assistance was found to result in a significant reduction in LV MVo_2, independent of the operating control mode. Moreover, regional organ blood flow distribution was independent of LVAD control mode.

Clinical complications

LV support in the presence of RV dysfunction

Right ventricular dysfunction is regarded as one of the most significant contraindications for use of left ventricular support. RV failure refractory to drug therapy has been reported to occur in up to 30% of candidates treated with an LVAD.[11] In our own experience approximately 20% of patients treated with LVAD support required right ventricular assistance.

Historically, RV function has been considered relatively unimportant in maintaining adequate flow provided that pulmonary vascular resistance remains within a normal range.[11-17] A number of studies using normal hearts have shown the right ventricle to be essentially a passive conduit with little need for active contractility as long as pulmonary vascular resistance remains normal.[17] Patients have been adequately supported despite ventricular fibrillation or stone heart syndrome.[18] Nevertheless, the mortality rate of patients in severe RV failure treated solely with univentricular LV assistance has been high.

A number of hypotheses have been advanced suggesting that decompression of the left ventricle during LV assistance can have a direct negative influence on the haemodynamic and anatomic performance of the right ventricle.[19,20] RV dysfunction in the presence of LVAD pumping has been attributed to mechanical uncoupling of the left and right ventricles and disruption of the normal biventricular geometric relations.[20] Volume unloading of the left ventricle has been shown to result in a deviation of the interventricular septum towards the free LV wall. Deviation of the septum accompanied by alterations in the relative volumes and compliances of the two ventricles has been regarded as significant due to direct mechanical ventricular interdependence.

Ventricular interdependence during diastole has been suggested to occur whenever the relative end-diastolic volumes of the two ventricles change disproportionately.[20] The diastolic compliance characteristics of the two ventricles may also be altered under these circumstances. The consequences of ventricular interaction during systole is less clear; however, it appears that a fall in right ventricular dP/dT associated with the leftward septal deviation results from LV unloading that may be due to loss of mechanical uncoupling across the septum.

Reductions in peak RV pressures and dP/dTs have led some to conclude that the right ventricular performance during LV decompression is diminished.[21] While peak RV pressures and dP/dTs are reduced, others have reported no change in RV performance based on RV energetic function and stroke-work/end-diastolic volume relationships between control and unloaded states. The apparent disparity between these reports has been suggested to be related to the methodology used in each study,[20] and in particular, issues related to load-dependence of the parameters used to assess RV function.

While it appears that unloading of the left ventricle can influence the haemodynamic and anatomic relations between the two ventricles due to direct mechanical ventricular interdependence, the significance of the effect is unclear. Recent reports suggest that the alterations in haemodynamics resulting from unloading of the LV play only a minor role in clinically significant RV failure.[20,22] A much more significant factor may involve the 'unmasking' of primary damage

to the RV once the right side is haemodynamically challenged due to increased flow provided by the LVAD. If the LVAD produces more flow than the RV can pump, and if the PVR is elevated, a vicious cycle leading to inadequate pulmonary venous return may ensue. The RV may then become refractory to pharmacological intervention once the primary disorder is unveiled.

Farrar and associates found, in the dog, that induction of ischaemic damage in the RV via coronary artery ligation produced a much more profound failure than direct decompression of the LV.[22] Chow,[23] on the other hand, using rapid ventricular pacing to induce heart failure, found that LV pressure reduction with an LVAD had a detrimental effect on the impaired RV, suggesting that anatomic ventricular interactions may have a more significant role in heart failure than in the normal heart in determining RV function during LV support. These experimental findings suggest that decompression of the left ventricle, as well as the primary disorder of the right ventricle, may both contribute to the deterioration of RV performance in the presence of an LVAD when operated in the synchronous counterpulsation mode of operation. The effect of LV decompression is even less clear when the LVAD is operated in an asynchronous mode.

Other studies have been performed to evaluate the potential of the RV to recover as a result of ventricular assistance. Bennick *et al.*[24] reported that the cardiac output and RV stroke work index [stroke volume index (mPaP–CVP) 0.0136] significantly increased in a series of 14 patients treated for between 4 and 233 days with the HeartMate 1000 IP LVAD. The improvement in right ventricular function was observed when the device was operated in an asynchronous mode of operation.

Conclusions

1. Left ventricular decompression due to LV assistance will lead to alterations in the mechanical coupling between the right and left ventricles, and therefore, influence RV pressure/flow relationships.
2. Adequate circulatory support with an LVAD is possible even in the presence of RV dysfunction providing PVR is not elevated.
3. Unmasking of RV pathology such as perioperative ischaemic damage may only be noted once the LVAD flows challenge the capability

of the RV *and if the PVR is elevated.*
4. Patients with elevated PVR (>5.0 wood units) and/or documented RV infarcts, particularly in the anterior free wall and interventricular septum, may be regarded as a criteria for exclusion from LVAD support.

Bleeding

Bleeding due to surgery, rheological abnormalities, or from the device itself, is a serious risk that must be anticipated when implanting a ventricular assist device. Bleeding has been reported to occur in approximately 40% of patients treated with these devices.[25,26] For reasons not completely understood, a small percentage of patients experience intraoperative coagulopathy that can pose a life-threatening condition if not managed properly.

Techniques currently used to minimize the risk of bleeding include meticulous surgical technique, and avoidance of pharmacological agents known to disrupt normal platelet function. Extreme caution in the use of anticoagulants, including antiplatelet agents, both preoperatively and during implantation, is also required.

Haemolysis

Destruction of red blood cells during mechanical circulatory support is generally considered significant if the plasma free haemoglobin values average greater than 10 mg/dl. Damage to red blood cells during ventricular assistance may occur due to a variety of mechanisms that include, but are not limited to, transfusion and/or drug reactions, complement activation, or mechanical stresses related to pumping.

The HeartMate 1000 IP LVAD has been observed to be associated with plasma free haemoglobin values that average approximately 8 mg/dl. However, individual patients have been treated having greater values, including one who was supported for 66 days with values that averaged 40 mg/dl and up to peak values of 112 mg/dl. These patients have been successfully supported as a bridge to transplant despite the existence of haemolysis.

Infection

Infection in the LVAD patient is difficult to assess owing to the lack of uniform reporting. Never-theless, it is generally agreed that end-stage cardiac patients who undergo implantation with a ventricular assist device are at significant risk for a variety of reasons. Infection may arise due to bacterial contamination at the time of surgery, via percutaneous leads, from vascular access or chest tube devices used in the treatment of the patient, or due to septicaemia. Typical infection rates for LVAD patients range from 20 to 75%.[25–27] However, only a fraction of these are regarded as true device-related events. In patients treated with the HeartMate device, the incidence of device-related events has been reported to be approximately 25%, with 85% of the patients with infections going on to be transplanted.[5]

Whereas mediastinal infection was the primary cause of death in 40% of patients receiving a total artificial heart as a bridge to transplant,[28,29] relatively few patients experience mediastinitis in the presence of an LVAD. Rooks *et al.*[30] recently reported a case involving a patient who experienced mediastinitis that was successfully treated during LVAD support; the patient was transplanted and went on to be a long-term survivor. In the HeartMate trial, there has been no significant difference in the rate of transplantation or survival for patients who did *versus* did not experience device-related infections.[5]

Thromboembolic complications

The risk of thromboembolic complications in patients supported with mechanical circulatory support devices has been a major preoccupation of many investigators using these devices.[26,27,31–34] Estimates of the frequency of embolic complications range from 2.8% for the HeartMate LVAD, to as high as 47% for other devices.[34] The low incidence of thromboembolic complications with the HeartMate device is attributed to the use of textured biomaterials that interface with the blood, as well as meticulous detail in the pump design to promote optimal flow patterns during actuation.

The textured surfaces encourage the formation of a biological lining that has proven to be highly haemocapatible. A number of studies have been reported summarizing the nature of this surface following long-term implantation.[35,36]

It is essential that any device intended for long-term implantation is designed to encourage optimal flow patterns within the pump chamber. The

HeartMate LVAD accomplishes this goal by promoting the formation of a wandering vortex within the pump chamber that continually washes the blood contacting surfaces and minimizes areas of stasis.

Three of 107 patients treated with the Heart-Mate LVAD have had embolic events. The first event occurred in a patient who had a mechanical aortic valve in the native heart. The patient experienced transient, reversible neurological dysfunction during support that was attributed to thrombus that was liberated from the valve (not the LVAD). Thrombus was visualized on the valve during support and at the time of transplantation. A second patient developed apical thrombus during support due to stasis within an extremely dilated left ventricle. Because the patient had experienced gastric bleeding that originated preoperatively, no anticoagulants were administered. This patient eventually experienced a CVA that was thought to be due to thrombus liberated by the inflow conduit that appeared to originate in the left ventricle. The final patient had positive antigens for candida. Following approximately three months of support, the patient experienced a renal infarct attributed to the septic emboli.

While the results with the HeartMate LVAD have been encouraging, it is clear that embolic complications can be expected even with the best of devices. Thromboembolism is a common complication for patients with dilated cardiomyopathy not treated with such devices.[37] Up to 60% of patients with dilated cardiomyopathy have either clinical or autopsy evidence of emboli.[38] Thrombus within the poorly contracting heart has been cited as being the source of such embolic complications.[39,40] It is also well known that patients in atrial fibrillation are at great risk of thromboembolism. We must, therefore, be realistic in our expectations with such devices and realize that thromboembolism will occur even with an optimally designed device.

Pathophysiological observations

The early literature devoted to characterizing the physiological responses to total heart replacement in animals described a number of transient events following implantation of a TAH. These included elevated CVPs, increased circulating blood volume, and high- as well as low-output syndrome.[41] Most of the investigations designed to study this syndrome focused on the role of neu-rohumoral mechanisms in the response. In reviewing the literature, as well as our own results, there does not appear to be any evidence of this phenomenon in LVAD patients.

An interesting observation in the HeartMate LVAD trial has been that patients with sepsis achieve exceptionally high flows (8–10 l/min) during support. Equally interesting is that many of these patients respond to IV antibiotics, with flows eventually declining to normal prior to transplantation. Considerable debate has existed regarding whether it is necessary to provide patients with flows of up to 10 litres per minute. Based on the favourable response of septic patients to high-flow conditions, it appears that it may be advantageous to have pumps capable of producing high flows during active infection.

End-stage cardiac patients often have a long history of poor peripheral perfusion that may have a deleterious effect on peripheral organ function. Long-term use of high-dose inotropes may also have a noxious effect on renal and/or hepatic function. Recent experience with mechanical circulatory support devices suggests that there may be transient reperfusion effects on renal function if restoration of flow occurs too rapidly.

Selected cases have been reported recently where LVADs have been implanted in patients with mechanical aortic valves in the native heart. The experience in these patients has been less than satisfactory owing to the risk of thromboembolism. The HeartMate LVAD was used in two such patients: one for 15 days and the other for 173 days. Although both patients were successfully transplanted and discharged, both had thrombus on the aortic valve at explant. Furthermore, one of the patients experienced a cerebral vascular accident during the period of support. The risk of thrombus on a mechanical aortic valve is increased because a properly performing LVAD will capture most of the ventricular output, leaving the aortic valve closed for the majority of the time. Any condition resulting in the opening of the mechanical aortic valve creates the potential for an embolic episode.

Autopsy observations

Performance of an autopsy following ventricular assistance is critical to obtain vitally needed information regarding the effectiveness of a device as well as its safety. Gross inspection of all the pump components, along with each of the individual organs, is essential to assess whether adequate perfusion was provided, to evaluate anatomical fit and fixation, and to examine the thromboembolic risk associated with use of the device.

Routine examination of the heart, lungs, brain, kidneys, liver, spleen, pancreas, gastrointestinal tract, and vessels, both grossly and microscopically, is required. Individual organs must be examined for any thrombus or vegetation and any emboli noted. Particular attention must be directed towards determining the possible relationship between any thrombus that is observed, and the presence of infarcts. If possible, it is valuable to date the thrombus to ascertain whether it may have antedated the device, or if it occurred within the period of support. The findings must be correlated with a detailed history of the patient to determine if other devices may have been used that could complicate conclusions pertaining to any adverse observation.

Pump retrieval analyses

Observations to be noted in pumps at the time of retrieval include thrombus, pannus, calcification, vegetation, and fresh coagulum. Thrombus is most frequently noted at junctions between pump components, and in areas favouring stasis. In patients with a history of sepsis, there may be focal vegetation. Occasionally the vegetation is associated with thrombus, which has led to numerous studies devoted to evaluating the relationship between infection and thrombosis.[27]

Pannus is classically identified in regions near anastomoses. Firmly adherent deposits of fibrinous material have been observed that can potentially proliferate to the point of totally occluding the cannulae. Pannus is most frequently observed in the inflow cannula of a VAD, but has been observed in association with the outflow cannula as well.

It is important to note that patients can be adequately supported without embolic complications despite the presence of thrombus and/or tissue deposition. Icenogle *et al.*,[34] for example, reported that 7 of 11 patients supported with the Symbion VAD had thrombus on the device, yet only 3 experienced thromboembolic complications.

A key area of concern in the explanted pump is the valves. For those devices utilizing bioprosthetic valves it is essential to examine the integrity of the leaflets and to determine whether calcification has occurred. The design of the valve with respect to flow patterns is critical to avoid areas of focal stasis.[42]

Continuous *versus* pulsatile flow

The literature is replete with articles aimed at determining the physiological responses to pulsatile *versus* non-pulsatile flow. For a thorough review of this topic the reader may wish to examine the works of Hickey and colleagues[43] and of Mavroudis.[44] The results from different investigations comparing the two perfusion states appear to be contradictory and confusing; however, as suggested by Philbin[45] and later by Wright and Furness,[46] the apparently conflicting results stem from the lack of adequate definition of pulsatile flow. Whereas non-pulsatile devices produce a uniform, monolithic form of pressure, pulsatile systems produce a waveform that is polymorphic and dependent upon both the device (pulse source) and the viscoelastic properties of the vascular system being perfused. Since different devices have been utilized that produce pulses of different amplitude and morphology, it has been difficult to compare results from one laboratory to the next. Nevertheless, the following discussion summarizes some of the salient results.

Haemodynamic responses to continuous *versus* pulsatile flow

Adequate flows and pressures can be achieved with either non-pulsatile or pulsatile perfusion. However, reflex responses to each type of perfusion reportedly differ. For example, the peripheral vascular resistance (PVR) has been shown to increase during non-pulsatile cardiopulmonary bypass (CPB).[43] When the PVR was measured during pulsatile flow, it was found to increase,[47] decrease,[48–51] or remain the same[52,53] compared with non-pulsatile flow. The consensus, however, appears to be that the PVR is lower during pulsatile flow.[43]

In key animal studies reported by Golding and colleagues, the early postoperative period during non-pulsatile pumping was characterized by a low cardiac output, high systemic and pulmonary vascular resistances, and a marked increase in circulating catecholamine.[54,55] These results are consistent with reports that non-pulsatile perfusion of the carotid sinus and aortic arch baroreceptors may cause an increase in symphatoadrenergic activity, systemic vascular resistance, and mean arterial pressure.[56,57] These effects were found to be transient, with the circulating catecholamine returning to normal within 14 days.[58,59] In studies performed for longer periods up to 99 days, normal physiological function returned, provided the flow was maintained high enough, with renal, endocrine and hepatic function remaining within normal limits.[58] These results suggest that a period of approximately two weeks is required following implantation of a non-pulsatile device for the body to accommodate to the altered perfusion. Beyond this time, non-pulsatile flow appears to be associated with normal haemodynamic and humoral responses.

To circumvent the problem of having to distinguish perfusion effects from those of anaesthesia and surgery, recent studies have been performed in chronic, awake, unanaesthetized animals.[60] After two weeks of pulsatile support utilizing an LV assist device, non-pulsatile pumping with a centrifugal pump was instituted. The pump was adjusted to maintain a comparable mean aortic pressure. Unlike the transient changes in cardiac output and humoral factors noted in the first two postoperative weeks, the central venous pressure, cardiac output, and systemic vascular resistance remained unchanged compared with pulsatile pumping. Moreover, the plasma catecholamine and renin angiotensin levels remained at control levels. This was an interesting study which demonstrated that if sufficient time is allowed to get over the transient effects of surgery, and if the mean pressure is held constant with adequate flows, both pulsatile and non-pulsatile perfusion are well tolerated.

Conclusions

The basic engineering principles required to assist the natural circulation for prolonged periods have been reduced to practice with a variety of existing devices. We now enter a whole new era of physiology devoted towards further investigating the host response to ventricular assistance, on improving our understanding of fundamental principles of cardiovascular physiology, and on reducing the incidence of clinical complications.

There are at present a variety of different LVADs that have been shown to provide adequate haemodynamic support for patients in severe LV failure. Some, especially the extracorporeal devices, are ideally suited for brief support for patients in acute LV failure. Postcardiotomy patients as well as individuals with acute myocardial infarction are best served with the least expensive, least invasive technology that can be used for uni- or biventricular support until the patient is stabilized. In the future, it is anticipated that if such patients fail to recover fully, but are stable, they may be weaned from extracorporeal support on to one of the implantable devices until transplantation.

Preliminary results with the HeartMate and Novacor devices have been highly encouraging for long-term support. In the near future, it can be expected that one or both of the devices will be used as an alternative to transplantation utilizing a simplified vented approach. A completely sealed system, without percutaneous access and/or a compliance chamber, is still under development.

It is clear, based on the present results that implantable LVADs provide adequate haemodynamic support. Now that there is confidence in the ability of these devices to improve survival, more interesting research is under way. Programmes are in progress to study neurohumoral reflex responses to ventricular support, and to assess exercise tolerance in the LVAD patient. Quality of life indices are being developed to evaluate LVAD candidates during long-term support. Critical studies are also in progress to improve patient selection, and to determine factors that may preclude patients from benefiting from such technology.

The clinical experience with the HeartMate LVAD has been highly rewarding. Patients have been supported for periods as long as 324 days on the pneumatic system and 460 days with the electromechanical device. Sixty-four per cent of the patients treated with the pneumatic LVAD as a bridge to transplant have been successfully transplanted, with an overall survival of approximately 55%. (For a more detailed overview of the results the reader is referred to Chapter 26.) Considering the high mortality rate for this patient population, these devices are proving to offer significant clinical utility in a safe and effective manner.

The next step towards realizing the true goal of this technology, to employ LVADs as an alternative to transplantation, has been taken by allowing qualified patients to be released from the controlled clinical environment to the home setting. Thermo Cardiosystems Inc. is currently studying patients released from the hospital on day trips with the hope of eventually supporting patients on an outpatient basis. As we gain longer term experience, and demonstrate that the device is safe and reliable in the home environment, sufficient data will be obtained to justify using these devices as an additional therapeutic option for patients either ineligible for cardiac transplantation, or for candidates for whom a donor heart does not exist.

References

1. Weber K, Janiki JS, Maskin CS. Pathophysiology of cardiac failure. *Am J Cardiol* 1985; **56**, 3B–7B.
2. Kanter KR, Swartz MT, Pennington G, Rusevich SA, Madden M, McBride LR, Termuhlen DF. Renal failure in patients with ventricular assist devices. *ASAIO Trans* 1987; **33**, 426–427.
3. Dasse KA, Frazier OH, Lesniak JM, Myers T, Burnett CM, Poirier VL. Clinical responses to ventricular assistance *versus* transplantation in a series of bridge to transplant patients. *ASAIO Trans* 1992; **38**, M622–626.
4. Friedel N, Viazis P, Schießler A, Warnecke H, Hennig E, Trittin A, Bottner W, Hetzer R. Recovery of end-organ failure during mechanical circulatory support. *Eur J Cardiothorac Surg* 1992; **6**, 519–523.
5. Frazier OH, Rose EA, Macmanus Q, Burton NA, Lefrak EA, Poirier VL, Dasse KA. Multicenter clinical evaluation of the HeartMate® 1000 IP left ventricular assist device. *Ann Thorac Surg* 1992; **53**, 1080–1090.
6. Scheinin S, Capek P, Radovancevic B, Duncon JM, McAllister HA, Frazier OH. The effect of prolonged left ventricular support on myocardial histopathology in patients with end-stage cardiomyopathy. *ASAIO J* 1992; **38**, M271–274.
7. Baldwin RT, Duncan JM, Radovancevic B, Frazier OH, Abou-Awdi NL. Recovery of pulmonary function in patients undergoing extended left ventricular assistance. *Chest* 1992; **102**, 45–49.
8. Loisance DY. Mechanical circulatory support in the 1990s. *Eur J Cardiothorac Surg* 1992; **6**(suppl 1), S107–112.
9. Myers TJ, Hare WD, McGee MG, Frazier OH, Dasse KA. LVAD automatic mode response to exercise. *ASAIO Abst* 1991; **20** 48.
10. Pantalos GM, Marks JD, Riebman JB, Everett SD, Burns GL, Burton NA, FePaulis R. Left ventricular oxygen consumption and organ blood flow distribution during pulsatile ventricular assist. *ASAIO Trans* 1988; 356–360.
11. DeBakey ME. Left ventricular bypass pump for cardiac assistance. *Am J Cardiol* 1971; **27**, 3–11.
12. Starr I, Jeffers WA, Meade RH. The absence of conspicuous increments of venous pressure after severe damage to the right ventricle of the dog, with a discussion of the relation between clinical congestive failure and heart disease. *Am Heart J* 1943; **26**, 291–301.
13. Rodbard S, Wagner D. Bypassing the right ventricle. *Proc Soc Exp Biol Med* 1949; **71**, 69–70.
14. Donald DE, Essex HE. Pressure studies after inactivation of the major portion of the canine right ventricle. *Am J Physiol* 1954; **14**, 155–161.
15. Dalta-Volla S, Battaglia G, Zerbini E. 'Auricularization' of right ventricular pressure curve. *Am Heart J* 1961; **61**, 25–33.
16. Sarwatani S, Mandell G, Kusaba E, Schraut W, Cascade P, Wajszczuk WJ, Kantrowitz A. Ventricular performance following ablation and prosthetic replacement of right ventricular myocardium. *ASAIO Trans* 1974; **20**, 629–635.
17. Jett GK, Applebaum RE, Clark RE. Right ventricular assistance for experimental right ventricular dysfunction. *J Thorac Cardiovasc Surg* 1986; **92**, 272–278.
18. Solomon AR, Sturm JT, Massin EK, Norman JC. Sequential electrocardiographic analyses of stone heart syndrome in a patient supported six days with an abdominal left ventricular assist device (ALVAD). *Cardiovasc Dis Bull, Texas Heart Inst* 1979; **6**, 173–180.
19. Farrar DJ, Compton PG, Hershon JJ, Foner JD, Hill JD. Right ventricular pressure–dimension relationship during left ventricular assistance in dogs. *ASAIO Trans* 1984; **30**, 121–123.
20. Elbeery JR, Owen CH, Savitt MA, Davis JW, Feneley MP, Rankin S, VanTrigt P. Effects of the left ventricular assist device on right ventricular function. *J Thorac Cardiovasc Surg* 1990; **99**, 809–816.
21. Miyamoto AT, Tanaka S, Matloff JM. Right ventricular function during left heart bypass. *J Thorac Cardiovasc Surg* 1983; **85**, 49–53.
22. Farrar DJ, Chow E, Compton PG, Foppiano L, Woodward J, Hill JD. Effects of acute right ventricular ischemia on ventricular interactions during prosthetic left ventricular support. *J Thorac Cardiovasc Surg* 1991; **102**, 588–595.
23. Chow E, Farrar DJ. Right heart function during prosthetic left ventricular assistance in a porcine model of congestive heart failure. *J Thorac Cardiovasc Surg* 1992; **104**, 569–578.
24. Bennick GB, Noda H, Duncan JM, Frazier OH. Clinical evaluation of right ventricular function in patients with left ventricular assist device (LVAD). *Int J Artific Organs* 1992; **15**, 109–113.
25. Portner PM, Oyer PE, Pennington DG, *et al.*

Implantable electrical left ventricular assist system: bridge to transplantation and the future. *Ann Thorac Surg* 1989; **47**, 142–150.

26. Pennington DG, McBride LR, Kanter KR, *et al.* Bridging to heart transplantation with circulatory support devices. *J Heart Transplant* 1989; **8**, 116–123.

27. Didisheim P, Olsen DB, Farrar DJ, *et al.* Infections and thromboembolism with implantable cardiovascular devices. *ASAIO Trans* 1989, **35**, 54–70.

28. Griffith BP, Kormos RL, Hardesty RL, Armitage JM, Dummer JS. The artificial heart: infection-related morbidity and its effect on transplantation. *Ann Thorac Surg* 1988; **45**, 409–414.

29. Rice LB, Karchmer AW. Artificial heart implantation: what limitations are imposed by infectious complications? *JAMA* 1988; **259**, 894–895.

30. Rooks JR, Burton NA, Lefrak EA, Macmanus Q. Mediastinitis complicating successful mechanical bridge to heart transplantation. *J Heart Lung Transplant* 1992; **11**, 261–264.

31. Levinson MM, Smith RG, Cork RC, *et al.* Thromboembolic complications of the Jarvik-7 total artificial heart: case report. *Artif Organs* 1986; **10**, 236–244.

32. DeVries WC, Anderson JL, Joyce LD, *et al.* Clinical use of the total artificial heart. *New Engl J Med* 1984; **310**, 273–278.

33. Termuhlen DF, Swartz MT, Pennington DG, *et al.* Thromboembolic complications with the Pierce–Donachy ventricular assist device. *ASAIO Trans* 1989; **35**, 616–618.

34. Icenogle TB, Smith RG, Cleavinger M, *et al.* Thromboembolic complications of the Symbion AVAD system. *Artif Organs* 1989; **13**, 532–538.

35. Dasse KA, Chipman SD, Sherman CN, Levine AH, Frazier OH. Clinical experience with textured blood contacting surfaces in ventricular assist devices. *ASAIO Trans* 1987; **33**, 418–425.

36. Graham TR, Dasse KA, Coumbe A, Salih V, Marrinan MT, Frazier OH, Lewis CT. Neo-intimal development on textured biomaterial surfaces during clinical use of an implantable left ventricular assist device. *Eur J Cardiothorac Surg* 1990; **4**, 182–190.

37. Fuster V, Gersh B, Giuliani AJ, Brandenburg RO, Frye RL. The natural history of idiopathic dilated cardiomyopathy. *Am J Cardiol* 1981; **47**, 525–535.

38. Gottdiener JS, Gay JA, Van Vorhees L, Dibianco R, Fletcher RD. Frequency and embolic potential of left ventricular thrombus in dilated cardiomyopathy: assessment by 2-dimensional echocardiography. *Am J Cardiol* 1983; **52**, 1281–1285.

39. Roberts WC, Siegel RJ, McManus BM. Idiopathic dilated cardiomyopathy: analysis of 152 necrosis patients. *Am J Cardiol* 1987; **60**, 1340–1355.

40. Maze SS, Kotler MJ, Parry WR. Flow characteristics in the dilated left ventricle with thrombus: qualitative and quantitative Doppler analysis. *Am J*

Cardiol 1989; **13**, 873–881.

41. Murakami T, Ozawa K, Harasaki H, Jacobs G, Kiraly R, Nose Y. Transient and permanent problems associated with the total artificial heart implantation. *ASAIO Trans* 1979; **25**, 239–247.

42. Wagner WR, Johnson PC, Winowich S, Pristas J. Evaluation of LVAD inflow and outflow valves and comparison between thromboembolic event and non-event patient groups. *Proc Cardiovasc Sci Tech Conf (AAMI)* 1991; 127.

43. Hickey PR, Buckley MJ, Philbin DM. Pulsatile and nonpulsatile cardiopulmonary bypass: review of a counter-productive controversy. *Ann Thorac Surg* 1983; **36**, 720–737.

44. Mavroudis C. To pulse or not to pulse. *Ann Thorac Surg* 1978; **25**, 259.

45. Philbin DM. Should we pulse? *J Thorac Cardiovasc Surg* 1982; **84**, 805.

46. Wright G, Furness A. What is pulsatile flow? *Ann Thorac Surg* 1985; **39**, 401–402.

47. Ogata T, Ida Y, Nonoyama A, *et al.* A comparative study of the effectiveness of pulsatile and nonpulsatile flow in extracorporeal circulation. *Arch Jpn Clin* 1960; **29**, 59.

48. Nakayama K, Tamiya T, Yamamoto K, *et al.* High-amplitude pulsatile pump in extracorporeal circulation with particular reference to hemodynamics. *Surgery* 1963; **54**, 798.

49. Mandelbaum I, Berry J, Silbert M, *et al.* Hemodynamic effects of pulsatile and nonpulsatile flow. *Arch Surg* 1965; **9**, 771.

50. Mandelbaum I, Burns WH. Pulsatile and nonpulsatile blood flow. *JAMA* 1965; **191**, 657.

51. Shepard RB, Kirklin JB. Relation of pulsatile flow to oxygen consumption and other variables during cardiopulmonary bypass. *J Cardiothorac Surg* 1969; **58**, 694.

52. Wesolowski SA, Sauvage LR, Pinc RD. Extracorporeal circulation: the role of the pulse in maintenance of the systemic circulation during heart lung bypass. *Surgery* 1955; **37**, 663.

53. Boucher JK, Rudy LW, Edmunds LH. Organ blood flow during pulsatile cardiopulmonary bypass. *J Appl Physiol* 1974; **36**, 86.

54. Golding LR, Jacobs G, Murakami T, *et al.* Chronic nonpulsatile blood flow in an alive, awake animal: 34-day survival. *ASAIO Trans* 1980; **26**, 251–254.

55. Golding LR, Murakami G, Harasaki H, *et al.* Chronic nonpulsatile blood flow. *ASAIO Trans* 1982; **28**, 81–85.

56. Angell-James JE, DeBurgh DM. Effects of graded pulsatile pressure on the reflex vasomotor responses elicited by changes of mean pressure in the perfused carotid sinus-aortic arch regions of the dog. *J Physiol (London)* 1971; **214**, 51.

57. Harrison TS, Chawla RC, Seaton JF, Robinson BH. Carotid sinus origin of adrenergic responses compromising the effectiveness of artificial circu-

latory support. *Surgery* 1970; **68**, 29.

58. Golding LR. Centrifugal pumps. In: Unger F (ed), *Assisted Circulation*. Berlin: Springer-Verlag, 1984: 142–152.

59. Valdes F, Takatani S, Jacobs G, Murakami T, Harasaki H, Golding LR, Nose Y. Comparison of hemodynamic changes in a chronic nonpulsatile biventricular bypass and total. artificial heart. *ASAIO Trans* 1980; **26**, 455–460.

60. Taenaka Y, Tatsumi E, Sakaki M, *et al*. Peripheral circulation during nonpulsatile systemic perfusion in chronic awake animals. *ASAIO Trans* 1991; **37**, M365–370.

3

The biomaterial–blood interface in circulatory support devices: a cardiac surgeon's view

Jack Copeland

Introduction

The biomaterial–blood interface has for years been the focus of much attention in devices for supporting the circulation.[1] In 1964, the US National Heart Lung and Blood Institute (NHLBI) initiated an artificial heart programme that had invested $264.4 million up to 1989.[2] (See also Fig. 20.1 in Chapter 20.) As a product of this investment, the money of numerous private sector investors, and the hard work of many investigators, several devices are at advanced stages of development. This development of devices for human use has, since the Medical Devices Amendments of 1976 and the Safe Medical Devices Act of 1990, been influenced to a great extent by the Food and Drug Administration (FDA). By law, they must review and approve devices and require a demonstration of safety, effectiveness and clinical utility before a device may be marketed.[3]

The intellectual, technical, financial and legal forces present in the United States and worldwide have resulted over a number of years in the development of several types of devices. Each of these has a history of extensive *in vitro* and preclinical animal testing. Most have also been tested in humans in ongoing clinical investigations. Industrial sponsors, faced with the reality of a restrictive medico-legal environment, have (with support from the NHLBI and their investors) endured over 17 years of high-cost research and development.[3] The cost of as much as $25 million

to bring a device to this stage has had profound effects upon those who drive the research and development effort. One of the most prominent effects has been to 'lock in' the design and components of each device for the future. Thus, the chance of a major change in any of the devices that are being developed is small because of the potential need to return to the extremely high-cost and long period of *in vitro* and preclinical testing currently required by the FDA. We therefore have a limited number of devices and materials (all of the linings are at least part polyurethane) to consider, particularly if we restrict our attention to those that are intended for extended use—as in the bridge-to-transplant, semi-permanent, or permanent implant applications (Table 3.1).

Definition of the problem

Each of the devices currently under investigation is the equivalent of an organ that performs the function of pumping blood. It is composed of 'tissues', some that contact the blood. Our concern is to infer from available evidence the clinical effectiveness and safety of these blood-contacting tissues.

One inclination might be to attribute all strokes to the lining of the device. Numerous authors of clinical articles have made incriminating references to the Biomer lining of the Jarvik-7 based

Table 3.1 Intermediate and long-term circulatory support devices.

Device	Polyurethane lining
Artificial heart	
Jarvik-7/CardioWest C-70	Biomer
Penn State Total Artificial Heart	Pellathane
Implantable ventricular assistance	
Novacor	Biomer
TCI (Thermo Cardiosystems Inc.)	Textured polyurethane/ sintered titanium
Extracorporeal pneumatic assistance	
Thoratec	'Biomer' (Thoratec BPS-215M polyurethane elastomer)
Symbion/CardioWest	Biomer
Nippon–Zeon	Cardiothane
Toboyo	Cardiothane
Cleveland Clinic	Biolysed polyurethane
Abiomed	Angioflex polyurethane

Source: reference 4.

upon the experience of DeVries with his series of four 'permanent' implants.[5] The explant evaluation of these hearts, however, in all cases failed to find any thrombi on the pumping chamber surfaces. In case 1 (a 112-day implant) and case 4 (a 10-day implant) there was no evidence of thrombosis or fibrin deposition. In case 2 (a 620-day implant) and case 3 (a 488-day implant) there was endoprosthetic infection of all valves and all anastomoses. In the two patients who had strokes, there was a temporal association between stroke and positive blood cultures suggestive of endoprosthetic infection. Is it possible that the Biomer had nothing to do with those strokes? Could they have been produced by embolization from a 'prosthetic endocarditis'? We know from extensive experience with valves and Dacron grafts that infections are not uncommonly related to valves and suture lines. There is no need to incriminate the Biomer from this experience. It appears that the sources of emboli were more likely vegetations.

The complexity of the clinical setting and of the device and our limited means for diagnosing intra-device thrombosis and embolic events challenge us to careful evaluation of available data. In a recent autopsy study of patients following centrifugal assist, it was found that the clinically diagnosed rate of thromboembolism was 2.3% in 35 patients. In five of eight patients (63%) in whom there was no clinical suspicion of emboli,

acute thromboembolic infarcts were found at autopsy.[6] We are probably 'under-reading' the clinical setting. If we could identify the precise location of a clot and track it to its destination we would have a perfect answer to this problem. In reality we must track all the evidence and draw conclusions.

Historical evidence regarding just the presence of a thromboembolic event is imperfect and probably underestimates the extent of the problem while only giving a hint as to the mechanism. One of the major problems we have experienced is in the setting of the operation to implant a device. If a neurological or other thromboembolic event occurs, is it related to the operation or caused by the device? What about the patient who has an embolic event and at explant has a perfectly clean device? In our experience with the Symbion BIVAD, multiple tiny thrombi could be seen through the translucent housing of the ventricle. Using transillumination, we observed and plotted the position of these foci daily. We documented changes in the patterns nearly every day, but there was no associated clinical embolic event that coincided with a change in the pattern of what must have been aggregated platelets.[7] Further, we noted that these foci were seen on the pump housing in an area near the outflow valve where the diaphragm hardly moved from systole to diastole. This was a very low flow area in a device with maximal mean flows of 4.5–5 l/min. We also found that we could avoid this problem either by positioning the ventricles more laterally, near the mid-axillary line, or having the patient sit upright. In both of these situations we observed improved diaphragmatic excursion and the absence of these 'platelet aggregates'. We presumed that this was simply due to the effect of position with respect to gravity on diaphragm excursion. The improved diaphragmatic excursion correlated with improved flow rate. I am unaware of any other chronic model in humans that provides the opportunity to observe the biomaterial–blood interface *in vivo*. It has confirmed animal studies that indicate thrombus generation tends to occur in areas of turbulence and of stagnation.[8]

Another aspect of historical evidence that warrants careful assessment is the disparity in investigational conditions and reported incidences of emboli. The permanent implant experience with the Jarvik-7 is not directly comparable to the Jarvik registry that found only nine of 171 patients bridged-to-transplant (5.3%) with a stroke and seven (4.1%) with a transient ischaemic attack,[9] or with the Jarvik-7 series from La Pitie Hospital with no clinical emboli in 58 patients, including one with the device in place for 602 days.[10] The median implant time from the registry was about two weeks and there were many anticoagulation regimens; whereas the meticulous system at La Pitie of monitoring and treating the haemostatic system is unlike any other in the world. Similarly the Texas Heart Institute experience with the TCI assist device has been outstanding. They have used aspirin and low-dose dipyridamole with their device and had no emboli in 18 patients with a mean duration of implant of 80 days. Such good results seem to have been attributed to the unique textured lining.[11]

Two other types of evidence may be of some benefit in sorting out the biomaterials problem in a clinical setting. Examination of the explanted device may be important, but also misleading. Sometimes it is more confounding to find tiny clots than not. Unfortunately, there is no common protocol for explant analysis. We know that stagnation may predispose to clot formation. Such stagnation in the presence of an air–blood–device interface may occur within a few minutes after explantation, confusing everyone including the team that examines the device after months of storage in preservative. The technique described by the Utah team in animals of flushing heparinized saline via a catheter into the pumping device avoids stasis and an air interface, and provides a gentle washing of the device.[12] Unfortunately, this would be impossible in most human cases. A reasonable approach in clinical situations might be immediate submersion of the explanted device in saline, followed by very gentle irrigation and then by examination of the entire device by the explanting surgeon. This might produce reliable and reproducible results for macroscopic examination. Microscopic examination (light, electron, scanning) could be completed later.

Autopsy reports provide a third type of clinical evidence for evaluation of the blood–biomaterial situation. Unfortunately, this information is often missing from clinical reports.

Mechanisms

It is important to remember that the biomaterial–blood interface is not just the lining of the device. For instance, in the CardioWest heart (see Fig.

19.3 in Chapter 19), blood flowing through an implanted ventricle must pass from atrium across a suture line joining atrium to a Biomer-covered Dacron mesh. It then passes through a quick-connect/valve-mount junction known to have some crevices[13] and next through a Medtronic–Hall valve. From there it is exposed to the Biomer lining on both the semi-rigid housing and the diaphragm. Finally, it exits by passing a somewhat irregular and creviced valve-mount/Medtronic–Hall valve/quick-connect complex, a Dacron graft and a graft–aorta anastomosis.

Blood–surface contact

We know that after instantaneous redistribution of interfacially bound water and ions at the blood–polymer interface, the first event that occurs is adsorption of plasma proteins and the formation of a protein layer. Platelets do not begin adhering for about one minute, by which time the protein layer is 0.02 μm thick.[14] The type of protein adsorbed to the surface greatly influences the degree of thrombogenesis. Albumin decreases the possibility of platelet adhesion and thrombogenesis or 'passivates' the surface. Fibrinogen and gamma globulin 'activate' the surface, enhancing platelet deposition and thrombogenesis. Adsorbed clotting factors (XII and XI) are also felt to be important in this activation. Polyurethane surfaces have been shown in many studies to adsorb relatively more albumin than other more thrombogenic surfaces such as glass, polyethylene, and polyvinyl chloride. *In vitro* studies have shown that Biomer and other polyurethanes tend to be more blood-compatible than most other polymer materials. Among the polyurethanes, those characterized by more soft segments and by hydrophilic properties seem to be more compatible.[14] Incorporation of heparin into Biomer ('heparin-immobilized Biomer') has in *ex vivo* experiments resulted in further reduction in fibrin deposition, platelet aggregation, and thrombus formation.[15]

In contrast to the smooth polyurethane surface is the textured blood contacting surface used in the TCI left ventricular assist device. An integrally textured polyurethane that is a one-piece polyurethane cast of a silicone mould serves as the flexing diaphragm. The surface is covered with fibrils 15 μm in diameter. The rigid side of the pumping chamber is covered with titanium microspheres 75–100 μm in diameter in a thickness of 3–4 spheres.[16–18] Early after implantation, a pseudo neo-intimal lining forms that consists of fibrin, platelets, red blood cells, and white blood cells. Later, at around 40 days, spindle-shaped cells and collagen are seen in addition to compacted fibrin mesh forming a denser lining. From what we know of activation of haemostatic mechanisms, this surface should cause continuous activation. The possibility of seeding this type of device with cells that may then develop a more cellular and adherent neo-intima has been successful in the laboratory.

A third type of surface, not yet tested clinically, has been developed by coating textured surfaces of the diaphragm and housing with gelatin that is then crosslinked by gluteraldehyde treatment. It is hoped that this type of surface might eliminate the need for anticoagulants.[19]

Flow

Contact of blood even with endothelium, the most perfect and thromboresistant surface known,[20] may produce thrombosis under conditions of low enough flow. Patients with cardiomyopathy and extremely low cardiac output are commonly found to have pulmonary embolism from blood clots formed in low-flow veins. Spontaneous clot formation within some low-flow ventricles can nearly be witnessed in real time with transthoracic or transoesophageal echocardiography. Animal and human experiences have documented this phenomenon in circulatory support devices. It is also well known that coagulation mechanisms account for clot formation in low-flow situations as opposed to platelet adherence and aggregation in higher flow settings (white thrombus formation in arteries). Careful experimental studies have substantiated these clinical observations, demonstrating a tendency for fibrin deposition at low shear rates and platelet adherence at higher shear rates.[21]

Activation of haemostatic systems

At the time of device implantation a major disturbance of the normal haemostatic equilibrium occurs. Surgical trauma liberates tissue factor III. Foreign surfaces, referring to any non-endothelial surface, stimulate factor XII and may adsorb factor XI which in turn may stimulate coagulation activity. Turbulence, shear forces, eddy currents, and non-endothelial surfaces activate platelets,

leading to degranulation and release of proaggregants. Thrombin is formed in large amounts leading to fibrin formation and to stimulation of fibrinolysis. If this activation were either not controlled or in the presence of sepsis, diffuse intravascular coagulopathy might result in consumption of all coagulation systems, formation of platelet aggregates, capillary occlusion, low perfusion, and death due to haemorrhage.

Is it possible to imagine any of the currently tested devices not causing some stimulation of, or 'strong and permanent aggression'[22] against, the haemostatic system? From everything we know about valves, conduits, anastomoses, apical cannulation, and the activation of the haemostatic as well as other systems, there must be some stimulation. Detailed documentation of the haemostatic status of implanted patients is most often absent or limited in clinical reports. Documentation in detail of the activation of the platelet, procoagulant, and fibrinolytic systems in the Jarvik-7 heart is available.[22] I am not aware of any other clinical study of this kind.

Clinical evidence exonerating the lining of artificial ventricles

I believe that most of the clinical evidence suggests that current artificial hearts are all potentially thrombogenic, but that it is not the lining that is incriminated in most studies. Valves, anastomoses, stagnation, turbulence, native heart to conduit connections, and inflow and outflow conduits and their connections are more suspect (Fig. 3.1).

The Jarvik-7 data offers considerable evidence. As previously mentioned, DeVries documented embolic strokes in two of his patients. Most occurred in close temporal relation to positive blood cultures. Case 2 had strokes on post-implant days

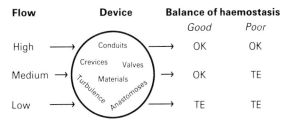

Fig. 3.1 Relationship of flow to thromboembolism (TE) and the haemostatic systems.

19, 94, 163, 352 and 620 and was found to have his first positive blood culture on day 21.[23] He was diagnosed as having prosthetic endocarditis from day 150 onward. Case 3 had a stroke on day 107 and positive blood cultures on days 39, 130 and many days thereafter. He was felt to have endocarditis from day 120 onward. At post mortem in these patients and the other two (case 1 was 112 days, case 4 was 10 days), there was no thrombosis of the Biomer linings in any of the hearts. There were vegetations typical of endocarditis on all valves and anastomoses in cases 2 and 3. This experience must be considered the 'worst case' scenario for any device since it was the first and the longest.

The registry for bridge-to-transplant experience with the Jarvik-7 has been briefly mentioned. Individual institutional experiences are also of interest. Besides having no neurological embolic events in 58 patients, including one with an implant time of 602 days, the La Pitie group reported no embolic events in a series of 18 autopsy cases post-Jarvik implantation. I have personally reviewed all interpretable explant evaluations of their devices, including 14 devices that were scored by Symbion (SOP scores) and 5 devices opened by Dr Gregorio Rabago, Jr, and myself. The SOP scores averaged 95% of the perfect score and the devices we examined were entirely free of thrombus except for two tiny white thrombi on the outflow valve of the right ventricle. These were not examined microscopically.

At Loyola in a 19-patient Jarvik-7 experience with 9.8 day mean implant time, they had one death from multiple cerebral infarcts that occurred on the tenth post-transplant day.[24] They had no thrombi on the ventricles or cuffs. They did have eight reoperations for bleeding and anticoagulated with heparin and low-dose dipyridamole. Pittsburgh reported on 16 patients with an average implant time of 9 days who were also anticoagulated with heparin and low-dose dipyridamole. They had one embolic stroke and reported that on post-explant examination most devices showed some tiny thrombi around the valve mount crevices. In addition they reported two large red thrombi, one associated with a left atrial line and a second in the diaphragm housing junction on the left side.[25] Our experience at the University of Arizona Heart Center in eight patients with a mean implantation time of 60 days, including one patient with 244 days of implantation utilizing heparin or warfarin plus low-dose

dipyridamole, revealed one stroke and one TIA.[26] The stroke occurred on implant day 218 in a patient with positive blood cultures. In the device from that patient there were two thin thrombi 5 mm in length in the diaphragm housing junction, one in each ventricle. There were also some scattered calcific deposits on electron microscopy. The patient with the TIA at 7 days, also the first to be bridged to transplantation with a TAH, was found to have tiny thrombi in the valve mount crevices. The remainder of our patients had no strokes and the devices revealed either no thrombi (2 cases) or tiny (<1 mm) white thrombi at the de-airing port perforation of the Biomer lining or in the diaphragm-housing junction.

The evidence with implantable LV assist systems regarding blood and biomaterials again is quite good. The Novacor experience that now exceeds 125 patients with 60% of the total surviving to transplantation has resulted in 89% survival of those transplanted. At Pittsburgh, in 11 patients with a mean duration of implantation of 38 days and an anticoagulation protocol of heparin or warfarin plus low-dose dipyridamole, there were two deaths from multi-organ failure. All nine of those transplanted survived. There were three TIAs and two strokes.[27] Bleeding was a problem intraoperatively, with a mean blood loss of 5300 ml and cardiac tamponade, eight episodes in 11 patients. At the University of Arizona Heart Center, of 13 implanted, seven died (3 of right heart failure, 2 of stroke, 1 of multiple organ failure, and 1 of late (40 days) tamponade). All six who were transplanted survived and among those there were no embolic events. Explant analysis in the two patients dying from stroke revealed in one case a 30% obstruction of the inflow conduit by an LV travecuulation. The other had evident thrombus on the distal side of the inflow valve and a history of inadequate anticoagulation. Our patients, who were anticoagulated with the same agents used at Pittsburgh, had no thrombus on the smooth Biomer lining and had some pseudo neo-intima in two inflow and three outflow conduits. There was a little fibrinous deposit on the inflow valves that was more apparent on the distal sides than on the proximals.

The implantable left ventricular assist experience using the Thermo Cardiosystems textured-surface device was reported in 18 patients.[28] The mean duration of support was 80 ± 77 days. Anticoagulation was with dextran early after implantation, followed by low-dose aspirin and dipyridamole. There have been only three deaths since 1988 in 14 patients, one from OKT3 reaction, one from air embolus, and one from right heart failure. There were no strokes. On explant analysis there was 'no evidence of thrombus in the pump, on the valves, or at the conduit connection sites'.

The major experience with extracorporeal pneumatic pulsatile devices is with univentricular and biventricular support with the Thoratec device using a sack-type pumping chamber of polyurethane made by the Thoratec company (BPS-215M polyurethane elastomer).[29] One hundred and twenty of the 154 patients had biventricular devices for a mean time of 17.5 days (range 0.3 to 226). Anticoagulation in this multicentre group was variable. There were 19 nonthromboembolic neurological events, including four cases of brain death believed to have occurred before implantation. Embolic events were found in 11 patients (8%), eight of whom had simultaneous infection. In the St Louis experience with 54 Pierce–Donachy pump implants, dextran followed by heparin or warfarin and low-dose dipyridamole was used for anticoagulation. In 27 patients supported for <4 days, none had thrombus in the device on explant analysis. Of the 27 supported for >4 days, nine devices (17% of the total, 33% of those implanted for >4 days) implanted for 4–27 days were found to have some visible thrombus in the device at explant. The other 18 devices with a mean implant time of 22 days were free of thrombus. Four of the nine patients with thrombus identified in their devices had cerebral or peripheral injuries, of which two were definitely embolic and two possibly embolic.[30] At the University of Arizona Heart Center, in 13 implants of the Symbion AVAD in a biventricular configuration, we had six deaths. The other seven were transplanted and all survived. We used heparin or warfarin and low-dose dipyridamole in this group that had a mean implant time of 55 days (range 10–166). Among the survivors, there were two strokes with minimal residual and one TIA. Among those that died, four had evidence on autopsy of emboli that included splenic and/or renal infarct in three, and cerebral infarct in one. Those four patients all had risk factors for stroke; two presented to our hospital on post-cardiotomy centrifugal pump support and two were found to have clots in the left sides of the hearts[31] at autopsy. As mentioned earlier, we found an area of stagnation in this device, but we also found means for preventing this from occurring.

Conclusions

From a clinician's view the blood–material interface is extremely complex. Molecular engineering of better surfaces or seeding with fibroblasts or autologous endothelium, better designs, higher flows, better valves and conduits, and improved techniques for anastomosis and apical or atrial insertion may be valuable in the future. We are at present, however, locked in by resource limitation and our medico-legal environment to the clinical study of just a few types of devices. These devices each have unique characteristics of design, flow, conduits and valves, but share in common a smooth polyurethane lining with the exception of the textured TCI lining.

From clinical studies that are known to underestimate the incidence of emboli, have inconsistent methods of explant analysis, and often fail to include autopsy data, it is difficult to know what happens between the complex blood-contacting surfaces and the even more complex haemostatic system. We have, however, in attempting to review current devices, found that current results with respect to thromboembolism and device thrombosis are good.

I believe the data from La Pitie hospital on activation of the platelet, procoagulant and fibrinolytic systems with the Jarvik-7 has general applicability. When taken with what is known about blood–polyurethane interactions and the effects of valves and turbulence on blood, there is little doubt that all the devices and blood-contacting surfaces currently under study are innately thrombogenic. They must, however, be evaluated in the context of design and flow. In searching for the explanation for the cause of embolic events in a certain device or institutional series, I would caution the tinkerers, inventors and engineers not to be too hasty in blaming the device or its blood-contacting materials. I would caution the clinicians not to underestimate the complexity of the haemostatic mechanism.

The data reviewed here show clearly that smooth polyurethane surfaces in most currently tested devices are, under the conditions of limited control of the haemostatic system, minimally implicated in thrombogenesis. During conditions of exquisite diagnostic and therapeutic control of the haemostatic system, such as practised by the La Pitie group, I would guess that any of the devices in use would have a near perfect record for absence of emboli. The records for devices presently suggest that the valves and perivalvular areas are the most likely sites for the genesis of emboli. There is evidence from my own series that, given an area of stagnation, thrombi will form. My guess is that with currently used flow rates and current intra-device flow characteristics most of the risk for thrombosis has been avoided.

The absence of embolic events from both La Pitie with the Jarvik-7 and from Texas with the TCI must currently be considered the best obtainable results. Can one say that since only aspirin and dipyridamole is used with the TCI that it is inherently less thrombogenic? Or might one focus on the short inflow conduit, and intradevice flow patterns? Given our current understanding of valves, conduits, and non-endothelialized surfaces on blood, it would seem too much to assume without more information that the textured surface is any better than polyurethane. Attention to further developments with the lining of the TCI device and duplication of the Texas experience in other institutions is warranted. The haemostatic testing and treatment techniques used at the La Pitie hospital also deserve further multi-institutional testing to validate their usefulness.

In summary, from a clinician's viewpoint we have some very promising devices and techniques that are of proven value in prolonging life. We have made considerable progress in the past eight years in making these devices work. I believe that for the next few years we need to continue to focus on better understanding and controlling the haemostatic system in implanted patients. In the interim, current devices with respect to blood contacting materials are well designed and do not require major changes.

Acknowledgement

The work upon which this chapter is based was supported by the University Medical Center, the Marshall Foundation and the University Heart Center, Arizona.

References

1. Pennington DG. Circulatory support at the turn of the decade. *ASAIO Trans* 1990; **36**, M136–131.
2. *The Artificial Heart: Prototypes, Policies and Patients.* The Institute of Medicine, National Academy Press, Washington, DC, 1991.
3. Hill JD, Lemperle B, Levinson M, Poirier VL, Griffith BP. FDA regulatory issues session: how much do we need to know before approving a ventricular assist device? *Ann Thorac Surg* 1993; **55**, 314–328.
4. Graham TR, Lewis CT. Lining artificial ventricles—status 1990. In *Heart: Harnessing Skeletal Muscle Power for Cardiac Assistance*, Salmons S, Jarvis JC (eds). Commission of the European Communities, secretariat: CCBMT, University of Twente, Box 217, 7500 AE Enschede, Netherlands.
5. DeVries WC. The permanent artificial heart. *JAMA* 1988; **259**, 849–859.
6. Curtis JJ, Walls JT, Boley TM, Schmaltz RA, Demmy TL. Autopsy findings in patients on postcardiotomy centrifugal ventricular assist. *ASAIO J* 1992; **38**, M688–690.
7. Icenogle TB, Smith RG, Cleavinger M, Vasu MA, Williams RJ, Sethi GK, Copeland JG. Thromboembolic complications of the symbion AVAD system. *Artif Organs* 1989; **13**, 532–538.
8. Olsen DB, Unger F, Oster H, Lawson J, Kessler T, Kolff J, Kolff WJ. Thrombus generation within the artificial heart. *J Thorac Cardiovasc Surg* 1975; **70**, 248–255.
9. Johnson KE, Prieto M, Joyce LD, Pritzker M, Emery RW. Summary of the clinical use of the Symbion total artificial heart. *J Heart Lung Transplant* 1992; **11**, 103–116.
10. Portner PM, Baumgartner WA, Cabrol C, Frazier OH. Circulatory support: 'How To' panel; Internal pulsatile circulatory support. *Ann Thorac Surg* 1993; **55**, 261–265.
11. Frazier OH, Duncan M, Radovancevic B, Vega DJ, Baldwin RT, Burnett CM, Lonquist JL. Successful bridge to heart transplantation with a new left ventricular assist device. *J Heart Lung Transplant* 1992; **11**, 530–537.
12. Nojiri C, Sung WK, Jacobs HA, Pantalos GM, Olsen DB. Scanning and transmission electron microscopic evaluation of the U–100 total artificial heart blood connecting surface. *ASAIO Trans* 1989; **35**, 679–683.
13. Levinson MM, Smith RG, Cork RC, Gallo J, Emery RW, Icenogle TB, Ott RA, Burns GL, Copeland JG. Thromboembolic complications of the Jarvik-7 total artificial heart: case report. *Artif Organs* 1986; **10**, 236–244.
14. Lelah MD, Cooper SL. *Polyurethanes in Medicine.* Boca Raton: CRC Press, 1986: 125.
15. Nojiri C, Okano T, Park KD, Kim SW. Suppression mechanisms for thrombus formation on heparin-immobilized segmented polyurethane-ureas. *ASAIO Trans* 1988; **34**, 386–398.
16. Dasse KA, Chipman SD, Sherman CN, Levine, Frazier OH. Clinical experience with textured

blood contacting surfaces in ventricular assist devices. *ASAIO Trans* 1987; **33**, 418–425.

17. Graham TR, Dasse K, Coumbe A, Salih, Marrinan MT, Frazier OH, Lewis CT. Neo-intimal development on textured biomaterial surfaces during clinical use of an implantable left ventricular assist device. *Eur J Cardiothorac Surg* 1990; **4**, 182–190.

18. Bernhard WF. A fibrillar blood–prosthetic interface for both temporary and permanent ventricular assist devices: experimental and clinical observations. *Artif Organs* 1989; **13**, 255–271.

19. Nose Y, Jacobs G, Kiraly RJ, Golding L, Harasaki H, Takatani S, Murabayashi S, Sukalac RW, Kambic H, Snow J. Experimental results for chronic left ventricular assist and total artificial heart development. *Artif Organs* 1983; **7**, 55–63.

20. Shepro D, D'Amore PA. Physiology and biochemistry of the vascular wall. In: *Handbook of Physiology— The Cardiovascular System IV*. Bethesda: American Physiology Society, 1984: 103–164.

21. Weiss HJ, Baumgartner HR, Turitto VT. Regulation of platelet-fibrin thrombi on subendothelium. *Ann NY Acad Sci* 1987; **516**, 380–397.

22. Bellon JL, Szefner J, Cabrol C. *Coagulation et Coeur Artificial*. Paris: Masson, 1989.

23. Kunin CM, Dobbins JJ, Melo JC, Levinson MM, Love K, Joyce LD, DeVries W. Infectious complications in four long term recipients of the Jarvik-7 artificial heart. *JAMA* 1988; **259**, 860–864.

24. Lonchyna VA, Piffarre R, Sullivan H, Montoya A, Bakhos M, Grieco J, Foy B, Blakeman B, Altergott R, Calandra D, Hinkamp T, Istanbouli M, Sinno J, Bartlett L. Successful use of the total artificial heart as a bridge to transplantation with no mediastinitis. *J Heart Lung Transplant* 1992; **11**, 803–811.

25. Griffith BP. Interim use of the Jarvik-7 artificial heart: lessons learned at Pittsburgh. *Ann Thorac Surg* 1989; **47**, 158–166.

26. Copeland JG, Smith R, Icenogle T, Vasu A, Rhenman B, Williams R, Cleavinger M. Orthotopic total artificial heart bridge to transplantation: preliminary results. *J Heart Transplant* 1989; **8**, 124–138.

27. Kormos RL, Borovetz HS, Gasior T, Antaki JF, Armitage JM, Pristas JM, Hardesty RL, Griffith BP. Experience with univentricular support in mortally ill cardiac transplant candidates. *Ann Thorac Surg* 1990; **49**, 261–272.

28. Frazier OH, Duncan JM, Radovancevic B, Vega JD, Baldwin, Burnett CM, Lonquist JL. Successful bridge to heart transplantation with a new left ventricular assist device. *J Heart Lung Transplant* 1992; **11**, 530–537.

29. Farrar DJ, Hill JD. Univentricular and biventricular Thoratec VAD support as a bridge to transplantation. *Ann Thorac Surg* 1993; **55**: 276–282.

30. Termuhlen DF, Swartz MT, Pennington G, McBride LR, Szukalski EA, Reedy JE, Ruzevich SA. Thromboembolic complications with the Pierce–Donachy ventricular assist device. *ASAIO Trans* 1989; **35**, 616–618.

31. Lick S, Copeland JG, Smith RG, Cleavinger M, Rosado LJ, Huston CL, Sethi GK, Molloy T. Use of the Symbion biventricular assist device in bridging to transplantation. *Ann Thorac Surg* 1993; **55**: 283–287.

4

The development of biomaterials for cardiovascular prostheses

DL Bader and SL Gigg

Introduction

This chapter concentrates on the mechanical and physical properties of the biological tissues and the biomaterials used in arterial prostheses. Of the several review articles in this field, the reader is referred to excellent recent contributions from How et al.[1] and Aebischer et al.[2] for specific details.

The blood vessel wall and other biological tissues of the body are structural materials in the same sense as many engineering materials. This has led to attempts to characterize the properties of biological tissues in a similar way to the properties of more standard engineering materials. Many of the properties may be related, but care should be taken as the biological tissues generally comprise several constituent materials and thus will exhibit complex mechanical behaviour.

When relating the properties of biological tissues to standard engineering concepts, care must be taken to define terms used. A review of the literature reveals that a wide variety of terms have been used to describe the properties of blood vessels and some will undoubtedly cause confusion to the non-specific engineer. An example of this is the definition of the term 'elastic', which describes the property of a material which enables it to deform when it is subjected to an applied load and return to its original form, with no associated release of energy or permanent deformation, when the load is removed. Young's modulus is the parameter which is a measure of the resistance to deformation and should only be employed with linear, isotropic and homogeneous materials. However, as will be described later in the chapter, blood vessel walls exhibit non-linear, anisotropic and non-homogeneous behaviour. Thus the reported values of Young's modulus for blood vessel walls are strictly incorrect and should be replaced by the term 'stiffness modulus'. Definitions of terms used in the text are given in the glossary (page 44).

Biomaterial considerations

When deciding on a material to be used as a replacement for a biological tissue, there are a few important factors to consider as summarized in Table 4.1.

Table 4.1 General specification for biomaterials.

Property	Characteristics
Chemical	Chemically inert
	Free from leachable impurities
	Minimal environmental degradation and ageing
	Sterilizable
Biological	Non-toxic
	Non-carcinogenic
	No teratological effects
Mechanical	Adequate strength
	Processable
	Properties matching those of body and surrounding tissue

Mechanical compatibility involves characterizing the important mechanical properties of the biological tissues and attempting to match them with synthetic analogues. This is particularly important if the implant materials are subjected to mechanical stresses and the implant is designed with specific mechanical functions. An example involves matching the compliance of vascular prostheses to those of the adjacent host vessels which has both mechanical and haemodynamic implications. Thus, matched materials will minimize the incidence of turbulence near to the anastamosis. This, in turn, will improve flow rates in the region of the graft and also reduce shear-induced neo-intimal injury and platelet activation. In addition, if the substrate material is matched to that of the biological wall then the endothelial cells will be subjected to a normal mechanical environment and display normal function.

Vascular prostheses must also provide a degree of flexibility and ease of surgeon handling. This will aid the precise surgical fitting of the grafts to the host vessels, with minimum disturbance of the blood path as well as minimum difficulty for the surgeon.

Having selected certain mechanical properties such as stiffness modulus, failure stress, and fatigue strength, these properties should remain constant within the lifetime of the implant. This is particularly important when considering that the prostheses will be required to withstand years of pulsatile blood pressure with absolute security. However, this requirement for constant properties is not always attainable as many biomaterials are susceptible to long-term attack from hostile body fluids. This results in common chemical processes involving, for example, swelling and leaching of polymeric biomaterials and corrosion of metallic implants. Polymers in particular, with their inherently weak covalent bonds, may experience profound changes in stiffness modulus in response to the internal environment. The tensile strengths of polymeric biomaterials are also affected in a variety of ways after prolonged contact with body fluids and tissues. For example, natural silk and polyglycolic acid gradually lose their strength *in vivo* and therefore are ideal suture materials, whilst polypropylene and polyester monofilaments demonstrate minimal strength changes during long-term implantation.

The host tissue response to the medical implant is also critical in determining the overall performance of the implant. In all cases an acute response associated with inflammation is provoked by the presence of the implant. The chronic response, which may occur at any time from a few months to over 10 years after implantation, is highly variable and is dependent upon both external and intrinsic factors. An undesirable response may lead to ultimate rejection of the implant. By comparison, long-term responses can provide overall stability of the implant where the host tissue adapts to the presence of the biomaterial. It is the objective of the biomaterials scientist to design implants made of advanced materials which can provide this adaptation response.

Structure and function of blood vessels

The structure and the function of the arterial system are inextricably linked as in any well designed system. The systemic blood supply system can be divided into four main sections according to its function, as illustrated in Table 4.2. The differences in the functions of these four sections give rise to different vessel structures. The mechanical properties of the vessels are dependent on both the relative proportion of the different components in the vessel walls and the orientation of these components.

The blood vessels consist of three distinct coats or tunics, whose proportions vary throughout the cardiovascular system.

1. The *tunica intima* is the innermost coat of the vessel wall and is lined by a layer of endothelial cells, which are water-repellent and help prevent intravascular thrombosis[3] and which sit on a basement membrane consisting of

Table 4.2 Classification of vessels in the cardiovascular system.

Vessel	Function	Description
Large elastic arteries	Conductive	Dampen the large pressure surges from the heart
Muscular arteries	Resistive	Contract to control the blood supply
Capillaries	Capacitive	Allow exchange of gases, nutrients and waste between tissue cells and blood
Veins	Reservoir	Conduit for blood back to heart and store for surplus load

collagenous-rich material associated with gly-cosaminoglycans and proteoglycans. This layer is separated from the next by the internal elastic lamina composed of collagen, elastin and reticular fibres.

2. The *tunica media* contains elastic tissue and smooth muscle arranged in circular laminae. The larger arteries contain more elastic tissue than the muscular arteries. Further down the arterial tree there is a greater smooth muscle component which regulates blood flow by sympathetic nerve supply.

3. The *tunic adventitia* comprises mainly intermingled collagen fibres and elastin fibres which surround the media and merge with the adjacent connective tissues. An outer elastic membrane may separate the tunica media from the tunica adventitia.

The structural and viscoelastic properties of the vascular tissues are determined largely by the fibrous proteins collagen and elastin and, to a lesser extent, by the contractile proteins and the proteoglycans of the ground substance.[4] Each of these four components will be discussed separately.

Collagen

Collagen is a fibrous protein with high tensile strength and low distensibility. Much of the function of collagen in the body is concerned with providing a strong though flexible framework to contain cells and tissue. A third of total body mass is collagen.

The collagen molecule is composed of linear, unbranching sequences of 20 or more naturally occurring amino acids.[5] One-third of the amino acid residues are composed of the small molecule glycine. Of the remainder there are large quantities of proline and hydroxyproline. The precise sequence of amino acids determines the type of collagen present. The collagen molecule consists of three chains of amino acids, each chain forms a left-hand helix, the three chains wind to form a right-hand triple helix. These form rods that are 300 nm long and 1.5 nm in diameter with frayed ends that are non-helical in configuration. This molecule is thus ideally suited to resist tensile forces but will buckle under compressive loads. The collagen fibres show a banded pattern under light and electron microscopy with a periodicity of 67 nm.

Collagen exhibits both intra- and intermolecu-

lar cross-links, involving both helical and non-helical portions of the protein. These cross-links and the tight helical bonding of collagen are important to the overall tensile strength and stability of the collagen fibre. The destruction of these cross-links will reduce the integrity of the fibre structure and therefore its mechanical characteristics. A diagram of the collagen molecule and its packing arrangement in a collagen fibril is shown in Fig. 4.1.

Vascular tissue contains several forms of collagen including types I, III and IV. The main site of collagen deposition in the blood vessels is within the adventitia. The fibres are located longitudinally to resist longitudinal strain. Collagen fibres are also present within the media of the muscular arteries. Within this layer it is laid down circumferentially to resist dilatation.

Collagen has a high stiffness modulus and tensile strength which resist overstretching of the arteries and protect against rupture at high pressures in the lumen. The proportion of collagen within the blood vessels increases with distance

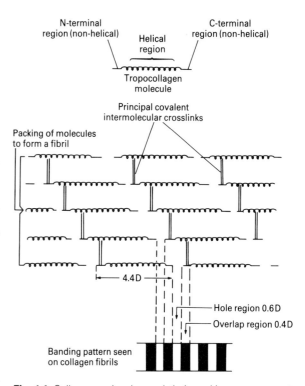

Fig. 4.1 Collagen molecules and their packing arrangement in a collagen fibril (D is the periodicity seen in the native fibril).

from the heart, and this change is associated with increased stiffness in the more distal arteries.[6]

Elastin

When extracted from tissue by biochemical methods, elastin appears as a yellow-brown sticky material with properties similar to those of rubber. In common with collagen, elastin is a protein containing 2–4% hydroxyproline. The protein chain also contains a high proportion of non-polar amino acids. There is debate as to the precise structure of the fibres in a 3-D network.[7]

Elastin occurs as a series of concentric fenestrated tubes extending along the length of the vessels,[8,9] with more elastic tissue in the proximal arteries than in the distal muscular arteries. Elastin provides a readily deformable, highly compliant honeycomb of material that encircles the vessel lumen. It is capable of returning to its original shape once the load is removed. Elastin exhibits a low stiffness modulus and low tensile strength, but a high strain to failure. The role of elastin is to distribute the load across the collagen fibre matrix in the blood vessel walls, thus maintaining a uniform state of tension.[10]

Smooth muscle

The tunica media of the vessel walls contains the largest proportion of smooth muscle. The smooth muscle cells are angled obliquely in the lamellae and can increase the thickness of the vessel wall as well as the diameter of the lumen itself.[11] The muscle cells are activated by sympathetic nervous impulses and are laid down in lamellae separated by layers of elastic tissue. Generally the smooth muscle is assumed to have a modulus of stiffness similar to that of elastin although its exact value depends on the degree of physiological action.[10] The physiological nature of smooth muscle and its stimulation by the sympathetic nervous system make it difficult to quantify exact mechanical properties owing to involuntary contraction and excitation. Smooth muscle is thought to be a major contributant to the viscous component responsible for the viscoelastic behaviour of the blood vessel walls.[12] The larger elastic artery walls show less viscoelastic behaviour than the muscular arteries.

The smooth muscle component along with the elastin have been described as a two-phase system,[13] which provides a graded response to the action of smooth muscle contraction. The relative contributions of the structural components on the mechanics of the vascular system are represented diagrammatically in Fig. 4.2.

Ground substance

The ground substance provides the main constituents of the extracellular matrix. The ground substance contains glycosaminoglycans and proteoglycans. They consist of unbranching chains of disaccharides; for example, hyaluronic acid and heparan sulphate. These molecules with their sulphate groups may be electrostatically attached to the positive groups associated with the fibres in the matrix.

Changes associated with ageing

The changes associated with ageing on the structural components of the vessel walls can have a dramatic effect on their properties and on the properties of the blood vessel as a whole. One noticeable ageing effect is the general increase in the complexity of the collagen networks, including an increase in the number of cross-links, and the decrease in the number of elastin fibres. While collagen fibres can be generated throughout life, elastic fibres cannot be replaced to any extent in the adult human.[14] These changes can lead to stiffer arteries, which in turn can lead to further problems associated with the cardiovascular system.[15]

The established changes in blood pressures associated with ageing will lead to a decrease in the effectiveness of the arteries in damping the pressure surges from the heart. This is reflected in an increase in the pulse wave velocity which has been measured at 8 m/s compared with the normal value of 5 m/s.

It is essential that these ageing changes be taken into account when designing arterial prostheses.

Mechanical testing of blood vessels

In vitro and *in vivo* testing

The mechanical properties of the blood vessel walls can be characterized using *in vitro* or *in vivo* methods.

In vitro testing is generally performed on either

cylindrical segments of arterial wall, sections of intact arterial wall or prepared strips which can be orientated in any direction with respect to the longitudinal axis of the vessel. These specimens can be loaded in a variety of ways ranging from uniaxial quasistatic tests to multiaxial dynamic tests. The simple uniaxial test involves parallel-sided strips of tissue which are suitably gripped and mounted in a standard material testing machine. These tests will provide stress–strain characteristics and establish material properties such as stiffness modulus, strength and strain to failure. A commonly used multiaxial test involves the inflation of segments of vessels providing relationships between pressure and volume in radial or longitudinal directions. These pressure–volume characteristics are generally expressed as a value of compliance of the blood vessel. Testing may also involve cyclic loading of specimens to determine the fatigue characteristics over a simulated lifetime. This factor is important in the design of vessel prostheses as it is desirable to achieve a material with fatigue properties match

ing those of the original vessel. The vessel can expect to experience approximately 5×10^7 load cycles each year.

In vitro testing is more straightforward to perform, and parameters, such as smooth muscle contraction, can be controlled; but it is important to take into account boundary conditions and other effects when extrapolating data to physiological conditions. This form of testing can also examine the effects of the structural components on the mechanical properties of vascular tissues using specific enzymes or their inhibitors. For example, Greenwald and Berry[15] used an enzyme inhibitor to reduce the degree of scleroprotein cross-linking and deposition and this resulted in a decrease in the stiffness modulus at both low and high stress levels.

In vivo methods can be non-invasive or invasive. Non-invasive methods include measurement of dimensions of vessels using angiography, echocardiography or ultrasound. Invasive methods have included the suturing of low-mass callipers to the blood vessel wall with attached strain

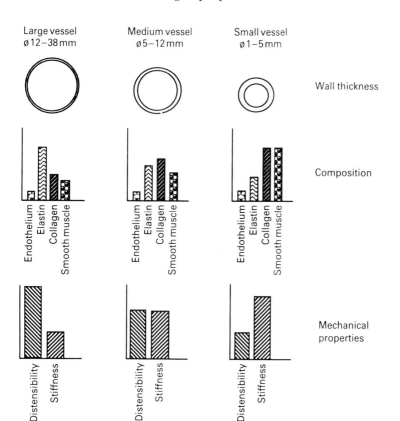

Fig. 4.2 Diagrammatic representation of changes in composition and mechanical properties of blood vessels of different size.

gauges[16] and the simultaneous measurement of pressure using a catheter transducer to record pressure–volume changes.

Laboratory modelling

An alternative approach is to establish a laboratory model of the cardiovascular system. This can include a reservoir, pump, conduits and representation of blood flow. The model can be used to examine the flow and impulse propagation characteristics of normal vessels and changes associated with ageing and pathological conditions, such as arterial stenoses and aneurysms.[17] It may also be used to assess the performance of a range of biomaterial grafts in terms of blood flow and biocompatibility.

Mechanical properties of blood vessels

Static properties

From experiments to observe the static elastic properties of blood vessel walls, the most noticeable observation is the non-linearity of the stress–strain or pressure–volume characteristic curve, as illustrated in Fig. 4.3. This non-linearity is characteristic of many soft biological tissues, such as tendon and articular cartilage. The curve can be divided into three regions: an initial region of low modulus known as the toe-in, a transition region, and a final region of much higher modulus. The region of the curve at which physiological conditions occur is within the transition region. Since the stress–strain curve is non-linear it is not possi-

ble to define a single discrete value for the modulus of stiffness for the blood vessel wall. The term 'incremental modulus' has been coined to describe the modulus over very small increments of stress or strain over which the modulus can be assumed to be constant. The incremental modulus[18] can be described by the following equation:

$$E_{inc} = \frac{\Delta P R_o R_i^2 2(1 - \nu^2)}{\Delta R_o (R_o^2 - R_i^2)} \qquad (1)$$

where R_o is the outer radius, R_i is the inner radius, ΔP is the pressure change, and ν is Poisson's ratio, taken as 0.5 for artery wall.

The direction of applied loading will influence the mechanical characteristics of the specimens. Arteries *in vivo* are tethered longitudinally and are therefore prestressed to some extent because of the restriction of longitudinal movement. Stress–strain curves for circumferential and longitudinal specimens show slightly different characteristics, as illustrated in Fig. 4.4. This is also due

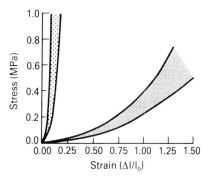

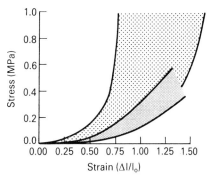

Fig. 4.4 Comparative form of stress–strain curves in (top) circumferential and (bottom) longitudinal directions for (*dark areas*) synthetic graft materials including woven and knitted PET and PTFE, and (*light areas*) proximal and distal sections of canine arteries. These curves are based on data from reference 18.

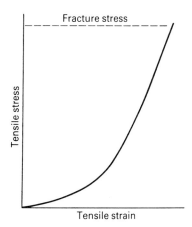

Fig. 4.3 Typical stress–strain behaviour of soft tissues subjected to an axial tensile force.

Table 4.3 Range of mechanical properties for blood vessels.

Mechanical property (MPa)	Vessel	Reported value
Tensile stiffness modulus	Thoracic aorta	0.30–0.94
	Abdominal aorta	0.98–1.42
	Iliac artery	1.10–3.50
	Femoral artery	1.23–5.50
Ultimate tensile strength	Artery*	
	longitudinal	1.7
	radial	1.4
Ultimate shear strength	Artery*	
	longitudinal	6.2
	radial	5.4

*Vessel not specified
Source: reference 19

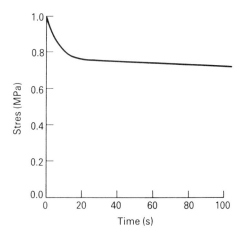

Fig. 4.5 Normalized stress relaxation curve for a porcine aortic specimen.

to the anisotropic nature of the vessel wall. Specific values for mechanical properties vary considerably owing to the biological variability of tissues and the test conditions, as evidenced by the data collected by Duck[19] and summarized in Table 4.3. What is clear, however, is that the smaller more distal arteries have a higher stiffness modulus than the elastic arteries but show less distensibility on their stress–strain curves. This can be related to their structural components (Fig. 4.2).

Preconditioning and hysteresis

When subjecting specimens of blood vessel to cyclic loading, it is interesting to note that the first few cycles give stress–strain characteristics different from those of later cycles. It is thought that by precycling or preconditioning the specimens they are being returned to a state more closely resembling that *in vivo*, where they may experience some longitudinal and radial stresses at all times. Preconditioning usually requires about ten cycles to ensure adequate repeatability.

Viscoelasticity

A complication in applying general elastic theory to blood vessel walls is that they exhibit viscoelastic behaviour. This characteristic is observed in all biological soft tissues. Thus when soft tissues are subjected to a constant load they exhibit an initial, almost elastic, deformation followed by a creep deformation, due to their viscous components, until a steady-state equilibrium value is attained. The viscoelastic behaviour is also demonstrated in stress relaxation tests. When specimens of porcine aorta were subjected to a

constant deformation, the resulting relaxation in stress followed the curves illustrated in Fig. 4.5.[20] These curves, which are similar to those obtained by Fung from rabbit mesentary,[21] indicate an initial region of rapid decrease in stress followed by a much slower decrease in stress relaxation.

Models of viscoelastic materials behaviour have been based upon systems of springs and dashpots in series or parallel or combinations of both. Two basic models are shown in Fig. 4.6. These models only apply strictly to linear materials experiencing small strains, and therefore cannot exactly replicate the behaviour of vessel walls. Indeed, no arrangement of dashpots and springs has yet been found to represent this complex behaviour.

Dynamic properties

The cardiovascular system is dynamic in form with the blood vessels undergoing a pulsatile loading

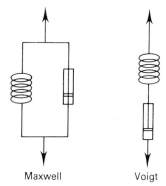

Maxwell   Voigt

Fig. 4.6 Common models of spring and dashpot elements to describe simple viscoelastic behaviour.

pattern at a frequency equivalent to the heart beat of about 1 Hz. Thus it is important to establish dynamic mechanical properties. The dynamic stiffness modulus can be represented by a complex number consisting of a real component, the stiffness modulus, and an imaginary component, describing a combination of the viscous components and the frequency. Thus:

$$E_{\text{dyn}} = E_{\text{stat}} + i\eta\omega \quad (2)$$

For the large elastic arteries near the heart, the viscous component is small and the dynamic modulus approximates to the static modulus. The viscous component becomes more significant in the distal arteries containing a higher proportion of smooth muscle. Viscoelastic materials which follow the behaviour governed by equation (2) generally show a continual rise in dynamic modulus with frequency. However, it has been shown that arteries follow this trend in dynamic modulus only up to frequencies of 2 Hz, at which point the dynamic stiffness modulus remains fairly constant with frequency.[22]

Pulse wave velocity

Pulse or pressure waves caused by the beating of the heart are propagated along the length of the vessel at a particular velocity. This pressure wave velocity can be measured experimentally. The measured velocity usually consists of the velocity of the generated wave superimposed on that of the reflected wave. By using high-frequency waves to measure the propagation, the reflected waves are attenuated to such an extent that they can be ignored.[23] The velocity of propagation of pressure waves, c', is usually calculated using the modified Moens–Korteweg equation,[24] given by:

$$c' = \sqrt{\frac{Eh}{2\rho R(1 - v^2)}} \quad (3)$$

where h is the wall thickness, ρ is the density, R is the radius of the vessel and v is Poisson's ratio.

For other dynamic test methods to examine the mechanical behaviour of both blood vessels and their anastomoses with biomaterial grafts, the reader is referred to a recent paper.[25]

Cardiovascular biomaterials

The repair of arterial defects by synthetic materials has been facilitated by advances in medical science, including the reliable use of anaesthetics, blood transfusion and vascular surgery. Early synthetic repair materials were diverse in nature, ranging from paraffin-lined silver, glass, vitallium and polyethylene. The prostheses, in the form of rigid tubes, had usually failed at their junction with the host tissue where the sutures, made from natural silk fibres, were slowly degraded within the body. The use of freshly harvested autologous vein grafts had been more effective as prostheses in replacing small arteries and major veins. However as surgeons began to require solutions to treat abdominal aneurysms, it soon became apparent that the relative large diameter of these vessels could not be matched by an autogenous vein. The use of freeze-dried human cadaveric arteries was attempted with limited success and long-term complications involving localized dilatations or aneurysms and some rupture of the vessel walls.

A major breakthrough in cardiovascular biomaterials occurred in the 1950s. In particular an American team led by Voorhees introduced woven tubes of porous synthetic materials to bridge gaps of several centimetres.[26] They observed that the interstices of the tube became blocked with fibrin and platelets and their lumen lined with a thin layer of tissue. The earliest grafts were made from a commercial fabric known as Vinyon-N®, which is similar in terms of its polymeric structure and fabrication technique to woven polyethylene terephthalate (PET) grafts that are in current use.

Current vascular prostheses can be classified according to their materials of construction, methods of construction and their diameter. The size criterion is somewhat arbitrary but is based on the degree of blood compatibility. The diameters are most conveniently divided into three groups, each with its own design specifications and optimum biomaterials.

1. Large-diameter prostheses

These may be defined as those replacements with diameters in the range 12–38 mm which are commonly required to replace the aorta and its immediate branches, the arteries arising from the aortic arch and the iliac arteries. Nearly all large-diameter vascular prostheses are made of poly-ethylene terephthalate, which is marketed as Dacron® by companies such as Bard and Meadox Medical. Over 70% of these prostheses are bifur-cated and are used to replace, for example, the abdominal aorta where it branches into the iliac arteries. The remaining 25% are straight prosthe-ses. Large-diameter vascular grafts are supplied in both porous and non-porous forms. The patency rate for these large-diameter prostheses is 95% for at least 5 years.[27] This relative success is probably due to a high blood velocity in the appropriate vessel and the fact that only a small proportion of blood actually makes contact with the walls of the large-diameter tube.

2. Medium-diameter prostheses

These may be defined as those prostheses with a diameter of 5–12 mm. About 70% of these are made from polytetrafluorethylene (PTFE), mar-keted by Gore and Associates. The remainder are made from Dacron, amounting to about 25% of the market, and those originating from biological tissues.

3. Small-diameter prostheses

These may be defined as those prostheses with a diameter of less than 5 mm. Traditionally these vessels have been replaced by autologous grafts, but if these fail or are unavailable, biomaterial solutions are required. Microporous expanded PTFE is currently used with a pore size of 20–30 μm. Currently only a small percentage of the small-diameter market is held by synthetic grafts, owing to their general failure to meet the strict requirements of an extreme level of blood compatibility.

Porosity

Most successful vascular prostheses that are used clinically are based on the concept of a porous conduit. The prosthetic structure behaves as a framework to support the host tissue within which blood clots and becomes entrapped. Tissue ingrowth occurs through the porous structure to form a compact fibrin layer, or neo-intima, on the internal surfaces of the prosthesis. The ultimate non-thrombogenic surface is one that is covered with endothelial cells, although a complete neo-intima has not been demonstrated in humans.

This process is an interesting example of vas-cular tissue adaptation. The adaptive mechanism is dependent on the porosity of the prosthesis. This porosity is defined as the ratio of the volume of void space to the total volume of porous material. The porosity is given in units of ml/min/cm^2 of water expressed from the lumen through the wall of an unclotted non-blood-exposed graft subjected to a transmural pressure of 120 mmHg (16 kPa). Most uncoated prosthe-ses display porosities greater than 2000/ml/min/cm^2. The distribution of pore size is also an important determinant in controlling tissue response and the overall compliance of the pros-thesis. Fabrics with pores less than 45 μm in diameter generally promote tissue ingrowth and rapid wound healing with minimal fibrous tis-sue.[1]

Graft preparation

Vascular grafts composed of Dacron are made using a wide variety of processes, including fibre extrusion and fabric formation using knitting and weaving techniques.[28] Fabrics composed of woven and non-woven yarns are made using standard textile manufacturing processes. The properties of the fabric reflect the individual yarns, whose properties depend on the number and twist of individual fibres as well as the material properties of the base polymer.

Fibres can be heat-processed to form a regular zig-zag or crimp that results in a low-modulus region in the stress–strain curves similar to that observed in the biological tissues, as indicated in Fig. 4.3. Although annular crimping will reduce kinking at the time of implantation and prevent buckling when the prosthesis is bent, it also significantly disturbs the inner flow surface of the graft.

Woven prostheses are constructed of longitudi-nal (warp direction) and circumferential (weft) yarns. The yarns pass over and under each other at right angles, creating inter-fibre friction which increases the bending stiffness of the fabric, but the prostheses do have a tendency to fray at the cut ends. This construction imparts a low porosity to the fabric (typical porosity values of 0.5) and the woven prosthesis can be implanted without preclotting. The ability of a fabric to drape or lie smoothly over a surface is related to the diameter or denier and the fibre stiffness.

In contrast, knitted structures are prepared by

looping yarns around needles and then inter-connecting the loops to form a continuous struc-ture. The number and size of the needles and the yarn size determines the spacing between the yarns and therefore the fabric porosity. Generally knitted fabrics tend to be highly porous (typical porosity values of 0.8) and have lower ultimate tensile strengths and stiffness compared with woven ones.[18] They are also less susceptible to fraying and are better at retaining sutures.

Polytetrafluorethylene grafts for both large- and small-diameter applications are generally made in an expanded porous form, known as expanded PTFE or more frequently referred to by the trade names of Goretex® and Vitagraft®. The technique that is used involves transforming melt extruded PTFE tubes by a process of heating and mechanical stretching into porous, flexible, non-woven fabric vascular grafts, with a high per-centage of transmural void spaces.[2] The structure consists of circumferentially orientated solid bands of the polymer, known as nodes, with a typical spacing of 30 μm, linked together at right-angles by numerous fine filaments. Expanded PTFE grafts are manufactured in a range of diameters from 4.5 mm to 30 mm and may include tapered and bifurcated sections. The material is flexible and easy to manipulate, but like PET it shows minimal elastic behaviour as a vascular graft. These grafts are impervious to blood and do not require preclotting or applica-tion of a coating material. Present grafts are extremely biodurable and resist bursting pres-sures in excess of 3600 mmHg (480 kPa). Expan-ded PTFE grafts do, however, have a tendency to allow prolonged bleeding around suture holes where the material is incapable of collapsing around oversize holes. Despite the relatively poor patency rates of, for example, about 55% at 3 years following reconstruction of the femoral and popliteal vessels adjacent to the knee,[29] expanded PTFE is still the most widely used material for salvage procedures in the lower extremities on occasions when there is no alternative to the use of a prosthetic graft.

The mechanical properties of these synthetic graft materials can be compared with those of appropriate biological tissues. Fig. 4.4 indicates stress–strain curves when the materials are tested in two specific directions. It is clear that in the circumferential direction the synthetic materials display a significantly higher stiffness modulus than blood vessels, particularly at low stress levels up to the transition region where physiological loading conditions apply. By comparison, the synthetic materials demonstrate a similar behav-iour, indicating reasonable mechanical matching to host tissues, when tested in the longitudinal direction.

Design modifications

Cast or extruded polypropylene and the related fluorinated ethylene propylene, with their inher-ent mechanical rigidity, are currently used in several graft designs to provide mechanical sup-port and prevent compression of grafts made of expanded PTFE and PET. The material is often bonded as a helical, external stent to the outer surface of segments of the graft that are intended to cross joints or other areas of anticipated kink-ing and compression. When used with PET grafts it obviates the need for annular crimping. Another application of polypropylene in vascular grafts is to form the rigid, PET-fabric covered support for the anastomosis ring in sutureless, intraluminal grafts.[2] In both cases the polypropyl-ene will not be in contact with blood.

Graft treatment

Preclotting is required prior to the implantation of porous knitted textile polyester prostheses.[30] When blood flow is restored, no blood should escape through the wall. In totally heparinized patients, as in graft replacement with cardio-pulmonary bypass, preclotted woven grafts are necessary to reduce the blood loss. An alternative to both preclotting and tightly woven grafts is the use of double velour PET grafts impregnated with collagen,[31] an example of which is the product Hemashield®, marketed by Meadox Medical. It does not require any processing in the operating room and is therefore less likely to be colonized by bacteria. The presence of the collagen coating, which is made of a formaldehyde cross-linked bovine skin tissue softened by exposure to glyc-erol, has a dramatic effect on the water permeability—reducing it to 9 ml/min/cm² at a pressure of 120 mmHg (16 kPa). However, the dissolution rate of collagen is unpredictable, and the overall healing schedule of this graft follows the same pattern as in any preclotted grafts.

Albumin-coated polyester arterial grafts are also employed. These have been shown to give a satisfactory healing performance *in vivo* and no bleeding at implantation.[32] The albumin pretreatment was shown to reinforce the graft structure, imparting slightly stiffer characteristics than the preclotted polyester control graft. This produced a reduced tendency of the coated prosthesis wall to stretch and dilate under the mechanical stresses of implantation, thus making the graft less likely to leak.

New generation materials

Polyurethanes have received much recent discussion as new candidate materials for small vascular grafts. The polyurethanes are usually block copolymers which consist of alternating blocks of hard and soft segments.[2] The hard hydrophillic segments generally consist of aromatic diisocyanates with chain extenders of either a diol, a diamine or water. The soft hydrophobic segments consist of hydroxyl-terminated polyesters or polyethers. Polyurethanes in cardiovascular prostheses include the trade names of Biomer®, Cardiothane® and Pellethane®. The advantages of these materials include relatively good haemocompatibility, a high modulus and elastomeric properties which can match those of the host tissues. However, polyurethanes are prone to hydrolytic degradation, particularly when they are used to fabricate porous prostheses.

Further directions in cardiovascular biomaterials involve the surface treatments of grafts with polymeric phospholipids, which are designed to mimic the lipid surfaces of blood cells,[33] and the improvement of techniques for seeding the surface of currently available graft materials with endothelial cells.

In the last four decades there has been considerable success in the development of cardiovascular biomaterials. However, problems still remain, particularly with respect to small-vessel prostheses, where mechanical matching and biocompatibility are critical factors. These can only be addressed by a combined approach involving the biomaterial scientist and cardiovascular surgeon.

Glossary

STRESS (σ)   The load divided by the area over which it is carried, with units of $N\ m^{-2}$ or Pa. Can be given as true stress, where area is taken as instantaneous area, or engineering stress where original area is used.

STRAIN (ϵ)   The ratio of extension (Δl) of the specimen to the original length (l_0).

STIFFNESS   The ratio of load to extension, with units of $N\ m^{-1}$

STIFFNESS MODULUS   The ratio of stress to strain at a prescribed stress level, with units of $N\ m^{-2}$ or Pa. For a linear, orthotropic material this property is known as the Young's modulus.

FATIGUE   The failure of a material under cyclic loading conditions. This occurs at a load lower than its tensile strength. The fatigue limit is the predicted number of cycles at a particular load before failure occurs.

COMPLEX NUMBER   An expression in the form $X = a + ib$, where a and b are real numbers and i is the imaginary unit. Used to describe time-varying quantities which are characterized by a modulus or magnitude together with a phase relationship with some time reference. They may be visualized as vectors in a cartesian coordinate system.

COMPLIANCE (DISTENSIBILITY)   A measure of the ability of a hollow structure to change its volume, generally the ratio of volume change to internal pressure change. The inverse of compliance is *elastance.*

ELASTICITY   A measure of a material's resistance to deformation.

VISCOELASTICITY   A material property where strain and strain rate are a function of the imposed stress.

VISCOSITY   Property of resisting deformation in a fluid.

POISSON'S RATIO   The ratio of strains in three orthogonal directions. For an incompressible isovolumetric material, such as a blood vessel wall, Poisson's ratio has a value of 0.5.

References

1. How TV, Guidoin R, Young SK. Engineering design of vascular prostheses. *Engng Med* 1992; **206**(H2), 61–72.
2. Aebischer P, Goddard M, Galletti PM, Lysaght M. Biomaterials and artificial organs. In: Williams DF (ed), *Medical and Dental Materials.* New York: VCH, 1992.
3. Green JF. *Mechanical Concepts in Cardiovascular and*

Pulmonary Physiology. Philadelphia: Lea & Febiger, 1977.

4. Nimni ME. Collagen in cardiovascular tissues. In: Hastings GW (ed), *Cardiovascular Biomaterials.* London: Springer-Verlag, 1992: 81–141.

5. Woodhead-Galloway J. *Collagen: the Anatomy of a Protein.* London: Edward Arnold, 1976.

6. Harkness MLR, Harkness RD, McDonald DA. The collagen and elastin content of the arterial wall in the dog. *Proc Roy Soc B* 1957; **146B**, 541–551.

7. Gotte L, Mammi M, Pezzin G. Some structural aspects of elastin revealed by X-ray diffraction and other physical methods. In: Crewther WG (ed), *Symposium on Fibrous Proteins.* Sydney: Butterworth, 1968: 236–245.

8. Cliff WJ. Aortic tunica media of ageing rats. *Exper Molec Pathol* 1970; **13**, 172–189.

9. Cliff WJ. *Blood Vessels.* Cambridge: Cambridge University Press, 1976.

10. Burton AC. The relationship between structure and function in the tissues of the blood vessel wall. *Physiol Rev* 1954; **34**, 619–642.

11. Wolinsky H, Glagov S. The structural basis for the static mechanical properties of the aortic media. *Circul Res* 1964; **14**, 400–413.

12. Caro CG, Pedley TJ, Shroter RC, Seed WA. Solid mechanics and the properties of blood vessel walls. In: Caro CG, Pedley TJ, Shroter RC, Seed WA (eds), *The Mechanics of the Circulation.* Oxford: Oxford University Press, 1978: 86–105.

13. Wolinsky H, Glagov S. The media as a two phase material. *Nature* 1963; **199**, 606–608.

14. Jacobsen W. Histological survey of normal connective tissue. In: Randall JT (ed), *Nature and Structure of Collagen.* London: Butterworth, 1953: 6–13.

15. Greenwald SE, Berry CL. The effect of alterations in scleroprotein content on the static elastic properties of the arterial wall. In: Kovach A, Monos E, Rubanyi G (eds), *Cardiovascular Physiology: Heart, Peripheral Circulation and Methodology.* Budapest: Pergamon, 1981: 203–212.

16. Peterson LM, Jensen RE, Parnell J. Mechanical properties of arteries in vivo. *Circul Res* 1960; **8**, 622–628.

17. Greenwald SE, Newman DL, Moodie TB. Impulse propagation in rubber-tube analogues of arterial stenoses and aneurysms. *Med Biol Engng Comp* 1985; **23**, 150–154.

18. How TV. Mechanical properties of arteries and arterial grafts. In: Hastings GW (ed), *Cardiovascular Biomaterials.* London: Springer-Verlag, 1992: 1–35.

19. Duck FA. *Physical Properties of Tissue: a Comprehensive Reference Book.* London: Academic Press, 1990: 152.

20. Gigg SL. The mechanical properties of porcine descending aorta. MSc Thesis, University of Surrey, 1992.

21. Fung YC. Elasticity of soft tissues in simple elongation. *Am J Physiol* 1967; **213**, 1532–1544.

22. Patel DJ, Vaishnav RN. The rheology of large blood vessels. In: Bergel DH (ed), *Cardiovascular Fluid Dynamics.* London: Academic Press, 1972: 1–64.

23. Anliker M, Histand MB, Ogden E. Dispersion and attenuation of small artificial pressure waves in the canine aorta. *Circul Res* 1968; **23**, 539–551.

24. Bergel DH. The dynamic elastic properties of the blood vessel walls. *J Physiol* 1961; **156**, 458–469.

25. Yokobori AT, Yokobori T. The mechanical test method of cardiovascular and related biomaterial. *Bio-Med Mat Engng* 1991; **1**, 25–43.

26. Voorhees AB, Jaretski A, Blakemore AH. The use of tubes constructed from Vinyon-N cloth in bridging arterial defects. *Ann Surg* 1952; **135**, 332–336.

27. Charlesworth D. Synthetic arteries. In: Williams D (ed), *Concise Encyclopaedia of Medical and Dental Materials.* Oxford: Pergamon, 1990: 34–39.

28. Silver FH, Douillon CJ. Biocompatibility: Interactions of biological and implantable materials. In: Silver FH, Douillon CJ (eds), *Biocompatibility.* New York: VCH, 1989.

29. Rutherford RB. In: Rutherford RB (ed), *Vascular Surgery.* Philadelphia: WB Saunders, 1989.

30. Yates SG, Barros AAB, Berger K, *et al.* The preclotting of porous arterial prostheses. *Ann Surg* 1978; **188**, 611–622.

31. Guidoin R, Rao T-J, Roy P-E, *et al.* Postoperative thrombocytopenia and haemolytic anaemia in peripheral arterial reconstruction involving collagen-impregnated grafts. *Clin Mater* 1988; **3**, 103–118.

32. Guidoin R, Marois Y, Rao T-J, *et al.* An albumin-coated polyester arterial prosthesis made ready to anastomose: *in vivo* evaluation in dogs. *Clin Mater* 1988; **3**, 119–131.

33. Chapman D, Charles SA. A coat of many lipids—in the clinic. *Chem Brit* 1992; **28**, 253–256.

Section II _____

Advanced Respiratory Support

5

The need for advanced respiratory support in the intensive care unit

Stephen Cockroft

Introduction

The first documented use of respiratory support, expired-air ventilation, may well date to the Old Testament (800 BC): 'The prophet Elisha went up and lay upon the child, and put his mouth on his mouth, and his eyes on his eyes . . . and the flesh of the child became warm' (2 Kings 4: 34). Paracelsus (1530) first performed intermittent positive-pressure ventilation (IPPV) using a pair of fire bellows, a technique later utilized by Robert Hooke (1667) to perform the first successful experimental thoracotomy.

The earliest widespread use of IPPV for therapeutic purposes occurred during the 1952 Copenhagen polio epidemic. During this period, a total of 12 722 patients were admitted to the Blegdam Hospital, with 70 requiring respiratory support. Over 1400 medical students were recruited for the task of manual ventilation via a tracheostomy tube and an overall 75% survival was achieved.

With the subsequent widespread introduction of therapeutic IPPV, respiratory care units were established in the early 1960s, from which intensive care units subsequently developed. These units achieved dramatic reductions in the hospital mortality for acute respiratory failure (e.g. from 63% to 8.6%).[1]

Acute respiratory failure remains one of the leading indications for admission to intensive care facilities within the United States. Annually 150 000 patients are estimated to develop acute hypoxic respiratory failure which results in 40 000 deaths.[2,3] Individual centres report mortality rates of between 20% and 80%,[4-8] with variability arising because acute respiratory failure may occur as a consequence of other systemic pathology (e.g. adult respiratory distress syndrome).[9]

It is certain that, in order to improve outcome in such patients, effective pulmonary support is required to maintain adequate tissue oxygen delivery and therefore tissue viability.[10] However, many currently available respiratory support techniques actually contribute to patient morbidity and mortality.

Oxygen therapy and toxicity

Oxygen is an elementary principle, largely distributed in nature. It exists in the air, in all the oxides and in vegetable and animal substances. Although oxygen, in the state of admixture in which it is found in the atmosphere is of vital importance, it cannot be respired in a pure state with impunity. Animals die in it long before the whole of the oxygen is consumed.

A Dictionary of Medical Science, 1874[11]

Profound arterial hypoxaemia results in the cessation of tissue oxidative phosphorylation and causes an increase in the rate of anaerobic metabolism. This change occurs when mitochondrial Po_2 falls below a critical level (0.3 kPa); oxygen consumption then falls and the various members of the electron transfer chain revert to their reduced states, mitochondrial NADH/ NAD$^+$ and lactate/pyruvate ratios rise with concomitant falls in ATP/ADP ratios. This results in a rapid reduction in the level of all high-energy compounds within the most rapidly metabolizing tissues (e.g. cortical grey matter), whereas tissues with lower energy requirements continue to function for longer. When this arterial hypoxaemia persists, irreversible cellular damage occurs.[12]

Arterial hypoxaemia is to be anticipated in most patients with respiratory failure breathing room air, and as tissue oxygen delivery is directly dependent on arterial oxygen saturation, it is imperative that this is corrected. The main therapeutic objective remains treatment of the primary cause of the hypoxaemia, but when this is not immediately possible the administration of an increased inspired oxygen fraction (Fio$_2$) will elevate alveolar Po$_2$ and hence improve arterial oxygen saturation.[12]

However, Paul Bert and Lorrain-Smith were the first to recognize that oxygen in high concentrations was potentially toxic to mammalian lung. Furthermore Bert proved that it was the partial pressure of oxygen, rather than its concentration, that was responsible for this toxic effect.[13] As the lung parenchymal Po$_2$ is directly dependent on alveolar Po$_2$, irrespective of arterial Po$_2$, it is the lung tissue that is most immediately susceptible to oxygen toxicity. Pulmonary oxygen toxicity may therefore occur, even in the presence of arterial hypoxaemia.[14]

With the widespread introduction of therapeutic mechanical ventilation, it was noted that many patients deteriorated after a period of ventilator support. Nash reported that 70 patients, receiving an Fio$_2$ of at least 0.9, developed lung consolidation with histological evidence of increased fibrin deposition and evidence of pulmonary fibrosis. Two phases for this process were described. There was an early exudative phase, characterized by congestion, alveolar oedema, alveolar haemorrhage, fibrinous exudation and hyaline membrane thickening within the alveoli. Later a proliferative phase occurred with alveolar and septal oedema, fibroblast proliferation coupled with fibrosis and hyperplasia of the alveolar lining cells. These changes were not dependent on the duration of mechanical ventilation, but were correlated with higher Fio$_2$ values.[15] Similar studies have since confirmed these histological changes[16] which mimic those previously seen after

thermal injury, smoke inhalation, influenza pneumonia and paraquat toxicity.[17]

The actual cellular injury is thought to be mediated by free radicals of oxygen, reactive intermediates of oxygen reduction processes.[18–21] From its ground state, molecular oxygen (O$_2$) may undergo a series of reductions in the presence of catalysts to form: superoxide radicals (O$_2$·), hydrogen peroxide (H$_2$O$_2$), hydroxyl radicals (·OH) and singlet oxygen (^{1}O$_2$). These free radicals are all products of normal cellular oxidation/reduction processes,[19] but their production increases under conditions of hyperoxia, and pulmonary parenchymal cells, phagocytes and capillary endothelium have all been traced as sources.[22–24] These species, especially singlet oxygen and hydroxyl radicals, are capable of a variety of toxic effects, including lipid peroxidation, depolymerization of mucopolysaccharides, sulfhydryl oxidation of proteins, and nucleic acid damage.[25–27]

As a consequence of increased production of these oxygen radicals it is believed that release and metabolism of arachidonic acid is initiated. Arachidonic acid metabolites are known to have biological properties which mimic those produced by pulmonary oxygen toxicity, and it has recently been shown that activation of the lipoxygenase pathway may be integral in generating these toxic mediators.[28–31]

These metabolic cascade reactions can theoretically be blocked by a variety of agents in an attempt to prevent pulmonary damage. Bacterial endotoxin has been shown to increase oxygen tolerance in rats,[32,33] which may be mediated via an increase in intracellular levels of superoxide dismutase, an antioxidant enzyme.[34] Tumour necrosis factor, interleukin-1 and interferon inducers have all similarly been demonstrated to provide protection against oxygen-induced lung injury.[35,36] In addition, antioxidants such as cysteamine, N-acetylcysteine and the leukotriene synthesis inhibitor AA861 exert similar effects in experimental models.[37,38]

Human volunteer studies have been conducted in an attempt to measure the safe upper limit for oxygen concentrations. However, this limit for pulmonary Po$_2$ is likely to be influenced by many factors such as concomitant disease, age, nutrition and presence of infection.

A latent period of several hours is known to occur before signs of oxygen toxicity manifest. This was demonstrated in a study of volunteers who remained asymptomatic whilst breathing 100% oxygen for 6–12 hours. During this time, no radiographic changes or changes in alveolar–arterial O_2 gradient (A–ao_2), pulmonary arterial pressure, total pulmonary vascular resistance, cardiac output or pulmonary extravascular water occurred.[39] After 12–22 hours of receiving 100% oxygen, tracheobronchial irritation and retrosternal pain coupled with the development of impaired tracheal ciliary clearance of mucus has been described.[40,41]

Two prospective clinical studies have attempted to quantify pulmonary oxygen toxicity. One study revealed no differences in dead space, pulmonary shunt fraction, or compliance in patients receiving at least 21 hours of mechanical ventilation with either 42% or 100% oxygen.[42] However, another prospective study randomized 10 patients with irreversible head injuries into two groups; five received 100% oxygen and the remainder air. Increases in dead space occurred in the former group after 30 hours, and at 40 hours increased shunt fraction occurred with radiological evidence of pulmonary oedema.[43]

Vital capacity is known to decrease in patients breathing high oxygen concentrations over periods in excess of 24 hours.[40] These observations have been quantified as 'unit pulmonary toxicity dose' in an attempt to predict the onset and severity of pulmonary oxygen toxicity. These concepts are still used by diving institutions worldwide.[13] However, the indices have been criticized as the measurement of vital capacity is known to be effort-dependent and therefore poorly reproducible.[44] Many other indicators of pulmonary damage have been studied and linked with the pathogenesis of pulmonary oxygen toxicity. These include reductions in tracheal mucus velocity,[41] increases in albumin and transferrin in bronchopulmonary alveolar lavage fluid, and increases in the release of fibronectin and alveolar growth factor from aspirated alveolar macrophages.[45,46]

It can be concluded that oxygen toxicity is unlikely to occur with alveolar P_{O_2} values below 0.5 atmospheres absolute (ATA) and ventilation for up to 24 hours with 1.0 ATA is likely to be safe.[47,48] In addition it is unlikely that pre-existing pulmonary diseases increase susceptibility to pulmonary oxygen toxicity. In clinical practice the dilemma remains, to avoid hyperoxia and yet maintain arterial oxygen content. In the future it is possible that pharmacological agents may well be proven to be of clinical use in blocking the development of pulmonary oxygen toxicity, allowing the safe administration of higher F_{IO_2} values to preserve arterial oxygen content.[13]

Negative pressure ventilation

Negative pressure ventilation was introduced in 1864 by Alfred F Jones of Lexington, Kentucky, who patented the 'barorespirator'. This was a large box in which the subject was placed with the head protruding through a hole in the top. The device applied alternately negative and positive pressure to the external body surfaces and augmented inspiration and expiration respectively. The year 1928 marked the commissioning of Philip Drinker, by the New York Consolidated Gas Company, to develop an artificial respirator device for longer term use. This 'iron lung' device remained in widespread clinical use until the 1950s and achieved patient inspiration by intermittently lowering the pressure on the surface of the chest wall to sub-atmospheric pressure.[49] The usefulness of these iron lung devices is limited by their size, obstruction of patient access and failure to ensure airway patency.

However, small cuirass and shell ventilators remain in clinical use for the intermittent respiratory support of patients with neuromuscular disease and chest wall abnormalities. Difficulties remain in obtaining an adequate seal around these devices, and even with reduced size, access to the patient is restricted.

Intermittent positive pressure ventilation

The introduction of anaesthetic agents during the late nineteenth century permitted increasingly complex surgery, with the exception of thoracotomy, to be conducted. It was found that whenever the chest wall was perforated and the parietal pleura opened, the resulting pneumothorax invariably proved fatal. It was the development of endotracheal intubation techniques (Macewan 1880) and laryngoscopy (Jackson 1895) that enabled Tuffier (1896) to perform the first successful lung resection using a non-rebreathing device to provide positive pressure ventilation.

Modern positive pressure ventilation devices evolved from the work of V Ray Bennett. He originally developed a breathing valve for the administration of supplementary oxygen to US aircrew and then designed the first commercial intermittent positive pressure ventilation (IPPV) device, the Puritan–Bennett PR1, which was released in 1956.

The use of IPPV in respiratory failure is undoubtedly beneficial. An increase in carbon dioxide elimination is achieved rapidly and it is quite possible, by adjusting tidal volume and respiratory rate, to compensate for changes in CO_2 production and physiological dead space. An increase in arterial oxygenation is achieved as a consequence of the reduced alveolar Pco$_2$, which may be further increased by application of positive end-expiratory pressure (PEEP) and increased Fio$_2$.[50] The commencement of mechanical ventilation achieves further increases in patient oxygenation as the work of breathing is significantly reduced. It has been shown that, in subjects with reduced pulmonary compliance, IPPV reduces overall oxygen consumption, thus permitting mixed venous oxygen tension, and consequently arterial oxygen saturation, to increase.[51]

However, these immediately beneficial effects are not achieved without potentially adverse side-effects.

Cardiac output and IPPV

As a consequence of the reversal of intrapleural pressure gradients, the venous return to the heart is reduced with the commencement of IPPV, an effect accentuated in the hypovolaemic or sedated patient.[52] The compliance of both lung and chest wall are additional factors that further influence the development of positive intrapleural pressures, with the combination of highly compliant lung and non-compliant chest wall resulting in the largest increases in pressure.[53]

By increasing the duration of the inspiratory phase of ventilation, and thereby shortening the duration of the expiratory phase, air trapping in alveolar units may occur. This will further increase mean intrapleural pressures and lead to greater impedance to venous return.

Direct cardiac tamponade, as a consequence of bilateral lung compression of the pericardial sac, has also been suggested as an additional factor reducing the efficiency of cardiac function.[54]

Organ perfusion and IPPV

In addition to reducing cardiac output, the commencement of IPPV is known to reduce cerebral, splanchnic and renal blood flow as a result of increased venous pressure leading to reduced perfusion pressures.[55]

Further impairment of renal function with IPPV occurs as a consequence of redistributed intrarenal blood flow. Diversion of blood from the outer cortical areas, to the inner renal cortex and medullary tissue, results in an overall reduction in urine output, creatinine clearance and sodium excretion.[56]

Left atrial volume receptors, in addition to carotid sinus and aortic arch baroreceptors, are influenced by the intrathoracic pressure changes that occur with the commencement of IPPV. Consequently, increased antidiuretic hormone is secreted from the posterior pituitary, with resulting oliguria.[57,58]

Pulmonary gas transfer and IPPV

During spontaneous ventilation the greatest alveolar ventilation occurs within the dependent lung regions, a phenomenon reversed with the commencement of IPPV. As the distribution of pulmonary blood flow remains unchanged, increased dead space ventilation and increased intrapulmonary shunt will limit the therapeutic benefits achieved.[59–61]

Pulmonary barotrauma

Macklin (1944) described the development of 'malignant interstitial emphysema' in spontaneously breathing patients, the earliest description of pulmonary barotrauma; but the introduction of mechanical ventilatory support has since altered the significance of this pathological process.[62]

It was originally demonstrated that alveolar rupture occurred at the junction between the alveolar bases and the adjacent vascular sheaths.[62] From these sites, air tracks via the perivascular sheaths to the great vessels and subsequently to the mediastinum, resulting in mediastinal emphysema. Subcutaneous emphysema results from tracking of this mediastinal air along the lines of least resistance within fascial planes, into the neck, thoracic and abdominal walls.[63,64] Air may gain entry into the pericardial cavity, resulting in pneumocardium,[65,66] or may track through the diaphragmatic hiatus into the peritoneal cavity.[67-69] Of most significance, however, is entry of air into the pleural cavity, resulting in pneumothorax.[70-74]

Macklin hypothesized that alveolar rupture occurred in response to the pressure gradient developed between the alveolus (influenced by airway pressure) and the vascular sheath (influenced by pulmonary capillary pressure). Hence alveolar rupture was more likely to occur in association with pulmonary hyperinflation and hypovolaemia.[62] Caldwell subsequently confirmed the role of pulmonary hyperinflation in the pathogenesis of interstitial emphysema but the role of reduced pulmonary capillary pressure remained unproved.[75]

More recently it has been suggested that the term 'volotrauma' may more accurately describe the pathogenesis of this mechanical lung injury.[76] It has been shown that when normal lung tissue is over-distended, interstitial and alveolar oedema develop, which may then lead to alveolar rupture.[77,78] Lung injury has been shown not to occur in experimental animal models ventilated with high airway pressures with external thoracic wall bindings to limit lung expansion.[79]

High peak airway pressures (PAP) are known to be a predisposing factor for the development of pulmonary barotrauma. It is generally recognized that higher PAP values are associated with an increased incidence of barotrauma, but an absolute value for safe upper limit has yet to be determined.[80] For example, Peterson reported a 43% incidence in patients exposed to PAP in excess of 70 cmH$_2$O. With PAP values of between 50 and 70 cmH$_2$O, an 8% incidence of barotrauma was noted and no barotrauma occurred with PAP values below 50 cmH$_2$O.[72] Yet other studies have reported a range of PAP values between 25 and 50 cmH$_2$O to be clinically safe.[71,81] In contrast, barotrauma has occurred in animal models at much lower PAP values (30 cmH$_2$O).[82]

No direct relationship has been proven between mean airway pressure (MAWP) values and the incidence of pulmonary barotrauma. However, intermittent mandatory ventilation (IMV) has been shown to minimize MAWP values compared with conventional ventilation, and Mathru and colleagues retrospectively established that only 7% of patients receiving IMV developed barotrauma compared with 22% of patients receiving conventional mechanical ventilation.[83,84]

Positive end-expiratory pressure increases lung functional residual capacity and may improve ventilation of previously poorly ventilated or collapsed alveolar units, and thereby reduce intrapulmonary shunt. This may achieve an immediate improvement in arterial oxygen saturation.[85,86] However, some reports have suggested that PEEP is associated with an increased risk of barotrauma,[68,72,87,88] whereas other studies have failed to demonstrate a causal relationship.[89,90] It is probable that high (>15 cmH$_2$O) PEEP levels are associated with increased risk, but these may be offset by advantageous reductions of Fio$_2$, minimizing pulmonary oxygen toxicity.[91]

The coexistence of alveolar pathology (ARDS, asthma, emphysema) has been shown to predispose to the development of barotrauma with an incidence ranging from 13% to 83%.[71,74,92,93] Certainly, with pathology confined to discrete bronchopulmonary segments, one would expect preferential distribution of ventilator breaths to these abnormally compliant areas to result in excessive pulmonary distension, gas trapping and consequent barotrauma. For example, necrotizing staphylococcal and pseudomonal pneumonia was associated with a 90% incidence of bronchopleural fistula amongst 19 military casualties in whom PAP values did not exceed 30 cmH$_2$O.[70] In another series, 40% of patients with aspiration pneumonitis developed pulmonary barotrauma, resulting from gastric acid-induced lung parenchymal necrosis.[87]

The earliest clinical manifestation of barotrauma may be pneumothorax. Sixty per cent are diagnosed clinically as a result of tachycardia, hypotension, diminished breath sounds and unilateral chest wall hyper-resonance.[74] Where clinical diagnosis is made quickly, the mortality is reduced (from 31% to 7%).[74] Other reports have suggested that higher mortality rates (58–77%) are to be expected for pneumothorax occurring whilst receiving IPPV.[87,89,92,93]

Chest radiography may be an early method of predicting occurrence of pneumothorax. Parenchymal air cysts, subpleural air and hilar air streaking may appear up to 12 hours in advance of pneumothorax development. These may be apparent only after careful examination of a magnified chest radiograph, and so a high index of suspicion is required to detect these subtle changes.[94] In addition, palpation of the cervical, supraclavicular and anterior chest wall may indicate the presence of surgical emphysema prior to development of pneumothorax.[74]

In addition to catastrophic cardiovascular collapse, pneumothorax may result in a persistent pulmonary air leak with eventual bronchopleural fistulae formation. These air leaks are associated with a high mortality and effective pulmonary ventilation may prove impossible.[95–98]

As PAP has been proven to influence the development of barotrauma, it has been suggested that limiting ventilator tidal volumes to 5–10 ml/kg may reduce PAP and hence minimize barotrauma.[80,99] Certainly in one series of CMV-induced pneumothoraces, 62 out of 74 patients were receiving a mean tidal volume of 18 ml/kg.[74]

Although asynchronous mechanical ventilation with a spontaneously breathing patient has yet to be proven to contribute to barotrauma, the use of sedation and muscle relaxants has been advocated.[100] These minimize the work of breathing and thereby reduce overall oxygen requirements. However, the use of muscle relaxants during respiratory support has been associated with an increased incidence of pulmonary embolus, in addition to the increased risks of accidental ventilator malfunction or disconnection.[101–104]

An alternative approach has been described by Darioli and Menitove which permits intentional hypoventilation in order to minimize PAP in conjunction with sedation, paralysis and maintenance of arterial oxygenation. No mortality was reported for either study population.[105,106]

High-frequency jet ventilation (HFJV) relies on the delivery of smaller tidal volumes at high rates (1–15 Hz) and was introduced as a means of administering IPPV whilst minimizing airway pressures. Although PAP and MAP are known to be reduced, HFV has yet to be shown to reduce the incidence of pulmonary barotrauma in clinical trials.[107–109]

Inverse ratio ventilation, prolonging the inspiratory phase of IPPV to exceed expiration (I:E ratios of up to 4:1), is a further method of reducing PAP. Depending on the expiratory time selected and the time constants for passive expiration of the various alveolar units, significant gas trapping may occur with this technique and depression of cardiac output may result. Certainly arterial oxygen content may be improved with IRV, but no evidence exists that the incidence of pulmonary barotrauma is reduced.[110,111]

Independent lung ventilation with selective application of two differing ventilatory patterns to each lung has been advocated for the treatment of unilateral lung disease. Differences in compliance, perfusion and dead space between the two lungs can thereby be correlated with appropriate ventilation of each side with minimal barotrauma to the normal lung. The therapeutic benefits of this technique remain unproven.[112–115]

Conclusions

Experimental models of pulmonary oxygen toxicity and barotrauma, despite their physiological simplicity relative to clinical situations, provide some insight into the predisposing factors for these conditions. It would certainly seem appropriate to extrapolate such findings into clinical practice in an attempt to minimize the adverse sequelae of conventional respiratory support techniques.

However, proving clinical effectiveness of any respiratory support technique is an immensely difficult task. Primary respiratory failure rarely occurs[116,117] and more often is associated with a multitude of coexisting pathological conditions making simple randomized clinical trials impossible. Consequently, large numbers of patients, in several clinical centres, have to be studied over significant time periods in order to prove any beneficial therapeutic effect.

Furthermore it is well documented that, within the intensive care unit, patients with acute respiratory failure rarely die as a direct result of hypoxaemia or hypercapnia.[116–118] More commonly other organ systems fail as part of a more global complex disorder which is likely to involve many differing pharmacological and cellular inflammatory mediators.[119] It is therefore unlikely that any therapeutic strategies for advanced respiratory support will, by themselves, achieve significant improvements in patient outcome without consideration of the more basic underlying pathophysiology.

References

1. O'Donoghue WJ, Baker JP, Bell GM. The management of acute respiratory failure in a respiratory intensive care unit. *Chest* 1970; **58**, 603.
2. Murray JF. Mechanisms of respiratory failure. *Am Rev Resp Dis* 1977; **115**, 1071.
3. Ashbaugh DG, Petty TL. Sepsis complicating the

acute respiratory distress syndrome. *Surg Gynecol Obst* 1972; **135**, 865–869.

4. Hill RN, Shible EM, Spragg RG, Moser KM. Adult respiratory distress syndromes: early predictors of mortality. *ASAIO Trans* 1975; **21**, 199–205.

5. Lutch JS, Murray JF. Continuous positive-pressure ventilation: effects on systemic oxygen transport and tissue oxygenation. *Ann Intern Med* 1972; **76**, 193–202.

6. McMahon SM, Halprin GM, Sieker HO. Positive end-expiratory airway pressure in severe arterial hypoxaemia. *Am Rev Respir Dis* 1973; **108**, 526–535.

7. Lamy M, Fallot RJ, Koeniger E, Harm-Petter D, Ratliff JL, Eberhart RC. Pathological features and mechanisms of hypoxaemia in adult respiratory distress syndrome. *Am Rev Respir Dis* 1976; **144**, 267.

8. Bartlett RH, Gazzaniga AB, Wilson AF, Geraghty T, Wetmore N. Mortality prediction in adult respiratory insufficiency. *Chest* 1975; **67**, 680.

9. Balk R, Bone RC. Classification of acute respiratory failure. *Med Clin N Am* 1983; **67**, 551–556.

10. Allen SJ, Tonnesen AS. Advanced respiratory life support. In: Hoyt JW, Tonnesen AS, Allen SJ, *Critical Care Practice*. Philadelphia: WB Saunders, 1991: 49–80.

11. Dunglison RT. Oxygen. In: *A Dictionary of Medical Science*. Philadelphia: Henry C Lea, 1874: 743.

12. Nunn JF. Oxygen. In: Nunn JF (ed), *Applied Respiratory Physiology*. London: Butterworths, 1987: 235–283.

13. Klein J. Normobaric pulmonary oxygen toxicity. *Anesth Analg* 1990; **70**, 195–207.

14. Nunn JF. Hyperoxia and oxygen toxicity. In: Nunn JF (ed), *Applied Respiratory Physiology*. London: Butterworths, 1987: 478–494.

15. Nash G, Blennerhassett JB, Pontoppidan H. Pulmonary lesions associated with oxygen therapy and artificial ventilation. *New Engl J Med* 1967; **276**, 368–374.

16. Gould V, Tosco R, Wheelis R. Oxygen pneumonitis in man: ultrastructural observations on the development of alveolar lesions. *Lab Invest* 1972; **26**, 499–508.

17. Katzenstein A, Bloor C, Leibow A. Diffuse alveolar damage: the role of oxygen, shock and related factors. *Am J Path* 1976; **85**, 210–228.

18. Clark J, Lambertson C. Pulmonary oxygen toxicity: a review. *Pharmacol Rev* 1971; **23**, 37–133.

19. Fridovich I. The biology of oxygen radicals. *Science* 1978; **201**, 875–880.

20. Haugaard N. Cellular mechanisms of oxygen toxicity. *Physiol Rev* 1968; **48**, 311–373,

21. Mustafa M, Tierney D. Biochemical and metabolic changes in the lung with oxygen, ozone and nitrogen dioxide toxicity. *Am Rev Respir Dis* 1978; **118**, 1001–1090.

22. Jamieson D, Chance B, Cadenas E, Boveris A. The relation of free radical production to hyperoxia. *Ann Rev Physiol* 1986; **48**, 703–719.

23. Rodell TC, Cheronis JC, Ohnemus CL, Piermattei DJ, Repine JE. Xanthine oxidase mediates elastase-induced injury to isolated lungs and endothelium. *J Appl Physiol* 1987; **63**, 2159–2163.

24. Saugstad OD, Hallman M, Abraham JL, Epstein B, Conchrane C, Gluck L. Hypoxanthine and oxygen induced lung injury: a possible basic mechanism of tissue damage? *Ped Res* 1984; **18**, 501–504.

25. Brown K, Fridovich I. DNA strand scission by enzymatically generated oxygen radicals. *Arch Biochem Biophys* 1981; **206**, 414.

26. Slater TF. Overview of methods used for detecting lipid peroxidation. *Meth Enzymol* 1984; **105**, 283.

27. Johnson KJ, Fantone JC, Kaplan J, Ward PA. *In vivo* damage of rat lungs by oxygen metabolites. *J Clin Invest* 1981; **67**: 983–993.

28. Sporn HS, Peters-Golden M, Simon RH. Hydrogen peroxide induced arachidonic acid metabolism in rat alveolar macrophage. *Am Rev Respir Dis* 1988; **137**, 49–56.

29. Farrukh IS, Michael JR, Peters SP. The role of cycloxygenase and lipoxygenase mediators in oxidant induced lung injury. *Am Rev Respir Dis* 1988; **137**, 1343–1349.

30. Jackson RM, Chandler DB, Fulmer JD. Production of arachidonic acid metabolites by endothelial cells in hyperoxia. *J Appl Physiol* 1986; **61**, 584–591.

31. Tate RM, Morris HG, Schroeder WR, Repine JE. Oxygen metabolites stimulate thromboxane production and vasoconstriction in isolated saline-perfused rabbit lungs. *J Clin Invest* 1984; **74**, 608–613.

32. Frank L, Neriishi K. Endotoxin treatment protects vitamin E deficient rats from pulmonary oxygen toxicity. *Am J Physiol* 1984; **247** (3, Pt 2): R520–526.

33. Frank L, Roberts RJ. Endotoxin protection against oxygen induced acute and chronic lung injury. *J Appl Physiol* 1979; **47**, 577–581.

34. Frank L, Summerville J, Massaro D. Protection from oxygen toxicity with endotoxin: role of the endogenous antioxidant enzymes of the lung. *J Clin Invest* 1980; **65**, 1104–1110.

35. White CW, Ghezzi P, Dinarello CA, Caldwell SA, McMurtry IF, Repine JE. Recombinant tumour necrosis factor/cachectin and interleukin-1 pretreatment decreases lung oxidized glutathione accumulation, lung injury and mortality in rats exposed to hyperoxia. *J Clin Invest* 1987; **79**, 1868–1873.

36. Kikkawa Y, Yano S, Skoza L. Protective effect of interferon inducers against hyperoxic pulmonary damage. *Lab Invest* 1984; **50**, 62–71.

37. Taniguchi H, Taki F, Takagi K, Satake T,

Sugiyama S, Ozawa T. The role of leukotriene B4 in the genesis of oxygen toxicity in the lung. *Am Rev Respir Dis* 1986; **133**, 805–808.

38. Patterson CE, Butler JA, Byrne FD, Rhodes ML. Oxidant lung injury: intervention with sulfhydryl reagents. *Lung* 1985; **163**, 23–32.

39. Van de Water JN, Kagey KS, Miller IT. Response of the lung to six to 12 hours of 100 per cent oxygen inhalation in normal man. *New Engl J Med* 1970; **283**, 621–626.

40. Comroe JH, Dripps RD, Dumke PR, Deming M. Oxygen toxicity: the effect of inhalation of high concentrations of oxygen for twenty-four hours on normal man at sea level and at a simulated altitude of 18,000 feet. *JAMA* 1945; **128**, 710–717.

41. Sackner MA, Landa J, Hirsch J, Zapata A. Pulmonary effects of oxygen breathing: a 6-hour study in normal men. *Ann Intern Med* 1975; **82**, 40–43.

42. Singer MM, Wright F, Stanley L, Roe BB, Hamilton WK. Oxygen toxicity in man: a prospective study in patients after open heart surgery. *New Engl J Med* 1970; **283**, 1473–1478.

43. Barber RE, Lee J, Hamilton WK. Oxygen toxicity in man: a prospective study in patients with irreversible brain damage. *New Engl J Med* 1970; **283**, 1478–1484.

44. Widell PJ, Bennet PB, Kivlin P, Gray W. Pulmonary oxygen toxicity in man at 2 ATA with intermittent air breathing. *Aerosp Med* 1974; **45**, 407–410.

45. Davis WB, Rennard SI, Bitterman PB, Crystal RG. Pulmonary oxygen toxicity: early reversible changes in human alveolar structures induced by hyperoxia. *New Engl J Med* 1983; **309**, 878–883.

46. Griffith DE, Holden WE, Morris JF, Min LK, Krishnamurthy GT. Effects of common therapeutic concentrations of oxygen on lung clearance of 99mTc DPTA and bronchoalveolar lavage albumin concentration. *Am Rev Respir Dis* 1986; **134**, 233–237.

47. Bostek CC. Oxygen toxicity: an introduction. *J Am Assoc Nurse Anesth* 1989; **57**, 231–237.

48. Jackson RM. Molecular, pharmacologic and clinical aspects of oxygen-induced lung injury. *Clin Chest Med* 1990; **11**, 73–86.

49. Drinker P, McKhann C. The use of a new apparatus for the prolonged administration of artificial respiration. *JAMA* 1929; **92**, 1658–1660.

50. Hall JR. Techniques of ventilation and oxygenation. In: Kaplan JA (ed), *Thoracic Anesthesia*. New York: Churchill Livingstone, 1983: 701–742.

51. Wilson RS, Sullivan SF, Malm JR, Bowman FO. The oxygen cost of breathing following anesthesia and cardiac surgery. *Anesthesiology* 1973; **39**, 387–393.

52. Cournand A, Motley HL, Werko L. Physiologic studies of the effects of intermittent positive pressure breathing on cardiac output in man. *Am J*

Physiol 1948; **152**, 162–174.

53. Qvist J, Pontopiddian H, Wilson RS, Lowenstein E, Laver MB. Haemodynamic responses to mechanical ventilation with PEEP. *Anesthesiology* 1975; **42**, 45–55.

54. Tyler DC. Positive end expiratory pressure: a review. *Crit Care Med* 1983; **11**, 300–308.

55. Manny J, Justice R, Hechtman HB. Abnormalities in organ blood flow and its distribution during positive end-expiratory pressure. *Surgery* 1979; **85**, 425–432.

56. Marquez JM, Douglas ME, Downs JB, Wu WH, Mantini EL, Kuck EJ, Calderwood HW. Renal function and cardiovascular responses during positive airway pressure. *Anesthesiology* 1979; **50**, 393–398.

57. Hemmer M, Viquerat CE, Suter PM, Vallotton MB. Urinary antidiuretic hormone excretion during mechanical ventilation and weaning in man. *Anesthesiology* 1980; **52**, 395–400.

58. Kumar A, Pontopiddan H, Falke KJ, Wilson RS. Inappropriate response to increased plasma ADH during mechanical ventilation in acute respiratory failure. *Anesthesiology* 1974; **40**, 215–221.

59. Westbrook PR, Stubbs SE, Sessler AD. Effects of anesthesia and muscle paralysis on respiratory mechanics in normal man. *J Appl Physiol* 1973; **34**, 81–86.

60. Landmark SJ, Knopp TJ, Rehder K, Sessler AD. Regional pulmonary perfusion and V/Q in awake and anesthetised-paralysed man. *J Appl Physiol* 1977; **43**, 993–1000.

61. Dueck R, Wagner PD, West JB. Effect of positive end-expiratory pressure on gas exchange in dogs with normal and edematous lungs. *Anesthesiology* 1977; **47**, 359–366.

62. Macklin MT, Macklin CC. Malignant interstitial emphysema of the lungs and mediastinum as an important occult complication in many respiratory diseases and other conditions: an interpretation of the clinical literature in the light of laboratory experiments. *Medicine* 1944; **23**, 281–353.

63. Maunder RJ, Pierson DJ, Hudson LD. Subcutaneous and mediastinal emphysema. *Arch Intern Med* 1984; **144**, 1447–1453.

64. Zimmerman JE, Dunbar BS, Klingenmaier CH. Management of subcutaneous emphysema, pneumomediastinum and pneumothorax during respirator therapy. *Crit Care Med* 1975; **3**, 69.

65. Hurd TE, Novak R, Gallagher J. Tension pneumocardium: a complication of mechanical ventilation. *Crit Care Med* 1984; **12**, 200–201.

66. Alpan G, Goder K, Glick B. Pneumopericardium during continuous positive pressure in respiratory distress syndrome. *Crit Care Med* 1984; **12**, 1080–1081.

67. Beilin B, Shulman DL, Weiss AT. Pneumoper-

itoneum as the presenting sign of pulmonary barotrauma during artificial ventilation. *Inten Care Med* 1986; **12**, 49–51.

68. Hillman KM. Pneumoperitoneum—a review. *Crit Care Med* 1982; **10**, 476–481.

69. Stringfield JT, Graham JP, Watts C. Pneumoperitoneum: a complication of mechanical ventilation. *JAMA* 1976; **235**, 744–746.

70. Fleming WH, Bowen JC. Early complications of long term respiratory support. *J Thorac Cardiovasc Surg* 1972; **64**, 729–737.

71. Kumar A, Pontoppidian H, Falke KJ, Wilson RS, Laver MB. Pulmonary barotrauma during mechanical ventilation. *Crit Care Med* 1973; **1**, 181–186.

72. Peterson GW, Horst B. Incidence of pulmonary barotrauma in a medical ICU. *Crit Care Med* 1983; **11**, 67–69.

73. Pingleton SK. Complications associated with the adult respiratory distress syndrome. *Clin Chest Med* 1982; **3**, 143–155.

74. Steier M, Ching N, Roberts ER, Nealon TF. Pneumothorax complicating continuous ventilatory support. *J Thorac Cardiovasc Surg* 1974; **67**, 17–23.

75. Caldwell EJ, Powell RD, Mullooly JP. Interstitial emphysema: a study of physiologic factors involved in experimental induction of the lesion. *Am Rev Respir Dis* 1970; **102**, 516–525.

76. Zapol WM. Volotrauma and the intravenous oxygenator in patients with adult respiratory distress syndrome. *Anesthesiology* 1992; **77**, 847–849.

77. Parker JC, Townsley MI, Rippe B, Taylor AE, Thigpen J. Increased microvascular permeability in dog lungs due to high peak airway pressures. *J Appl Physiol* 1984; **57**, 1809–1816.

78. West JB, Tsukimoto K, Mathieu-Castello O, Prediletto R. Stress failure in pulmonary capillaries. *J Appl Physiol* 1991; **70**, 1731–1742

79. Dreyfuss D, Soler P, Basset G, Saumon G. High inflation pressure pulmonary edema: Respective effects of high airway pressure, high tidal volume and positive end-expiratory pressure. *Am Rev Respir Dis* 1988; **137**, 1159–1164.

80. Haake R, Schlichtig R, Ulstad DR, Henschen RR. Barotrauma: pathophysiology, risk factors and prevention. *Chest* 1987; **91**, 608–613.

81. Nennhaus HP, Javid J, Julian OC. Alveolar and pleural rupture, hazards of positive pressure ventilation. *Arch Surg* 1967; **94**, 136–141.

82. Tsuno K, Prato P, Kolobow T. Acute lung injury from mechanical ventilation at moderately high airway pressures. *J Appl Physiol* 1990; **69**, 956–961.

83. Kirby RR, Perry JC, Calderwood HW, Ruiz BC, Lederman DS. Cardiorespiratory effects of high positive end-expiratory pressure. *Anesthesiology* 1975; **43**, 533–539.

84. Mathru M, Venus B. Ventilator-induced barotrauma in controlled mechanical ventilation versus intermittent mandatory ventilation. *Crit Care Med* 1983; **11**, 359–361.

85. Nunn JF. Artificial ventilation. In: Nunn JF (ed), *Applied Respiratory Physiology*. London: Butterworths, 1987: 392–422.

86. Ashbaugh DG, Petty TL, Bigelow DB, Harris TM. Continuous positive pressure breathing (CPPB) in adult respiratory distress syndrome. *J Thorac Cardiovasc Surg* 1969; **57**, 31–41.

87. de Latorre F, Tomasa A, Klamburg J, Leon C, Soler M, Rius J. Incidence of pneumothorax and pneumomediastinum in patients with aspiration pneumonia requiring ventilatory support. *Chest* 1977; **72**, 141–144.

88. Powner DJ, Snyder JV, Morris CW. Retroperitoneal air dissection associated with mechanical ventilation. *Chest* 1976; **69**, 739–742.

89. Cullen DJ, Caldera DL. The incidence of ventilator-induced pulmonary barotrauma in critically ill patients. *Anesthesiology* 1979; **50**, 185–190.

90. Kirby RR, Downs JB, Civetta JM. High-level positive end-expiratory pressure (PEEP) in acute respiratory insufficiency. *Chest* 1975; **67**, 156–163.

91. Weisman JM, Rinaldo JE, Rogers RM. Positive end-expiratory pressure in adult respiratory failure. *New Engl J Med* 1982; **307**, 1381–1384.

92. Rolfing BM, Webb WR, Schlobohm RM. Ventilator-related extra-alveolar air in adults. *Radiology* 1976; **121**, 25–31.

93. Woodring JH. Pulmonary interstitial emphysema in the adult respiratory distress syndrome. *Crit Care Med* 1985; **13**, 786–791.

94. Albelda SM, Gefter WB, Kelley MA. Ventilator-induced subpleural air cysts: clinical, radiographic and pathological significance. *Am Rev Respir Dis* 1983; **127**, 360–365.

95. Downs JB, Chapman RL. Treatment of bronchopleural fistula during continuous positive pressure ventilation. *Chest* 1976; **69**, 363–366.

96. Pierson DJ. Persistent bronchopleural air leak during mechanical ventilation. a review. *Respir Care* 1982; **27**, 408–416.

97. Powner DJ, Grenvik A. Ventilatory management of life threatening bronchopleural fistula: a summary. *Crit Care Med* 1981; **9**, 54–58.

98. Pierson DJ, Horton CA, Bates PW. Persistent bronchopleural air leak during mechanical ventilation: a review of 39 cases. *Chest* 1986; **90**, 321–323.

99. Suter PM, Fairley HB, Isenberg MD. Effect of tidal volume and positive end-expiratory pressure on compliance during mechanical ventilation. *Chest* 1978; **73**, 158–162.

100. Heenan TJ, Downs JB, Douglas ME, Ruiz BC, Jumper L. Intermittent mandatory ventilation: is synchronization important? *Chest* 1980; **77**, 598–602.

101. Willatts SM. Paralysis of ventilated patients. Yes or

no? *Inten Care Med* 1985; **11**, 2–4.

102. Myllynen P, Kammonen M, Rokkanen P, Bostman O, Lalla M, Laasonen E. Deep venous thrombosis and pulmonary embolism with acute spinal cord injury: a comparison with non-paralyzed patients immobilized due to spinal fractures. *J Trauma* 1985; **25**, 541–543.

103. Coon WW. Venous thromboembolism: prevalance, risk factors and prevention. *Clin Chest Med* 1984; **3**, 391–401.

104. Jenkins J, Keep P. Fatal embolism despite low dose heparin. *Lancet* 1976; **i**, 544.

105. Darioli E, Perret C. Mechanical controlled hypoventilation in status asthmaticus. *Am Rev Respir Dis* 1984; **129**, 385–387.

106. Menitove SM, Goldring RM. Combined ventilator and bicarbonate strategy in the management of status asthmaticus. *Am J Med* 1983; **94**, 898–901.

107. Sladen A, Gantupalli K, Klain M. High-frequency jet ventilation versus intermittent positive pressure ventilation. *Crit Care Med* 1984; **12**, 788–790.

108. Carlon GC, Howland WS, Ray C, Miodownik S, Griffin JP, Groegner JS. High-frequency jet ventilation: a prospective randomized evaluation. *Chest* 1983; **84**, 551–559.

109. Hurst JM, Branson RD, Davis K, Barrette RR, Adams KS. Comparison of conventional mechanical ventilation and high frequency ventilation. *Ann Surg* 1990; **211**, 486–491.

110. Gurevitch MJ, VanDyke J, Young ES. Improved oxygenation and lower peak airway pressure in severe adult respiratory distress syndrome: treatment with inverse ratio ventilation. *Chest* 1986; **89**, 211.

111. Macintyre NR. New forms of mechanical ventilation in the adult. *Clin Chest Med* 1988; **9**, 47–54.

112. Graziano CC, Khan R, Howland WS, Baron R, Ramaker J. Acute life-threatening ventilation perfusion inequality: an indication for independent lung ventilation. *Crit Care Med* 1978; **6**, 380–383.

113. Carlon GC, Ray C, Klein R, Goldiner PL, Miodownik J. Criteria for selective positive end-expiratory pressure and independent synchronized ventilation of each lung. *Chest* 1978; **74**, 501–507.

114. Hillman, Barber JD. Asynchronous independent lung ventilation (AILV). *Crit Care Med* 1980; **8**, 390–395.

115. Gallagher TJ, Banner MJ, Smith RA. A simplified method of independent lung ventilation. *Crit Care Med* 1980; **8**, 396–399.

116. Bartlett RH, Morris AH, Fairley HB, Hirsch R, O'Connor N, Pontopiddian H. A prospective study of acute hypoxic respiratory failure. *Chest* 1986; **89**, 684–689.

117. Gillespie DJ, Marsh HMM, Divertie MB, Meadows JA. Clinical outcome of respiratory failure in patients requiring prolonged (>24 hours) mechanical ventilation. *Chest* 1986; **90**, 364–369.

118. Cockroft S, Baxter MK, Goldhill DR, Withington PS. Acute respiratory failure in the ITU and quality of life after hospital discharge. *Clin Inten Care* 1993; **4**, 99.

119. Lamy M, Deby-Dupont G, Deby C, Faymonville M, Damas P. Why is our present therapy for adult respiratory distress syndrome so ineffective? *Inten Crit Care Dig* 1992; **11**, 6–12.

6

Technical overview of advanced respiratory support

Dereck Wheeldon

Introduction

There have been significant technical advances since the first application of extracorporeal membrane oxygenation (ECMO) in the early 1970s. Ventilation techniques have improved considerably, with modern computer controlled machines allowing optimal gas exchange with minimal baro/volutrauma. Novel methods employing high-frequency and tracheal ventilation promise further improvements. The experimental use of liquid ventilation shows promise, as does the use of exogenous surfactants. Mechanical ventilation, however sophisticated and innovative, will not always suffice to keep a patient alive or, more commonly, will exacerbate the lung injury, in the process, and ultimately lead to the demise of the patient.

Early extracorporeal systems employed oxygenators with large surface areas and priming volume such that bleeding was a major complication. Oxygenators and circuitry have been miniaturized and gas exchange membranes improved. Today, surface coatings allow minimal anticoagulation and stimulation of the immune system.

The original veno-arterial support modes paid scant attention to the necessity for maintaining pulmonary blood flow, a factor now known to impede lung healing. New high-performance membranes have made it feasible to use intravascular designs which are showing real promise.

The development of thin-walled percutaneous cannulae has made access much less complicated and facilitated high-flow techniques, when required.

Further development of this technology will involve the generation of automated, low-prime, high-efficiency, simple-access systems which will not require any anticoagulation. This will encourage much earlier intervention, especially with the identification of early markers for developing adult respiratory distress syndrome (ARDS). While applications in acute respiratory support have provided the proving grounds for the technology, there is a much larger potential application in chronic conditions, cardiorespiratory resuscitation and as a surgical support tool. The development of this technology will ultimately lead to a totally implantable artificial lung.

The aetiology of acute respiratory failure is diverse.[1] Until the early 1970s, forced mechanical ventilation provided the only means of supporting gas exchange with the hope that the lung injury would resolve. There is now an increasing array of devices, technologies and techniques available to support 'at risk' patients from respiratory failure. However, the search for a common causative pathway, and hence definitive treatments, continues.

The techniques can be differentiated into those which augment gas exchange via the natural lung, and those which employ alternative non-pulmonary gas exchange.

Augmented pulmonary gas exchange

Early mechanical ventilators employed negative pressure applied around the entire body, in the belief that this was more physiological. Modern machines make greater use of endotracheal positive-pressure modalities, and the advent of computer controlled systems has allowed greater interaction between machine and patient. Approaches that have been proposed for use in adult patients include:

1. External ventilation (iron lung or cuirass).
2. Negative-pressure ventilation.
3. Positive-pressure ventilation with independent pressure, volume and rate controls.
4. Inverse-ratio ventilation.
5. Jet ventilation.
6. Intratracheal pulmonary ventilation.

Constant flow, and a variant of this called 'tracheal insufflation of oxygen', has been proposed, based on experimental work, but has yet to show clinical value. For neonatal patients a more limited range of novel ventilator strategies have been reported. However, there is to date no compelling evidence that any one of these strategies has resulted in an improved outcome.[2]

A more recent adaptation of mechanical ventilation involves high-frequency ventilation. In essence, the concept is mechanical ventilation at supra-physiological rates and low tidal volumes. The types of machines can be classified as oscilators, jets or flow interrupters, and then subclassified in terms of whether the expiratory phase is active or passive. In terms of efficacy, it would seem probable that high-frequency ventilation offers advantages over conventional positive-pressure ventilation in conditions of homogenous lung injury, whilst patchy lung injury is less susceptible to successful treatment by this method.[3]

Gattinoni has proposed that the ARDS lung be regarded as a 'baby lung' and that the remaining volume of lung taking part in gas exchange can be estimated by measuring static compliance.[4] A compliance below 25 ml/cmH$_2$O makes the use of some form of artificial lung mandatory, whilst a patient with a compliance greater than 30 ml/cmH$_2$O can tolerate spontaneous breathing. Generally, when the residual normally inflated lung is smaller than 20% of the expected, any form of mechanical ventilation alone may induce irreversible lung damage.

Ventilation techniques to facilitate permissive hypercapnia ($P\text{CO}_2 = 9$–12 kPa) result in lower ventilator settings and higher gradients across the oxygenator, so improving gas exchange.[5]

The critical role of substances which decrease the surface tension at the alveolar lining has been known for some time. Trials of exogenous surfactant administration in neonates and adults have been encouraging, but relatively large doses are required and current preparations are prohibitively expensive in the dosage required.[6]

Since the 1920s efforts have been made to exchange gas by ventilation with a liquid medium. Perfluoro chemicals have a number of useful characteristics for this purpose, including high oxygen and carbon dioxide transport capacity (50 and 160 dl respectively) and a low surface tension. A few isolated case studies have been very promising.[7]

Non-pulmonary gas exchange

Most equipment used for extracorporeal life-support (ECLS) is borrowed from cardiopulmonary bypass (CPB) applications, and is therefore designed for short-term use. It is useful to understand the limitations of each of the devices when applied to long-term use (Table 6.1).

Oxygenators

The impetus for extracorporeal methods of respiratory (and cardiac) support was provided by the desire to repair cardiac lesions. In the early 1950s a number of methods were used, including profound hypothermia, cross circulation and in 1953 the first mechanical 'oxygenator'. These early artificial lungs involved the direct contact of gas with blood and were therefore limited to relatively short-term use (hours) because of the associated blood trauma. In the 1960s membrane lungs were developed from the recently discovered polymer of methylsiloxane (silicon rubber) which had the unique characteristic of selective gas permeability when fabricated as a thin sheet. Whilst oxygen and carbon dioxide transfer across the material itself was more than adequate, it soon became apparent that the limiting factor is the time taken for oxygen to diffuse across plasma to bind haemoglobin. In practical terms this means that the blood film thickness becomes the limiting factor to oxygen exchange (Fig. 6.1).

The challenge was, therefore, to produce devi-

Table 6.1 The major ECLS components, their design specifications and the manner in which they are used for ECLS applications.

Device	Design application	ECLS application
Roller pump	Intermittent use (<6 h) Manual regulation	Continuous use (weeks) Requires servo-regulation Frequent tubing 'Walking' Requires power back-up
Centrifugal pump	Intermittent use (<6 h) Blood flow monitoring	Continuous use (weeks) Blood flow monitoring Head changes: 3–5 days
Collin Cardio Pump	Intermittent pulsatile Blood flow monitoring	Continuous use (weeks) Automatic valving Inlet–outlet pressures Blood flow monitoring Requires power back-up
Bubble trap	Single use (<6 h)	Single use (weeks)
Oxygen sensor	Single use (<1 day)	Single use (weeks)
Air bubble detector	Intermittent use (<1 day)	Continuous use (weeks)
Water circulator	Intermittent use (days)	Continuous use (weeks)
Bladder box	NA	Specific design

ces which have minimal blood film thickness (or a method of mechanical agitation of the blood film) whilst still maintaining maximum transmembrane gas concentration gradients and a minimal resistance to blood flow. In 1971 the first successful prolonged ECLS patient was supported on a Bramson membrane lung by the Pacific Medical team for 3 days.[8] The Bramson was one of a number of early membrane oxygenators containing 14 blood cells fabricated with alternate siloxane, blood, oxygen and water screens. The priming volume was one litre and the surface area 5.6 m[2]. This oxygenator and a number of similar

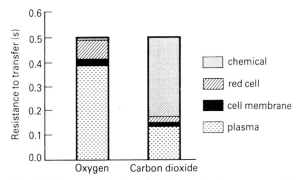

Fig. 6.1 Oxygen and carbon dioxide transfer times compared in terms of *resistance*. It is clear that the major barrier to oxygen transfer is diffusion through plasma, whilst with carbon dioxide the chemical reactions within the red cell are the most time-consuming. This means that the effective depth of the blood path adjacent to a membrane plays the most important part in oxygen transfer.

designs were subsequently manufactured in a disposable format.[9] The most notable of these was the spirally wound siloxane envelope device designed by Kolobow and manufactured by SciMed which has become the workhorse of extracorporeal membrane oxygenation.[10]

Hollow-fibre technology has provided the possibility of reducing oxygenator size by virtue of the increased gas transport across porous polymeric membranes. Gas transport across these membranes is not selective and increases with an increasing pressure gradient and greatly decreases with increasing temperature. Microporous membranes that exhibit virtually no gas transport can be produced from polymers as a solid sheet. Membrane thickness can be increased, thereby augmenting its strength. The micropores range from 0.01 to 1.0 µm and have heterogeneous shapes. They can be round or oval, slit-like or fibrillar passages. The hydrophobic nature of many microporous membranes prevents the passage of plasma and water across the pores. However, there is always a critical pressure beyond which plasma and water will pass through the micropores, causing a precipitous loss of gas transport. This has recently been shown to be associated with the lipid content of the plasma.[11] It has also recently become possible to coat these membranes with heparin using an end-point attached covalent bonding, so making systemic heparinization less important and reducing the bleeding complications.[12] A number of alternative strategies for rendering prosthetic surfaces more biocompatible are also in use or under development, including the addition of surface modifying agents (SMAs) to the base polymer. Coating microporous membranes with an ultra-thin layer of a gas-selective polymer such as silicone or polysulphone[13] produces a composite membrane with the benefits of both.

It remains impossible to produce prosthetic capillary networks similar to the human lung, which has a blood film thickness in the order of one red blood cell and a length of under 1000 μm. In plate and sheet membrane lungs as well as in capillary-type membrane lungs, the usual width of the blood flow channel is near 200 μm with a 20–40 cm blood path length. This yields a compromise between blood layer thickness, gas transport and resistance to blood flow. In order to avoid the boundary layer effect, a number of designs include a thin fabric mesh, or introduce pulsatile motion, or create secondary blood flow patterns. Unlike with oxygen transport, the movement of CO_2 from red blood cells to plasma and across the polymeric membrane is much less impaired by the presence of a boundary layer. As with the natural lung, CO_2 removal primarily depends on the ventilation rate of the membrane lung.

Membrane lungs are rated by their O_2 and CO_2 transport under standard input and output conditions; this is the 'reference blood flow'.[14] In practice this defines the maximum blood flow providing an outlet blood oxygen saturation above 95%, with a venous saturation of 65%. In long-term clinical perfusion, it is worthwhile choosing a membrane lung with excess gas transport capacity to compensate for any increased

metabolic demands, and to compensate for any deterioration of membrane lung performance.[15] The use of permissive hypercapnia and negative pressure on the expiratory side of the lung can further enhance CO_2 exchange. Table 6.2 gives some comparisons for gas exchange in a variety of membrane systems.

The coiled silicone sheet oxygenator remains the device of choice for most ECLS applications, but there is increased use of heparin-coated hollow-fibre devices. Silicone membranes can be heparin bonded, but a commercial system is not yet available.

A number of alternative extracorporeal techniques have been proposed over the last few years. These include pumpless arteriovenous shunts,[16] PA to LA shunts,[17] haemodialysis for CO_2 removal,[18] and peritoneal lavage with perfluorocarbon. All these techniques are in preclinical stages of development.

Blood pumps

Three types of blood pump are in use with ECLS systems. The traditional De Bakey type of roller pump has the advantages of simplicity and low cost. For long-term use the tubing insert needs to be moved at frequent intervals to prevent wear and subsequent rupture, and the drive control needs to be servo-regulated to some measure of input flow, usually via a small reservoir and pressure sensor, to prevent high levels of negative pressure being generated[19] (Fig. 6.2).

Centrifugal pumps, on the other hand, have the advantage of being interactive to input and output pressures, but require flow monitoring and are not really suited to the low flows used in neonatal ECMO. However, the pump consoles do

Table 6.2 Comparison of a variety of gas exchanging devices.

Oxygenator	Membrane material	Type	Surface area (m²)	Oxygen transfer (dl/min/m²)	CO_2 transfer (dl/min/m²)
Human	Alveolus	Capillary	>120.0	44	31
CML-2	Polypropylene	Sheet	3.0	37	31
HF-4000	Polyethylene	HF-E	4.5	38	29
Maxima	Polypropylene	HF-E	2.0	63	48
Oxy-51	Polypropylene	HF-1	5.2	31	26
IVOX #7	Polyprop/silox	HF-E	0.21	247	229

CML-2 to Oxy-51 are all conventional CPB oxygenators. The hollow-fibre devices have blood either external or internal to the fibre lumen. Whilst the human lung has the largest capacity, this is by virtue of the huge surface area which can be recruited. The combination of hollow-fibre and siloxane membrane employed in IVOX makes it much more efficient, limited only by the surface area which can be deployed.

have the advantages of built-in alarms, pressure, flow and temperature displays, and battery back-up. The disposable pumping heads usually require changing at intervals of 3–5 days[20] (Fig. 6.3).

The Collin Cardio pump is a derivative of the roller pump that uses large-bore compliant elliptic tubing inserts which can be variably tensioned across three rollers. This gives a system which is sensitive to both preload and afterload and which uses the pump insert as a small reservoir.[21] The pump control is, as yet, not commercially available as a complete system and has primarily been used in association with the AREC technique (see later) for infants and children, but it could theoretically be expanded to adult use[22] (Fig. 6.4).

Circuits

Two major types of ECLS circuit are in use: venovenous (VV) and venoarterial (VA). There are advantages and disadvantages to both approaches (Table 6.3), but there is now a definite swing towards VV systems in both adults and children (other than for cardiac assist applications).

Table 6.3 Comparison between venovenous and venoarterial ECLS.

Venovenous	Venoarterial
Advantages	
Sparing the carotid	Cardiac support
Avoidance of oxygen toxicity	Rapid stabilization
Oxygenated Po perfusion	Extensive clinical experience
Oxygenated Cor perfusion	Excellent gas transfer
No systemic emboli	
Disadvantages	
No cardiac support	Carotid ligation
Partial recirculation	Non-pulsatile flow
Lower systemic Po_2	Reduced Po flow
Limited clinical experience	Potential for oxygen toxicity
Fluctuating pressures	Reduced myocardial oxygen

Po = pulmonary; Cor = coronary.

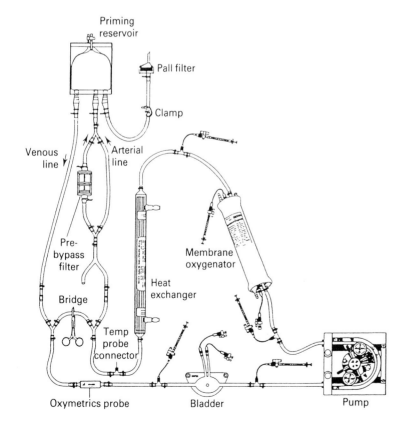

Fig. 6.2 A typical neonatal circuit employing a roller blood pump. Note that the use of this pump requires some device to control pump speed to venous return—the bladder box. The circuit is shown in its priming configuration. From Washington Childrens' Hospital, USA.

Venoarterial

VA bypass emerged as the dominant approach in early ECMO mainly because of its great effectiveness in terms of systemic oxygen delivery and the fact that the technique derived from conventional bypass. The main problem with this technique, from a respiratory standpoint, is the site of reinfusion of oxygenated blood. Femoro-femoral cannulation provides easy access to large vessels, but has the disadvantage of precluding perfusion of the thoracic aorta with well-oxygenated blood. The use of a femorally introduced long cannula extending to the aortic arch has been used, but high resistance limits the flow. Perfusion through the brachial, axillary, iliac or right common carotid artery overcomes the problem of distribution, but is also limited by size and a difficult

cutdown. Another solution is to use a mixed venous and arterial return, but this requires metering of the respective flows and a double cannulation.

The major advantage of VA bypass is the ability to provide cardiac as well as respiratory support. However, most investigators agree that the restoration of normal oxygenation is accompanied by rapid haemodynamic stabilization in those patients who do not have a primary cardiac problem. While high flows are achievable with VA bypass, there is evidence that extended reduction of pulmonary blood flow below about 25% of the total cardiac output is associated with pulmonary ischaemia, as blood is diverted away from areas of high pulmonary resistance, and leads to altered histology and eventual necrosis.[23]

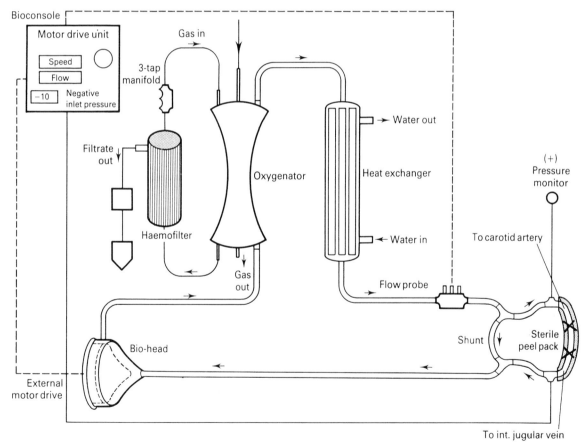

Fig. 6.3 A neonatal circuit employing a centrifugal pump. Because the pump is both preload and afterload sensitive, no reservoir is required. A flow transducer is, however, required. A haemofilter is placed in parallel to the oxygenator, as an optional extra. From Royal Childrens' Hospital, Victoria, Australia.

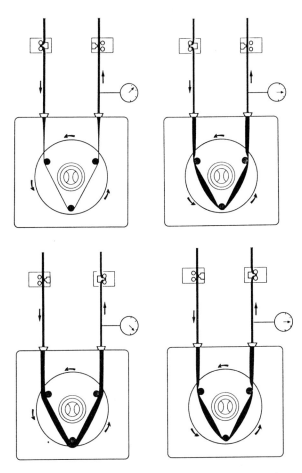

Fig. 6.4 The Collin Cardio pump operates through a four-stage cycle. At the *bottom right* the pump tube is filling, the inflow clamp is open and the outflow clamp is closed. The volume capacity depends on the tension set on the rollers. At the *bottom left* the pre-set pressure is about to be reached, at which point the outflow clamp opens and the inflow clamp is closed. *Top right* shows the eject phase taking place, and at the *top left* ejection is complete and the cycle restarts. Courtesy Professor Durandy, Paris.

Venovenous

There are a great many more variations possible with VV bypass. The negative findings from the National Institutes of Health (NIH) sponsored trial in 1974[24] prompted further laboratory investigations into CPB for respiratory support. Out of these efforts the concept of extracorporeal carbon dioxide removal was born. This recognizes that sufficient oxygen transfer can usually be accomplished by simple oxygen insufflation into the unventilated lung, whilst carbon dioxide can be removed by the extracorporeal circuit.[25] Using a flow of 25–30% of the total cardiac output, adequate CO_2 removal is possible (Fig. 6.5). A small subset of patients will require additional oxygen transfer from the extracorporeal circuit and therefore a higher flow.

Extracorporeal CO_2 removal has been implemented with a variety of cannulation schemes, including proximal and distal femoral and internal jugulars, double-lumen femoral and internal jugular and single- and double-lumen percutaneous options. One of the main problems associated with this technique is the avoidance of venous mixing and recirculation. With low-flow techniques this is only a minor problem, but with high-flow systems special cannulation options may be required to limit mixing. This could range from introducing the return catheter through the tricuspid valve, to using specially designed dual-lumen catheters.[26]

A variant of VV bypass, which makes use of a tidal flow, has been championed by Durand's group in Paris. This has become known as AREC after the French description of 'assistance respiratoire extracorporelle'.[22] The technique is currently limited to neonates and children and consists of a special double-lumen Teflon cannula with an eccentric septum creating a large lumen for drainage and a small blind-tipped lumen with side holes, directed towards the tricuspid valve, for reinfusion. A Collin Cardio pump is used with an occluding device borrowed from single-needle dialysis applications. Blood is alternately drained and reinfused with a cycle time of 6 seconds and a drainage to infusion time ratio of 2:1. The AREC flow is adjusted to about 30% of systemic blood flow. This system provides an extremely simple and safe solution to extracorporeal respiratory support and, with proper commercial development, would provide the basis for a totally automatic machine (Fig. 6.6). This technique can also be used with a conventional roller pump using inflow and outflow reservoirs with a synchronized occluding system.[26]

Choice of cannula

Blood flow out of the patient and the pressure required to reinfuse blood depend on the flow characteristics of the respective cannulae. Since ECLS techniques involve the use of a wide range of different cannula designs, simple use of cannula size and length is not particularly helpful when selecting an appropriate cannula. The Michigan group have developed the concept of impedance related to catheter performance in which the pressure–flow relationship can be characterized by an M number, derived from a nomogram (Fig. 6.7). Using this system, lower M numbers give higher flows for the same pressure differential.[27] The availability of thin-walled sophisticated cannulae which can be introduced percutaneously has had a major impact on the efficacy and safety of ECLS.

Safety

There is currently no specifically designed equipment produced for ECLS. This has given rise to a multitude of adaptations to meet the need, with many systems being unnecessarily complicated. In a 1990 survey of ECMO centres, Allison *et al.*[28] found that 28 manufacturers supplied 15 different types of devices for ECMO circuits. Current systems tend to require a large input of management by specially trained personnel and the techniques themselves produce multiple opportunities for misadventure. The Extracorporeal Life Support Organization (ELSO) reports a patient complication rate of one in every 81.7 hours of ECMO[29] and a mechanical complication rate of one in every 297.7 hours. Whilst the formation of ELSO in the USA and the European Extracorporeal Support Organization (EESO) has done much to promulgate safe operating practices, there is still a disturbingly high complication morbidity and mortality in what is otherwise one of the great success stories of modern medicine.

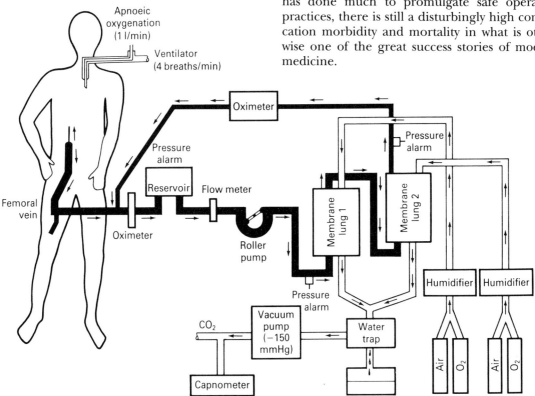

Fig. 6.5 The essential elements of the venovenous ECCO technique, popularized by Gattinoni, as used in Marberg. The extracorporeal circuit is used primarily to remove CO_2, which requires a membrane surface area of some 9 m^2 for an adult. The Scimed oxygenators are run under negative pressure and ventilated at a variable Fio_2. Cannulation is via a dual-lumen venous cannula in the IVC and an additional distal cannula. Oxygenation is via tracheal insufflation and a small amount of PEEP with a respiratory rate of 4 bpm. The EC flow is about 30% of systemic blood flow. Reprinted with permission from reference 33.

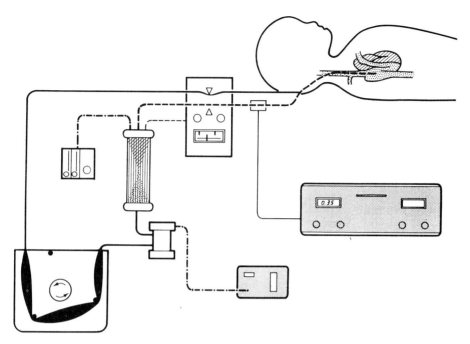

Fig. 6.6 The AREC technique employs tidal venovenous perfusion via a special dual-lumen catheter which aspirates blood from the caval junction and returns it in the direction of the tricuspid valve. The external occluders are borrowed from a dialysis machine together with the controller. The Collin Cardio pump provides both the pumping and the reservoir functions. Courtesy Professor Durandy, Paris.

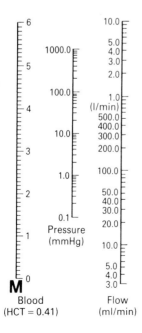

Fig. 6.7 This nomogram, developed by the Michigan group,[27] allows the pressure/flow characteristics of inflow and outflow cannula to be determined. The use of pure size and length is not a reliable method for determining these parameters because of the complex designs available for ECLS catheters. The **M** number can be regarded as a measure of hydraulic impedance, with a higher number depicting worse performance.

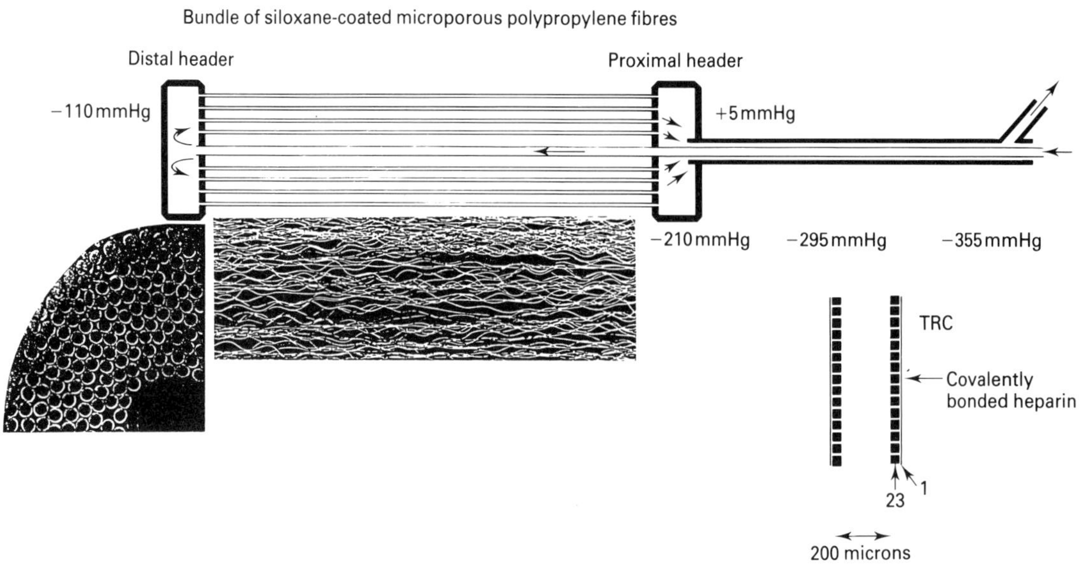

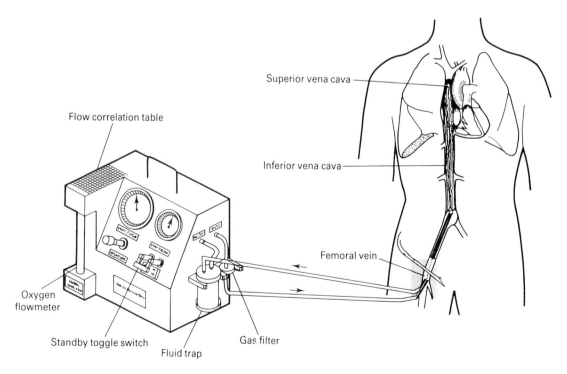

Bundle of siloxane-coated microporous polypropylene fibres

Distal header

Proximal header

−110 mmHg

+5 mmHg

−210 mmHg   −295 mmHg   −355 mmHg

TRC

Covalently
bonded heparin

23 1

200 microns

Fig. 6.8 The intravascular oxygenator is composed of a bundle of crimped polypropylene fibres covered with a very thin layer of siloxane, to which is bonded heparin as a thromboresistant coating (TRC). Pure oxygen is aspirated through the fibres, with a proximal pressure of about −350 mmHg, producing a distal header pressure of about −100 mmHg. This arrangement prevents the possibility of gas emboli.

Flow correlation table

Superior vena cava

Inferior vena cava

Femoral vein

Oxygen
flowmeter

Standby toggle switch

Fluid trap

Gas filter

Fig. 6.9 The IVOX in place in the cava, with connections to the gas controller. Four sizes are available to suit patients from about 30 kg to 90 kg bodyweight.

Intravascular oxygenation

It has been known for some time that the application of a thin layer of selective gas-permeable membrane over the supportive matrix of a hollow fibre provides for much enhanced gas transport.[13] Mortensen took this concept through to a design for a clinical implantable oxygenator[30] by constructing a bundle of crimped siloxane-coated hollow fibres designed to be placed in the vena cavae (Figs 6.8 and 6.9). Four sizes of IVOX® have been manufactured for clinical trials, providing 0.2–0.5 m² of surface area, without overt obstruction to the venous return. Oxygen is aspirated through the fibres at flows of up to 3.5 l/min. Whilst gas transfer across this system is up to six times greater than with conventional membranes, the actual total gas transfer is limited to about 130 ml/min, or roughly half the basal requirement, owing to limitations of size. The surface area could be increased by decreasing the fibre size, but there is a trade-off against resistance. Moreover, only a fraction of the total venous flow comes into contact with the entire membrane surface area.

Table 6.4 lists the comparative advantages and disadvantages of ECMO and IVOX®. It should be noted that the characteristics described are not fixed, in that ECMO is evolving rapidly now that fairly widespread clinical use is taking place. The advent of better cannulae and heparin-bonded circuits is also reducing the complication rate. However, IVOX is the first clinical version of a family of devices, and only a limited clinical experience has been gained to date.

There appears to be considerable scope to improve this approach and two further experimental designs have already emerged. One uses a modified pulmonary catheter with a 'bottle brush' array of fibres,[31] and another uses a balloon to induce secondary flow characteristics around the fibres.[32]

One of the major worries with the introduction of a large foreign surface area into the vascular system, in a group of patients who are critically ill and in whom a significant proportion have existing systemic infection, is one of overwhelming infection. However, this has not been a significant problem.

Conclusions

The last few years have seen considerable improvements in the sophistication of ventilators and the adoption of techniques to minimize volutrauma of the lung. The main developments in extracorporeal systems involve the availability of improved membrane oxygenators and the increasing availability of surface modified circuits. The Collin Cardio pump and associated controls opens up the possibility of a totally automated system, without overt complexity. The range of cannulae now available makes percutaneous placement a reality and minimizes the invasiveness of the procedure. However, a purpose-built machine and associated disposables is still not available on the market.

The intravascular approach has considerable promise in providing a simple and safe solution to temporary respiratory support and may even provide an alternative to mechanical ventilation in a range of clinical settings. Further development of this technology may also lead the way to the provision of devices for assisting patients with chronic respiratory disorders, and ultimately to the development of an implantable total artificial lung.

Table 6.4 Comparative advantages and disadvantages of ECMO and IVOX.

ECMO	IVOX
Advantages	*Advantages*
Capable of total respiratory support	Relatively simple (only minimal training)
Capable of cardiac support in V–A mode	Small surface area (no priming volume)
Flexible gas exchange characteristics	Safe (very low complication rate)
Equipment easily visualized	Low resource use
Disadvantages	*Disadvantages*
Relatively complex (trained staff needed)	Limited to approximately 30% respiratory support
Large surface area (priming volume)	Oxygenator difficult to visualize
Components require frequent change	No cardiac support capability
Complication rate relatively high	Gas exchange characteristics relatively fixed
Expensive (high resource use)	

References

1. Oh TE. Defining adult respiratory distress syndrome. *Br J Hosp Med* 1992; **47**, 350–353.
2. Wung JT, James LS. Optimizing conventional respiratory support. In: Arensman RM, Cornish JD (eds), *Extracorporeal Life Support*. Oxford: Blackwell Scientific, 1993: 51–67.
3. Keogh BF, Sim KM. High frequency ventilation in adult respiratory failure. *Br J Intens Care* 1993; **3**, 263–268.
4. Gattinoni L, Pesenti A, Bombini M, *et al*. Relationships between lung computed tomographic density, gas exchange and PEEP in acute respiratory failure. *Anesthesiology* 1988; **69**, 824.
5. Hickling KG, Henderson SJ, Jackson R. Low mortality with low-volume pressure-limited ventilation with permissive hypercapnia in severe adult respiratory distress syndrome. *Intens Care Med* 1990; **16**, 372–377.
6. Long W, Thompson T, Sundell H, *et al*. Effects of two rescue doses of a synthetic surfactant on mortality rate and survival without broncho-pulmonary dysplasia in 700- to 1350-gram infants with respiratory distress syndrome. *J Pediat* 1991; **118**, 595–605.
7. Greenspan JS, Wolfson MR, Rubenstein SD, Shaffer TH. Liquid ventilation of human preterm neonates. *J Pediat* 1990; **117**, 106–111.
8. Hill D, O'Brien TG, Murray JJ. Extracorporeal oxygenation for acute post-traumatic respiratory failure: use of the Bramson Membrane Lung. *New Engl J Med* 1972; **286**, 629–634.
9. Bramsom ML, Osborn JJ, Main FB, *et al*. A new disposable membrane oxygenator with integral heat exchange. *J Thorac Cardiovasc Surg* 1965; **50**, 391.
10. Kolobow T, Bowman RL. Construction and evaluation of an alveolar membrane artificial heart lung. *ASAIO Trans* 1963; **9**, 238.
11. Montoya JP, Shanley CJ, Scott I, Merz I, Bartlett RH. Plasma leakage through microporous membranes: role of phospholipids. *ASAIO J* 1992; **38**, M399–405.
12. Larm O, Larsson R, Olsson P. A new nonthrombogenic surface prepared by selective covalent binding of heparin via a modified reducing terminal residue. *Biomater Med Dev Artif Organs* 1983; **11**, 161–173.
13. Tsai CC, Huo HH, Kulkarni PV, Eberhart RC. Biocompatible coatings with high albumin affinity. *ASAIO Trans* 1990; **36**, M307–320.
14. Galletti PM, Richardson PD, Snider MT, Friedman J. A standardised method for defining the overall gas transfer performance of artificial lungs. *ASAIO Trans* 1972; **18**, 359–368.
15. Clayton RH, Pearson DT, Murray A. Assessment of oxygen transfer in membrane oxygenators during clinical cardiopulmonary bypass. *Clin Phys Physiol Meas* 1992; **13**, 167–177.
16. Awad JA, Deslauriers DM, Guojin L, Martin L. Prolonged pumpless arteriovenous perfusion for carbon dioxide extraction. *Ann Thorac Surg* 1991; **51**, 534–540.
17. Takinami M, Ishigami N, Suzuki K, Haraday. Experimental evaluation of pumpless ECMO by left pulmonary artery – left atrium bypass: comparative studies on Sarns 16310 and Masterflo 50 membrane oxygenator. *Japan J Artif Org* 1990; **19**, 600–603.
18. Gille JP, Sautegeau A, Schryem F, Munsch L, Tousseul B. Haemodialysis for extracorporeal CO_2 removal. *J Eur Soc Artif Org* 1986; **4** (suppl 2), 294–297.
19. Toomasian JM, Chapman RA, McCall M. Servoregulation for long term perfusion. *Proc Am Acad Cardiovasc Perf* 1988; **9**, 114–117.
20. Horton SB, Horton AM, Mullaly RJ, Butt WW, Mee RBB. Extracorporeal membrane oxygenation life support: a new approach. *Perfusion* 1993; **8**, 239–247.
21. Kezler M, Kolobow T. Venovenous ECMO. In: Arensman RM, Cornish JD (eds), *Extracorporeal Life Support*. Oxford: Blackwell Scientific, 1993: 51–67.
22. Durandy Y, Chevalier JY, Lecompte Y. Single cannula venovenous bypass for respiratory membrane lung support. *J Thorac Cardiovasc Surg* 1990; **99**, 404–409.
23. Koul B, Wollmer P, Willen H, Kugelberg J, Steen S. Venoarterial extracorporeal membrane oxygenation—How safe is it? *J Thorac Cardiovasc Surg* 1992; **104**, 579–584.
24. Extracorporeal support for respiratory insufficiency: a collaborative study in response to RFP-NHLI-73-20. US Dept Health Education and Welfare, National Institutes of Health, Bethesda, MD, 1979.
25. Kolobow T, Gattinoni L, Tomlinson T, White D, Pierce J, Iapichino G. The carbon dioxide membrane lung (CDML): a new concept. *ASAIO Trans* 1977; **23**, 17–21.
26. Kolobow T, Borelli M, Spatola R, *et al*. Single catheter venovenous membrane lung bypass in the treatment of experimental ARDS. *ASAIO Trans* 1988; **34**, 35–38.
27. Delius RE, Montoya P, Merz SI, McKenzie J, Snedecor S, Bove EL, Bartlett RH. New method for describing the performance of cardiac surgery cannulas. *Ann Thorac Surg* 1992; **53**, 278–281.
28. Allison PL, Kurusz M, Graves DF, Zwischenberger JB. Devices and monitoring during neonatal ECMO: survey results. *Perfusion* 1990; **90**, 193–201.
29. Extracorporeal Life Support Organisation (ELSO) Registry, Ann Arbor Michigan, 1992.
30. Mortensen JD. An intravenacaval blood gas exchange (IVCBGE) device: preliminary report.

ASAIO Trans 1987; **33**, 570–573.

31. Snider MT, High KM, Ultman JS, Panol GRJ, Richard RB, Stene JK, Russell GB, Campbell DB, Al-Mondhiry HAB, Keifer JC. Initial development of a miniaturized intrapulmonary arterial artificial lung. Abstracts of ASAIO 38th Annual Meeting, 1992 (abstract M65).

32. Hatler BG, Johnson PC, Sawzik PJ, Shaffer FD, Klain M, Lund LW, *et al*. Respiratory dialysis: a new concept in pulmonary support. *ASAIO J* 1992; **38**, M322–325.

33. Muller E. In: Arensman RM, Cornish JD (eds), *Extracorporeal Life Support*. Oxford: Blackwell Scientific, 1993.

7

The IVOX® intravascular gas-exchange device: current status*

P Stuart Withington and Timothy R Graham

Introduction

Adult respiratory distress syndrome (ARDS) remains a common problem in most intensive care units, the annual incidence varying between 1.5 and 75 per 100 000 population. The wide variation in incidence is due in part to the lack of any internationally agreed diagnostic criteria, and this in turn causes problems when trying to study the disease. The syndrome was originally introduced by Ashbaugh et al.[1] in 1971 to describe patients with severe dyspnoea, tachypnoea, refractory cyanosis and diffuse alveolar infiltration on the chest X-ray. Post mortem studies on patients dying with ARDS revealed pulmonary oedema, atelectasis, vascular congestion and alveolar hyaline membranes. Since the syndrome was first described the mortality rate has remained essentially unchanged in the range 50–75% when uncomplicated[2] and up to 90% when part complicated by sepsis. ARDS is a clinical condition: the term gives no indication of the diverse nature of the disease or of the varied underlying pathologies. The 'trigger mechanism' for ARDS can be due to a direct or an indirect pulmonary insult.[3] Direct disorders include those caused by aspiration; inhalation; drugs; lung contusions; diffuse pneumonia and embolic phenomena. It is also recognized that ARDS can be caused indirectly and form part of a much wider syndrome of multiorgan dysfunction (MODS), a common pathway for which is thought to be a systemic inflammatory response syndrome[4] (SIRS) caused by release of various cytokines that activate macrophages. The causes of SIRS include shock from any cause; infection; major trauma; and haematological, metabolic and drug-induced disorders.

In patients with severe pulmonary dysfunction, endotracheal intubation and mechanical positive pressure ventilation remains the most common method for trying to maintain adequate gas exchange. However, there is an increasing body of evidence to demonstrate that mechanical ventilation in patients with ARDS can cause further lung injury. The main mechanisms for this damage appear to be oxygen toxicity from high inspired levels, barotrauma from high airway pressures,[5] and volotrauma[6] due to overdistention and tearing of the residual lung tissue. As a result of a better understanding of the deleterious effects of mechanical ventilation, a variety of new ventilatory techniques have appeared. These include: low-tidal-volume intermittent mandatory ventilation; pressure controlled ventilation; reverse I:E (inspiratory:expiratory time) ratio ventilation; pressure release ventilation; and high-frequency jet ventilation. New ideas to help reduce the degree of mechanical ventilation and oxygen toxicity include permissive hypercapnoea[7] and permissive hypoxaemia, the limits for which have still to be determined. Newer pharmacological therapies include those directed at the mediators

*Since preparing this chapter, the IVOX device has been withdrawn following the merger of CardioPulmonics.

of inflammation such as monoclonal antibodies targeted against endotoxin, interleukin-1, tumour necrosis factor,[8] and those to help improve pulmonary function such as artificial surfactant.[9]

An artificial gas exchange surface

A different strategy to help reduce the damaging effects of mechanical ventilation is to take over part or all of the lung gas exchange function using an artificial gas exchange surface. The equipment to perform this type of therapy usually consists of a membrane oxygenator placed in a pumped extracorporeal circulation. There have been many reports on the use of extracorporeal gas exchange for pulmonary support. Early trials in the late 1970s[10] failed to show any improvement in survival when compared with conventional methods of therapy. A more recent study by Morris[11] reached a similar conclusion. However, many European centres performing extracorporeal gas exchange are reporting more encouraging figures.[12] Despite the fact that extracorporeal gas exchange is of unproved benefit in ARDS, many centres continue to use and develop the technology. The techniques involved are complicated, of relatively high risk and expensive in terms of equipment and personnel.

Recently introduced is the IVOX® device (CardioPulmonics Inc., Salt Lake City, Utah). This is an intravenous membrane oxygenator which is currently undergoing multicentre clinical trials under an investigational device exemption certificate issued by the US Food and Drug Administration. This equipment has been developed by Mortensen[13] to augment the gas exchange provided by conventional mechanical ventilation.

The device (Fig. 7.1) consists of multiple microporous hollow polypropylene fibres in an elongated arrangement placed in the vena cava for prepulmonary gas exchange. The surface of each fibre is coated with a layer of a siloxane that is less than 1 μm thick; this forms the blood–gas interface. All blood-contacting surfaces of the device are covered with a thromboresistant coating of covalently bonded heparin. Owing to the coaxial construction, insertion is via a single surgical venotomy in either the femoral or jugular veins on the right side of the body (see Fig. 6.9 in Chapter 6).

The device is available in four sizes: 7, 8, 9 and 10 mm transverse diameter. The largest that will fit into the venous system is chosen, to maximize the area available for gas exchange and minimize the amount of blood streaming around the device

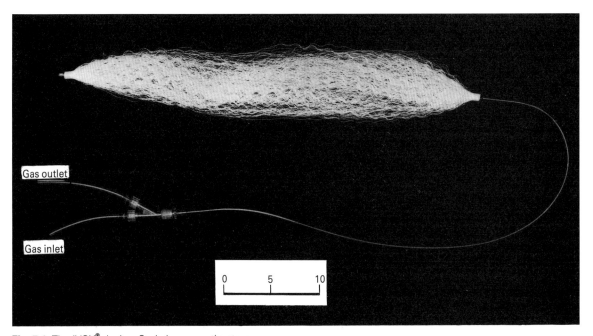

Gas outlet

Gas inlet

0   5   10

Fig. 7.1 The IVOX® device. Scale bar = centimetres.

and therefore not exposed to the exchange surface. To further minimize blood streaming, the individual fibres are crimped to encourage turbulent flow and hence mixing of blood around the device.

Once the appropriate size of device has been selected an introducer is placed in the chosen vein. The device is tested for leaks within the fibres and de-aired in a fluid-filled tube prior to insertion. Placement of the device via the introducer is guided by X-ray screening to ensure the device lies well within the caval system. Problems observed at the time of insertion have been blood loss, arrhythmias and cardiovascular instability. During insertion the patients are heparinized to an activated clotting time (ACT) of 600 s, and thereafter the ACT can be maintained at 180–200 s. A controlled vacuum of about 300 mmHg draws oxygen through the device at 1–3 l/min. Sub-atmospheric pressure is used to avoid the problem of gas emboli should any of the hollow fibres break. Gas exchange occurs by diffusion across the membrane driven by the partial pressure gradients of O_2 and CO_2. The total volume exchanged also depends on the permeability of the membrane and the surface area available for exchange. The surface area of the device varies between 0.21 and 0.5 m^2 depending on the size selected. Maximum estimated gas transfer for oxygen and carbon dioxide is 140–260 ml/m^2/min. The maximum oxygen delivery for the largest device is therefore approximately 130 ml/min, which represents about half of an adult's basal oxygen requirements.

Early animal experiments demonstrated the device to be safe and to provide potentially clinically useful gas exchange. This led to a phase I clinical trial in 1990. Several individual centres have now started to publish their own early results.

Phase I study

The entry criteria for the phase I study (Table 7.1) resembled those previously used for the collaborative ECMO study by Zapol *et al.*[10] Patients meeting these criteria have a predicted mortality of 60–90% with conventional therapy.[14]

Jurmann *et al.*[15] reported one survivor out of three patients. Gas transfer (CO_2) for the three devices varied from a minimum of 64 ml/m^2/min to a maximum of 179 ml/m^2/min, this being well

Table 7.1 Entry criteria for the phase I study.

Endotracheal intubation with mechanical ventilation for >24 h
Arterial Po_2 less than 8 kPa
Fio_2 greater than 0.5
PEEP greater than 10 cmH$_2$O

PEEP = positive end-expiratory pressure.

below the maximum capacity for the device (reasons for this are discussed later). High *et al.*[16] reported one survivor out of five patients, gas transfer varying between 66 and 256 ml/m^2/min.

The full results of the phase I study have been published by Zwischenberger and Cox.[17] Thirty-four patients completed the study, the overall mortality being 73.5%. From the summary data, 26% of patients had reversal of their lung dysfunction and survived, 58% showed some improvement in gas exchange though died from other causes, and 16% received no benefit and died in respiratory failure.

Phase II study

From the phase I study it was apparent that the device used could contribute to overall gas exchange and did not lead to any directly related major complications. Subsequent on these findings a phase II multicentre trial commenced in 1991, the entry criteria being as listed in Table 7.2 (the conditions to be fulfilled on three occasions at least one hour apart).

As well as conducting an implantation study, all centres also carried out a prospective survey of acute respiratory failure (ARF) within their own institutions. Entry criteria for the prospective survey are that the patients must be receiving IPPV with an $Fio_2 > 0.5$ for at least 24 hours. Fio_2

Table 7.2 Entry criteria for the phase II study.

Ventilation:	Patients receiving IPPV
	Minute volume >150 ml/kg
	PEEP >10 cmH$_2$O
	or MAP >30 cmH$_2$O
	or PIP >45 cmH$_2$O
Gas exchange:	Fio_2 >0.5
	and $Paco_2$ >5.3 kPa
	and Pao_2 <8.0 kPa

IPPV = intermittent positive-pressure ventilation; MAP = mean airway pressure; PIP = peak inspiratory pressure.

administration is regulated to maintain an adequate arterial oxygen saturation (>90%).

Twenty-four clinical centres are participating in the phase II implantation study and the prospective survey, eight in the USA and 14 in Europe. In the prospective survey, figures from the Royal London Hospital demonstrate that over an 18-month period (1 April 1991 to 30 September 1992) a total of 108 patients fulfilled the entry criteria (6.5% of admissions). The ARF patients had an ITU mortality of 47.2% and a hospital mortality of 56.5%. Preliminary results from the whole group have been collated and presented by Vasilyev *et al.*[18] A total of 1426 patients have so far been entered with a hospital mortality rate of 44.4%. If the patients were hypoxaemic ($Pao_2 < 8.0$ kPa with $Fio_2 > 0.5$) or hypercabic ($Paco_2 > 5.3$ kPa) at the time of entry into the survey, then mortality increased to 66.7%. This survey indicates the serious nature of ARF and the fact that, despite recent advances in intensive care management, the condition still carries a high mortality rate. However, even though the entry criteria for the survey rely on parameters of ARF, figures from the Royal London Hospital demonstrate that the mode of death is only occasionally attributed to failure of gas exchange; the most common cause of death being multiorgan failure related to sepsis syndrome. Again this illustrates the systemic nature of the disease state and it has yet to be demonstrated that by augmenting gas exchange the overall outcome can be improved.

By 1991 the device had been used in 64 patients with a 38% survival rate (data from CardioPulmonics). This survival rate does not appear to differ significantly from rates quoted for conventional therapy. At the Royal London Hospital we have implanted five devices into four patients fulfilling the agreed entrance criteria and have had no survivors, the gas transfer achieved being similar to that reported by Jurmann and co-workers.

To date approximately 150 devices have been implanted clinically. Preliminary analysis of the multicentre data has been performed using patients from the prospective survey as comparisons matched with those patients receiving the IVOX device therapy. As a measure of the efficacy of therapy, ventilator settings have been examined at 20 hours after implantation, particular emphasis being placed on the Fio_2, minute ventilation and amount of PEEP. Early results indicate that patients with intrapulmonic aetiologies to their underlying disease (pneumonia, pneumonitis, etc.) have a significantly greater reduction in the above mentioned ventilator settings compared with the matched comparison patients. This improvement is less marked when the underlying disease state is of a systemic or catastrophic nature. It must, however, be stressed that these findings are preliminary and a full analysis has not yet been performed.

Complications of IVOX

Haemodynamic instability, usually at the time of insertion of the device, has been reported. The most common cause for this was blood loss during insertion occurring in an already compromised patient. It would appear that there is a learning curve for the insertion procedure, because in those centres performing many implantations the blood loss and degree of haemodynamic instability was much reduced. Other causes of haemodynamic instability might be related to some degree of venous obstruction within the caval system or liberation of vasoactive substances from the vessel walls.

Thrombogenic occurrences have been noticed, the majority being thrombi found attached to the device at the time of removal. Two embolic events have been reported where an association with the device could not be ruled out.

Anticoagulation problems occurred in a few patients, being mainly bleeding from the insertion site or other areas of injury. In a few cases the bleeding was so severe that the device had to be removed in order to stop heparin therapy.

Mechanical complications have been reported with the device. These complications included malfunction of the device, broken fibres such that blood appeared in the gas conduit, and failure to unfurl during implantation. Another 'complication' has been the failure to achieve maximum expected gas transfer. Many users have reported gas exchange (mainly for CO_2 as this is easier to measure) that has fallen well below expectations. This may be due to a variety of physical factors including failure to unfurl, malpositioning of the device, and thrombus or coagulum forming on the device. Physiological factors such as cardiac output and mixed venous gas tensions may also contribute to a lower than expected gas transfer.

Other complications reported included possible device-related infection, venous damage such as vessel laceration or erosion, and vascular obstruction with swelling of the lower limb.

Discussion

It would appear, taking acute respiratory failure patients as a whole, that IVOX therapy does not greatly influence outcome despite proven gas exchange capabilities. However, as mentioned previously, ARDS is not a single homogeneous disease but a manifestation of a variety of insults, some localized to the lung and others part of a more generalized systemic upset.

An explanation for these findings may lie with the pattern of disease leading to pulmonary failure. Many authors[19] have reported an increased oxygen demand during sepsis, which may be due to a variety of factors such as peripheral A–V shunting, histotoxic injury uncoupling oxidative phosphorylation, impairment of ATP regeneration, peripheral oedema or simply an increased oxygen requirement of inflammatory cells. Whatever the mechanism there would appear to be a supply-dependent oxygen utilization in patients with sepsis and MODS. Shoemaker *et al.*[20] have demonstrated that critically ill surgical patients are more likely to survive if they have a cardiac index of over $4.5 \, l/min/m^{-2}$, an oxygen delivery (D_{O_2}) of $>600 \, ml/m^{-2}/min$ and an oxygen consumption (V_{O_2}) of $>170 \, ml/m^{-2}/min$. Furthermore, when these figures are actually achieved by therapeutic manoeuvres, the mortality rate could be reduced from approximately 29% to 4%. For the average 70 kg adult this equates to a D_{O_2} of over $1000 \, ml/min$. Other workers[21] have found that even higher levels of D_{O_2} can further improve outcome. Also of note is the finding of a supply-dependent V_{O_2}.

Weg[22] has reviewed the literature on the subject. Normal individuals have a physiological dependence on V_{O_2} at very low levels of D_{O_2} ($300 \, ml/min$), but at delivery rates above this consumption is independent of delivery. In critically ill patients with ARDS or sepsis this pattern is no longer seen; V_{O_2} varies directly with D_{O_2} over a wide range and tissue oxygen extraction is compromised. Given the high rates of delivery apparently needed during sepsis and ARDS, it is hardly surprising that the addition of an extra 5–10% by the IVOX device appears to make

relatively little difference to overall mortality.

Another phenomenon associated with the sepsis syndrome is the reduction in the oxygen extraction ratio. The patient therefore suffers not only from supply-dependent oxygen utilization, but also from the reduced ability to extract the supplied oxygen from the arterial blood. This reduction in oxygen utilization is manifest by an abnormally high mixed venous oxygen tension, and as the device is situated in the venous system any increase in venous oxygen tension will decrease the diffusion gradient for oxygen and so reduce the amount of gas exchange.

In patients with respiratory failure that is not accompanied by SIRS and its deleterious effects on V_{O_2} (that is in patients without an increased D_{O_2}) the picture may be quite different. The amount of O_2 and CO_2 exchanged by the device might represent a significant contribution to whole-body requirements and enable a useful reduction in the intensity of mechanical ventilation. The changes in gas exchange needed across the spectrum of disease states causing ARF or ARDS may in part explain some of the findings regarding patients with pulmonic or systemic aetiologies. The device has been used to good effect in at least two patients with acute severe asthma who could not be maintained with conventional therapy. Presumably these patients had isolated ARF without systemic problems.

A full analysis of the data collected so far will be needed to determine which patients and which types of ARF may benefit from therapy with the IVOX device. In order to establish a clinical role, a randomized trial comparing current recognized critical care practice with and without the device will be needed. This may be extremely difficult given the rapidly changing therapeutic alternatives for the treatment of ARF and its related conditions. Further progress in the design and manufacture of the device promise decreased complications, a more 'user friendly' system and increased gas transfer capabilities which in theory should offer benefits to a wider range of patients.

References

1. Asbaugh DG, Bigelow DB, Petty TL, Levine BE. Acute respiratory distress in adults. *Lancet* 1967; **ii**, 319–323.
2. Petty TL. Indicators of risk, course and prognosis

in adult respiratory distress syndrome (ARDS). *Am Rev Respir Dis* 1985; **132**, 471.

3. Oh TE. Defining adult respiratory distress syndrome. *Br J Hosp Med* 1992; **47**, 350–353.

4. Bone RC, *et al.* American College of Chest Physicians/Society of Critical Care Medicine consensus conference: Definitions for sepsis and organ failure and guidelines for the use of innovative therapies in sepsis. *Crit Care Med* 1992; **20**, 864–890.

5. Kolobow T, Moretti MP, Fumagalli R, Mascheroni D, Prato P, Chen V, Joris M. Severe impairment in lung function induced by high peak airway pressure during mechanical ventilation: an experimental study. *Am Rev Respir Dis* 1987; **135**, 312–315.

6. Dreyfuss D, Soler P, Basset G, Saumon G. High inflation pressure pulmonary edema: respective effects of high airway pressure, high tidal volume and positive end-expiratory pressure. *Am Rev Respir Dis* 1988; **137**, 1159–1164.

7. Hickling KG, Henderson SJ, Jackson R. Low mortality associated with low-volume pressure-limited ventilation with permissive hypercapnia in severe adult respiratory distress syndrome. *Intens Care Med* 1990; **16**, 372–377.

8. Exley AR, Cohen J, Buurman W. Monoclonal antibody to TNF in severe septic shock. *Lancet* 1990; **335**, 1275–1277.

9. Robertson B. Surfactant replacement in neonatal and adult respiratory distress syndrome. *Eur J Anaesth* 1984; **1**, 335–343.

10. Zapol WM, Snider MT, Hill JD, Fallat RJ, Bartlett RH, Edmunds LH, Morris AH, Pierce EC, Thomas AN, Proctor HJ, Drinker PA, Pratt PG, Bagniewski A, Miller RG. Extracorporeal membrane oxygenation in severe acute respiratory failure. *JAMA* 1979; **242**, 2193–2196.

11. Morris AH. Protocols, ECCO₂R and the evaluation of ARDS therapy. *Japan J Intens Care Med* 1992; **16**, 61–63.

12. Firmin RK. Extracorporeal membrane oxygenation in the 90s: a personal view. *Perfusion* 1990; **5**, 161–166.

13. Mortensen JD, Berry G. Conceptual and design features of a practical, clinically effective intravenous mechanical blood oxygen/carbon dioxide exchange device (IVOX). *Int J Artif Org* 1989; **12**, 384–389.

14. Montgomery AB, Stager MA, Carrico CJ, *et al.* Causes of mortality in patients with the adult respiratory distress syndrome. *Am Rev Respir Dis* 1985; **132**, 485–489.

15. Jurmann MJ, Demertzis S, Schaefers H, Wahlers T, Haverich A. Intravascular oxygenation for advanced respiratory failure. *ASAIO Trans* 1991; **38**, 120–124.

16. High KM, Snider MT, Richard R, Russell GB, Stene JK, Campbell DB, Aufiero TX, Thieme GA. Clinical trials of an intravenous oxygenator in patients with adult respiratory distress syndrome. *Anaesthesiology* 1992; **77**, 856–863.

17. Zwischenberger JB, Cox CS. A new intravascular membrane oxygenator to augment blood gas transfer in patients with acute respiratory failure. *Texas Med* 1991; **87**, 60–63.

18. Vasilyev S, Schaap RNS, Mortensen JD. Survival rates of patients with acute respiratory failure in 1991–1992 utilising mechanical ventilator augmentation of blood gas transfer: a multicentre prospective survey. Second European Congress on Extracorporeal Lung Support, Marburg, September 1992 (abstract L30).

19. Tuchschmidt J, Oblitas D, Fried JC. Oxygen consumption in sepsis and septic shock. *Crit Care Med* 1991; **19**, 664–671.

20. Shoemaker WC, Montgomery ES, Kaplan E. Physiological patterns in surviving and non-surviving shock patients. *Arch Surg* 1973; **106**, 630.

21. Hankeln KB, Senker R, Shwarten JU. Evaluation of prognostic indices based on haemodynamic and oxygen transport variables in shock patients with adult respiratory distress syndrome. *Crit Care Med* 1987; **15**, 1.

22. Weg JG. Oxygen transport in adults with respiratory distress syndrome and other acute circulatory problems: relationship of oxygen delivery and oxygen consumption. *Crit Care Med* 1991; **19**, 650–657.

8

Extracorporeal membrane oxygenation for neonates and older children

RK Firmin, J Waggoner and GA Pearson

Introduction

Extracorporeal membrane oxygenation (ECMO)[1,2] is a technique for providing life support for days or weeks using an adaptation of conventional cardiopulmonary bypass technology. The first heart–lung machine developed by Gibbon[3] in 1951 was suitable only for short periods of support sufficient to perform simple intracardiac surgical procedures. Prolonged life support was not possible until improvements in oxygenator technology had been achieved. Prolonged life support using a bubble oxygenator was attempted in 1965 by Rashkind et al.[4] Low blood flow circuits with a high gas sweep rate using rotating disc oxygenators were successfully introduced for CO_2 removal in 1966.[5] However, excessive blood trauma was a feature of bubble and disc oxygenators and prolonged support was not viable clinically. The membrane oxygenators developed by Bramson, Kolobow, Lande and others[6,7] overcame this problem by separating the gas and blood phases with a silicone membrane which is freely permeable to the respiratory gases but prevents direct contact between gas and blood. A high membrane surface area is achieved by using a spirally wound silastic membrane (Kolobow).

ECMO was first applied to adult patients with severe respiratory failure in the 1970s, with the first successful case being reported by Hill et al. in 1972.[8] Despite the initial enthusiasm for the technique, a multicentre trial conducted by the National Institute of Health (NIH) in the USA did not indicate significant benefit in this group of patients,[9] and adult ECMO was largely abandoned. The exception was Gattinoni, working in Italy, who developed a low-flow venovenous perfusion technique he called $ECCO_2R$ (extracorporeal CO_2 removal).[10]

In parallel with the evaluation in adults, ECMO was applied to neonates by Bartlett and his colleagues with more success.[11–14] As a result of remarkable improvements in survival compared with historical controls, and two modified-design randomized trials, both of which showed benefit,[15,16] neonatal ECMO became accepted as a standard treatment for mature neonates with refractory respiratory failure in the 1980s, at least in the USA. However, the adaptive designs of these trials has meant that their results have not been universally accepted[17] and debate continues.[18] Nevertheless, with the increasing clinical experience of ECMO in neonates and the greater understanding of how to manage and apply it, the role of ECMO in older children and adults is currently being re-evaluated.[19–22] The results in these groups are now far better than in those reported in the earlier NIH study. Although the number of older patients undergoing ECMO is much lower than for neonates, it is already clear that there is a clinical role for the technique outside the neonatal period in selected patients.[20] Just as there is renewed interest in ECMO in older patients, there is also interest in applying it to preterm infants.[23,24]

ECMO is, therefore, an effective life support technique for selected neonates and older children. With modern circuits and circuit management protocols it has become increasingly safe. In the modern era no infant with cardiopulmonary failure or child with isolated pulmonary failure should be allowed to die without the use of ECMO support being carefully considered.

Indications for ECMO

Theoretically, ECMO can be offered to any patient with potentially reversible pulmonary, cardiac or cardiopulmonary failure. In practice one has to define groups of patients who are sick enough to justify extracorporeal life support, whilst excluding those whose outcome is inevitably hopeless. The selection criteria for neonatal ECMO have been reasonably defined both in terms of the conditions for which it is appropriate and the point of disease severity at which to intervene[1] (see below). Such clear guidelines are not available for those trying to select older patients. However, in general terms, the principles for selecting a potential ECMO candidate of any age are the same:

1. Does the patient have a potentially reversible pulmonary, cardiac or cardiopulmonary problem?
2. Are the neurological status and the function of other organs consistent with a reasonable outcome?
3. Is even limited heparinization contraindicated?
4. Is there anything to be gained by further pursuit of conventional treatment?

Selection for neonatal ECMO

The indications for neonatal ECMO have become relatively standardized. Again the selection criteria are designed to define infants sick enough to warrant invasive life support, without expecting unacceptable morbidity. In practice, ECMO is therefore reserved for those patients in whom there remains a possibility of satisfactory outcome despite a failure to respond to maximal conventional techniques.

Firstly, the exclusion of patients with irreversible disease precludes the treatment of patients with severe chromosomal abnormalities or other congenital malformations that are incompatible with a reasonable quality of life (e.g. hypoplastic left heart). Similarly, babies who have suffered a severe hypoxic injury and who have associated hypoxic–ischaemic encephalopathy or established brain damage are excluded. The clinical evaluation must include cranial ultrasound looking specifically for lesions involving the brain parenchyma, which may be associated with a poor neurological outcome. Additionally cranial ultrasound is required to detect haemorrhage in the lateral ventricles extending beyond the subependymal or choroidal regions. Significant intraventricular haemorrhage (by this definition) may extend catastrophically after even limited heparinization.

A history of prolonged high-pressure mechanical ventilation (with high fractional inspired oxygen concentrations) is likely to be associated with bronchopulmonary dysplasia. This will eventually reach a level that delays lung recovery beyond the realistic time limits of ECMO perfusion (although these are not well defined). In clinical terms this means that patients mechanically ventilated at high pressures for more than 10 days are excluded on the expectation of irreversible pulmonary disease.

Infants are required to be of sufficient size to allow cervical cannulation—the vascular access of choice. Vascular access becomes progressively more difficult below a birthweight of 2 kg. However, smaller infants have been treated successfully by experienced teams. A predisposition towards intraventricular haemorrhage (significantly aggravated by the systemic heparinization necessary for ECMO circuits) in preterm infants, means that only mature infants (>34 weeks) are generally considered.[25] Recently ECMO has been applied successfully using even lower levels of heparinization than in standard practice. This is one reason why, in some American institutions, there has been a successful return of interest in the treatment of more preterm infants.[23,24]

Patients with severe coagulopathy prior to ECMO are avoided, although it is a matter of clinical judgement what 'cut off' levels are employed. Our own practice has been to pay less attention to the pre-ECMO platelet count (as this will be supplemented by regular transfusion) and to accept patients even with profound thrombocytopenia. We tolerate mild disseminated intravascular coagulation but are cautious when patients have a persistent elevation of the INR to a value of >2.5 which is not correctable by the administration of vitamin K, or the infusion of fresh frozen plasma and of cryoprecipitate.

These criteria define a group of mature infants who are a relatively small sub-population of neonatal intensive care (NICU) patients (approximately 5 per 1000 NICU admissions).[26] The most common causes of severe cardiopulmonary failure in this group are meconium aspiration syndrome, congenital diaphragmatic hernia, sepsis (including pneumonia) and respiratory distress syndrome.

All these conditions may be complicated by a high pulmonary vascular resistance.[27] This is recognized as a persistent fetal circulation (PFC), more correctly described as persistent pulmonary hypertension of the newborn (PPHN). When perinatal/neonatal illness or hypoxia is superimposed upon the transitional circulation, the pulmonary vascular resistance remains elevated. The pressures on the right side of the circulation reach levels that may cause right to left shunting through persistent fetal connections despite the fact that systemic vascular resistance is higher than in the fetal circulation. The extent of the contribution of this pathophysiology varies among cases. A significant proportion of otherwise normal neonatal ECMO candidates present with isolated severe PFC following a history of perinatal or neonatal asphyxia. The condition responds well to oxygenation.

Since ECMO is more invasive than most conventional therapy, it is customary to reserve treatment for situations when other therapeutic options have failed or are inappropriate. Attempts to introduce uniformity to these decisions have led to the use of numerical criteria, as an adjunct to (but not a replacement for) clinical decision-making. Using historical controls, a number of ventilatory indices have been applied and found to distinguish infants otherwise likely to die on conventional treatment.[28] Although survival rates based on historical data may not represent the current status, this standardization remains useful in comparing the outcome of patients either referred for ECMO at different points in their illness or not referred at all.

Indices that relate the extent of ventilation to the resultant blood gases, particularly the post-ductal Po_2, have found the widest application. The oxygenation index (OI)[29] is calculated as a fraction. The numerator is derived by multiplying the mean airway pressure by the fractional inspired oxygen concentration and consequently is a numerical expression of the level of ventilatory support being provided. The denominator is the value of post-ductal Pao_2 expressed in mmHg and represents a measure of how much oxygenation is being achieved. Although the OI does not represent a physiological quantity, its value in retrospective discrimination of neonatal data has led to its common usage in prospective patient selection.

A more physiological measure of effective ventilation is the alveolar arterial oxygen difference. This is obtained by subtracting the arterial Pao_2 from the so-called 'ideal' alveolar Po_2 (defined as the Po_2 that the lung would have if there were no ventilation/perfusion inequalities and perfect gas exchange were occurring; it is derived from the alveolar gas equation[30]). Values of 610 mmHg or more, for more than 8 hours, have defined a 79% mortality in retrospective study.[31]

Neonates (particularly those with congenital diaphragmatic hernia) may also require extracorporeal support on the basis of intractable carbon dioxide retention. Attempts to standardize the severity of such problems have also used numerical formulae. Bohn *et al.*[32] attempted to define a population of patients with pulmonary hypoplasia who would prove irretrievable on the basis of an index, similar to the oxygenation index, but calculated by multiplying the mean airway pressure by the respiratory rate and dividing the result by the $Paco_2$.

Congenital diaphragmatic hernia is the condition in which decision-making is perhaps most difficult. These patients are notoriously labile and the values of predictive indices can vary greatly with time. Hence some babies require consideration for ECMO preoperatively and others may only deteriorate postoperatively. There is evidence to suggest that the relative merits of early/delayed repair are less significant if ECMO is available in each case as a rescue therapy.[33] The liability of these patients is due to the interaction of three components in the aetiology of their cardiopulmonary failure:

1. Pulmonary hypertension and persistent fetal circulation.
2. Pulmonary hypoplasia secondary to lung compression *in utero*.
3. The compression of existing lung tissue by hernial contents, particularly if the baby has

been allowed to self-ventilate or has been inappropriately resuscitated.

As a consequence, alternative predictors of outcome have been sought for use in these patients. The presence of a honeymoon period[34] or of a normal preductal blood gas at any stage of the illness[35] have been suggested to indicate that the pulmonary hypoplasia is not so severe as to be incompatible with life. The justification of the latter is that a preductal measurement lessens the distortion created by a right to left ductal shunt. However, clinical experience in our own and other centres includes many cases where a favourable outcome has been achieved despite poor prognostic indicators.[36,37] Since there are no sound criteria for reliably distinguishing patients with an inevitably fatal degree of pulmonary hypoplasia, maximal therapy is recommended for all of these patients. This is reflected by their lower survival rate (Table 8.1) and higher morbidity when compared with other neonatal ECMO patients.

Selection of older patients

Selection of patients for paediatric and adult ECMO uses the general principles outlined above. However, the data on which to base such decisions is not as plentiful or clear as it is for neonatal patients.[38] In addition, instead of presenting with 'cardiopulmonary failure', older patients are more easily considered in two groups: patients with mainly pulmonary failure, and those in whom ECMO is primarily indicated for cardiac support. Both groups require assessment of the potential reversibility and degree of severity of presentation. In some instances (such as the postoperative cardiac surgical patient with pulmo-

nary hypertension) the two components may still be difficult to separate.

In assessing those patients with respiratory failure for ECMO, the principal difficulties lie in judging the appropriate timing of referral and separating the assessment of the reversibility of the primary pulmonary pathology from that of secondary barotrauma, the consequence of conventional ventilation.[39] In this context, lung biopsy may be indicated.[40] In terms of primary diagnosis, patients with pulmonary trauma, viral and bacterial pneumonia, acute (or adult) respiratory distress syndrome (ARDS), asthma, drowning, hypothermia, pulmonary sickle cell sequestration crisis, poisoning (e.g. with tricyclic antidepressants) and other less common pathologies can all be considered.

Careful consideration must be given to the underlying diagnosis to avoid placing a patient with a progressive or irreversible disease on ECMO. Again, lung biopsy may prove useful but it is also necessary to understand the likely natural history of each condition. For example, varicella pneumonia in a previously healthy patient is a different order of problem from cytomegalovirus infection after a bone marrow transplant. Both present as viral pneumoniae but the prognosis is good with ECMO in the first and very poor in the second case with or without ECMO. It may be difficult to turn some patients down, but the decision-making may become even more difficult four weeks into an ECMO run.

In terms of assessing the severity of secondary barotrauma due to positive-pressure mechanical ventilation, its duration, pressure and inspired oxygen concentration (Fio_2) all have to be considered. In general, in the older patient, ventilation at high pressures and Fio_2 for more than 7 days tends to lead to progressive fibrosis[40] and is

Table 8.1 Summary of experience with ECMO in neonates (1992).

Diagnosis	Number of patients	Outcome (% survival)	ELSO number	Outcome (% survival)
MAS	16	15 (94%)	2611	2440 (93%)
PFC	14	10 (71%)	859	728 (85%)
CDH	9	8 (89%)	1318	785 (60%)
Sepsis	6	2 (33%)	984	756 (77%)
RDS	4	2 (50%)	900	754 (84%)
Others	8	5 (62%)	253	195 (77%)
Totals	57	42 (74%)	6925	5658 (82%)

MAS = meconium aspiration syndrome; PFC = persistent fetal circulation;
CDH = congenital diaphragmatic hernia; RDS = respiratory distress syndrome.

therefore a contraindication to ECMO.

In terms of the severity at which to recommend ECMO in a patient with a particular condition, clinical judgement is important.[20] The lack of uniformity, and indeed diversity, of presentation differentiates this decision process from that involved in neonates and standardization is less easily applied. The assessment of bullae, pneumothoraces and air leaks with different pulmonary pathologies may heavily influence decision-making. In some of these cases conventional treatment may be contraindicated as it may be actively damaging. Objective numerical indices are available to imply poor prognosis with conventional treatment,[38,41] but their ratification is less extensive than for neonates. The degree of pulmonary dysfunction may be measured in terms of:

1. Transpulmonary shunt (>30% of the measured cardiac output indicates severe ventilation perfusion mismatch).
2. Static compliance (<0.5 ml/cmH$_2$O/kg indicates severe non-compliance).
3. Pulmonary artery pressure–pulmonary hypertension (>50 mmHg systolic) secondary to lung disease[42] may also be an indicator of poor prognosis.

ECMO supports cardiac function best when right heart failure is a consequence of pulmonary hypertension. In biventricular failure, ventricular assist devices or total artificial hearts are likely to be more appropriate. A standard venoarterial ECMO cannulation may need supplementing with the addition of a left atrial vent for such patients. The difficulty, as in previous situations, is to intervene with appropriate technology in cases in which there is a potentially reversible problem before multisystem failure is established. The main indications for cardiac support have been:

1. After cardiac surgery, usually for congenital heart disease.
2. As a bridge to cardiac or cardiopulmonary transplantation.
3. To support myocarditis, or after heart transplant rejection.

ECMO can be used following cardiac surgery in an attempt to salvage patients who do not wean from cardiopulmonary bypass in the operating theatre or to support those whose heart and pulmonary function deteriorates in the intensive care unit. The majority of these patients (and the most responsive) are those who have had surgery for congenital heart disease. Those with prior myocardial dysfunction fare less well.

With modern surgical techniques and methods of myocardial protection, low-output states which do not respond to inotropic support are not common and often reflect an undiagnosed or uncorrected problem. A careful appraisal of the cardiac repair therefore needs to be made before embarking on ECMO. This will involve a combination of intracardiac pressure and saturation measurements (either at operation or at cardiac catheterization) and echocardiography. The principal aim is to detect unrelieved outflow tract obstructions and/or residual shunts. With the increasing sophistication of both hand-held and transoesophageal echo/Doppler probes, an accurate assessment of ventricular function and the quality of the repair is usually possible.

Failure to wean from cardiopulmonary bypass is a fairly clear-cut end-point. The decision towards ECMO support is then precipitated by an overt failure of conventional treatment. However, the outcome for this group has often been poor with ECMO and the continued use of direct cannulation via sternotomy is associated with excessive blood loss. In a later phase of the recovery, decision-making may be more difficult. Bartlett's group have used persistent low output—defined as a mixed venous saturation of <50% and cardiac index of <2 l/m^2/min on full pharmacological and mechanical (intra-aortic balloon pump) support for more than 2 hours—as an indication for ECMO. With increasing experience and confidence in ECMO, many programmes now intervene earlier in postoperative patients than was formerly the case. The improving results of ECMO as cardiac support reflect this fall in the threshold for treatment.

The place of ECMO to support myocarditis and transplant patients is controversial, both in terms of using mechanical support at all and in terms of whether ECMO or biventricular support techniques are more appropriate.

It can be argued that the correct location of an ECMO programme is in a cardiothoracic centre as the success of prolonged extracorporeal life support in salvaging any of these patients is partly due to the fact that the technique is then routine.[43]

Components of the ECMO circuit

Successful ECMO in the modern era reflects the refinement of the circuit design. The relatively benign effects on the blood during passage through an extracorporeal circuit, and the reliability and stability of the circuit in routine operation, enable prolonged perfusion, sufficient to establish native organ recovery. The choice of circuit components and the apparent, but deceptive, simplicity of the design of an ECMO circuit are fundamental to this. ECMO circuits differ from conventional peroperative cardiopulmonary bypass in both design and application.

The main components of both cardiopulmonary bypass circuits and ECMO circuits are similar: an oxygenator, heat exchanger, pump, and reservoir. In the ECMO circuit, the components are designed to maintain normothermia and to remain stable and functional for extended periods. Areas of stasis are avoided so that low-level heparinization can be used. Prolonged support requires some form of servo-regulation. The circuit configuration is therefore significantly different from peroperative bypass and is relatively standardized following the Bartlett design.

The oxygenator

The membrane oxygenator is the device which all the circuit supports. It is designed as a silicone envelope with a fine wire mesh in between. This membrane is tightly wound around a polycarbonate spool and covered in a tight multilayer protective sleeve. Blood enters from the bottom of the oxygenator and the sweep gas from the top. Gas exchange occurs very efficiently across the silastic membrane, driven by diffusion gradients which are maximized by the resultant counter-

current. The 'gold standard' oxygenating device is the Avecor ECMO oxygenator (formerly SciMed). Unlike the microporous membrane oxygenators commonly used in cardiopulmonary bypass, these devices rarely develop plasma leakage and may be used for periods of a month or more. They are available in sizes from 0.4 m^2 membrane surface area up to 4.5 m^2. A newer version (Ultrox series) has an integral stainless steel heat exchanger. The size of oxygenator required depends on the size of the patient and whether venoarterial or venovenous ECMO is being used. In general, the membrane surface area required for a venovenous perfusion is approximately twice that needed for venoarterial perfusion (see Table 8.2).

Newer devices are being developed, notably heparin-bonded hollow-fibre oxygenators and newer configurations of silastic membrane oxygenators. With the exception of the Medtronic heparin-bonded oxygenators which have been used clinically in adult ECMO, these oxygenators have usually been used in open-heart surgery or experimentally in the laboratory.

The heat exchanger

Since the circuit is exposed to ambient temperatures and cold gases via the oxygenator, blood temperature regulation is necessary to avoid the deleterious effects of prolonged hypothermia. Placing the heat exchanger in a post-oxygenator position reverses the overall cooling effect of passage through the circuit and warms the blood just prior to its return to the patient. The common preference is for heat exchangers that are constructed from stainless steel, not aluminium as is commonly the case for CPB. Aluminium tends to oxidize and fragment when used

Table 8.2 Choice of ECMO circuit components.

Patient weight	<2 kg	2–8 kg	8–12 kg	12–20 kg	20–35 kg	35–70 kg	>70 kg
Diameter of tubing	$\frac{1}{4}$ in	$\frac{1}{4}$ in	$\frac{1}{4}$ in (VA); $\frac{3}{8}$ in (VV)	$\frac{3}{8}$ in	$\frac{3}{8}$ in	$\frac{3}{8}$ in	$\frac{3}{8}$ in
Diameter of raceway	$\frac{1}{4}$ in	$\frac{1}{4}$ in	$\frac{3}{8}$ in	$\frac{3}{8}$ in	$\frac{3}{8}$ in	$\frac{1}{2}$ in	$\frac{1}{2}$ in
Oxygenator size	0.4 m^2 (Avecor)	0.8 m^2 (Avecor)	1.5 m^2 (Avecor)	2.0 m^2 (Ultrox)	2.5 m^2 (Ultrox)	3.5 m^2 (Ultrox 1)	$2 \times 3.5 \text{ m}^2$ (Ultrox 1)
Arterial cannula size	8–10 F	8–14 F	14–16 F	16–20 F	20–22 F	22–24 F	24 F
Venous cannula size	8–10 F	10–16 F	16–18 F	18–22 F	20–27 F	29 F	29 F
Priming volume	400 ml	500 ml	800 ml	1100 ml	1300 ml	1500 ml	1500 (–2500) ml

for extended periods.[44] A separate stainless steel heat exchanger is marketed with Avecor oxygenators. It is a highly efficient heat exchanger and, if located after the oxygenator in a vertical position, also functions as a highly efficient bubble trap. It is a cylindrical polycarbonate shell with stainless steel tubes. Heat transference occurs rapidly between blood flowing through the stainless steel tubes and the thermoregulated water jacket flowing in counter-current to the direction of blood flow. A water heater and pump circulates water at a preset temperature (Seabrook, Cincinnati Sub Zero), which, combined with the overhead heating of the cot, maintains normothermia.

The pump

A roller pump

Most centres performing neonatal ECMO use roller pumps. With Super Tygon® tubing in the raceways, these pumps are very reliable and may be used for prolonged periods with little haemolysis. The particular model of pump (e.g. Sarns, Polystan, Cobe Stockert) is less important than the accuracy with which it is set up and monitored.

The electronic ECMO roller pump generates the forward propulsion necessary to circulate venous blood through the high-resistance membrane oxygenator. To accomplish this, the rotating roller heads tightly compress (but do not occlude) a length of blood-filled tubing against a fixed, circular stainless steel 'well'. The resultant flow is essentially non-pulsatile. When calibrated to the diameter of the tubing, the pump displays the (calculated) litres per minute blood flow which can be adjusted as clinically indicated.

Most roller pumps have the capability to accommodate a wide range of tubing sizes and desired flow rates. Some have additional features which integrate computer-aided blood flow systems, sophisticated flow sensors and bubble detectors. In the absence of this type of servo-regulation, a bladder box controller is required (see later). All have a back-up manual handcrank in the event of power or electrical failures.

Long-term exposure to the compression from the roller heads results microscopically in spallation and macroscopically in alteration of the tubing's shape and eventually visible damage. Even the most durable tubing type on the market

(Super Tygon) is susceptible to rupture. Constant tubing inspection and surveillance cannot be over-emphasized, and periodic 'walking' of the raceway (moving a different section of tubing into the pump head) is considered essential by most units.

A centrifugal pump

Centrifugal pumps, which may be of the constrained vortex (Biomedicus) or impeller (Delphin, St Jude) type, are favoured by some as they are at less risk with respect to pumping air and do not require a bladder. Each requires an electromagnetic flowmeter and alarms to monitor flow, as the revolutions per minute of the centrifugal head do not necessarily translate into effective forward flow. In centrifugal pumps the propulsion is provided by a magnetic cone or impeller rotating on an external electrical drive motor. The impeller heads have vanes to facilitate propulsion but the biomedicus pumps rely on the centrifugal effect of a rotating concentric cone.

The operation of a centrifugal pump is dependent upon an adequate venous return. At high blood flow rates or in situations where venous drainage is reduced, the heads will develop high levels of suction and gross haemolysis may occur. This may be protected against by monitoring the venous inlet pressure. Furthermore, centrifugal pump heads are not licensed beyond 72 hours. This, the increased risk of haemolysis and their greater cost has prevented their widespread application for ECMO, although they have been used more frequently as ventricular assist devices. Malfunction of the magnetic heads may occur abruptly and clotting within the pump heads has also been reported. Equipment failure of the pump head is made more serious if manual operation is not possible.

Perhaps the best ECMO-related use for this type of pump is for patient transfer, as the circuit can be compacted more than is possible with a roller pump design and venous drainage is less dependent on gravity syphon.

A peristaltic pump

A third type of pump, which has been used in France for many years for CPB and more recently for single-cannula, tidal-flow venovenous ECMO (or AREC—assistance respiratoire extracorporeale[45]), is the peristaltic Rhône Poulenc pump.

This combines the best characteristics of the other two types, although the raceway, as currently designed in silastic, is not robust enough for very prolonged use. With this pump a bladder/reservoir is unnecessary, it is almost impossible to pump air, and both inflow and outflow can be occluded without raceway rupture. Development of this pump by modification of the raceway and other minor adjustments should lead to a device superior to both roller and centrifugal pumps.

The reservoir

The large-volume reservoirs used in CPB favour clot formation in areas of stasis when used with low levels of heparinization for prolonged extracorporeal support. The Avecor bladders used for ECMO are small-volume (30–50 ml) and made of silastic. Their ovoid design minimizes areas of stasis. They fit into a bladder box which is used in the servo-regulation of the roller pump. The top of the bladder tends to trap air which may be aspirated from the infusion ports. As the bladders were originally designed for use in supporting infants, they have a $\frac{1}{4}$-inch connector fitting on inflow and outflow. If a $\frac{3}{8}$-inch or $\frac{1}{2}$-inch tubing set is indicated by the size of the patient (see Table 8.2), a bypass loop can be placed across the bladder. This allows for adequate flow but still allows the bladder to function as the servo-regulator of the pump. Bladders with larger connectors are now becoming available.

Servo-regulation

The bladder box assembly is an electronic device which functions as the monitor and servo-regulator of the quantity of venous blood diverted through the circuit. It houses the distensible reservoir bladder between a fixed front plate and a retractable rear switch which electronically connects to the roller pump control system.

With adequate venous drainage to the circuit, and a pump flow rate less than that rate, the distended blood-filled bladder exerts sufficient pressure to keep the switch fully retracted, thus allowing continuous operation of the pump at a preset flow. Should insufficient venous drainage occur (e.g. from hypovolaemia or an upstream obstruction in the circuit) the bladder will collapse and the switch will move forward, thereby halting the roller pump's operation. Designed as a safety mechanism, the bladder box prevents the pump from collapsing the tubing and potentially causing cavitation and air embolism or micro-emboli formation. It is therefore imperative that the perfusionist or ECMO specialist routinely check the bladder box assembly to ensure that the switch and alarm system are functioning.

Circuits

Pre-assembled sterile circuits are generally standard for neonatal patients but may be custom-designed, by each ECMO centre, for larger patients. Such customization must still adhere to the prerequisites of minimizing opportunities for stasis and maintaining normothermia. Tubing material, overall dimensions, component compatibility, priming ease, and innovative additions (e.g. Galveston diamonds) are considered when designing the tubing pack. Super Tygon tubing can be used throughout, or limited to the raceway as it is more expensive than standard PVC tubing.

In-line blood gas monitoring

Continuous measurement of circuit blood gases provides valuable information relative to the patient's minute-to-minute response to ECMO support. Of particular importance is the measurement of mixed venous blood saturation ($S\mathrm{vo}_2$) measured proximal to the oxygenator.[46] During venoarterial ECMO, the $S\mathrm{vo}_2$ reflects the adequacy of oxygen delivery. During venovenous ECMO, however, the $S\mathrm{vo}_2$ is influenced by recirculation and becomes less useful clinically. Measurement of 'arterialized' blood gases measured distally within the ECMO circuit may provide information relative to the performance of the oxygenator.

Several types of in-line continuous blood gas monitoring systems are available which utilize optical fluorescence technology via sensors either directly located in the blood path or separated by a membrane-lined flow-through cell inserted in the circuit. A variety of models are available (e.g. CDI, Baxter). In addition to providing clinical data, they are generally accepted as cost-efficient by decreasing the number of blood gases taken from the patient. However, periodic checking of their calibration with laboratory samples is recommended.

Pressure monitoring systems

Continuous monitoring of the pressure at the blood entry and exit ports around the oxygenator will alert the ECMO specialist to impending malfunction. Standard pressure transducers can be attached to the circuit and attached to single- or multichannel monitors. Rises in both pre- and post-oxygenator pressures occur in the event of a downstream obstruction, and obstruction to flow within the oxygenator (e.g. from clot formation) widens the gap between these pressures. It is also wise to monitor the pressure in the gas phase of the oxygenator, particularly if it is being run close to its recommended maximum. The pressure in the gas phase should be maintained below that in the blood phase so that air or gas embolism is less likely in the event of membrane rupture.

Portable/back-up power system

A portable battery-operated power source is essential if mobility on ECMO is anticipated or is wise as insurance against the event of mains power disruption. Several powerful yet compact power sources with variable wattage capacity, multiple electrical outlets, and low-battery alarm systems are available on the market. It is recommended that all electrical ECMO equipment be plugged into the power source which is then plugged into the main power outlet so that when not in use, it remains fully-charged.

The activated clotting time system

The need for continuous anticoagulation during ECMO makes bedside monitoring of the activated clotting time (ACT) necessary. Several systems are available to perform the ACT testing (e.g. Haemochron, Haemotech) which are easy to use, provide immediate and reliable results, and are relatively inexpensive. Given that the integrity of the circuit is at stake, the perfusionist or ECMO specialist must be familiar with the ACT system used and remain accurate and consistent in performing the ACT test. When working at low levels of heparinization it is essential for the calibration of the sensor to be checked regularly.

The neonatal ECMO bed

When a roller pump system is being used, pump flow is dependent upon gravity-assisted venous drainage. Accordingly, patients on ECMO often require elevation to enhance the venous syphon. Several neonatal beds are available with an adjustable mattress height. Additional features include an oversized mattress, open access to the patient, and overhead heating system.

The ECMO cart

The ECMO equipment should be arranged on a sturdy, compact and mobile cart. Desired features include IV infusion pump pole mounts, adjustable shelves, locking wheels, and lighting. An additional mobile fully-stocked supply cart is essential to provide ready access to all ECMO-related items.

Priming protocols

Individual centres commonly adhere to their own protocols with regard to priming. A typical example is described here.

Appropriate sizes of sterile packed circuit components are assembled according to the circuit design. The choice of circuit components depends upon the size of patient, the style of support required and the mode of cannulation. Venous cannulae and drainage tubing must be of sufficient calibre to allow the required flow without inordinate suction. The return circuit tubing and cannula may be of smaller bore but must be large enough to tolerate the anticipated flow without generating excessive pressure[47,48] (<300 mmHg proximal to the membrane lung). The primary importance of reducing suction and pressure is that they threaten circuit integrity and cause haemolysis.

The sash that will be used at the bedside during cannulation is replaced by a bubble filter and the prime also allowed to flow through the bridge which connects the afferent and efferent limbs of the circuit. Once assembled, larger circuits require flushing with carbon dioxide prior to liquid priming. The greater solubility of this gas compared with the constituents of room air or oxygen makes bubble formation less likely during liquid priming. The carbon dioxide can be administered into the bladder and 'walked' around the circuit using clamps, or alternatively distributed throughout the circuit by using it as the sweep gas across the membrane oxygenator prior to liquid priming.

Liquid priming proceeds in phases. It is customary to introduce each phase into the bladder so that it can be guided around the whole circuit driving the previous phase ahead of it. Excess volume during this process is released from the pre-bladder pigtail and the tubing connecting this area to the bladder is clamped. The first fluid phase is a 20% albumin solution. This will coat tygon, any competitive PVC tubing, and silicone with a layer of protein. The intention is to reduce later platelet aggregation and, more immediately, minimize microbubble formation at the liquid/tubing interface. The second liquid phase is a crystalloid solution with physiological levels of electrolytes in solution (Plasmalyte A or Hartmanns). Once the entire circuit is fully liquid-primed and all air pockets have been removed, the circuit is transferred to the bedside and blood priming proceeds during cannulation. The internal volume of the circuit varies according to the size of the components selected. For a neonate a typical priming volume is 450 ml, and such a circuit will require only one unit of donated blood. Larger circuits, for older children and adults, rarely require more than two units. Prior to commencing bypass, the acid–base and electrolyte balance of the prime are determined. Hyperkalaemia may be counteracted by the addition of calcium to the prime and acidosis adjusted by the addition of bicarbonate. Extreme disturbances of acid–base and electrolyte composition may be associated with the use of old blood in the prime and ultimately can be treated with ultrafiltration of the circuit prior to commencing bypass.

Cannulation for ECMO

See Chapter 40.

ECMO management

About 80% of the work done on an ECMO patient relates to the function of the extracorporeal circuit. The remainder consists of nursing care. This has led to the development of ECMO specialists who manage the technical aspects of patient care. ECMO specialists are usually either nurses, respiratory therapists or perfusionists.

Successful ECMO management requires teamwork and adherence to well tried protocols. Continual audit and revision are a natural necessity. The basic starting points of bedside protocols are listed in Table 8.3.

Gas exchange and haemodynamics

Comprehensive accounts of the physiology of extracorporeal life support are widely available, but some key issues bear repetition. ECMO interacts with the native circulation in ways that distinguish it from peroperative cardiopulmonary bypass. During convention CPB, the extracorporeal circuit is used to replace the function of the heart and lungs. During ECMO, the circuit is a closed system which runs in parallel to the circulation to produce degrees of support that rarely need to reach total CPB. This frequently gives a circulation with near normal pulsatility. When managing patients on ECMO it is rare to require blood flow rates that match or exceed the native cardiac output. The principal aim is usually to ensure adequate systemic oxygen delivery.

During venoarterial (VA) ECMO the delivery of oxygenated blood to the tissues can be visualized as the sum of the cardiac output and the extracorporeal blood flow. If the systemic delivery of blood is largely fixed by the extracorporeal blood flow (as it is when operated close to full CPB) the best way to guarantee adequate peripheral oxygen delivery is to maintain high mixed venous oxygen saturations, using values that incorporate fluctuations in peripheral oxygen demand.[46] Arterial blood gases lose their usefulness as they are more a measure of membrane oxygenator function than patient status. Larger patients may be able to accommodate pulmonary arterial catheters during ECMO, but in their absence the right atrial drainage provides a useful approximation to mixed venous blood and it is routine to monitor this saturation continuously during venoarterial ECMO.

During venovenous (VV) perfusion, the potential for a variable degree of recirculation and venous mixing within the atrium means that the mixed venous oxygen saturation is a misleading measurement. Useful data may be derived from cephalad venous drainage, but the atrial blood draining to the circuit represents a mixture of oxygenated blood from the circuit and systemic venous blood. Blood entering the pulmonary artery is, similarly, a mixture of systemic venous

Table 8.3 Bedside ECMO protocols (see text)*.

Blood gas parameters	
To clear more CO_2	Increase the sweep gas flow rate
To clear less CO_2	Decrease the sweep gas flow rate
To improve oxygenation	Increase the blood flow through the circuit
To wean from ECMO support	Decrease the blood flow through the circuit and proportionately wean the gas (sweep) flow
'Full flow' ECMO support (VA)	100 ml/kg/min
'Full flow' ECMO support (VV)	120 ml/kg/min
Anticoagulation	
Heparin infusion	20–40 units/kg/h
Monitor anticoagulation	Hourly, whole-blood ACT
Older children	180–200 s
Neonates	160–180 s
Bleeding patient (or surgery)	140–160 s
Platelet supplements	
Older children	To maintain count >75 000/mm^3
Neonates	To maintain count >100 000/mm^3
Bleeding or surgery	To maintain count >150 000/mm^3
Fluid restriction	
Neonates	50–80 ml/kg/day
Older children	30–60 ml/kg/day

* Release and reposition bridge clamp every 15 minutes.

and ECMO circuit return. In the absence of pulmonary function, systemic arterial blood is little different. A degree of systemic desaturation is therefore to be expected during VV perfusion. Oxygen delivery under these circumstances relies upon a rise in the resting cardiac output. Cardiac function must therefore be reliable or remediable to permit VV cannulation. Myocardial dysfunction secondary to hypoxia may improve when venovenous ECMO is established because of improvements in myocardial oxygenation.

Within limits dictated by the internal surface area of the membrane oxygenator, the thickness of the blood phase within it and the haemoglobin concentration, oxygen delivery can be titrated by adjusting the extracorporeal blood flow. Increases in blood flow across the oxygenator will increase oxygenation except in the circumstances of significant recirculation during VV bypass. The degree of recirculation under these circumstances will increase with increasing circuit blood flow.

Carbon dioxide clearance, by contrast and because of its greater solubility, is a function of the minute volume of the oxygenator. Effective CO_2 clearance requires much lower blood flows than oxygenation. The 'sweep gas' (usually 100% oxygen) passing in counter-current through the oxygenator maximizes diffusion gradients between the gas and blood phases, making CO_2 removal very efficient. Occasionally, carbogen gas (95% oxygen and 5% carbon dioxide) is used as a sweep gas to inhibit CO_2 removal when it becomes excessive.

The haemodynamic effects of ECMO support are partly determined by the mode of cannulation. The degree of haemodynamic change induced by the introduction of ECMO will depend acutely upon the extracorporeal blood flow, at least in venoarterial ECMO. The longer-term effects result from a sustained fall in pulmonary vascular resistance.

Venoarterial support provides right ventricular assist and produces mixed changes in left ventricular loading conditions. In the absence of an anatomic left-to-right shunt, the LV preload is reduced but afterload is probably significantly increased.[49–51] As ECMO blood flow rates are increased and approach the native cardiac output, the pulse pressure dwindles. It is customary to describe 'full flow' as a blood flow rate equivalent to the resting cardiac output (100 ml/kg/min for VA and 120 ml/kg/min for VV). Total CPB may be achieved, however, and a virtually non-pulsatile circulation results. This causes difficulty in assessing cardiac function. During such profound alteration in loading conditions apparent LV function (as measured by simple LV ejection phase indices) is inversely related to the extracorporeal blood flow rate.

If LV function is truly compromised (for example in the case of a postoperative cardiac surgical patient or in situations of myocardial stun[52,53] it may become necessary to drain the left atrium directly to the circuit or indirectly across the atrial septum. In such circumstances a VA cannulation is essential. However, for lesser degrees of cardiac dysfunction the necessity for VA cannulation may be debatable. In addition to increasing LV afterload, there is evidence to suggest that myocardial oxygenation may be inferior compared with VV cannulation.[54] Certainly, in venoarterial ECMO, coronary blood flow is still, for the most part, derived from blood ejected from the left ventricle in systole. In the absence of native pulmonary function this may be the most deoxygenated blood in the body.

Venoarterial ECMO in neonates can be associated with very different haemodynamic effects. The persistence of a ductus arteriosus in the context of a falling pulmonary vascular resistance may allow a left-to-right shunt that increases in significance as the pulmonary vascular resistance falls.[55] The pulmonary blood flow under such circumstances can be significantly elevated. The result of an increase in LV preload and afterload may be LV dilatation and mitral regurgitation. High pulmonary blood flow like this carries a risk of pulmonary oedema and/or haemorrhage. If spontaneous ductal closure does not occur at an appropriate time, it may be necessary to perform surgical ductal ligation during ECMO.

Management of the lung

One of the major differences between modern ECMO and practice in the era of the NIH study[9] is the recognition of the importance of lung rest.[39] The extreme examples are patients who are referred because of severe barotrauma and multiple air leaks. In these patients it is difficult to envisage any form of positive-pressure ventilation achieving any more than further lung damage. The extreme 'rest setting' that can be employed is an apnoeic perfusion during VA bypass (or apnoeic oxygenation during extracorporeal CO_2 removal).

Since the patients are largely independent of their own pulmonary function, endotracheal tubes can be changed at will and bronchoscopy or total bronchopulmonary lavage performed for prolonged periods. This provides therapeutic options that would not exist without extracorporeal support.[56] Similarly it becomes far easier to perform extensive, more classical, physiotherapy and endotracheal toilet than would otherwise be possible.

It is routine to keep patients intubated during ECMO but ventilation settings are not designed primarily to provide gas exchange. The main considerations are:

1. The minimization of pulmonary oedema and atelectasis.
2. The prevention of further barotrauma.

There are additional considerations such as the optimizing of pulmonary blood flow. Good pulmonary care also involves fluid restriction and the correction of the oedema with which most patients present.

These aims are usually approached by ventilation settings designed to reduce the mean airway pressure but to maintain some distending pressure in the airways. Hence a relatively low peak inspiratory pressure but long inspiratory time, high end-expiratory pressure and low rates are employed.[57,58] Classical settings for a neonate would be an inspiration time of one second, fractional inspired oxygen of 25–30%, pressures of 20 cm of water over 10 or 12 PEEP and a rate of 10 breaths per minute.

Duration of ECMO

When the clinical status, chest X-ray and blood gas data start to improve, the patient is weaned off ECMO gradually. During ECMO the blood flow to the circuit and the gas composition and flow ('sweep') across the oxygenator are the variables routinely adjusted in response to patient requirements. Thus the return of native lung function naturally stimulates a gradual reduction in these parameters. When the circuit no longer seems to be making a significant contribution (i.e. the blood flow through the circuit and gas flow are low) a formal 'trial-off' ECMO is performed. The point at which to choose to attempt this must also be determined by the safety limits of the circuit. It is our practice to avoid blood flow rates through a neonatal circuit of less than 100 ml/min for fear of creating areas of relative stasis and allowing clots to form.

A 'trial-off' in a patient who is VA cannulated will necessarily involve clamping the afferent and efferent limbs of the circuit and opening the bridge to allow the circuit to cycle, independent from the patient. It is therefore preceded by the rationalization of ventilation settings to promote pulmonary gas exchange and the provision of adequate venous access to supply fluids, calories and any critical drug infusions. Serial blood gas measurements from the patient are necessary to monitor this period of the perfusion which, if successful, proceeds to decannulation.

The haemodynamic effects of venovenous ECMO are far less significant than those of VA and so a 'trial-off' need involve no more than removing the gas source from the oxygenator. The composition of the gas phase of the oxygenator then gradually equilibrates with the venous blood over 15–20 min and the results are assessed by analysis of the patient's arterial blood gas levels.

Decannulation

See Chapter 40.

Results

Although the widespread acceptance of ECMO has been impeded by a lack of comparative data with conventional treatment, there is no lack of data surrounding the outcome of ECMO treated patients. Practising ECMO centres contribute data to a central registry at the offices of the Extracorporeal Life Support Organisation (ELSO) in Ann Arbor, Michigan, USA. This is thought to be a near-complete record of neonatal and paediatric ECMO as practised throughout the world. Records of adult patients are regrettably less complete and the ELSO registry in this regard largely represents American experience.

In the neonatal population, historical controls exist with which these results can be compared. Even without these the survival data are impressive when one takes into account that the ECMO candidates are selected by their severity of presentation. However, without a valid control population there is no frame of reference with which to interpret this information objectively. Attempts to gather reliable comparative data necessitate prospective randomization because of the necessary selection criteria employed in assessing ECMO candidates.

In October 1992 there were 94 ELSO-registered practising ECMO centres worldwide. Almost all (the majority exclusively) treat neonates. Close to 7000 neonates have received ECMO with an overall survival rate of 82%. Within the different common neonatal diagnostic groups the survival rates vary, infants with pulmonary hypoplasia or established parenchymal lung damage fairing worst (Table 8.1). British experience in neonatal ECMO was until recently limited to one centre. There are now five practising neonatal ECMO centres in the UK, coordinated by the steering group of a collaborative trial of neonatal ECMO *versus* conventional treatment. ECMO has only recently been introduced into this country[59] and referrals are made comparatively late by American standards. A total of 90 neonates have been treated with survival rates that match the ELSO registry (Table 8.1).

Paediatric and adult patients are a far more diverse group in terms of diagnostic categorization. In general, ECMO has been used to support either isolated pulmonary failure or cardiac failure, often following cardiac surgery. We have treated 31 patients with pulmonary failure and 10 patients with cardiac failure whose specific diagnoses are shown in Tables 8.4 and 8.5. These are compared with the ELSO registry which contains data on fewer patients than the neonatal registry (474 paediatric pulmonary and 760 paediatric cardiac against over 7000 neonates). Our results with pulmonary failure have been excellent, with an overall survival of 84% (compared with 48% in the registry). This probably reflects differences in case selection between ours and the pooled data. Particularly impressive results were seen when ECMO was used for single-system failure in viral pneumonias with or without secondary bacterial infection.

Our results with cardiac failure are similar to those of the registry in the 40–50% survival range. The best results in the cardiac failure situation are in patients with postoperative pulmonary hypertension. Those who require ECMO having failed to be weaned from conventional CPB have a worse prognosis, although some do survive.

Patient-related complications

The morbidity and quality of the outcome of neonatal ECMO survivors has also never been subjected to prospective comparative assessment

Table 8.4 Results of paediatric pulmonary support.

Diagnosis	Leicester number	Survival (%)	ELSO number	Survival (%)
Bacterial Pneumonia	7	100	34	47
viral	10	90	136	51
ARDS	5	100	125	44
Aspiration	5	60	48	56
Pneumocystis	0		7	29
Intrapulmonary haemorrhage	0		7	71
Other	4	50	117	45
Totals	31	84	474	48

against non-ECMO treated patients surviving similar degrees of illness. Even less data is available on older children and adults.

Neurological disorders

From a neurological viewpoint a significant handicap rate is to be expected when candidates have been selected by their severity of presentation and a demonstrable failure to respond to maximal conventional treatment. Existing follow-up studies confirm a significant handicap rate of 15–35% in neonatal ECMO survivors. Figures for completely normal survivors are in the range 50–85%.[60–62] Follow-up studies on similar infants treated conventionally are fewer in number but suggest that the handicap rate is not significantly different.[63] Data from older children who have had a severe respiratory insult and have survived with conventional treatment show a similar handicap rate.[38] Our own patients have fared at least as well as that, with only one having significant handicap (which had been suspected prior to ECMO referral). Additionally we have observed a number of patients with a choreiform movement disorder. In each case dystonic movements were apparent immediately after ECMO and resolved

over days to weeks. Despite giving rise to concern, in each case the signs have resolved without obvious residual sequelae. The aetiology is suspected to be a variant of the central anticholinergic syndrome.[64,65]

Respiratory disorders

A degree of respiratory morbidity is also to be expected in candidates who prior to ECMO were frequently subjected to the extremes of positive-pressure mechanical ventilation. Again, prospective comparative data with other forms of treatment are not available, though one would expect the use of 'rest settings' and modest ventilation to produce less barotrauma and a lower incidence of chronic lung disease in an ECMO treated group. A small number of infants (particularly some of the patients with congenital diaphragmatic hernia) survive the neonatorum with the help of ECMO but have, what could retrospectively be termed, 'inevitably fatal' degrees of pulmonary hypoplasia or pulmonary hypertension. A respiratory morbidity follows ending in death, usually before the first birthday. It could be argued that the treatment achieves little; however, since there is no satisfactory way of predicting

Table 8.5 Results of paediatric cardiac ECMO.

Diagnosis	Leicester number	Cannulation	Survival	ELSO class and number	Survival (%)
Fallots	3	VA	1	Cardiac surgery (657)	44
Truncus	2	VA	2	Transplant (34)	29
AV canal	2	VA	0	Myocarditis (21)	62
TGA (atrial)	1	VA	0	Cardiomyopathy (29)	62
TGA (switch)	1	VA + LAV	0	Other (19)	74
Interrupted arch	1	VA	1		
Totals	10		4	(760)	46

which patients will inevitably have a poor outcome, no infants are excluded by severity of presentation.

In the paediatric age-group there are few data. Our own experience[20] has been encouraging, however, with abnormal lung function being present only in those with pre-existing lung disease. Pre-existing pulmonary damage or bronchopulmonary dysplasia was present in some patients with respiratory syncytial virus (RSV) pneumonia and was reflected in post-ECMO respiratory function tests.

Bleeding

Bleeding complications are some of the most serious of the patient-related complications. This is particularly true of intracranial haemorrhage which is an important cause of neurological morbidity and mortality. The other common sites of bleeding are cannulation sites, the gastrointestinal tract, chest drain sites, surgical incisions and needle punctures. Haemothorax, intrapulmonary haemorrhage and cardiac tamponade may all occur.

Bleeding in ECMO patients is related to several factors and not just the use of heparin. Many complex reactions are initiated when blood interfaces with the artificial surfaces in the circuit—the tubing, the oxygenator and the heat exchanger. These surfaces include PVC, silastic, polycarbonate, polyurethane, other plastics and stainless steel. The albumin and blood used in the prime do coat and 'pacify' these surfaces to some extent. However, during perfusion further blood proteins, including clotting factors, tend to adhere roughly in proportion to their concentration in plasma. In addition to the soluble clotting factors, platelets also adhere as microaggregates, usually in relation to fibrinogen molecules. Frank thrombus formation may also occur in areas of stasis. When these factors are combined with the dilution of the patient's own blood on the initiation of ECMO, the overall effect is for the platelet count and the level of soluble clotting factors to fall. In many patients the severity of illness prior to ECMO may mean that the coagulation system is already abnormal.

As well as the more obvious haematological abnormalities, there are changes in the local tissues and microcirculation which predispose to bleeding. These include sepsis, hypoxia, hypovolaemia and reperfusion. Hypertension, which is a possible sequel to venoarterial ECMO, may also predispose to bleeding, particularly intracerebral. In addition there may be local factors in particular organs. Prior administration of tolazoline and the occurrence of 'stress ulcers' predispose to gastrointestinal bleeding. Obstruction of the left internal jugular vein due to neck position may predispose to posterior fossa intracerebral haemorrhage. A patent ductus arteriosus may predispose to pulmonary haemorrhage. There are other examples.

Surgical sites, particularly cannulation incisions, chest drain tracks and needle sticks may all bleed. However, in most cases haemorrhage can be prevented by careful technique. During surgery on ECMO, generous use of fibrin glue and electrocautery are customary. Chest drains (particularly those inserted prior to referral for ECMO) should be left *in situ* to avoid bleeding from the chest wall or to allow drainage of blood from the penetrating lung injuries incurred at their insertion.

Management of bleeding during ECMO (see also Chapter 35)

Bleeding complications may be reduced by maintaining the levels of soluble clotting factors as near normal as possible. This is achieved by the periodic infusion of fresh frozen plasma and cryoprecipitate as required and by maintaining a platelet count above $100\,000/mm^3$. The ACT should be controlled as close to the limits of safety as is possible, although these are not well defined and it is certainly possible to maintain patients without heparin for limited periods. The generally accepted, appropriate ACT level has fallen over recent years but is currently 160–180 s. Many centres, however, still run a little higher than this (ACT 180–200).

On occasion there may be excessive consumption of clotting factors mirroring disseminated intravascular coagulopathy (DIC). This may reflect systemic sepsis or other patient causes, but may also reflect progressive thrombosis within the oxygenator. We have seen this on two occasions during prolonged paediatric ECMO cases before oxygenator function had deteriorated perceptively. The state may be reversed by changing the oxygenator (or circuit) and administering further clotting factors.

When active bleeding occurs or a surgical procedure is necessary, it is again necessary to use fresh frozen plasma, cryoprecipitate and platelets. The platelet count should be elevated further to 150 000/mm³. The heparin infusion should be reduced so that the ACT is close to 160 s. If the site of haemorrhage is a surgical one or there is bleeding into the pericardium or pleura, early consideration should be given to surgical exploration. Antifibrinolytic drugs, notably epsilon amino caproic acid (EACA), have been shown to have a beneficial effect in some patients. Aprotonin is another agent, which amongst other properties, is an antifibrinolytic. This has not been subject to controlled trial in ECMO, but has dramatic effects on bleeding after cardiac surgery. Paradoxically, it elevates the ACT so that when it is started the ACT which had been stable at 180 s increases to about 220 s without change in the heparin dose. We have used aprotonin in the event of haemorrhage during ECMO and in the context of surgery. Our subjective impression is favourable but our data insufficient to constitute proof.

Circuit-related complications

Patients, selected for ECMO because of failing conventional treatment, are totally dependent on the circuit for life support for part of their ECMO run. Particularly during the early phases of a perfusion, any circuit failure or operator error cannot be effectively compensated by an alteration of, or return to, conventional ventilation. Technical emergencies therefore carry a high risk of mortality and morbidity, and so it is customary to have someone at the bedside who is capable, in the event of an emergency, of resuscitating the circuit in order to save the patient (an ECMO specialist). Fortunately major mechanical complications are rare so that the training of ECMO specialists for these emergencies needs to be done in the laboratory. In over 15 000 hours we have had only five mechanical failures. All but one were successfully corrected without compromise to the patient.

Future trends

Technological advances in oxygenator design and the biocompatibility of artificial surfaces should lead to improved long-term perfusion, with fewer patient complications related to anticoagulant. Venovenous cannulation by percutaneous techniques is likely to replace venoarterial cannulation for isolated pulmonary failure. Newer pumps, probably of the peristaltic type, should make for fewer circuit-related complications. It is likely that the whole system will become more compact, in-line monitored and auto-regulated.

Patient selection will remain a critical issue not least with changes in conventional management. Ventilation strategies are continuously being refined and new modalities assessed as the technology improves. Potentially promising also are pharmacological advances in the development and use of selective pulmonary vasodilators such as nitric oxide. Controlled trials may play an important part in this debate. However, it should be remembered that there are significant problems in applying standard randomization protocols to life support techniques, as the history of the evolution of ECMO has shown.

References

1. Bartlett RH. Extracorporeal life support for cardiopulmonary failure. *Curr Prob Surg* 1990; **27**, 621–705.
2. Arensman RM, Cornish JD (eds). *Extracorporeal Life Support*. Oxford: Blackwell Scientific, 1993
3. Gibbon JH. Application of a mechanical heart and lung apparatus to cardiac surgery. *Minn Med* 1954; **37**, 171.
4. Rashkind WJ, Freeman A, Klein D. Evaluation of a disposable plastic low volume pumpless oxygenator as a lung substitute. *J Paed* 1965; **66**, 94–102.
5. Yoshinaga N, *et al.* Application of assisting extracorporeal circulation to a patient with severe carbon dioxide intoxication. *Masui* 1966; **15**, 1041–1043.
6. Kolobow T, Hayano F, Weathersby PK. Dispersion-casting thin and ultrathin fabric-reinforced silicone rubber membrane for use in the membrane lung. *Med Instrum* 1975; **9**, 124–128.
7. Lande AJ, Dos SJ, Carlson RG, Perschau RA, Lange RP, Sonstegard LJ, Lillehei CW. A new membrane oxygenator–dialyzer. *Surg Clin N Amer* 1967; **47**, 1461–1470.
8. Hill JD, O'Brien TG, Murray JJ, Dontigny L, Bramson ML, Osborn JJ, Gerbode F. Prolonged extracorporeal oxygenation for acute post-traumatic respiratory failure (shock-lung syndrome): use of the Bramson membrane lung. *New Eng J Med* 1972; **286**, 629–634.
9. Zapol WM, Snider MT, Hill JD, Fallat RJ, Bartlett RH, Edmunds LH, Morris AH, Pierce E, Thomas AN, Proctor HJ, Drinker PA, Pratt PC, Bagniewski A, Miller RJ. Extracorporeal membrane oxygenation in severe acute respiratory failure: a randomized prospective study. *JAMA* 1979; **242**, 2193–2196.

10. Gattinoni L, Pesenti A, Mascheroni D, Marcolin R, Fumagalli R, Rossi F, Iapichino G, Romagnoli G, Uziel L, Agostoni A, *et al.* Low-frequency positive-pressure ventilation with extracorporeal CO_2 removal in severe acute respiratory failure. *JAMA* 1986; **256**, 881–886.

11. Bartlett RH, Gazzaniga AB, Jefferies R. Extracorporeal membrane oxygenation (ECMO) cardiopulmonary support in infancy. *ASAIO Trans* 1976; **22**, 80–88.

12. Bartlett RH, Andrews AF, Toomasian JM. Extracorporeal membrane oxygenation (ECMO) for newborn respiratory failure: 45 cases. *Surgery* 1982; **92**, 425–433.

13. Bartlett RH, Gazzaniga AB, Toomasian J, Coran AG, Roloff D, Rucker R, Corwin AG. Extracorporeal membrane oxygenation (ECMO) in neonatal respiratory failure. 100 cases. *Ann Surg* 1986; **204**, 236–245 (erratum: *Ann Surg* 1987; **205**, 11A).

14. Toomasian JM, Snedecor SM, Cornell RG, Cilley RE, Bartlett RH. National experience with extracorporeal membrane oxygenation for newborn respiratory failure: data from 715 cases. *ASAIO Trans* 1988; **34**, 140–147.

15. Bartlett RH, Roloff DW, Cornell RG, Andrews AF, Dillon PW, Zwischenberger JB. Extracorporeal circulation in neonatal respiratory failure: a prospective randomized study. *Pediatrics* 1985; **76**, 479–487.

16. O'Rourke PP, Crone RK, Vacanti JP, Ware JH, Lillehei CW, Parad RB, Epstein MF. Extracorporeal membrane oxygenation and conventional medical therapy in neonates with persistent pulmonary hypertension of the newborn: a prospective randomized study. *Pediatrics* 1989; **84**, 957–963.

17. Elliott SJ. Neonatal extracorporeal membrane oxygenation: how not to assess novel technologies (see comments). *Lancet* 1991; **337**, 476–478.

18. Lantos JD, Frader J. Extracorporeal membrane oxygenation and the ethics of clinical research in pediatrics (see comments). *New Eng J Med* 1990; **323**, 409–413.

19. O'Rourke PP, Crone RK. Pediatric applications of extracorporeal membrane oxygenation (editorial; comment). *J Pediat* 1990; **116**, 393–394.

20. Pearson GA, Grant J, Field D, Sosnowski A, Firmin RK. Extracorporeal life support in paediatrics. *Arch Dis Child* 1993; **68**, 94–96.

21. Adolph V, Heaton J, Steiner R, Bonis S, Falterman K, Arensman R. Extracorporeal membrane oxygenation for non-neonatal respiratory failure. *J Pediat Surg* 1991; **26**, 326–330.

22. Kolobow T. An update on adult extracorporeal membrane oxygenation—extracorporeal CO_2 removal. *ASAIO Trans* 1988; **34**, 1004–1005.

23. Levy FH, O'Rourke PP, Crone RK. Extracorporeal membrane oxygenation. *Anesth Analg* 1992; **75**, 1053–1062.

24. Bui KC, LaClair P, Vanderkerhove J, Bartlett RH. ECMO in premature infants: review of factors associated with mortality. *ASAIO Trans* 1991; **37**, 54–59.

25. Cilley RE, Zwischenberger JB, *et al.* Intracranial haemorrhage during extracorporeal membrane oxygenation. *Pediatrics* 1986; **78**, 699–704.

26. Bartlett RH. UK First National ECMO Conference, 1991 (unpublished).

27. Pearson GA, Firmin RK, Sosnowski A, Field D. Neonatal extracorporeal membrane oxygenation: review. *Br J Hosp Med* 1992; **47**, 646–653.

28. Wetmore NE, McEwen D, O'Connor MJ. Defining indications for artificial organ support in respiratory failure. *ASAIO Trans* 1979; **25**, 459–461.

29. Hallman M, Merritt TA, Jarvenpaa AL, Boynton B, Mannino F, Gluck L, Moore T, Edwards D. Exogenous human surfactant for treatment of severe respiratory distress syndrome: a randomised prospective clinical trial. *J Pediat* 1985; **106**, 963–969.

30. West JB (ed). *Best and Taylor's Physiological Basis of Medical Practice.* Baltimore: Williams & Wilkins, 1985: 572–585.

31. Beck R, Anderson KD, Pearson GD. Criteria for extracorporeal membrane oxygenation in a population of infants with persistent pulmonary hypertension of the newborn. *J Pediat Surg* 1986; **21**, 297–302.

32. Bohn D, Tamura M, Perrin D, Barker G, Rabinovitch M. Ventilatory predictors of pulmonary hypoplasia in congenital diaphragmatic hernia, confirmed by morphologic assessment. *J Pediat* 1987; **111**, 423–431.

33. Coughlin JC, Drucker DEM, Klein MD. Delayed repair of congenital diaphragmatic hernia. *Proc Third Annual Meeting of the Extracorporeal Life Support Organisation,* 1991: 23.

34. Johnston PW, Liberman R, Gangitano E, Vogt J. Ventilation parameters and arterial blood gases as a prediction of hypoplasia in congenital diaphragmatic hernia. *J Pediatr Surg* 1990; **25**, 496–499.

35. Stolar C, Dillon P, Reyes C. Selective use of extracorporeal membrane oxygenation in the management of congenital diaphragmatic hernia. *J Pediatr Surg* 1988; **23**, 207–211.

36. Bailey PV, Connors RH, Tracy TJ, Stephens C, Pennington DG, Weber TR. A critical analysis of extracorporeal membrane oxygenation for congenital diaphragmatic hernia (see comments). *Surgery* 1989; **106**, 611–615.

37. Adolph V, Arensman RM, Falterman KW, Goldsmith JP. Ventilatory management casebook: congenital diaphragmatic hernia meeting criteria for extracorporeal membrane oxygenation. *J Perinatol* 1990; **10**, 202–205.

38. Rivera RA, Butt W, Shann F. Predictors of mortality in children with respiratory failure: possible indications for ECMO. *Anaesth Intens Care* 1990; **18**, 385–389.

39. Kolobow T. Acute respiratory failure: on how to injure healthy lungs (and prevent sick lungs from recovering). *ASAIO Trans* 1988; **34**, 31–34.

40. Pratt PC, Vollmer RT, Shelburne JD, Crapo JD. Pulmonary morphology in a multihospital collaborative extracorporeal membrane oxygenation project. I: Light microscopy. *Am J Pathol* 1979; **95**, 191–214.

41. Gattinoni L, Pesenti A, Marcolin R, Mascheroni D, Fumagalli R, Rossi F, Avalli L, Giuffrida A, Baglioni S, Coffano B. Extracorporeal support in acute respiratory failure. In: Artigas A, Lemaire F, Suter P, Zapol WM (eds), *Adult Respiratory Distress Syndrome.* Edinburgh: Churchill Livingstone, 1992: 469–475.

42. Barth PJ, Knoch M, Muller E, Sangmeister C, Bittinger A. Morphometry of parenchymal and vascular alterations in ARDS after extracorporeal carbon dioxide removal therapy. *Pathol Res Pract* 1992; **188**, 653–656.

43. Pearson GA, Underwood M, Chan KC, Firmin RK. Extracorporeal membrane oxygenation and paediatric cardiology. *Cardiol Young* 1993; **3**, 197–201.

44. Vogler C, Sotelo AC, Lagunoff D, Braun P, Schreifels JA, Weber T. Aluminium-containing emboli in infants treated with extracorporeal membrane oxygenation. *New Engl J Med* 1988; **319**, 75–79.

45. Chevalier JY, Durandy Y, Batisse A, Mathe JC, Costil J. Preliminary report: extracorporeal lung support for neonatal acute respiratory failure. *Lancet* 1990; **335**, 1364–1366.

46. Bartlett RH, Cilley RE. Physiology of extracorporeal life support. In: Arensman RM, Cornish JD (eds), *Extracorporeal Life Support.* Oxford: Blackwell Scientific, 1993: 89–104.

47. Montoya JP, Merz SI, Bartlett RH. A standardized system for describing flow/pressure relationships in vascular access devices. *ASAIO Trans* 1991; **37**, 4–8.

48. Sinard JM, Merz SI, Hatcher MD, Montoya JP, Bartlett RH. Evaluation of extracorporeal perfusion catheters using a standardized measurement technique—the M number. *ASAIO Trans* 1991; **37**, 60–64.

49. Seo T, Ito T, Iio K, Kato J, Takagi H. Experimental study on the hemodynamic effects of veno-arterial extracorporeal membrane oxygenation with an automatically driven blood pump on puppies. *Artif Organs* 1991; **15**, 402–407.

50. Bavaria JE, Ratcliffe MB, Gupta KB, Wenger RK, Bogen DK, Edmunds LJ. Changes in left ventricular systolic wall stress during biventricular circulatory assistance. *Ann Thorac Surg* 1988; **45**, 526–532.

51. Axelrod HI, Baumann FG, Galloway AC. Left ventricular stress during extracorporeal membrane oxygenation (letter). *Ann Thorac Surg* 1989; **47**, 330.

52. Braunwald E, Kloner RA. The stunned myocardium: prolonged, postischemic ventricular dysfunction. *Circulation* 1982; **66**, 1146–1149.

53. Hirschl RB, Heiss KF, Bartlett RH. Severe myocardial dysfunction during extracorporeal membrane oxygenation. *J Pediat Surg* 1992; **27**, 48–53.

54. Kinsella JP, Gerstmann DR, Rosenberg AA. The effect of extracorporeal membrane oxygenation on coronary perfusion and regional blood flow distribution. *Pediat Res* 1992; **31**, 80–84.

55. Burch KD, Covitz W, Lovett EJ, Howell C, Kanto WJ. The significance of ductal shunting during extracorporeal membrane oxygenation. *J Pediat Surg* 1989; **24**, 855–889.

56. Hiratzka LF, Swan DM, Rose EF. Bilateral simultaneous lung lavage utilizing membrane oxygenator for pulmonary alveolar lipoproteinosis in an 8-month-old infant. *Ann Thorac Surg* 1983; **35**, 313–317.

57. Keszler M, Subramanian KN, Smith YA, Dhaniseddy R, Mehta N, Molina B, Cox CB, Moront MG. Pulmonary management during extracorporeal membrane oxygenation. *Crit Care Med* 1989; **17**, 495–500.

58. Keszler M, Ryckman FC, McDonald JJ, Sweet LD, Moront MG, Boegli MJ, Cox C, Leftridge CA. A prospective, multicenter, randomized study of high versus low positive end-expiratory pressure during extracorporeal membrane oxygenation. *J Pediat* 1992; **120**, 107–113.

59. Sosnowski AW, Bonser SJ, Field DJ, Graham TR, Firmin RK. Extracorporeal membrane oxygenation (see comments). *Br Med J* 1990; **301**, 303–304.

60. Glass P, Miller M, Short B. Morbidity for survivors of extracorporeal membrane oxygenation: neurodevelopmental outcome at 1 year of age. *Pediatrics* 1989; **83**, 72–78.

61. Adolph V, Ekelund C, Smith C, Starrett A, Falterman K, Arensman R. Developmental outcome of neonates treated with extracorporeal membrane oxygenation. *J Pediat Surg* 1990; **25**, 43–46.

62. Hofkosh D, Thompson AE, Nozza RJ, Kemp SS, Bowen A, Feldman HM. Ten years of extracorporeal membrane oxygenation: neurodevelopmental outcome. *Pediatrics* 1991; **87**, 549–555.

63. Brett C, Dekl M, *et al.* Developmental outcome of hyperventilated neonates: preliminary observations. *Pediatrics* 1981; **65**, 588–591.

64. Schneck HJ, Rupreht J. Central anticholinergic syndrome (CAS) in anesthesia and intensive care. *Acta Anaesth Belgica* 1989; **40**, 219–228.

65. Rupreht J, Dworacek B. Central anticholinergic syndrome during postoperative period. *Ann Franc Anesth Reanim* 1990; **9**, 295–304.

9

Extracorporeal venovenous long-term bypass for lung assist (ELA) in adults

H Lennartz

Introduction

The first extracorporeal long-term bypass (ECMO) for lung support in adults was carried out by Hill and associates.[1] The subsequent results of the multicentre study were, however, disappointing.[2] The survival rate of patients undergoing ECMO was no higher than that of patients who were treated with mechanical ventilation. In both groups the mortality rate was about 90%.

Adult respiratory distress syndrome (ARDS) has been defined by Ashbaugh et al.[3] as an acute arterial hypoxaemia. There is a progressive lung failure (Fig. 9.1) which can result from the aspiration of gastric contents, inhalation of toxic fumes, from pneumonia, or by capillary leak into the lung following shock or sepsis. The main reason for lung destruction in ARDS during mechanical ventilation is the hypoxic damage of the lung followed by liberation of numerous mediators and oxygen radicals. The patient becomes hypoxic and hypercapnic. Mechanical ventilation leads either to healing or to a further deterioration of gas exchange (Fig. 9.2). Increased ventilation leads to a vicious circle, which finally reaches a point of no return and causes the death of the patient from the complications of mechanical ventilation. Numerous studies based on animal experiments have proved that mechanical ventilation alone may be the reason for barotrauma and lung destruction, and may even be the reason for multiple organ failure.[4,5]

The method of bypass

Since 1985, our institution has treated 137 patients suffering from ARDS with a technique of extracorporeal lung assist (ELA) which was developed by Kolobow and Gattinoni.[6] We use a venovenous bypass technique. The venous blood is drained from the inferior vena cava into a reservoir via a double-lumen catheter.[7] From the inferior vena cava the blood is passed via a roller pump through two silicone membrane gas-exchange devices (which each have a surface area of 4.5 m^2) to the patient through the interior lumen of the right atrial cannula. In order to improve the CO_2 elimination the gas exchange devices are connected in series. In counter-flow to the blood flow, oxygen or an oxygen–air mixture, which is warmed and moistened, is conducted through the membrane gas-exchange device with the help of a vacuum. The scheme is shown in Chapter 6 (Fig. 6.5).

Heparin is added continually during the bypass. The heparin dose is adapted to the activated clotting time (ACT) and the activated partial thromboplastin time (APTT). We keep the ACT at 180–200 s and the APTT at 50–60 s. During the bypass we carry out apnoic oxygenation with low-frequency positive-pressure mechanical ventilation of 4–5 l/min. In addition, the patient receives 0.5–1 litres of oxygen via a fine catheter which is sited in the trachea near to the bifurcation. In order to avoid barotrauma, the maximum pressure of the ventilator is limited to 35–40 cmH$_2$O. The priming volume of the bypass circuit is 2 litres and consists of 4 units of packed red blood cells and 4 units of fresh frozen plasma with 400 IU of heparin per unit.

Since September 1989 we have used a heparin-coated system with PVC tubing and microporous polypropylene membrane lungs. All tubes and connectors, as well as the membrane lung, are heparin-coated.

In collaboration with Stoeckert Instrumente GmbH, Munich, we have developed a system in which a bubble detector and a water circuit are integrated with a flowmeter for the mixing of oxygen and room air (Fig. 9.3). To cannulate the inferior vena cava, a 23–25 Charrier catheter is inserted to the atrial border through the femoral vein using the Seldinger technique. With the same technique, the right jugular vein is cannulated with a 17–19 Charrier catheter. The catheters are heparin-coated. With this new system, the priming volume of the extracorporeal circuit has been reduced to 1 litre. The priming volume consists of 2 units of packed red cells and 2 units

of fresh frozen plasma and 500 IU of antithrombin III. During bypass, heparin and AT-III are added continuously. The heparin dose is adapted to the APTT, and the AT-III dose is adapted to the serum AT-III level. We keep the APTT at 35–45 s and the AT-III above 100%.

Results

One hundred and thirty-seven patients (64 male, 73 female) suffering from ARDS stage 4 (according to the Morel classification[8]) were treated with extracorporeal bypass to assist lung function. The average age was 29.2 ± 12.2 years. The average pretreatment time was 15 ± 9 days and the average time of support was 12.5 ± 8 days. The underlying diseases were: multiple trauma 39%, pneumonia 23%, surgical and post-surgical complications 14%, complications during pregnancy and delivery 16% and others, including inhalation aspiration, 8%.

Ventilation scores were calculated for all

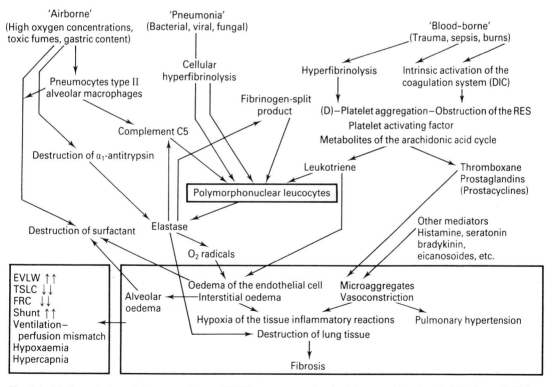

Fig. 9.1 Adult respiratory distress syndrome (ARDS): causes, pathophysiology and biochemical findings. EVLW = extravascular lung water; TSLC = total statistic lung compliance; FRC = functional residual capacity.

patients following the method of Smith and Gordon.[9] All scored more than 80 points. The expected mortality of this group, according to Smith and Gordon, was 100%.

All patients were treated for 12–24 hours with a conventional ventilation plan of treatment, including all therapeutic measures; i.e. inversed-ratio ventilation, high PEEP, haemodynamic stabilization, forced-fluid output, and cleaning of the respiratory tract. If there was no significant

improvement in the status of the patient following this, bypass was started.

Contraindications to extracorporeal ventilatory support were: craniocerebral trauma with fresh intracerebral bleeding, acute bleeding, large bronchopleural fistula, progressive fibrosis, cardiac lung oedema, lymphangitis carcinomatosis, immunosuppression including AIDS, and age greater than 65 years.

Sixty-seven patients were treated with the non-heparinized system; 70% showed an improvement in gas exchange and 52% survived. Seventy patients were treated with the heparinized system; 79% showed an improvement in gas exchange and 64% survived.

In 10 patients, gas exchange and static and dynamic lung volumes were measured one and two years after ELA (Fig. 9.4). By discharge, gas exchange showed a significantly decreased P_{O_2}. Dynamic lung volumes were 35% of the predicted values. Total lung capacity was reduced to 40% and vital capacity was reduced to 30%. Two years later all pulmonary function tests showed normal values.

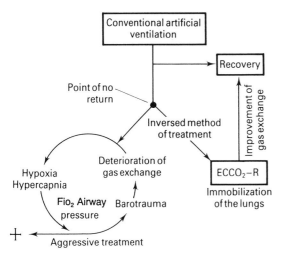

Fig. 9.2 Problems with mechanical ventilation in severe progressive ARDS.

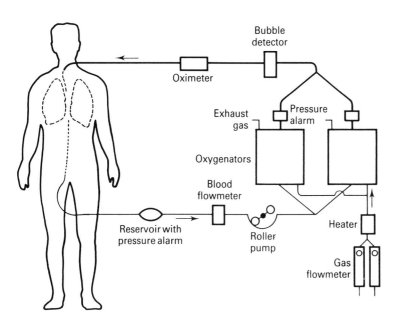

Fig. 9.3 Model of the Stoecker venovenous bypass system.

Complications

Complications included reduction of platelet numbers to under 50% of the starting value, bleeding around the surgical cannulae, and bleeding from the lung. In five cases we had to disconnect the patients from the bypass because of lung bleeding. The daily blood loss was 675 ml with the conventional system and 425 ml using the heparin-coated system.

On starting treatment with the heparin-coated system in patients with high levels of bilirubin, there were frequent plasma leakages. According to one theory (K. Motthagy, personal communication) this is due to the changed surface tension of the patient's plasma. After the development of

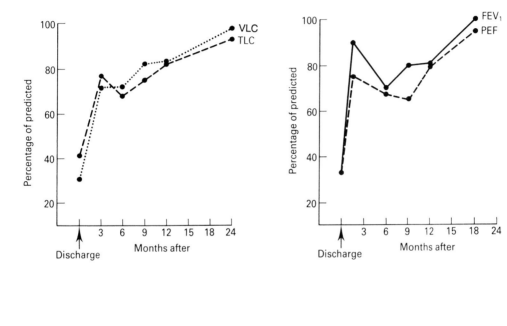

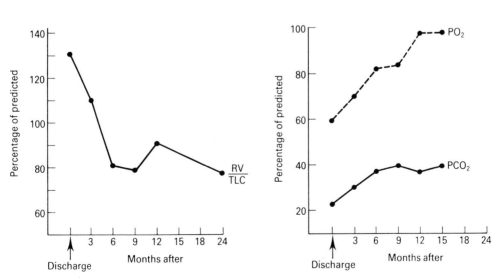

Fig. 9.4 (*Top left and right*) Static and dynamic lung volumes after extracorporeal CO_2 removal. (*Bottom right*) Arterial blood gas pressures. (*Bottom left*) Degree of emphysema (RV/TLC). TLC = total lung capacity; VLC = vital lung capacity; RV = residual volume.

'EKLA 3' by Carmeda AB, Sweden, the stability of the membrane lungs was considerably increased, with no decrease in gas exchange.

Discussion

Kolobow and associates have demonstrated the dissociation of respiratory function in animals,[6] and have suggested the concept of apnoeic oxygenation in extracorporeal CO_2 elimination. They demonstrated that ventilation is not necessary to maintain a normal oxygen partial pressure, if a quantity of oxygen corresponding to the oxygen required is delivered by a bronchoalveolar oxygen supply under conditions of normal pulmonary blood flow. Ventilation (i.e. the elimination of the metabolic CO_2) can then be performed by a venovenous bypass and a membrane lung. The reaction of Pv_{CO_2} and Pa_{CO_2} during ELA and the ventilation patterns (Fig. 9.5) prove that the method is really apnoeic oxygenation. During the non-physiological situation of a closed system, with insufflation of oxygen and reduced elimination of CO_2, the arterial Pco_2 can not only reach the mixed venous value but even surpass it. This is the so-called Christiansen–Douglas–Haldane effect.

The method of ELA with low-frequency positive-pressure ventilation (LFPPV) is different from ECMO in various ways (Table 9.1). The aim of ECMO is to overcome the breakdown in arterial oxygenation and to reduce the Fio_2 on the ventilator. ELA, however, serves to rest the lung and reverse the therapeutic principle from high-frequency ventilation and ventilation with high tidal volumes and high peak inspiratory pressure (PIP) to LFPPV with reduced pressure. Unlike ECMO, ELA is characterized by a venovenous bypass with a low blood flow and high gas flow; i.e.

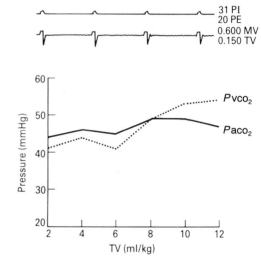

Fig. 9.5 Ventilation patterns (pressures and volumes) and inverse reaction of Pv_{CO_2} and Pa_{CO_2} independent of tidal volume. PI = inspiratory pressure; PE = terminal expiratory pressure; MV = minute volume; TV = tidal volume.

Table 9.1 Principal differences between ECMO (venoarterial bypass) and extracorporeal CO_2 removal (venovenous bypass—ELA).

	ECMO	ECCO$_2$-R
Purpose of treatment	Short-term oxygenation and reduction of Fio_2	Long-term repose of lung and reduction of PIP and Fio_2, but apnoeic oxygenation by the affected lung
Extracorporeal circulation	VA for oxygenation of arterial blood Substitution of oxygenation	VV to eliminate CO_2 Substitution of ventilation
Respiration	Conventional CPPV Frequency 8–15 Max pressure 50 cmH$_2$O PEEP 5–10 cmH$_2$O	LFPPV Frequency 2–4 Max pressure 35–40 cmH$_2$O PEEP 20–30 cmH$_2$O
Bypass flow	3–6 l/min	30% of cardiac output 1.5–2.5 l/min
Haemodynamics	Influenced by the VA bypass	Not influenced
Lung blood flow	10–20% of cardiac output	100% of cardiac output Increase of mixed venous O$_2$ saturation
Duration	2–10 days	Up to 25 days
Success	About 10% under comparable indication	About 50% under comparable indication

Table 9.2 Svo_2 in 10 patients during extracorporeal CO_2 removal, compared with 10 patients undergoing ECMO.

	Before bypass	During bypass
ECMO	56%	55%
ECCO$_2$-R	56.7%	79.8%

Source: reference 10.

high ventilation and perfusion ratio of the membrane lungs. During ELA, haemodynamics are not affected, the lung perfusion is not altered and, importantly for the healing of the lung, the mixed venous oxygen saturation is increased. On comparing the results of Jardin *et al.*[10] with the data from 10 of our patients (Table 9.2), there is no increase in Svo_2 with ECMO; but during ELA, Svo_2 increased from 56.7% to 79.8%. We consider this to be an important difference. The oxygen delivered via the bronchial arteries only reaches the bronchioles. The pneumocytes type I and II and the interstitial tissue of the lung receive oxygen only from the pulmonary artery. Owing to the reduction of lung perfusion during ECMO and the additional trauma of mechanical ventilation with high PIP, the lung becomes necrotic. At autopsy, Jardin and coworkers discovered that a generalized severe necrosis of the lungs had developed before death in all 10 patients who were treated with ECMO.

The reduction of mortality to below 50% in patients with severe progressive ARDS stage 4 argues strongly for the use of ELA. This technique seems to be superior to any other form of respiratory treatment currently available for these patients.

References

1. Hill JD, O'Brian TG, Murray JD. Prolonged extracorporeal oxygenation for acute post-traumatic respiratory failure (shock-lung syndrome). *New Engl J Med* 1972; **286**, 629–634.
2. Zapol WM, Snider MT, Hill JD. Extracorporeal membrane oxygenation in severe acute respiratory failure. *JAMA* 1979; **242**, 2193–2196.
3. Ashbaugh DG, Bigelow DB, Petty TL, Levine BE. Acute respiratory distress in adults. *Lancet* 1967; **2**, 319–323.
4. Kirby RR. Ventilatory support and pulmonary barotrauma. *Anesthesiology* 1979; **50**, 181–182.
5. Dreyfuss D, Basset G, Soler P, Saumon G. Permeability pulmonary edema due to ventilation with high peak airway pressure is related to changes in volume, not in pressure. *Am Rev Resp Dis* 1986; **133**, A266.
6. Kolobow T, Gattinoni L, Tomlinson T, Pierce JE. An alternative to breathing. *J Thorac Cardiovasc Surg* 1978; **75**, 261–266.
7. Pesenti A, Kolobow T, Biboni A, Gattinoni L, Damia G. Single vein cannulation for extracorporal respiratory support: life support system. *Proceedings of the Ninth Meeting of the European Society for Artificial Organs*, Brussels, 1982: 165–196.
8. Morel DR, Dargent F, Bachmann M, Suter PM, Junod AF. Pulmonary extraction of serotonin and propranolol in patients with adult respiratory distress syndrome. *Am Rev Resp Dis* 1985; **132**, 479–484.
9. Smith PEM, Gordon IJ. An index to predict outcome of adult respiratory distress syndrome. *Intens Care Med* 1986; **12**, 86–89.
10. Jardin F, Regnier B, Gastine H, Lemaire F. Pulmonary hemodynamics and gas exchange during veno-arterial bypass with membrane lung oxygenation. In: Unger F (ed), *Assisted Circulation*. Berlin: Springer Verlag, 1979: 258–266.

Section III

Cardiopulmonary Bypass

10

Pulsatile and non-pulsatile perfusion in cardiac surgery: the continuing controversy*

Kenneth M Taylor

Introduction

There are few more physiological concepts than that of pulsatile blood flow. It therefore seems strange that, when cardiac surgeons stop the heart and substitute artificial blood flow by extracorporeal circulation, the majority continue to use non-pulsatile arterial perfusion. In the earliest days of open heart surgery, the will to develop and use suitable pulsatile pump systems was much in evidence. The technological complexity of early systems, and the growing awareness that relatively short periods of smooth non-pulsatile perfusion were compatible with survival, encouraged the adoption of non-pulsatile flow as the accepted mode of perfusion. Yet this is surely a case of 'virtue out of necessity'. If pulsatile pumps could be developed which were simple, safe, reliable and cost-effective in use, would physiological superiority overcome traditional compromise?

Technology has now provided cardiac surgeons with the necessary pulsatile pumps which fulfil the above criteria. Nevertheless, the move towards pulsatile perfusion in routine cardiac surgery, while adopted enthusiastically by a minority, has evoked little or no response from the majority. The natural conservatism of many cardiac surgeons is understandable. At the heart of this issue, however, is the persistent confusion and uncertainty concerning the real benefit(s) of pulsatile perfusion. The published literature is extensive, but apparently contradictory. The confusion will persist as long as uncertainties exist regarding the primary effects of pulsatile and non-pulsatile perfusion in clinical cardiac surgery, and when surgeons are more convinced that the clinical benefits are real, quantifiable and understandable. In addition, such conviction must be sufficient to overcome the negative impact of issues of simplicity and reliability in day-to-day operation, cost implications, and the inevitable inertia of traditional practice.

This background may explain the continuing controversy relating to pulsatile perfusion. It is, apparently, an evergreen subject for further study and debate. Recent interest in the use of pulsatile perfusion in other areas of extracorporeal circulation has added fresh fuel to the fire (such as ECMO, ventricular assist, organ preservation). The author has had both a research and a clinical interest in this area for about 20 years. This chapter is written with the sure knowledge that, whatever else, it will not be the last word on this subject. It is written, however, as a trilogy—containing, as it must do whenever pulsatile perfusion is discussed, elements of physiology, technology and even psychology.

*This chapter is a modified version of a review article that appeared in *Perfusion* 1988; **3**, 1–16.

Vasoconstriction during cardiac surgery

The essential haemodynamic consequence of cardiopulmonary bypass (CPB) perfusion is the development of progressive systemic arterial vasoconstriction. Numerous studies have documented the progressive rise in vascular resistance index from the onset of artificial circulation, extending through into the early postoperative period following cardiac surgery.[1–6] The associated arterial hypertension has necessitated the widespread use of vasodilator agents such as sodium nitroprusside or GTN.[7]

The pathological consequences of vasoconstriction are two-fold:

1. Peripheral circulatory adequacy is reduced.
2. Vasoconstriction necessarily increases left ventricular work.

Where the elevation of vascular resistance is modest and myocardial contractile function is normal, increased peripheral resistance will be associated with a corresponding increase in myocardial performance and ventricular work.[8] Excessive elevation in peripheral resistance may, however, impose an excessive afterload on the left ventricle, with eventual reduction in cardiac pumping efficiency and fall in cardiac output. In patients whose ventricular function is already compromised and whose reserve is limited, even modest rises in vascular resistance may result in cardiac decompensation. Once vasoconstriction has been established, a vicious circle may develop with reduction in cardiac output leading to peripheral circulatory inadequacy with consequent release of peripheral vasoconstrictor substances which further raise vascular resistance and further diminish cardiac output.[6,9–11]

The pattern of vasoconstriction during and after open heart surgery is shown in Fig. 10.1. The progressive rise in vascular resistance index during the period of extracorporeal circulation and into the early postoperative period is well shown. It is obvious that such an elevation in peripheral vascular resistance will necessarily present the left ventricle at the end of the perfusion period with an obligatory increase in workload. This increased work is demanded at a time when the heart is recovering from the period of aortic cross-clamping and ischaemic arrest required during the cardiac surgical procedure. The vasoconstriction associated with extracorporeal circulation thus creates a detrimental haemodynamic envir-

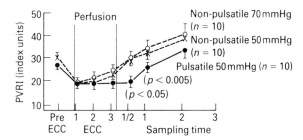

Fig. 10.1 Effect of pulsatile and non-pulsatile perfusion on peripheral vascular resistance index (PVRI). Note that both non-pulsatile groups show vasoconstriction during the perfusion period. Pulsatile perfusion maintains normal PVRI levels during perfusion. Reproduced by permission from reference 16.

onment (Fig. 10.2). The early days of cardiac surgery were marked by a high incidence of low cardiac output syndrome. Though myocardial preservation techniques have ensured substantially superior contractile function from the recovering myocardium,[12–14] it is logical that maintenance of normal vascular resistance index levels would be associated with superior cardiac performance in the recovery period. Subsequent studies have shown that where high PVRI levels are reduced following cardiac surgery (e.g. with vasodilator techniques such as epidural anaesthesia, sodium nitroprusside, etc.), a significant increase in cardiac performance is the inevitable result.[7,15]

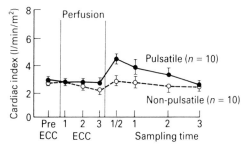

Fig. 10.2 Effect of pulsatile and non-pulsatile perfusion on cardiac index. These results are taken from the same experimental subjects as in Fig. 10.1. Note that cardiac index is significantly higher in the first hour postperfusion in the pulsatile group. Reproduced by permission from reference 16.

Vasoconstrictor mechanisms during cardiac surgery

Following the initial descriptions of the vasoconstrictive response to open heart surgery, a number of aetiological mechanisms have been proposed. These include:

1. Catecholamine release.
2. Activation of the renin–angiotensin system.
3. Increased secretion of vasopressin (ADH).
4. Local tissue vasoconstrictor agents (e.g. thromboxane A_2).

A number of reports have indicated that catecholamine secretion is increased during and after open heart surgery. This may be directly related to the use of hypothermia during surgery, but must also be a response to the altered perfusion associated with the use of non-pulsatile flow.[16] Both vasopressin/ADH and renin–angiotensin activation have been related directly to non-pulsatile perfusion. Lack of pulsatility in the arterial circulation appears to trigger both of these important vasoconstrictor mechanisms. The speed of response of vasopressin release[17] appears more rapid than that of renin–angiotensin activation which has been studied extensively by the author's group.[5,9,15] The potential role of thromboxane A_2 in the vasoconstrictive response to cardiac surgery has only recently emerged.[18] Increased thromboxane production appears to be a result of non-pulsatile perfusion, though the role of platelet activation, a major consequence of extracorporeal circulation, may be much more important.

Renin–angiotensin activation during cardiac surgery

It has been known for many years that loss of pulsatility in the renal arteries with maintenance of mean flow and pressure is associated with increased renin release.[19,20] The end-product of renin–angiotensin activation is the powerful vasoconstrictor, angiotensin II. Marked elevation of plasma angiotensin II has been demonstrated both during and after cardiac surgical procedures.[5,9,15] In addition to its vasoconstrictive action, angiotensin II has been shown to produce subendocardial ischaemia in the heart. Studies have shown a significant correlation between the increase in angiotensin II levels and the increase

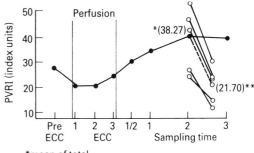

Fig. 10.3 Effect of angiotensin converting enzyme inhibitor (SQ14225) on vasoconstriction after non-pulsatile CPB. The mean levels of PVRI are shown for the placebo controls. The change in PVRI levels is shown for each individual subject at the start and end of the 20-minute infusion period. Note the rapid fall in PVRI levels to normal in the SQ14225 group. Reproduced by permission from reference 21.

in vascular resistance index during cardiac surgery.[9] The principal role of angiotensin II in postoperative haemodynamics has been shown when elevated angiotensin II levels were reduced rapidly using a specific angiotensin I/angiotensin II converting enzyme inhibitor. A highly significant fall in vascular resistance levels is seen with a simultaneous increase in cardiac index (Figs 10.3 and 10.4).[21]

Thus far we have identified vasoconstriction as the principal haemodynamic feature in cardiac surgery patients. The rise in vascular resistance begins at the onset of perfusion and continues

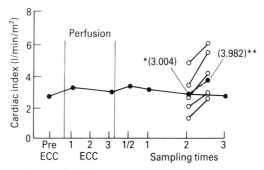

Fig. 10.4 Effect of angiotensin converting enzyme inhibitor (SQ14225) on cardiac index after non-pulsatile CPB. These results are taken from the same experimental subjects as in Fig. 10.3. Note the substantial rise in cardiac index in the SQ14225 group associated with the abolition of vasoconstriction. Reproduced by permission from reference 21.

into the early postoperative period. It threatens cardiovascular stability, first by compromising vital organ perfusion and second by increasing LV work. A number of vasopressor substances have been identified, all of which appear to be secreted in excess during cardiac surgery, specifically during the period of artificial circulation when perfusion is non-pulsatile.

Pulsatile and non-pulsatile perfusion during cardiac surgery

When cardiac surgery began, pioneering workers had, in many instances, attempted to develop pulsatile systems which would reproduce the pulsatile flow produced by the normal heart. The technological complexity of these systems proved, at that time, to be an insurmountable barrier and the use of short periods of non-pulsatile perfusion during cardiopulmonary bypass were found to be compatible with patient survival.[22] Confidence increased and non-pulsatile perfusion became established as the routine mode of perfusion. Over the years, and particularly in the last decade, however, studies have demonstrated, both in terms of metabolism and haemodynamics, that non-pulsatile flow has a potentially detrimental effect on cell metabolism and organ function. These pathological effects were either preventable or significantly diminished by substituting more physiological pulsatile flow during the period of artificial circulation. One of the principal theories proposed for the physiological effects of pulsatile arterial blood flow relates to neuro-endocrine reflex mechanisms triggered by baroreceptor discharge. Angell-James and de Burgh[23] have shown that carotid baroreceptors exhibit a marked increase in discharge frequency when arterial flow is changed from pulsatile to non-pulsatile, even for the same mean levels of flow and pressure. Other authors have suggested that this baroreceptor mechanism might induce reflex vasoconstriction in the peripheral circulation either by direct neural reflexes or stimulating the release of humoral vasoconstrictors (e.g. angiotensin, vasopressin or catecholamines).[24]

Haemodynamic effects of pulsatile perfusion

It is now generally accepted on the basis of numerous studies that pulsatile perfusion prevents vasoconstriction associated with non-pulsatile perfusion.[1,2,9,25–28] Similar results have been shown for plasma angiotensin II levels, indicating that pulsatile perfusion prevents the large and progressive rise in renin–angiotensin activation[9] and vasopressin release.[17] Philbin[18] has reported attenuation of the rise in the local vasoconstrictor thromboxane A_2 with the use of pulsatile perfusion. These results are interesting in that at least three known vasoconstrictor mechanisms appear to be significantly modified when pulsatile flow is used during the period of artificial circulation.

A number of groups using pulsatile perfusion in clinical practice have also reported improved haemodynamic status in the immediate postoperative phase after pulsatile flow. Some have reported a reduced requirement for circulatory support either with intra-aortic balloon counterpulsation or with inotropic drugs.[29–31] Reduced perioperative myocardial infarction has been reported with a significant reduction in haemodynamic related mortality and a lower incidence of intraoperative and low cardiac output associated deaths.[31] These clinical studies have demonstrated the haemodynamic superiority of pulsatile perfusion particularly in those patients with impaired LV function. In such patients, excessive vasoconstriction may exceed the already diminished reserve of LV function and so set up the essentials for a low cardiac output state in the postoperative period.

Organ function studies during pulsatile and non-pulsatile perfusion

Many studies have been reported in the literature concerning the metabolic effects of pulsatile and non-pulsatile perfusion during cardiac surgical procedures. These may be considered as studies concerned with cell metabolism in general and specific organ function studies including brain, kidney, liver and pancreas.

General cell metabolism

The basic processes of cell metabolism (in particular oxygen consumption and the development of metabolic acidosis) have been considered to reflect the overall state of capillary flow and adequacy of tissue perfusion.[1,2,32] Reduced oxygen consumption and increasing metabolic acidosis are accepted as the inevitable accompaniment of non-pulsatile perfusion.[1,2,33–35] Others have reported impaired uptake of energy substrates including glucose. These disturbances in general cell metabolism may well reflect the reduction in peripheral tissue perfusion in response to the vasoconstrictive effect of non-pulsatile flow. Though some authors have suggested that normal cell metabolism may be restored by raising flow rates above 110 ml/kg/min,[36–38] this remains both controversial and impractical in view of the excessively high flow rates it would entail. There is general agreement that at the customary flow rates of 60–100 ml/kg/min, the disturbance in cell metabolism may be prevented by using pulsatile perfusion.[1–4,2–28,32–35]

Vital organ function

Brain

Cerebral function during and after cardiac surgery is presently an area of particular interest and concern in view of the reported high incidence of cerebral dysfunction in cardiac surgical patients.[39–42] A number of studies have indicated that non-pulsatile perfusion is associated with haemodynamic and metabolic disturbance in the brain. Recent studies have shown a significant reduction in cerebral capillary diameter and cerebral blood flow levels during non-pulsatile perfusion. These changes were not observed during pulsatile flow for the same mean levels of flow and pressure.[43,44] Though brain cell death has been attributed to the use of non-pulsatile perfusion,[45] it is more generally accepted that non-pulsatile flow produces a functional disturbance in the brain and not a syndrome of irreversible cell structural damage unless severe carotid stenotic lesions coexist.[41,46]

The author's group has used the hypothalamic pituitary axis as a useful study model for cerebral function during open heart surgery.[47–54] The pattern of stress responses during surgical procedures is well described. During cardiac surgery using non-pulsatile perfusion, however, the normal hypothalamic pituitary stress response patterns are not seen. The anterior pituitary remains unresponsive to a trophic stimulus of thyrotrophin releasing hormone (TRH) in contrast to the normal response seen during major non-cardiac surgery.[51] This anterior pituitary hypofunction is also seen in the fall-off of ACTH secretion to substress levels and the consequent reduction in cortisol secretion by the adrenal cortex.[47,48] The abnormal hypothalamic–pituitary adrenal function which occurs during non-pulsatile perfusion returns rapidly to normal within 30 minutes of the end of the period of artificial circulation. The anterior pituitary TRH response returns to normal, ACTH and cortisol secretions return to stress levels.

In comparative studies of patients carefully matched and perfused at the same levels of mean flow and pressure, those patients perfused with pulsatile flow (Fig. 10.5) retained normal TRH response patterns and normal stress levels of ACTH and cortisol secretion (Fig. 10.6) during artificial circulation.[52,53] Similar results have been reported by Philbin's group in relation to the posterior pituitary secretion of vasopressin/ADH.[17]

Liver

Liver dysfunction following open heart surgery is a well-known phenomenon and is particularly

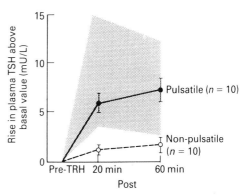

Fig. 10.5 Anterior pituitary responses to thyrotrophin-releasing hormone (TRH) during pulsatile and non-pulsatile perfusion. Note that the patients perfused with pulsatile flow in identical perfusion conditions exhibit restoration of a normal TRH test response (normal response range shown in cross-hatched area). TRH response during non-pulsatile perfusion is subnormal. Reproduced by permission from reference 53.

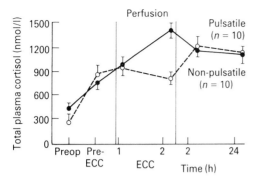

Fig. 10.6 Plasma cortisol levels corrected for haemodilution during pulsatile and non-pulsatile perfusion. Note that pulsatile perfusion preserves cortisol secretion during the perfusion period, in contrast to the fall in cortisol levels during non-pulsatile flow. Reproduced by permission from reference 52

seen in patients with preoperative hepatic dysfunction or pre-existing congestive cardiac failure.[55–57] Recent studies have been carried out to investigate the effects of pulsatile and non-pulsatile perfusion on liver haemodynamics and oxygen consumption.[58] The results of these studies have confirmed that pulsatile perfusion maintains significantly lower peripheral vascular resistance in the general circulation and that total liver blood flow is sustained more effectively by pulsatile perfusion due to specific preservation of hepatic arterial and portal venous flow (Fig. 10.7). In addition, hepatic oxygen consumption was better preserved during and after pulsatile perfusion. The authors concluded that the

improvement in total liver blood flow under pulsatile perfusion conditions related to the prevention of hepatic arterial vasoconstriction which was seen with non-pulsatile flow.[58] It must be said, however, that the liver has a different haemodynamic and metabolic environment by virtue of the contribution to total liver blood flow and oxygen availability of the portal venous component.

Pancreas

Ischaemic pancreatitis has been reported in a number of patients after open heart surgery.[59] Most authors believed the pancreatitis reflected impaired perfusion of the organ during the period of extracorporeal circulation and particularly where low cardiac output continued into the early postoperative period. In addition, isolated findings have suggested that plasma amylase levels are significantly increased after non-pulsatile perfusion.[60] The definitive study of Murray, using the amylase creatinine clearance ratio as a more accurate index of pancreatic exocrine function, showed a marked increase in ACCR values in patients perfused with non-pulsatile flow. Levels remained elevated over the first 48 hours following cardiac surgery. By contrast a matched set of patients perfused with pulsatile flow showed no ACCR elevation during or after the cardiac surgery procedure (Fig. 10.8).

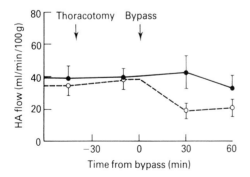

Fig. 10.7 Hepatic arterial flow measured during pulsatile and non-pulsatile CPB. The significant fall in flow during non-pulsatile perfusion (broken line) is associated with a simultaneous rise in hepatic arterial resistance. Pulsatile perfusion maintains constant hepatic arterial flow levels. Reproduced by permission from reference 58.

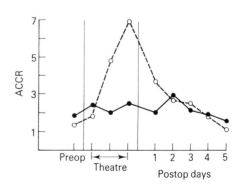

Fig. 10.8 Amylase creatinine clearance ratios (ACCR) in patients perfused with pulsatile (closed circles) and non-pulsatile perfusion (open circles) during open heart surgery. The ACCR is markedly elevated in the non-pulsatile group beginning at the onset of perfusion. The ACCR levels remain at control values in the pulsatile group. Reproduced by permission from reference 61.

Kidney

Despite the fact that many of the earliest studies into the pathophysiology of pulsatile and non-pulsatile perfusion focused on the kidney, the organ appears relatively resistant to the altered haemodynamics of cardiac surgery. Several authors have previously reported defects in renal excretory function during non-pulsatile flow.[62–66] In addition, a number of studies have demonstrated that pulsatile perfusion is associated with significantly higher blood flow levels than the corresponding figures for non-pulsatile flow.[63–67] It is the author's conviction, however, that renal vascular auto-regulation exerts a considerable protective mechanism by which the kidney is spared many of the deleterious effects of altered perfusion. In our experience, relatively sophisticated tests of renal tubular function have to be used before any significant differences may be demonstrated. It appears that the kidney is more resistant to the perfusion differences between pulsatile and non-pulsatile flow than are other organs.

It is important to gain a proper perspective in relation to the disturbances in vital organ function associated with conventional non-pulsatile CPB. The effect of the imperfect perfusion of non-pulsatile flow seems primarily to be a functional impairment which is fully reversible, assuming restoration of normal spontaneous pulsatile circulation in the cardiac recovery period and maintenance of optimal perfusion at least in the first 48 hours after surgery. In the vast majority of patients undergoing cardiac surgery, such restoration of optimal perfusion is the norm and, as has been shown, rapid functional recovery in vital organs may be demonstrated. There is a sense, however, in which the initial imperfect perfusion and functional disturbance 'prime' these vital organs, so that if an additional haemodynamic insult or period of severe cardiovascular instability occurs in the cardiac recovery period or within the first 24–28 hours following surgery, the additional haemodynamic insult will rapidly induce the full-blown picture of organ failure. This has been seen and reported in a number of situations (e.g. where the early postoperative period following cardiac surgery is complicated by a period of cardiac arrest or a period of extreme low cardiac output). In such circumstances complete renal failure, hepatic failure and the appearance of definitive ischaemic pancreatitis have all been reported. It is the author's firm belief that in routine cardiac surgical practice it is preferable to utilize pulsatile perfusion and so deliver optimal perfusion during the period of artificial circulation, thus preventing any of the attendant complications described.

Practical aspects of pulsatile perfusion during cardiac surgery

Reports of clinical use of pulsatile perfusion systems during cardiac surgery have not infrequently lacked adequate detail or basic understanding of practical issues.

Pulsatile flow delivery may itself be variable, depending on the type of pulsatile perfusion system employed. The use of modified roller pumps to deliver pulsatile flow has, in the author's opinion, been most successful in clinical practice. Modified roller pumps, usually based on a stepping motor which accelerates and decelerates the pump head, are simple, reliable and familiar in use, and require no modifications in cannulation techniques. Although more complex ventricular-type pumps have been developed, with claims that they provide more physiological waveforms than modified roller pumps, clinical experience with such pumps has been more limited. Those systems based on the intra-aortic balloon pump (e.g. the pulsatile assist device or PAD) place the pumping chamber in the arterial return line. Fears regarding possible gas embolism, and some reports of increased haemolysis, have raised concerns over these particular devices. Although claims have been made for the pulsatile capability of centrifugal pumps, the flat sinusoidal output of these pumps is not truly pulsatile when compared with modified roller or ventricular pumps.

There is a real need for investigators to provide clear data on flows, pressure, dP/dT and dFlow/dT generated by particular systems. Fourier analysis of pulsatile waveforms has been advocated by some experts.

It is also important to recognize that other components of the extracorporeal circuit may modify the pulsatility delivered into the patient's arterial circulation. In particular, membrane oxygenators exert a variable 'damping' effect, although arterial cannulae and arterial line filters may also be implicated.

Variability in anaesthetic technique may also be

important. High-dose narcotic anaesthesia may block the normal vasoconstrictive endocrine stress responses. Any anaesthetic or pharmacological regimen which is vasodilatory may reduce systemic vascular resistance levels substantially. Many units around the world undertake CPB at systemic vascular resistance (SVR) levels of less than 50% of accepted normal values. At such low levels of SVR, pulsatile pumps will not generate the pulsatile arterial pressure and flow patterns in the patient's circulation seen when pulsing at normal levels of vascular resistance.

The role of platelet and white cell activation in microembolic organ damage

If we have at least some understanding of the ways in which to optimize perfusion during cardiac surgery, there remains an area of pathophysiology which is as yet rather poorly understood. This relates to the response of blood cells, specifically platelet and white blood cell activation. Platelets and white cells may be activated by a number of stimuli.[68–72] During cardiac surgery, massive activation is induced by bringing the circulatory blood into contact with the artificial materials of the CPB circuit. The materials used in tubing, oxygenators, reservoirs, etc., are in no sense biocompatible. Though full heparin anticoagulation is employed, platelet and white blood cell activation and the formation of blood cell aggregates cannot yet be prevented.[73,74] Such blood cell responses to synthetic materials may be seen also in other situations (e.g. haemodialysis or haemofiltration). Microaggregates are also a feature of stored homologous blood and may be introduced into the patient's venous circulation during homologous blood transfusion.

Blood cell microemboli during cardiac surgery were initially thought to exert their pathologies simply by blocking the small blood vessels and creating subsequent ischaemia in vital organs (e.g. brain, kidney, etc.). Such an approach is now understood to be too simplistic, since studies have shown that the blood cells within cellular microaggregates are active and appear to liberate the contents of their secretory granules into the adjacent capillary or, alternatively, into the endothelium and interstitial space where the microaggregate has lodged. The contents of such granules include potentially pathological substances including histamine, serotonin, kinins, etc. There is convincing evidence that, at least during open heart surgery, such cellular aggregates lodge within the small vessels of the lung,[75,76] and the brain.[77] Studies of retinal angiography during cardiac surgery (Fig. 10.9) have shown retinal small vessel occlusion in 100% of patients undergoing conventional CPB.[77] It seems very unlikely that microembolic processes should affect only the lung and the brain. Rather, it seems likely that this is a generalized response, and presumably future studies will demonstrate similar changes in the liver, kidney, gut and other organs.

Studies of blood cell aggregation within the lung have shown a pattern of lung permeability defects which may be the precursor of the adult respiratory distress syndrome.[76] It appears that the timing of development of permeability defects across the alveolar capillary membrane is simultaneous with the trapping of activated white cells within the pulmonary capillaries. The whole subject of vascular permeability defects and the role of substances such as histamine and serotonin require much further investigation.

The role of the thromboxane/prostacyclin axis in both platelet activation and local vessel haemo-

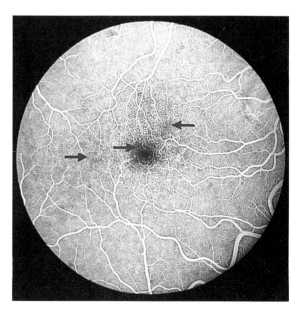

Fig. 10.9 Retinal angiogram (fluorescein) in a patient during conventional CPB. The retinal camera is focused on the macula. Embolic occlusions of arterioles are visible at the maculate border at 3 and 6 o'clock. Areas of non-perfusion are visible at 8 and 11 o'clock and in the peripheral retina.

dynamics is emerging as an important area for further research. It is now appreciated that during cardiac surgery[78] the axis orientates towards thromboxane with the appearance of vasoconstriction within the circulation and activation of platelets with the formation of platelet based microaggregates. Recent studies[18,79,80] show massive secretions of both thromboxane and prostacyclin during cardiac surgical procedures at levels substantially higher than those found during other major surgery. In addition, others have shown that while non-pulsatile perfusion produces a disproportionate rise in thromboxane over prostacyclin this rise is attenuated when pulsatile flow is substituted.[18] This suggests that impaired perfusion in the peripheral circulation may be associated with an increase in the local concentration of thromboxane, thus orientating the thromboxane/prostacyclin axis towards further vasoconstriction and platelet activation. It is not yet known whether the use of natural prostacyclin or its synthetic carbacyclin and oxycyclin derivatives may obviate those haemodynamic and haematological effects.[78,81–83] Early data suggest that, in addition to general platelet preservation effect, prostacyclin infusion during extracorporeal circulation reduces microaggregation present within the pulmonary circulation.[84]

The whole area of local vascular vasoactive substances is one which requires much further study. It is now clear that the walls of blood vessels, and indeed the walls of the heart itself, contain a large number of vasoactive substances, many with opposing haemodynamic actions, which will be released into the circulation in general and into local vasculature under a variety of stimuli. Disturbance in the physiological balance, either by local trauma or by some central pathology, may induce very marked haemodynamic effects mediated through these locally occurring vasoactive agents. Such substances include the previously discussed thromboxane and prostacyclin, endothelial relaxant factor (ERF), vasoactive peptides present in peripheral blood vessels and in the walls of the heart, particularly in the atrium, and leucotrienes (known to exert profound local vascular effects, but also to produce marked coronary artery vasoactivity).

Within the area of the haemodynamic effects of blood cell activation, the numerous mediators and pathways of the systemic inflammatory response are all believed to be of importance. Activation of the complement system and genera-

tion of histotoxic free radicals are involved. In this whole area of interest, one of the possibilities in the context of open heart surgery is that the inflammatory response, rather than being localized to the particular site of injury, becomes systemic and widespread.

Recognition of patient groups at particular risk of cardiovascular instability

Within the total population of patients undergoing cardiac surgery, a number of important high-risk groups have been identified. Ideally, in all patients, but particularly in the following subgroups, optimal perfusion is of paramount importance. It should be stressed that cardiovascular stability should exist in the period of surgery before the onset of CPB and that the achieving and maintenance of optimal cardiovascular stability should be the principal focus of postoperative care. The high-risk groups include:

1. Patients with occult coronary artery disease unable to equalize myocardial energy supply/demand, who become particularly at risk of myocardial ischaemia and infarction when LV work and cardiac output increase.
2. Patients with significant arterial disease, in particular where they have flow-limiting stenoses in the arterial supply to vital organs. In such patients, flow distal to the stenosis is pressure-passive and circulatory auto-regulation compromised. This can be seen in cardiac surgery patients (e.g. where significant carotid artery stenoses exist and the patient becomes at risk of sustaining a significant hypoperfusion defect of the brain).
3. Patients with chronic arterial hypertension. It is not well enough appreciated that, in such patients, the cerebral blood flow auto-regulation curve shifts to the right and that these patients require higher perfusion pressures in order to maintain cerebral blood flow auto-regulation.[85]
4. Patients with existing chronic vital organ insufficiency. Where chronic renal failure or chronic hepatic insufficiency exists, even modest reductions in perfusion during cardiac surgery may induce disproportionate organ dysfunction and damage. In this context, recent reports have stressed the importance of

using pulsatile perfusion during cardiac surgery in, for example, patients in chronic renal failure on dialysis programmes. In these patient groups, the maintenance of optimal perfusion prevents otherwise inevitable vital organ function deterioration.

Summary

Many of the advances in cardiac surgery in recent years have been refinements in the technology of our specialty. The systemic pathophysiology of CPB is now accepted as a major contributor to overall morbidity and even mortality. Although blood flow delivery during CPB is not the *only* contributing factor, it is nonetheless most important. If the pathological effects of CPB are to be minimized, perfusion and blood flow delivery to the patient's vital organs must be optimized. Avoidance of vasoconstriction is central to this philosophy. Although vasodilatory drugs and/or anaesthetic agents may, at least in part, counter such vasoconstriction, the ability to prevent it is conceptually more attractive. This is the foundation for the advocacy of pulsatile perfusion in cardiac surgery. Its physiological superiority rests primarily on its ability to provide superior blood flow delivery, not on the secondary benefits in vital organ function.

The argument is a haemodynamic argument— and it always has been.

References

1. Dunn J, Kirsh MM, Harness J, Carroll M, Straker J, Sloan H. Haemodynamic, metabolic, and haematologic effects of pulsatile cardiopulmonary bypass. *J Thorac Cardiovasc Surg* 1974; **68**, 137–147.
2. Jacobs LA, Klopp EH, Seamore W, Topas SR, Gott VL. Improved organ function during cardiopulmonary bypass with a roller pump modified to deliver pulsatile flow. *J Thorac Cardiovasc Surg* 1969; **58**, 703–712.
3. Takeda J. Experimental study of peripheral circulation during extracorporeal circulation with special reference to a comparison of pulsatile flow with nonpulsatile flow. *Arch Japan Chir* 1960; **29**, 1407–1412.
4. Hickey PR, Bockley MJ, Philbin DM. Pulsatile and nonpulsatile cardiopulmonary bypass: a review of a nonproductive controversy. *Ann Thorac Surg* 1983; **36**, 720–737.
5. Taylor KM, Bain WH, Morton JJ. The role of angio-

6. Estafanous FG, Tarazi RC, Viljoen JF, El Tanil MY. Systemic hypertension following myocardial revascularisation. *Am Heart J* 1973; **85**, 732–738.
7. Stinson EB, Holloway EL, Derby GC, *et al.* Control of myocardial performance early after open-heart operations by vasodilator treatment. *J Thorac Cardiovasc Surg* 1977; **73**, 523–528.
8. Sonnenblick EH, Downing SE. Afterload as a primary determinant of ventricular performance. *Am J Physiol* 1963; **204**, 604–608.
9. Taylor KM, Bain WH, Russell M, Brannan JJ, Morton JJ. Peripheral vascular resistance and angiotensin II levels during pulsatile and nonpulsatile cardiopulmonary bypass. *Thorax* 1979; **34**, 594–598.
10. Hoar PF, Hickey RF, Willyot DJ. Systemic hypertension following myocardial revascularization: a method of treatment using epidural anaesthesia. *J Thorac Cardiovasc Surg* 1976; **71**, 859–864.
11. Salerno TA, Henderson M, Keith FM, Charrette EJP. Hypertension after coronary operation: can it be prevented by pulsatile perfusion? *J Thorac Cardiovasc Surg* 1981; **81**, 396–399.
12. Hearse DJ, Braimbridge MV, Jynge P. Protection of the ischemic myocardium. In: *Cardioplegia 1981.* New York: Raven Press.
13. Buckberg GD. A proposed solution to the cardioplegic controversy. *J Thorac Cardiovasc Surg* 1979; **77**, 803–815.
14. Bretschneider HJ, Hubner G, Knoll D, Lohr B, Nordbeck H, Spieckermann PG. Myocardial resistance and tolerance to ischaemia: physiological and biochemical basis. *J Cardiovasc Surg* 1975; **16**, 241–260.
15. Taylor KM, Casals J, Morton JJ, Mittra S, Brannan JJ, Bain WH. The haemodynamic effects of angiotensin blockade after cardiopulmonary bypass. *Br Heart J* 1979; **41**, 380.
16. Taylor KM, *Cardiopulmonary Bypass.* London: Chapman & Hall Medical, 1986.
17. Levine FH, Philbin DM, Kono K, *et al.* Plasma vasopressin levels and urinary sodium excretion during cardiopulmonary bypass with and without pulsatile flow. *Ann Thorac Surg* 1981; **32**, 63–67.
18. Watkins DW, Peterson MB, Kong DI, *et al.* Thromboxane and prostacyclin changes during cardiopulmonary bypass with and without pulsatile flow. *J Thorac Cardiovasc Surg* 1982; **84**, 250–256.
19. Kohlstaedt KG, Page IH. The liberation of renin by perfusion of kidneys following reduction of pulse pressure. *J Exp Med* 1970; **72**, 201–205.
20. Many M, Soroff HS, Birtwell WC, Giron F, Wise H, Deterline RA. The physiologic role of pulsatile and nonpulsatile blood flow. II: Effects on renal function. *Arch Surg* 1967; **95**, 726–766.
21. Taylor KM, Casals JG, Brown JJ, *et al.* Haemody-

tensin II in the development of peripheral vasoconstriction during open-heart surgery. *Am Heart J* 1980; **100**, 935–937.

namic effects of SQ14225 after cardiopulmonary bypass. *Cardiovasc Res* 1980; **14**, 199–205.

22. Taylor KM. The present status of pulsatile perfusion. *Curr Med Lit—Cardiovasc Med* 1984; **3**, 66–69.

23. Angell-James JE, de Burgh Daly M. Effects of graded pulsatile pressure on the reflex vasomotor responses elicited by changes of mean pressure in the perfused carotid sinus-aortic arch regions of the dog. *J Physiol* 1971; **214**, 51–58.

24. Mavroudis C. To pulse or not to pulse. *Ann Thorac Surg* 1978; **25**, 259–271.

25. Clarke CP, Kahn DR, Dufek JH. The effects of nonpulsatile blood flow on canine lungs. *Ann Thorac Surg* 1968; **6**, 450–455.

26. Nakayama K, Tamiya T, Yamamoto K. High amplitude pulsatile pump in extracorporeal circulation with particular reference to haemodynamics. *Surgery* 1963; **54**, 798–802.

27. Mendelbaum I, Burns WH. Pulsatile and nonpulsatile blood flow. *JAMA* 1965; **191**, 121–123.

28. Trinkle JK, Helton NE, Wood RC. Metabolic comparison of a new pulsatile pump and a roller pump for cardiopulmonary bypass. *J Thorac Cardiovasc Surg* 1969; **58**, 562–566.

29. Bregman D, Bowman FO, Parodi EN, *et al.* An improved method of myocardial protection with pulsation during cardiopulmonary bypass. *Circulation* 1977; **56** (suppl 11), 157.

30. Maddoux G, Pappas G, Jenkins M, *et al.* Effect of pulsatile and nonpulsatile flow during cardiopulmonary bypass on left ventricular ejection fraction early after aortocoronary bypass surgery. *Am J Cardiol* 1976; **37**, 1000–1004.

31. Taylor KM. Why pulsatile flow during cardiopulmonary bypass? In: Longmore DB (ed), *Towards Safer Cardiac Surgery*. Lancaster: MTP, 1981: 481–500.

32. Shepard RB, Kirklin JW. Relation of pulsatile flow to oxygen consumption and other variables during cardiopulmonary bypass. *J Thorac Cardiovasc Surg* 1969; **58**, 694–698.

33. Ogata T, Ida Y, Nonoyama A. A comparative study on the effectiveness of pulsatile and nonpulsatile blood flow in extracorporeal circulation. *Arch Japan Chir* 1960; **29**, 59–62.

34. Steed DL, Follette DM, Foglia R, Maloney JV, Buckberg GD. Effects of pulsatile assistance and nonpulsatile flow on subendocardial perfusion during cardiopulmonary bypass. *Ann Thorac Surg* 1978; **26**, 133–141.

35. Chun-Hsiu Y, Bang-Yu C, I-Shan W. Preliminary observations on physiological effects of pulsatile cardiopulmonary bypass in animals. *ASAIO Trans* 1981; **27**, 480–484.

36. Boucher JK, Rudy LW, Edmunds LH. Organ blood flow during pulsatile cardiopulmonary bypass. *J Appl Physiol* 1974; **36**, 86–90.

37. Frater RWM, Wakayama S, Oka Y, *et al.* Pulsatile cardiopulmonary bypass: failure to influence hae-modynamics or hormones. *Circulation* 1980; **62** (suppl 1), 19–25.

38. Harken AH. The influence of pulsatile perfusion on oxygen uptake by the isolated canine hind limb. *J Thorac Cardiovasc Surg* 1975; **70**, 237–241.

39. Smith PLC, Treasure T, Newman SP, *et al.* Cerebral consequences of cardiopulmonary bypass. *Lancet* 1986; **i**, 823–825.

40. Treasure T. Cerebral complications of cardiac surgery (comment). *Curr Med Lit—Cardiovasc Med* 1985; **4**, 33–37.

41. Gardner TJ, Horneffer PJ, Manolio TA, *et al.* Stroke following coronary artery bypass grafting: a 10-year study. *Ann Thorac Surg* 1985; **40**, 574–581.

42. Shaw PJ, Bates D, Cartlidge NEF, Heaviside D, Julian DG, Shaw DA. Early neurological complications of coronary artery bypass surgery. *Br Med J* 1985; **291**, 1384–1387.

43. De Paepe J, Pomerantzeff PMA, Nakiri K, Armelin E, Verginelli G, Zerbini EJ. Observation of the microcirculation of the cerebral cortex of dogs subjected to pulsatile and nonpulsatile flow during extracorporeal circulation. In: *A Propos Du Debit Pulse*. Belgium: Cobe Laboratories Inc, 1979.

44. Matsumoto T, Wolferth CC, Perlman MH. Effect of pulsatile and nonpulsatile perfusion upon cerebral and conjunctival microcirculation in dogs. *Am Surg* 1971; **37**, 61–64.

45. Sanderson JM, Wright G, Sims FW. Brain damage in dogs immediately following pulsatile and non-pulsatile blood flows in extracorporeal circulation. *Thorax* 1972; **27**, 275–286.

46. Taylor KM. Pathophysiology of brain damage during open heart surgery. *Tex Heart Inst J* 1986; **13**, 91–96.

47. Taylor KM, Walker MS, Rao LGS, Jones JV, Gray CE. Plasma levels of cortisol, free cortisol and corticotrophin during cardiopulmonary bypass. *J Endocrinol* 1975; **67**, 29–30.

48. Taylor KM, Jones JV, Walker MS, Rao LGS, Bain WH. The cortisol response during heart–lung bypass. *Circulation* 1976; **54**, 20–26.

49. Taylor KMM, Bain WH, Jones JV, Walker MS. The effect of haemodilution on plasma levels of cortisol and free cortisol. *J Thorac Cardiovasc Surg* 1976; **72**, 57–61.

50. Bremner WF, Taylor KM, Baird S, Ratcliffe JG, Bain WH, Lawrie TDV. Hypothalamo–pituitary–thyroid axis function during cardiopulmonary bypass. *J Thorac Cardiovasc Surg* 1978; **75**, 392–399.

51. Taylor KM, Wright GS, Bremner WF, Bain WH, Caves PK, Beastall GH. Anterior pituitary response to TRH during open-heart surgery. *Cardiovasc Res* 1978; **12**, 114–119.

52. Taylor KM, Wright GS, Reid JM, *et al.* Comparative studies of pulsatile and nonpulsatile flow during cardiopulmonary bypass. II: The effects on adrenal

secretion of cortisol. *J Thorac Cardiovasc Surg* 1978; **75**, 574–578.

53. Taylor KM, Wright GS, Bain WH, Caves PK, Beastall GS. Comparative studies of pulsatile and nonpulsatile flow during cardiopulmonary bypass. III: Anterior pituitary response to thyrotrophin-releasing hormone. *J Thorac Cardiovasc Surg* 1978; **75**, 579–584.
54. Taylor KM. Hypothalamic and pituitary changes in relation to injury. *Ann Roy Coll Surg Engl* 1978; **60**, 229–233.
55. Collins JD, Bassendine MF, Ferner R. Incidence and prognostic importance of jaundice after cardiopulmonary bypass surgery. *Lancet* 1983; **1**, 1119–1122.
56. Olsson R, Hermodsson S, Roberts D, Waldenstrom J. Hepatic dysfunction after open-heart surgery. *Scand J Thor Cardiovasc Surg* 1984; **18**, 217–222.
57. Sanderson RG, Ellison JH, Benson JA, Starr A. Jaundice following open-heart surgery. *Ann Surg* 1967; **165**, 217–224.
58. Mathie RT, Desai JB, Taylor KM. The effect of normothermic cardiopulmonary bypass on hepatic blood flow in the dog. *Perfusion* 1986; **1**, 245–253.
59. Feiner H. Pancreatitis after cardiac surgery. *Am J Surg* 1976; **131**, 684–688.
60. Moores WY, Gago O, Morris JD, Peck CC. Serum and urinary amylase levels following pulsatile and continuous cardiopulmonary bypass. *J Thorac Cardiovasc Surg* 1977; **74**, 73–76.
61. Murray WR, Mittra S, Mittra D, Roberts LB, Taylor KM. The amylase creatinine clearance ratio following cardiopulmonary bypass. *J Thorac Cardiovasc Surg* 1982; **82**, 248–253.
62. Webber CE, Garnett ES. The relationship between colloid osmotic pressure and plasma proteins during and after cardiopulmonary bypass. *J Thorac Cardiovasc Surg* 1973; **65**, 234–237.
63. German JC, Chalmers GS, Hirai J, Mukherjee ND, Wakabayashi A, Connolly NE. Comparison of nonpulsatile and pulsatile extracorporeal circulation on renal tissue perfusion. *Chest* 1972; **61**, 65–69.
64. Johnston G, Hammill F, Marzec U, *et al.* Prolonged pulseless perfusion in unanaesthetized calves. *Arch Surg* 1976; **III**, 1225–1230.
65. Golding LR, Jacobs G, Murakami T, *et al.* Chronic nonpulsatile blood flow in an alive, awake animal: 34 days' survival. *ASAIO Trans* 1980; **26**, 251–255.
66. Many M, Giron F, Birtwell WC, *et al.* Effects of depulsation of renal blood flow upon renal function and renin secretion. *Surgery* 1969; **66**, 242.
67. Paquet KJ. Haemodynamic studies on normothermic perfusion of the isolated pig kidney with pulsatile and nonpulsatile flows. *J Cardiovasc Surg* 1969; **1**, 45–48.
68. Taylor KM. Heparin, protamine and prostacyclin therapy during cardiopulmonary bypass. In: Taylor KM (ed), *Cardiopulmonary Bypass: Principles and*

Management. London: Chapman and Hall, 1986: 277–288.
69. Edmunds LH. The sangreal (editorial). *J Thorac Cardiovasc Surg* 1985; **90**, 1–6.
70. Marcus AJ. Platelet function and its disorders: platelet aggregation. In: Colman RW, Hirsh J, Marder V, Salzman EW (eds), *Textbook of Haemostasis and Thrombosis*. Philadelphia: Lippincott, 1982: chap. 23.
71. Salzman EW, Lindon J, Brier D, Merril EW. Surface induced platelet adhesion, aggregation and release. *Ann NY Acad Sci* 1977; **283**, 114–119.
72. Wicher SJ, Brash JL. Platelet foreign surface interactions. *J Biomed Mater Res* 1978; **12**, 181–186.
73. Hennessey VI, Hicks RE, Niewiarowski S, Edmunds LH, Colman RW. Effects of surface area and composition on the function of human platelets during extracorporeal circulation. *Am J Physiol* 1977; **232**, H622–628.
74. Harker LA, Malpass TW, Branson HE, Hessel EA, Slichter SJ. Mechanisms of abnormal bleeding in patients undergoing cardiopulmonary bypass: acquired transient platelet dysfunction association with selective granule release. *Blood* 1980; **56**, 824.
75. Fessatidis ITh, Man WK, Brannan JJ, Taylor KM. Haemodynamic and haematological effects of prostacyclin infusion. In: Torino BP (ed), *Progress in Angiology*. Minerva Medica, 1986: 519–522.
76. Royston DJ, Fleming J, Desai JB, Taylor KM. Neutrophil activation and pulmonary injury during open-heart surgery. *J Thorac Cardiovasc Surg* 1986; **91**, 758–766.
77. Blauth C, Kohner EM, Arnold J, Taylor KM. Retinal microembolism during cardiopulmonary bypass demonstrated by fluorescein angiography. *Lancet* 1986; **ii**, 837–839.
78. Taylor KM. Prostacyclin therapy during cardiopulmonary bypass—is it beneficial? *Perfusion* 1987; **2**, 1–7.
79. Ritter JM, Hamilton G, Barrow SE, Taylor KM. Prostacyclin in the circulation of patients with vascular disorders undergoing surgery. *Clin Sci* 1986; **71**, 743–747.
80. Solis RT, Kennedy PS, Beall AC, *et al.* Cardiopulmonary bypass: microembolization and platelet aggregation. *Circulation* 1975; **52**, 103–108.
81. Longmore DB. The value of prostacyclins in cardiopulmonary bypass. In: Longmore DB (ed), *Towards Safer Cardiac Surgery*. Lancaster: MTP, 1981: 355–370.
82. Faichney A, Davidson KG, Wheatley DJ, Davidson JF, Walker ID. Prostacyclin in cardiopulmonary bypass operations. *J Thorac Cardiovasc Surg* 1982; **84**, 602–608.
83. Addonizio VP, Fisher CA, Jenkin BK, Strauss JF, Musial JF, Edmunds LH. Iloprost (ZK 36374), a stable analogue of prostacyclin, preserves platelets during simulated extracorporeal circulation. *J*

Thorac Cardiovasc Surg 1985; **89**, 926–933.

84. Fessatidis ITh, Brannan JJ, Taylor KM, Kanellaki-Kyparissi M, Olsen ECJ. Effect of prostacyclin PGI$_2$ on cardiopulmonary bypass-induced lung injury. *Perfusion* 1994; **9**, 23–33.

85. Graham DI, Brierley JB. Vascular disorders of the central nervous system. In: Adams JH, Corseltis JAN, Duchen LW (eds), *Neuropathology*, 4th edn. London: Edward Arnold, 1984: 157–207.

11

The choice of blood pump for cardiopulmonary bypass

J Kuo and Timothy R Graham

Introduction

Work on extracorporeal gas exchange within blood dates back to the last part of the nineteenth century when Frey and Gruber[1] worked on an oxygenator in 1885. However, it was not until the late 1930s that the most significant contribution to the advancement of cardiopulmonary bypass (CPB) came from Gibbon's pioneering work at the Massachusetts General Hospital. There he carried out the first elective CPB in the cat,[2] and in 1954 Gibbon reported the first successful CPB in a human when he repaired an atrial septal defect on a 18-year-old girl with a CPB time of 45 minutes.[3]

The development of blood pumps dates back to the end of the nineteenth century when Jacobj used a rubber bladder compressed by a motor-driven eccentric shaft.[4] Today the blood pump remains a vital component of the heart–lung machine. In 1954, Gibbon stated that one of the essential features of every mechanical heart–lung apparatus was a good method of pumping blood through the circuit which did not cause haemolysis. Despite modern engineering advances, a totally atraumatic blood pump is still not available.

In 1934, DeBakey designed the roller pump to facilitate rapid blood transfusion.[5] The roller pump was used by Gibbon in his pioneering work, and to this day it is still the most commonly used type of arterial perfusion pump within the CPB circuit. The first experimental use of a centrifugal pump was reported by Saxton and Andrews in 1960.[6] A combined effort to develop an implantable blood pump by the University of Minnesota, University of California, San Diego and Medtronic Inc. in 1964 led to development of the magnetically coupled centrifugal pump.[7]

There are currently two main categories of blood pump available to surgeons and perfusionists for routine cardiopulmonary bypass: the roller pump and the centrifugal pump. Three types of centrifugal pump are available: the Biomedicus constrained vortex, the Sarns Delphin, and the St Jude.

Pump mechanics

The roller pump (Fig. 11.1) is a positive-displacement type producing flow by compressing silastic tubing between the parallel wall of the roller and the backing plate. This system allows a constant delivery of blood volume despite minor variations of outlet pressure. The disadvantages of this system are that line obstruction upstream results in generation of gaseous microemboli (cavitation), whereas obstruction downstream may lead to line disruption. Careful monitoring therefore remains essential.

The centrifugal pump is a kinetic type which works by imparting kinetic energy to the blood through rapid rotation of an impella or rotor.

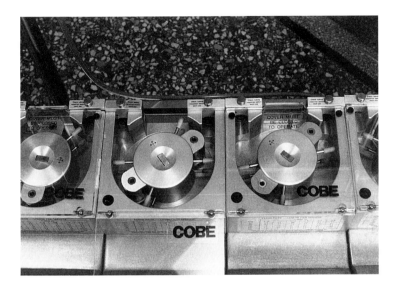

Fig. 11.1 The Cobe roller pump.

The Biomedicus pump (Fig. 11.2) operates on the constrained vortex principle. The rotating cones use viscous drag to induce a vortex which is constrained within the casing and therefore generates flow. The other two types of centrifugal pump use a bladed impella to propel blood from the inlet to the outlet port. The Sarns pump (Fig. 11.3) has a straight-fin impella design which generates pressure by spinning the liquid approximately as a solid body vortex within the casing. The St Jude pump (Fig. 11.4) has a curved-fin impella design which propels blood by maintaining a constant perpendicular force vector against the blood flow path. The design of this fin

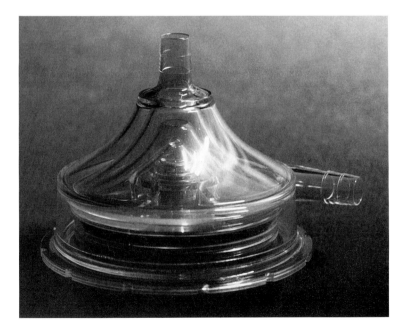

Fig. 11.2 The Biomedicus centrifugal pump.

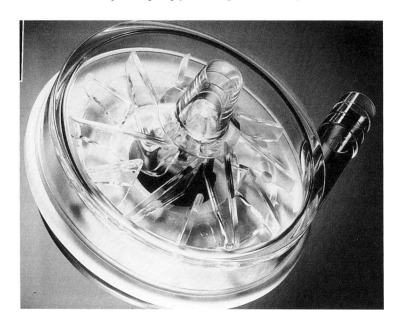

Fig. 11.3 The Sarns centrifugal pump.

attempts to match the shape of the moving fluid mass, thereby theoretically reducing turbulence.

The flow generated by the different pumps may be affected by changing fluid conditions such as temperature and viscosity. Temperature has a profound effect on flow from the roller pump: a lower temperature results in stiffer tubing and decreased compliance, thus causing a decrease in flow, whereas the centrifugal pump is unaffected. However, flow from the centrifugal pump is more dependent on fluid viscosity than is the roller pump. The centrifugal type is afterload-sensitive, and with increasing viscosity the outflow resistance is increased, resulting in decreased flow—as demonstrated by Landis *et al.*[8] When the line pressure (afterload) increases, the output falls

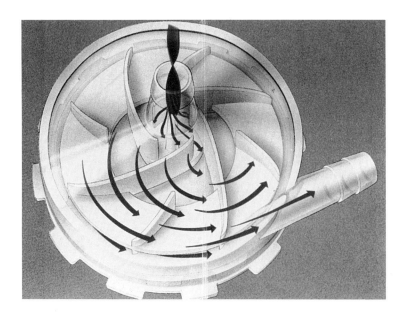

Fig. 11.4 The St Jude centrifugal pump.

steeply, preventing excessive build-up of pressure and thus avoiding line and pump disruption. A disadvantage of the centrifugal pump is its non-occlusive nature which provides no protection against retrograde flow when the pump stops. This may create a 'siphon' effect, sucking blood out of the aorta or air into the aorta from needle holes or around the pursestring holding the aortic cannula.[9] A one-way valve or judicious clamping should be used on the arterial line to prevent this occurring.

Evaluation of blood pumps *in vitro*

Centrifugal pumps differ in efficiency and subsequent heat generation within the pump. *In vitro* studies have shown that the cone type requires approximately 18% higher revolutions per minute than the bladed-impella type to generate a similar flow, which results in an overall 7% relative increase in temperature in the test circuit.[10] However, the significance of the need to dissipate the extra heat generated to the circulating blood during CPB remains to be established.

Haemolysis

In vivo assessment of blood cell trauma related to pumps is difficult because it has not been easy to separate the damage caused by other factors such as cardiotomy suction and the gas exchange device. Therefore most of the studies are *in vitro* evaluations. Koja *et al.*[11] demonstrated, using canine blood in an *in vitro* circuit for a period of 6 hours, that the mean hourly increment of plasma free haemoglobin for the roller pump was six times that of the Biomedicus centrifugal pump. Similarly, Oku *et al.*[12] reported a higher haemolytic index in the roller pump compared with the Biomedicus pump after 12 hours of blood pumping. Hoerr *et al.*[13] found no significant differences in haemolysis between the two pumps with up to 16 hours of test circulation, but after 16 hours the roller pump produced significantly more haemolysis. Although the bladed impella centrifugal pumps (Sarns and St Jude) have also been shown to be less haemolytic than the roller pump, comparison of these with the Biomedicus pump has produced no clear differences.[14–16]

Platelet dysfunction

The effects of the pump on platelets can be assessed by platelet numbers, degranulation and aggregation. An *in vitro* experimental test circuit using bovine blood showed no significant difference in platelet numbers between the centrifugal and the roller pump.[14] However, several animal studies have demonstrated that the Biomedicus pump has better preservation of platelet numbers than the roller pump.[17,18]

Gaseous microemboli

Microemboli, both gaseous and particulate, are generated during CPB. They have been implicated as an important cause of organ dysfunction, especially neuropsychological deficit.

The mechanisms of generation of gaseous microemboli during CPB are well documented: low filling volumes, agitation and mechanical disturbance of the oxygenator and arterial line filter, rapid refilling of the oxygenator, fast rewarming of the blood, and a high Po_2.[19] Once generated, these gaseous microemboli may be passed into the systemic circulation by the roller pump whereas the centrifugal pump has the ability to 'trap' them. If a large amount of air is accidentally introduced into the circuit, the centrifugal pump head will deprime itself and no flow results. Approximately 30–50 ml of air will deprime both the impella and the cone pumps. However, when a smaller amount of air is introduced, it becomes displaced to the centre of the vortex because of its low density.[20] This results in a reduction, though not complete elimination, of air embolisation. Wheeldon *et al.*[21] have demonstrated that during routine CPB there was a reduction in post-filter microbubble transmission (as measured by the TM8 ultrasound device) in a centrifugal pump group compared with a roller pump group.

Particulate microembolization

Particulate microemboli may be in the form of platelet, leucocyte and fibrin aggregates or foreign materials such as silicon and polyvinyl chloride (PVC) tubing fragments due to spallation. Fragmentation and shredding of the luminal surfaces of the PVC tubing occurred in areas exposed to the roller pump heads,[22,23] whereas no spallation has been demonstrated with the centrifugal pump.[16] These advantages may theoretically lead to better preservation of the neuropsychological function following CPB.

Clinical evaluation

In our institution, we performed recently a prospective randomized clinical study to evaluate the effects of CPB using the roller pump or the St Jude centrifugal pump. We recruited 50 patients who were undergoing routine coronary artery bypass surgery. All had good left ventricular function, with three-vessel coronary artery disease. (Patients with a history of haematological disorder or an impaired renal function were excluded.) The 50 subjects were then randomized into two equal groups. The components of the bypass circuit were identical in both groups except for the choice of pump. Myocardial preservation using the St Thomas' crystalloid cardioplegic solution was applied for all patients. The bypass time was kept to a minimum of 90 minutes and patients excluded from the study if it exceeded 120 minutes. None of these patients received dopamine or inotropic support during the perioperative period. Patient demographics and bypass data were similar for the two groups.

The areas of investigation in our study included assessment of blood cell trauma, renal perfusion and function, and the implication of haemolysis on renal perfusion.

Blood cell trauma

Use of the centrifugal pump for routine CPB was first reported in 1978 by Lynch *et al.*[20] They concluded that postoperative blood loss was significantly less with the Biomedicus pump than with a roller pump. Since then other clinical studies have reported that the centrifugal type is less traumatic to blood cells during clinical CPB. Jakob *et al.*[24] found that the peak plasma haemoglobin level in a roller pump group was twice that of a centrifugal pump group after 120 minutes of bypass. Our own clinical evaluation of the St Jude pump versus the roller type also demonstrated that the centrifugal pump was associated with significantly less haemolysis (Fig. 11.5).

Similarly, better platelet number preservation has been observed with the centrifugal pump.[21,25] We assessed platelet dysfunction by performing platelet aggregation studies using the Born

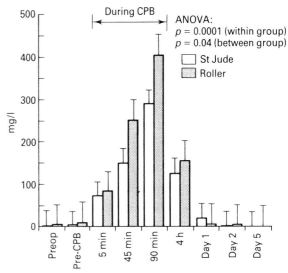

Fig. 11.5 Plasma free haemoglobin liberated during CPB.

method in platelet-rich plasma to 50 and 100 μmol/l adenosine diphosphate (ADP) at timed intervals: preoperative and 4 and 24 hours post-operative. The parameters measured were the time to maximum aggregation (t_{max}), the slope of the initial aggregation curve (S_{agg}), and the percentage change in maximum aggregation. As Table 11.1 shows, following CPB, t_{max} was significantly more prolonged with the centrifugal pump group.

Platelet aggregation induced with 50 μmol/l of ADP showed no significant changes in the slope of initial aggregation in either group, but with 100 μmol/l the slope fell by 17.1% in the centrifugal pump group compared with 26.6% in the roller pump group. The percentage change in maximum aggregation remained unchanged in both groups. This study confirmed that CPB adversely affects platelet aggregability and the centrifugal pump appears to cause less functional damage to platelets than does the roller pump. Furthermore, use of the roller type was associated with significantly greater platelet activation as assessed by peak plasma beta thromboglobulin level (Fig. 11.6).

Neutropenia is a well documented finding associated with bypass, and activation of polymorphonuclear granulocytes is probably complement-related.[26] Activated polymorphonuclear granulocytes then aggregate and become sequestrated in the pulmonary capillaries. This mechanism may be important in the pathogenesis

Table 11.1 Changes in platelet aggregation following CPB.

Group	Time to maximum aggregation (t_{max}) (s)			Significance
	Preop	4 h postop	24 h postop	
Roller pump	104 ± 20	129 ± 19*	162 ± 24**†	*p = NS **p = 0.03 †p = NS
Centrifugal pump	105 ± 14	170 ± 17*	236 ± 16**†	*p = 0.009 **p = 0.003 †p = 0.02

* and ** compared with preop; † compared with 4 hours.

of 'postperfusion lung'.[26] Driessen *et al.*[27] reported no decrease in the white cell count following bypass (after correction for haemodilution) with the centrifugal pump, whereas the roller pump produced a significant drop. They suggested that the lack of neutropenia with the centrifugal pump may indicate less neutrophil activation. Further studies are required to determine whether this is reflected in better preservation of lung function during CPB.

Systemic vascular resistance and organ perfusion

Use of a centrifugal pump in the pulsatile mode has been associated with a ten-fold lower dose of sodium nitroprusside to maintain systemic vascular resistance within physiological limits, compared to the roller pump.[27] However, it remains uncertain whether this difference is due to the pump type, the use of the pulsatile mode, or a combination of both. The pulsatile mode is unlikely to play an important role in this case because the amplitude of the pulse pressure is small (much lower than those produced by the roller pump in the pulsatile mode).

We measured the effective renal plasma flow using Wagoner's technique of single intravenous injection of [125]iodohippurate[28] in 20 patients (St Jude pump, $n = 10$; roller pump, $n = 10$). Renal blood flow and renal vascular resistance were calculated using standard formulae. There was no significant difference between the two groups in terms of demographic and bypass data (in particular, the CPB time and cross-clamp time). The effective renal plasma flow rose significantly at day 1 following CPB in both groups ($p = 0.003$) and returned to baseline level by day 7 ($p = 0.02$) (see Fig. 11.7). The renal blood flow showed no significant difference between the preoperative level and that at day 1 in both groups ($p > 0.05$) but fell significantly at day 7 ($p = 0.004$) (see Fig. 11.8). The renal vascular resistance corrected for haemodilution showed a significant rise following CPB in the roller pump group ($p = 0.01$) but no significant changes in the centrifugal pump group ($p > 0.05$) (see Fig. 11.9).

We hypothesize that this difference in the renal vascular resistance may be related to the differing

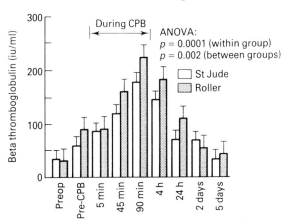

Fig. 11.6 Changes in plasma beta thromboglobulin level (mean ± SE) associated with CPB.

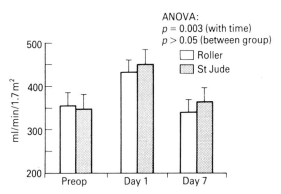

Fig. 11.7 Changes in effective renal plasma flow (mean ± SE) associated with CPB.

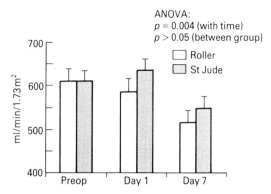

Fig. 11.8 Changes in renal blood flow (mean ± SE) associated with CPB.

degree of haemolysis associated with each pump type. As early as 1957, Nizat *et al.*[29] showed that a product released by lysis of red blood cells can produce profound renal vasoconstriction. However, it was only recently that endothelium-derived relaxation factor (EDRF), a potent vasodilator, was shown to play a role in the regulation of systemic and renal haemodynamics.[30,31] Plasma free haemoglobin is a known inhibitor of EDRF.[32]

We have investigated the effect of haemolysis during CPB on renal haemodynamics. In this study, 24 patients were divided into two groups: group A (plasma free haemoglobin >400 mg/l) and group B (<400 mg/l). At day 1, group A showed a 11.1% fall (median) in renal blood flow from the preoperative baseline value compared

with a 1.4% increase (median) in group B. This may be due to the corresponding change in renal vascular resistance corrected for haematocrit in these two groups of patients: a 32.5% increase from preoperative baseline value (group A) versus 5% increase (group B). These results suggest that plasma free haemoglobin may be one of the factors affecting peripheral vascular resistance and organ haemodynamics after CPB.

Conclusions

It is becoming increasingly evident that the centrifugal pump has several potential advantages over the conventional roller pump. The centrifugal pump has an improved blood handling capability, minimizes both particulate and gaseous microembolisation, and is associated with better systemic and renal haemodynamics.

However, no data are currently available to show whether these findings result in an improved clinical outcome, to justify the additional cost incurred with centrifugal pump systems. The use of a centrifugal pump may result in an overall reduction in hospital cost secondary to reduced postoperative blood product usage and a shorter stay in the intensive care unit. Prospective controlled clinical trials comparing the different types of blood pump for routine and non-routine CPB are required which have comparable outcome measures, both clinical and financial, in order to decide this important issue.

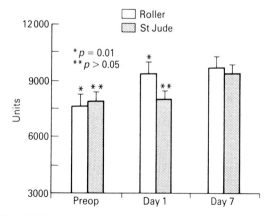

Fig. 11.9 Changes in corrected renal vascular resistance (mean ± SE) associated with CPB.

References

1. Frey MV, Gruber M. Untersuchungen über den Staffwechsel Isolierter Organe: Ein Respirations Apparat für Isolierte Organe. *Arch Physiol* 1885; **9**, 519.
2. Gibbon JHJ. Artificial maintenance of circulation during experimental occlusion of the pulmonary artery. *Arch Surg* 1937; **34**, 1105–1131.
3. Gibbon JHJ. Application of a mechanical heart and lung apparatus to cardiac surgery. *Minn Med* 1954; **37**, 171–185.
4. Jacobj C. Ein Beitrag zur Technik der künstlichen Durchblutung überlebender Organe. *Arch Exper Pathol Pharmakol* 1895; **31**, 330–348.
5. DeBakey ME. Simple continuous-flow blood transfusion instrument. *New Orl Med S J* 1934; **87**, 386–389.
6. Saxton GA, Andrews CB. An ideal heart pump with

hydrodynamic characteristics analogous to the mammalian heart. *ASAIO Trans* 1960; **6**, 288–291.

7. Bernstein EF, Cosentino LC, Reich S. A compact, low-haemolysis, non-thrombogenic system for non-thoracotomy prolonged left ventricular bypass. *ASAIO Trans* 1974; **20**, 643–653.

8. Landis GH, Mandl JP, Holt DW. Pump flow dynamics of the roller pump and constrained vortex pump. *Proc. AMSECT* 1979; **11**, 201–213.

9. Kolff J, McClurken JB, Alpern JB. Beware centrifugal pumps: not a one-way street, but a potential dangerous 'siphon'. *Ann Thorac Surg* 1990; **50**, 512.

10. Edelman W, Levendusky J, Lichenstein I. The impact of impella and bearing design on thermal concentration in a centrifugal pump. Pathophysiology & techniques of cardiopulmonary bypass proceedings 1992: 174.

11. Koja K, Kuniyoshi Y, Ikemura F, *et al.* Influence of the centrifugal pump (Bio-Pump) on blood components. *Japan J Artif Organs* 1986; **15**, 545–548.

12. Oku T, Harasaki H, Smith W, Nose Y. Hemolysis: a comparative study of four nonpulsatile pumps. *ASAIO Trans* 1988; **34**, 500–504.

13. Hoerr HR, Kraemer MF, Williams JL, *et al.* In vitro comparison of the blood handling by the constrained vortex and twin roller blood pumps. *J Extra-Corp Tech* 1986; **19**, 316–321.

14. Iatridis E, Chan T. An evaluation of vortex, centrifugal and roller pump systems. In: Schima TH, (ed.), *Proceedings of the International Workshop on Rotary Blood Pumps.* Obertauern, Austria, 1988: 76–81. Oxford: Blackwell Scientific.

15. Engelhardt H, Vogelsang B, Reul H, Rau G. Hydrodynamical and haemodynamical evaluation of rotary blood pumps. In: Schima TH (ed.), *Proceedings of the International Workshop on Rotary Blood Pumps.* Obertauern, Austria, 1988: 76–81. Oxford: Blackwell Scientific.

16. Noon GP, Sekela ME, Glueck J, Coleman CL, Feldman L. Composition of Delphin and BioMedicus pumps. *ASAIO Trans* 1990; **36**, M616–619.

17. Takeda H, Yamazaki R, Takahira M, Ishibashi Y, Sakai K, Tanabe T. Catecholamine and prostaglandin changes during early period of cardiopulmonary bypass: comparison between centrifugal and roller pumps. *Japan J Artif Organs* 1985; **14**, 1777–1781.

18. Matsukura H, Uzawa S, Goda T, *et al.* An experimental study of the preservation of platelets during extracorporeal circulation. *Japan J Thorac Surg* 1983; **36**, 890–892.

19. Demierre D, Maass D, Garcia E, Turina M. ECC source of gaseous microemboli. *J Extra-Corp Tech* 1985; **17**, 20–26.

20. Lynch MF, Peterson D, Baker V. Centrifugal blood pumping for open heart surgery. *Minn Med* 1978; **61**, 536–537.

21. Wheeldon DR, Bethune DW, Gill RD. Vortex pumping for routine cardiac surgery: a comparative study. *Perfusion* 1990; **5**, 135–143.

22. Orenstein JM, Noriko S, Aaron B, Buchholz B, Bloom S. Microemboli observed in deaths following cardiopulmonary bypass surgery: silicon antifoam agents and polyvinyl chloride tubing as sources of emboli. *Hum Pathol* 1982; **13**, 1082.

23. Uretzky G, Landsburg G, Cohn D, Wax Y, Borman JB. Analysis of microembolic particles originating in extracorporeal circuits. *Perfusion* 1987; **2**, 9–17.

24. Jakob HG, Hafner G, Thelemann C, Sturer A, Prellwitz W, Oelert H. Routine extracorporeal circulation with a centrifugal or roller pump. *ASAIO Trans* 1991; **37**(3), M487–489.

25. Parault BG, Conrad SA. The effect of extracorporeal circulation time and patient age on platelet retention during cardiopulmonary bypass: a comparison of roller and centrifugal pumps. *J Extra-Corp Tech* 1991; **23**, 34–38.

26. Hammerschmidt DE, Stroncek DF, Bowers TK, *et al.* Complement activation and neutropenia occurring during cardiopulmonary bypass. *J Thorac Cardiovasc Surg* 1981; **83**, 370–377.

27. Driessen JJ, Fransen G, Rondelez L, Schelstraete E, Gevaert L. Comparison of the standard roller pump and a pulsatile centrifugal pump for extracorporeal circulation during routine coronary artery bypass grafting. *Perfusion* 1991; **6**, 303–311.

28. Wagoner RD, Tauxe WN, Maher FT, Hunt JC. Measurement of effective renal plasma flow with sodium iodohippurate-131. *JAMA* 1964; **187**, 811–813.

29. Nizat A, Cuypers Y. Extraction: à partir des hématies de deux fractions douees d'activité vasoconstrictrice sur le rein. *Arch Int Physiol* 1957; **65**, 642.

30. Vallance P, Collier J, Moncada S. Effects of endothelium-derived nitric oxide on peripheral arteriolar tone in man. *Lancet* 1989; **ii**, 997–1000.

31. Tolins JP, Palmer RMJ, Moncada S, Raij L. Role of endothelium-derived relaxing factor in regulation of renal haemodynamic responses. *Am J Physiol* 1990; **258**, H655–662.

32. Edwards DH, Griffith TM, Ryley HC, Henderson AH. Haptoglobin–haemoglobin complex in human plasma inhibits endothelium dependent relaxation: evidence that endothelium-derived relaxing factor acts as a local autocoid. *Cardiovasc Res* 1986; **20**, 549–556.

Section IV _____

Short-Term and Medium-Term Support

12

Principles of intra-aortic balloon counterpulsation*

Malcolm J Underwood and Timothy R Graham

Introduction

The concept of mechanical circulatory support was devised three decades ago to treat cardiogenic shock, which had a mortality of nearly 100% even with medical therapy.[1] The field of temporary circulatory support has become well established and a wide array of support systems are available. Intra-aortic balloon counterpulsation (IABC) provides circulatory support for patients with severe but potentially reversible cardiac dysfunction. It has largely been confined to cardiac units, but with improving technology its use may extend to other specialities. Effective use requires an understanding of its physiological effects, knowledge of indications and contraindications for its use, and close cooperation between medical, nursing and technical personnel.

Counterpulsation was described by Harken in 1958.[2] He removed blood from the femoral artery during systole and rapidly reinfused it during diastole. This required bilateral femoral arteriotomies and haemolysis restricted its clinical use. Moulopoulos[3] used a balloon pump positioned in the descending aorta to accomplish the same purpose, but technological advances were not sufficient for clinical use until 1968.[4] One-hundred thousand new patients each year may benefit from IABC,[5] but with improving technol-

ogy, simple techniques of insertion and management, its use may now extend even further.

Physiological principles

Counterpulsation describes a technique which assists the heart in series with the cardiac cycle. The aim is to offload the ventricle in the ejection phase of the cardiac cycle and increase myocardial blood flow in the filling phase. IABC may achieve this but cannot augment a cardiac output that does not exist. IABC has been used in RV failure[6,7] using a balloon in the main pulmonary artery, but this application is limited. One of the commonest causes of RV failure is *left* ventricular failure, and *aortic* counterpulsation may improve RV function indirectly by reducing the left atrial filling pressure and the pressure gradient across the pulmonary vascular bed, and improving RV subendocardial blood flow.

To understand the physiological effects of IABC, an appreciation of myocardial oxygen supply and demand and the factors that regulate cardiac output is required.

Control of cardiac output

Cardiac output is the quantity of blood moved per minute by the heart from the great veins to the aorta and represents the product of the stroke volume and heart rate (Table 12.1).

Cardiac rate is primarily controlled by cardiac

* This chapter has been published as an article in the *British Journal of Hospital Medicine* 1993.

innervation; stimulation of sympathetic nerves increase the rate and parasympathetic stimulation decreases it. Stroke volume represents the amount of blood moved by the ventricle per ejection and for the left ventricle at rest is approximately 70–90 ml. This is determined in part by autonomic neural input, with sympathetic stimuli causing the myocardial fibres to contract with greater strength at any given length and parasympathetic stimulation having the opposite effect. Stroke volume also varies with the intrinsic length of the cardiac muscle fibres independently of neural input.

Table 12.1 Formulae for haemodynamic variables.

Cardiac output
  $SV \times HR$

Cardiac index
  $\dfrac{CO}{BSA}$

Systematic vascular resistance
  $\dfrac{MAP - CVP}{CO}$

Stroke volume
  $LVEDV - LVESV$

Stroke work
  $SV \times MAP$

Left ventricular stroke work
  $SV \times (MAP - PCWP) \times 0.316$

Left ventricular stroke work index
  $\dfrac{LVSW}{BSA}$

Left ventricular stroke volume index
  $\dfrac{SV}{BSA}$

Nomenclature	
HR	= Heart rate
SV	= Stroke volume
CO	= Cardiac output
BSA	= Body surface area
MAP	= Mean arterial pressure
CVP	= Central venous pressure
LVEDV	= Left ventricular end-diastolic volume
LVESV	= Left ventricular end-systolic volume
PCWP	= Pulmonary capillary wedge pressure
LVSW	= Left ventricular stroke work

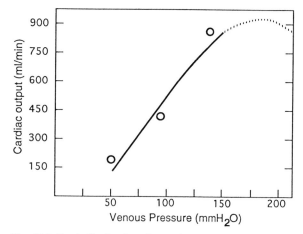

Fig. 12.1 Frank–Starling length–tension curve.

The force of contraction of the myocardium is dependent on 'preload' and 'afterload'. Preload is the degree to which the myocardium is stretched before contraction. It represents venous return, and the ability of the heart to accurately keep the stroke volume equal to the venous return is illustrated by the Frank–Starling length–tension curve (Fig. 12.1).[8] Afterload reflects the stress which develops in the left ventricular wall during systole between mitral valve closure and aortic valve opening and is a major determinant of myocardial oxygen consumption. This is affected by the pressure at which the aortic valve opens, and hence the lower the aortic pressure the lower the stress in the wall of the left ventricle and the greater the subsequent contraction of the muscle. If central aortic pressure is lowered, the afterload and oxygen consumption of the myocardium are reduced and cardiac output improved.

Myocardial oxygen consumption

Myocardial oxygen supply is chiefly determined by the integrity of the coronary arteries and is related to their patency, diastolic perfusion gradient and length of diastole. The principal determinants of myocardial oxygen demand are heart rate, myocardial contractility, ventricular volume and systolic blood pressure. Coronary blood flow occurs primarily in diastole and the coronary perfusion gradient is the difference between the aortic pressure and LV pressure throughout diastole. This is augmented or diminished by alterations in aortic diastolic pressure and changes in

LV diastolic pressure. Maintenance of an adequate perfusion gradient is particularly important in myocardial ischaemia.

Applied physiology of intra-aortic balloon counterpulsation

Treatment of myocardial ischaemia should augment oxygen delivery to the heart whilst reducing consumption. It should also support the systemic circulation. The IABP is a mechanical device which aims to meet these criteria.

Counterpulsation involves the phasic displacement of blood within a fixed intravascular space. Synchronized with the cardiac cycle it reduces the blood volume in the ascending aorta during ventricular systole and augments the volume of blood in the aortic root during diastole.

The balloon is positioned in the descending aorta (Fig. 12.2), usually via the femoral artery, and intermittently inflated and deflated with helium gas. The pump may be activated to inflate the balloon by an electrical signal from the R wave of the electrocardiogram, by the arterial pressure trace, or by a pacemaker, so that inflation occurs on the dicrotic notch of the arterial pulse wave and deflation just before the upstroke of the next waveform. The normal aortic root pressure pattern is modified with the systolic pressure now decreasing and diastolic pressure increasing (Fig. 12.3).

Oxygen demand of the myocardium in each cardiac cycle is reflected by the integral of systolic

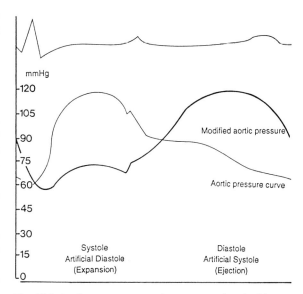

Fig. 12.3 Aortic root pressure changes associated with use of IABC.

pressure with respect to time (the tension–time index) and myocardial oxygen supply is related to the difference between the time integrals of diastolic pressure in the aorta (diastolic pressure–time index) and the left ventricle. Pressure changes invoked by counterpulsation favour an increase in the diastolic pressure–time index, thereby augmenting myocardial oxygen supply, and a decrease in the tension–time index, thus diminishing myocardial oxygen demand (Fig. 12.4). The decreased systolic pressure is reflected by a reduction in the LV afterload with an increase in stroke volume.

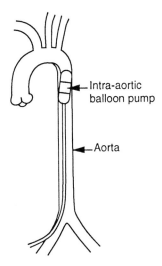

Fig. 12.2 Intra-aortic balloon pump positioned in the aorta.

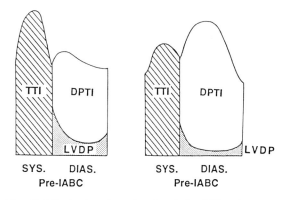

Fig. 12.4 Reduction of tension–time index (TTI) and augmentation of diastolic pressure–time index (DPTI) by intra-aortic counterpulsation.

In summary, IABC decreases the oxygen demands of the myocardium whilst increasing oxygen availability. Combined with the advantageous alteration of cardiac loading, this provides optimal conditions to alleviate myocardial ischaemia and support the circulation.

Clinical issues

IABC has been applied in a variety of conditions most commonly related to ischaemic heart disease. There is uncertainty over some indications for its use. A summary has been described by Kantrowitz[9] and a modification is shown in Table 12.2. Controversial indications include insertion as prophylaxis in high-risk patients undergoing cardiac catheterization (including coronary angioplasty) and major non-cardiac surgery.[10,11] In these situations an assessment of risk and potential benefit be made for each patient. IABC may be a valuable method of optimizing myocardial function in high-risk patients who need non-cardiac surgery, with a substantial reduction in the expected mortality.[12,13] It should be considered for patients who develop or have the potential to develop myocardial problems during the course of non-cardiac procedures.

Table 12.2 Indications for IABC.

ISCHAEMIC HEART DISEASE
1. Following acute myocardial infarction with cardiogenic shock
2. Following acute myocardial infarction associated with ventricular or papillary muscle rupture
3. In unstable angina pectoris

IN ASSOCIATION WITH CARDIAC SURGERY

Preoperative support
1. To support and provide time for diagnosis and management (e.g. post-infarct ventricular septal defect)
2. To improve myocardial function prior to definitive surgical procedure (e.g. transplantation, urgent surgery following failed angioplasty)

Postoperative support
1. For LV failure after CPB
2. For primary graft failure after transplantation
3. For intraoperative myocardial infarction

OTHERS
1. Intraoperative support for cardiac patients undergoing non-cardiac surgery
2. Patients who develop myocardial dysfunction following other procedures (e.g. general surgical patients)
3. Critically ill patients who develop myocardial dysfunction unrelated to their primary condition

Contraindications and complications

Aortic valve regurgitation is an absolute contraindication since augmentation of the diastolic pressure in this situation increases the LV afterload and LV diastolic volume, with detrimental effects. Tachydysrhythmias (e.g. SVT, AF) cause problems in regulating balloon inflation and deflation and should be controlled by appropriate means (e.g. drugs, pacing). Care should be taken in patients with peripheral vascular disease or prosthetic aortic grafts. Complications occur in up to 10% of patients[14] but are well recognized with careful monitoring.[15] They include limb ischaemia due to thrombosis or embolism (most notably in patients with pre-existing peripheral vascular disease), bleeding problems, infection, aortic dissection, and more rarely balloon rupture, gas embolism, or mesenteric and renal ischaemia.[14]

Technique of balloon insertion and removal

Insertion is carried out percutaneously via the femoral artery. Modern kits provide a balloon pre-wrapped around a central wire (Fig. 12.5) and this can be inserted into the artery via a previously positioned sheath (Fig. 12.6), although 'sheathless' balloons are now available. It can be removed without surgically exposing and repairing the femoral artery. A radiograph should be taken to confirm its position. Heparin is given (30 U/kg loading dose) and maintained at 500–1000 U every 2 hours, keeping the activated clotting time in the range 150–200 s.[16] Percutaneous techniques have enhanced the ease of application of the device, although in specialist centres insertion can be achieved via the iliac arteries and ascending or descending aorta at the time of cardiac surgery.

Removal is straightforward if certain principles are observed. The balloon should be completely collapsed by aspiration and pulled down into the sheath. The femoral artery distally is tightly compressed to prevent possible emboli, and balloon and sheath are removed together. Blood is allowed to spurt from the artery for a few seconds to allow extrusion of blood clots. Manual compression is applied over the insertion site for 30 minutes and a compression dressing for 24 hours. The insertion site and distal limb pulses are monitored for signs of haematoma formation or limb ischaemia.

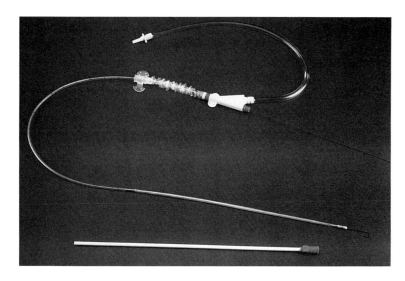

Fig. 12.5 Percor Stat-DL 9.5FG IAB pump with Stat Gard.

Patient management and device control

The need for IABC arises when the impaired ventricle cannot maintain adequate tissue perfusion despite an optimal circulating volume and appropriate inotropic support. All patients requiring IABP require a Swann Ganz catheter. This enables right atrial pressure, pulmonary arterial

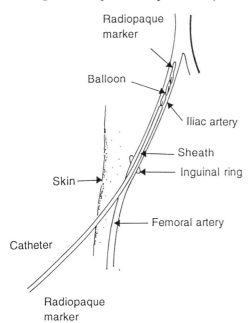

Fig. 12.6 Percutaneous transfemoral insertion of the intra-aortic balloon.

pressure, pulmonary capillary wedge pressure and cardiac output to be measured. The dynamic variables of systemic and pulmonary vascular resistances, stroke volume index and stroke index can also be calculated (Table 12.1) and the patient's response to pharmacological manipulation monitored. Blood taken via the catheter allows measurement of the mixed venous saturation. If, after insertion of a Swann Ganz catheter, achievement of adequate LV filling pressures and inotropic manipulation, the systolic blood pressure is below 90 mmHg, the cardiac index is less than $1.8 \, l/min/m^2$ and the mixed venous saturation is below 30%, the indications exist for mechanical support.[17]

Some patients may benefit from 'prophylactic' insertion (e.g. patients with impaired myocardial function who require non-cardiac surgery). A Swann Ganz catheter is still required to establish their initial haemodynamic status, determine any deterioration of myocardical function and monitor their response to IABC.

Timing of balloon inflation and deflation may be accomplished using the ECG or the arterial pressure waveform. Adjustment is easily made with modern consoles (Fig. 12.7). With ECG control, balloon inflation is set at the peak of the T wave and deflation within the PR interval. If the ECG is of poor quality or if large T waves, pacing spikes or intraoperative use of diathermy causes interference, inflation may be set to occur at the dicrotic notch of the arterial pressure trace with

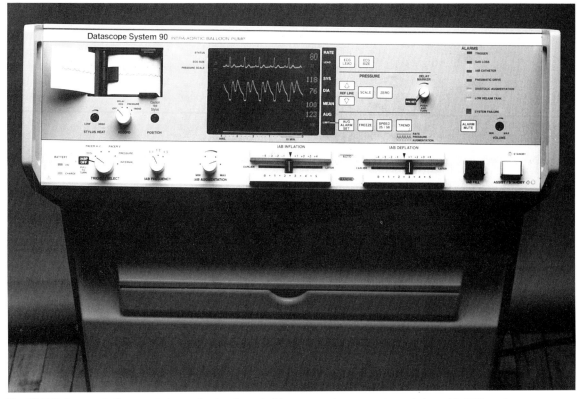

Fig. 12.7 Datascope balloon control console showing arterial pressure changes and correlation with ECG tracing.

deflation completed just before the onset of systole. Optimal haemodynamic effects are achieved by varying the inflation volume or timing of the inflation/deflation sequence; (i.e. the balloon can be set to inflate and deflate during every cardiac cycle (1:1), or every other cycle (1:2) up to a sequence of 1:8. The optimal setting is determined by the haemodynamic response, aided by measuring the parameters discussed previously using the Swann Ganz catheter.

The IABC should remain until haemodynamic function has recovered enough for support to be weaned off. As cardiac function improves, equalization of the peak aortic systolic pressure and balloon systole is observed. Pharmacological support should be minimized before removal so that it may be increased if deterioration subsequently occurs. Weaning is achieved by decreasing the frequency of counterpulsation (e.g. from 1:1 to 1:2) or by decreasing the volume of helium pumped per cycle. If a cardiac index of over $2\,l/min/m^2$, a pulmonary capillary wedge pressure below 18 mmHg and an LV stroke work index above $20\ \mathrm{g\text{-}m/m^2}$ can be maintained with progressive decreases in the frequency or volume of counterpulsation, weaning is likely to be successful.[17]

References

1. Amsterdam EA, DeMaria AN, Hughes JL, *et al.* Myocardial infarction: shock, mechanisms and management. In: Mason DT (eds), *Congestive Heart Failure.* New York: Yorke Medical Books, 1976.
2. Harken DE. Presentation at the International College of Cardiology, Brussels, Belgium, 1958.
3. Moulopoulos SD, Topaz S, Kolff WF. Diastolic balloon pumping (with carbon dioxide) in the aorta: a mechanical assist to the failing circulation. *Am Heart J* 1962; **63**, 669.
4. Kantrowitz A, Tjonneland F, Freed PS, *et al.* Initial clinical experience with intra-aortic balloon pumping in cardiogenic shock. *JAMA* 1968; **203**, 135.
5. Bregman D. Clinical experience with percutaneous intra-aortic balloon pumping. In: Unger F (ed), *Assisted Circulation*, vol 3. Berlin: Springer Verlag, 1989: 74–85.

6. Spence PA, Weisel RD, Easdown J, *et al.* The haemodynamic effects and mechanism of action of pulmonary artery balloon counterpulsation in the treatment of right ventricular failure during left heart bypass. *Ann Thorac Surg* 1985; **39**, 329–335.

7. Symbas PN, McKeown PP, Santora AH, Viasis SE. Pulmonary artery balloon counterpulsation for treatment of intraoperative right ventricular failure. *Ann Thorac Surg* 1985; **39**, 437–440.

8. Little RC, Little WC. The output of the heart and its control. In: Little RC, Little WC (eds), *Physiology of the Heart and Circulation*. Chicago: Year Book Medical Publishers, 1989: 221–222.

9. Kantrowitz A. Intra-aortic balloon counterpulsation: clinical aspects and prospects. In: Unger F (ed), *Assisted Circulation*, vol 3. Berlin: Springer Verlag, 1989: 52–73.

10. D'Agostino RS, Baldwin JC. Intra-aortic balloon counterpulsation: present status. *Compr Ther* 1986; **12**, 47–54.

11. Satler LF, Rackley CE. Assessment of adequate circulatory assist during intra-aortic balloon counter-pulsation. In: Brest AN (ed), *Advance in Critical Care Cardiology*. Philadelphia: Cardiovascular Clinics, 1986: 141–149.

12. Georgen RF, Dietrick JA, Pifarre R, *et al.* Placement of intra-aortic balloon pump allows definitive biliary surgery in patients with severe cardiac disease. *Surgery* 1989; **106**, 808–812.

13. Grotz RL, Yeston NS. Intra-aortic balloon counterpulsation in high risk cardiac patients undergoing non-cardiac surgery. *Surgery* 1989; **106**, 1–5.

14. Freedman RJ. The intra-aortic balloon pump system: current roles and future directions. *J Appl Cardiol* 1991; **6**, 313–318.

15. Glenville BE, Crokett J, Bennett JG. Compartment syndrome and intra-aortic balloon. *J Thorac Cardiovasc Surg* 1986; **34**, 292–294.

16. F. Guzman M, Hedley-Brown A (eds). *Cardiothoracic Handbook*. London: Butterworths, 1989: 60–61.

17. Lee ME. Mechanical support of the circulation. In: Gray RJ, Matloff JM (eds), *Medical Management of the Cardiac Surgical Patient*. Baltimore: Williams & Wilkins, 1990: 164–174.

13

The development and future of the Hemopump®

Richard K Wampler

Introduction

The Hemopump® is a catheter-mounted mechanical circulatory assist device that can support the majority of the circulation and significantly reduce left ventricular work. It can be introduced via a peripheral artery or the ascending aorta. This chapter presents an overview of the development and operation of this pump and the results of a clinical trial in which it was used to treat cardiogenic shock. New applications and second-generation technologies based on the principle of the Hemopump are discussed.

Cardiogenic shock is a life-threatening condition characterized by severe LV dysfunction, hypoperfusion and secondary organ failure. The strategy of current therapy is based on the premise that the heart often has the potential to recover from even severe acute myocardial dysfunction if it is relieved of the requirement to support the circulation and is effectively decompressed. The current therapy for cardiogenic shock combines pharmacological agents and temporary mechanical circulatory assistance (usually the intra-aortic balloon pump, IABP) to increase the cardiac output and decrease LV work until the heart recovers and is able to resume support of the circulation. However, this therapy has been of limited clinical utility in decreasing the high mortality (80–90%) associated with cardiogenic shock.[1-3] This failure may reflect the limitations of the therapeutic armamentarium rather than an error in the hypothesis. If, indeed, the heart has the potential to recover from acute myocardial dysfunction, it could be that these disappointing results are due to the fact that current therapy simply does not provide sufficient haemodynamic improvement and ventricular unloading to facilitate return of myocardial function.

It has been suggested that mechanical assist modalities more powerful than the IABP might provide the level of haemodynamic improvement needed to effect myocardial recovery and reduce the mortality of cardiogenic shock. Indeed, the notion of using LV assist devices (LVADs) to treat cardiogenic shock has a certain theoretical allure since LVADs have the potential to produce greater haemodynamic improvement and ventricular unloading than the IABP. In addition, LVADs have been shown to facilitate recovery of non-contractile but viable or 'stunned' myocardium in the setting of cardiogenic shock in experimental animals.[4-7] However, when one begins to contemplate the substantial barriers which must be overcome to use existing LVADs in the routine treatment of circulatory failure, discouragement cannot be too far behind.

Unfortunately, existing LVADs have not yet evolved to practical devices since current embodiments tend to be large, cumbersome, complicated experimental devices which have been adapted to limited use in surgical patients.[8-12] Although LVADs have demonstrated some limited clinical utility in patients who fail to wean from bypass and as bridges to cardiac transplantation, they are rarely used in the treatment of cardiogenic shock secondary to acute myocardial infarction. This is true because the major surgery needed to implant LVADs and the attendant risks has precluded their use in the treatment of acute myocardial infarction and seriously limited their use in surgical patients. It is, after all, one thing to plumb conduits of garden-hose size into the heart of a patient with an open sternum, and something altogether different to contemplate such a procedure on a patient with myocardial infarction. Clearly, a new approach was needed.

The genesis of the Hemopump

In order to exploit the theoretical benefits of LVADs in the treatment of cardiogenic shock, an 'ideal' device was needed which could combine the haemodynamic power of the LVAD and the simplicity and safety of the IABP. By the time I began thinking about circulatory assistance, the clinical stage had been set for the appearance of a radically different, practical LVAD which could be readily adapted to clinical use.

In 1981, armed with considerable naivety, I proposed a novel approach to the implementation of mechanical circulatory assistance. It seemed to me that existing LVADs with their large blood conduits, air hoses and the major surgery needed for their implantation could never evolve into a practical clinical device. For LVADs to be practical, I reasoned, the logistics of achieving circulatory access and implantation had to be simplified. An old Islamic proverb says: 'If you cannot bring Muhammad to the mountain, then bring the mountain to Muhammad'. When I began to think of the problem of circulatory access without the prejudice of previous approaches, and began to think of the pump as the mountain, the solution was not far away. The Hemopump solves the problem of circulatory access by taking the 'mountain to Muhammad'. Instead of pulling blood out of the heart and returning it to the circulation with external pumps and conduits, I thought, 'why not place the pump inside the arterial system?' The concept of positioning the pump inside the arterial system instead of outside the heart (or body) in a very real sense did 'deliver the mountain to Muhammad' and made it possible to avoid many of the

problems attendant with the use of existing LVADs.

This solution assumed that it would be possible to create a miniaturized catheter-mounted device that could be placed intra-arterially to remove blood directly from the left ventricle and pump it into the aorta. This pump would be remotely driven via an external motor. This first essential piece of the puzzle came to me as a result of my experience with submersible pumps with which I became familiar while working on village water supplies in rural Egypt in 1975.

The second essential piece of the puzzle was the pumping mechanism of the device. The blood pump would need to be no more than 8 mm in diameter and produce at least 2–3 litres of flow per minute. Given these constraints it seemed clear that only a miniaturized axial flow pump could be adapted to this purpose. Such pumps are descendants of the principle of the Archimedes screw originally developed by the ancient Egyptians to pump water from the Nile river for irrigation 2000 years before Christ. The Hemopump was born at the moment when I took the principle of the submersible pump and the Archimedes screw and adapted them to the problem of pumping blood.

The Hemopump provides an elegant solution to a very difficult problem. It is innovative because it combines simplicity and safety with great haemodynamic power. The pump has made it possible to provide a large degree of circulatory support and LV decompression with minimal risk. Given these unique attributes, the Hemopump seemed ideally suited for use in the treatment of cardiogenic shock.

System description

The Hemopump is a circulatory assist device capable of providing temporary support for the left ventricle without the need for a major surgical procedure.[13] It draws blood out of the left ventricle and expels it into the aorta (Fig. 13.1). It can be placed via a peripheral vascular access or by the ascending aorta, and can provide up to 4.7 l/min of flow without the need for a contribution from the left ventricle or synchronization. Since the inflow cannula is placed within the left ventricle, Hemopump assistance results in a significant degree of LV decompression and reduction in LV work.

The pump is currently available in three different models: 24F femoral, sternotomy, and 14F percutaneous (Fig. 13.2). Attached distally to the pump housing is an inflow cannula. During operation the inflow cannula resides in the left ventricle and the outlet of the pump in the ascending aorta. Proximal to the pump and inflow cannula is a 3 mm diameter (9.5F) flexible drive cable (107 cm long) which transmits rotary motion from an external drive motor to the pump.

The console (Fig. 13.3) is an integrated electronic controller incorporating all of the power, control and diagnostic/alarm systems required to operate the pump and supply it with purge fluid for the rotating shaft seal.

Blood is removed from the left ventricle and expelled into the aorta as a result of the hydraulic gradient produced by the spinning pump rotor. Blood flows from the tip of the inflow cannula, out of the left ventricular cavity, and into the systemic circulation.

Clinical trials

A clinical trial was conducted in the USA from April 1988 to November 1991 to study the use of the Hemopump in the treatment of cardiogenic shock.[14] The results of the FDA trial are summarized below.

Patients were recruited into the trial with the following diagnoses:

1. Acute myocardial infarction
2. Failure to wean from cardiopulmonary bypass
3. Low cardiac output syndrome following CPB
4. Other (i.e. donor graft rejection, cardiomyopathy, acute donor graft failure etc.

Patients were also intended to meet the following haemodynamic criteria:

1. Cardiac index of less than $2.0 \, 1/min/m^2$
2. Pulmonary capillary wedge pressure of greater than 18.0 mmHg
3. Systolic blood pressure of less than 90 mmHg.

In addition, patients were to be refractory to fluid challenge and drug therapy. Safety and effectiveness of the Hemopump was assessed by evaluation of the haemodynamic response, blood chemistries (including plasma free haemoglobin), weaning from support and 30-day survival.

One-hundred and fourteen patients were accepted into the study. The pump was successfully inserted in 88 (77.2%), of whom 76 (86.4%) were male. The mean age was 54 years (range 9–76). Shock was secondary to the following diagnostic aetiologies: acute myocardial infarction (AMI) 33%; failure to wean from cardiopulmonary bypass (FTW) 25%; post-cardiotomy low cardiac output syndrome (LCO) 16%; other 23%.

Haemodynamic response

The principal effect of the Hemopump should be improvement in the haemodynamic condition of the patient. Analysis of haemodynamic data has demonstrated a statistically and clinically significant improvement in haemodynamics when comparing the status of a patient prior to pump

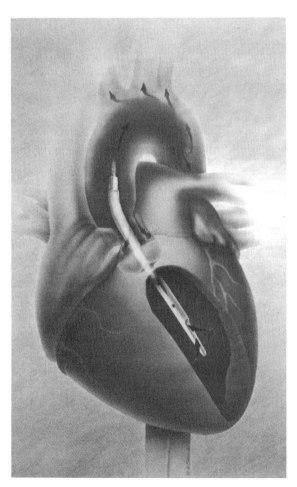

Fig. 13.1 The sternotomy Hemopump.

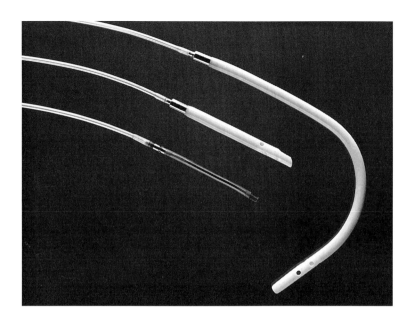

Fig. 13.2 Hemopump catheters.

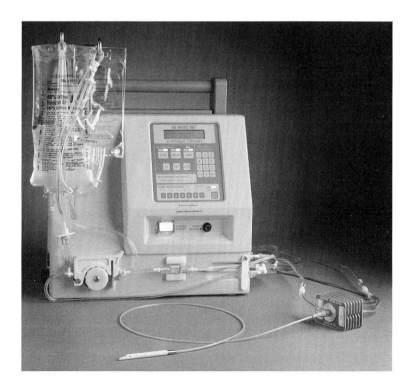

Fig. 13.3 The Hemopump console.

Table 13.1 Haemodynamic response following Hemopump insertion.

	Pre-insert	At 24 h	During operation
CI (l/min/m²)	1.72 ± 0.074	2.24 ± 0.08	2.16 ± 0.08
PCWP (mm Hg)	25 ± 1	16 ± 0.5	16 ± 0.6
SBP (mm Hg)	77 ± 2.1	74 ± 2.6	78 ± 2.6

CI = cardiac index; PCWP = pulmonary capillary wedge pressure; SBP =systolic blood pressure.

insertion versus during pump operation. The haemodynamic response for the patients in which values were available are summarized in Table 13.1.

Overall survival

The overall survival to weaning from support was 42% and to 30 days following pump removal was 27.3%. The survival by aetiology is included in Table 13.2.

Haematological effects

The mean levels of the plasma free haemoglobin and platelets during assistance are shown in Table 13.3.

Complications and device-related adverse events

The safety of the Hemopump was judged by an evaluation of blood trauma, anatomic compatibility, incidence of thromboembolism, leg ischaemia and related complications.

Table 13.2 Survival by aetiology.

Disease	Weaned		30 day survivor	
AMI	51%	(15/29)	34.5%	(10/29)
FTW	32%	(8/25)	24%	(6/25)
LCO	28.6%	(4/14)	14.3%	(2/14)
Other	50%	(10/20)	30%	(6/20)

AMI = acute myocardial infarction; FTW = failure to wean; LCO = low cardiac output.

Device-related adverse events

These included mechanical failure of the system, difficulty placing or removing the system, and loss of assistance. Non-insertion of the pump was reported in 22.8% (26/114) of the patients. There was loss of circulatory assistance secondary to ejection of the cannula from the ventricle in 12.5% (11/88), and from drive cable fracture in 9% (8/88).

Haematological complications

Blood loss of more than 500 ml was seen in 18.2% (16/88) of patients and was thought to be related to the Hemopump in six of these.

Thrombocytopenia (platelets <50 000/mm³) was reported in 18.2% (16/88) and was thought to be related to the Hemopump in five cases. Platelet levels quickly returned to normal after device removal.

Excessive haemolysis (at least one plasma free haemoglobin reading greater than 50 mg/dl) was reported in 10.2% (9/88) of patients. In two patients the haemolysis was related to aspirated material lodged in the pump rotor.

Infectious complications

Septicaemia was seen in 12.5% (11/88) of patients and was fatal in six. The Hemopump was not implicated as the source of sepsis in any case.

Infection at the insertion site was seen in three patients and resolved with treatment.

Vascular complications

Leg ischaemia was device-related in three of four reported cases. The overall incidence was 4.5% (4/88). All resolved with treatment, none required amputations.

Vascular injury was caused by the Hemopump in 7.9% (7/88). All were repaired without residual deficit.

Table 13.3 Laboratory values at admission and during pump operation.

	Pre-insert	At 24 h	During operation
Platelets (all) (× 1000/mm³)	207 ± 11.9	116 ± 8.1	122 ± 7.1
Free haemoglobin (all) (mg/dl)	18.49	34.97	44.9
Haemoglobin (all) (g/dl)	11.5 ± 0.24	10.4 ± 0.20	10.4 ± 0.17

Thromboembolism was reported in 9% (8/88) of patients, either as a focal neurologic deficit or loss of a peripheral pulse. These cases were all associated with pre-existing mural thrombus.

Valvular injuries

Autopsy finding of valve abnormality was present in two cases. These were one minor abrasions and haemorrhage and one tear. Neither was considered to be haemodynamically significant.

Clinical evidence of valve injury or haemodynamic insufficiency/stenosis was not observed in any patient.

Death

Death occurring during assistance was reported in 58% (51/88) of patients. One of these was related to excessive blood loss during insertion.

Death following weaning was reported in 35.1% (13/37) of patients. None of these deaths were attributed to the Hemopump.

Discussion of results

The results of the phase I trial demonstrated that the Hemopump was haemodynamically effective and was capable of supporting the circulation of a large number of patients with cardiogenic shock. Furthermore, those patients who demonstrated a significant haemodynamic improvement in response to assistance often experienced LV recovery and long-term survival. In spite of these successes, however, the outcome of the phase I trial was disappointing in that the improvement in survival was not as dramatic as we had hoped. Consequently, we were not able to build a compelling argument in support of filing for a premarket approval application with the FDA. The approval application based on the phase I trial has been withdrawn pending approval of a phase II trial.

Some of the reasons for the non-filing of the phase I study are as follows. With the benefit of hindsight it seems clear that the phase I trial was doomed from the start because the Hemopump was used in critical patients who were *expected to die*, rather than in less critical patients. Unfortunately, the survival of patients proved to be more dependent upon the severity of shock and the timing of intervention than on the effect of the Hemopump. The decision to treat patients with

essentially 'irreversible' shock proved beyond a doubt that such shock is, usually, truly irreversible.

Our clinical experience to date demonstrates that the Hemopump is safe and effective and may offer significant clinical benefit to patients with cardiogenic shock secondary to *potentially reversible* acute LV dysfunction. The single greatest factor influencing survival is the timing of intervention. If the pump is not used aggressively, early in the course of shock, nearly all of the opportunity for survival will be lost because of secondary organ failure and sepsis.

Future technology and trials

In response to the painful lessons of the phase I trial we have changed our regulatory and marketing strategy. A number of changes have been made in the design to improve its safety and effectiveness, and a new clinical protocol for the phase II study has been developed.

A sternotomy Hemopump device with a short (10.5 cm) inflow cannula has been introduced to facilitate intra-operative insertion through a median sternotomy. This pump has improved hydraulics which results in flows of approximately 4.7 l/min. In addition, a number of design and manufacturing changes have been introduced to improve durability and reliability. This device is in clinical use in Europe and will be evaluated in the USA under an Investigational Device Exemption.

For medical patients a small version of the Hemopump has been developed which is intended for percutaneous femoral insertion. The percutaneous Hemopump is 14F in size and is intended for wire-guided insertion under fluoroscopic imaging. The percutaneous pump is capable of 2.2 l/min of flow at 70 mmHg. It is intended for 7 days of use. It is anticipated that this device will be evaluated for use in supported high-risk angioplasty and in the setting of acute intervention following acute myocardial infarction.

Phase II trial with the sternotomy Hemopump

Although the pump was originally conceived for use in the treatment of cardiogenic shock, we have come to the conclusion that the difficulties of conducting a study of cardiogenic shock that would pass the scrutiny of the FDA may well be insurmountable. Substantial resources have therefore been invested in a search for the ideal clinical trial, and it is now our proposal that the phase II trial for the sternotomy Hemopump will study its clinical utility for intra-operative non-oxygenator support during aortocoronary bypass (ACB) surgery.

The purpose of this clinical investigation is to show that the pump system is equivalent to, or better than, conventional extracorporeal CPB when used to support a subset of patients who would normally be candidates for isolated aorto-coronary bypass graft surgery. It is our belief that such a study can demonstrate significant reductions in blood transfusions, complications, recovery time and cost. Recent experience with surgery on the beating heart and the historical development of ACB surgery supports this hypothesis.

Background to the phase II trial

When direct coronary artery surgery was introduced during the late 1950s in the form of patch plasty and endarterectomy, it was performed on the beating heart without CPB.[15,16] Shortly thereafter, aortocoronary bypass grafts using the saphenous vein and the internal mammary artery were successfully placed to the left anterior descending and the right coronary artery with CPB.[17] However, complete revascularization was not always achievable because the circumflex and posterior vessels were inaccessible in the non-decompressed beating heart. In order to place grafts to these vessels, some means of ventricular decompression and circulatory support was necessary. CPB with an artificial oxygenator was used successfully to complete revascularization for segmental disease by Favaloro and others in 1968.[18–23]

However, even with low mortality, the morbidity of revascularization with CPB is still significant, particularly in those patients who undergo revascularization in unfavourable clinical situations and in older patients. This morbidity may be related to CPB where, for a period of time, conditions of non-physiological circulation exist. If, indeed, CPB and the artificial oxygenator contribute to the mortality and morbidity of coronary artery surgery, it is possible that the avoidance of CPB and the artificial oxygenator could benefit patients.

Motivated by the desire to avoid the complications of CPB and the artificial oxygenator, a number of investigators have reported successful results. In 1975, Trapp and Bisarya[24] and Ankeney[25] published their experiences with non-oxygenator and non-CPB ACB surgery. Buffalo *et al.*[26] and Benetti *et al.*[27] have recently published their results with patients (593 and 700 respectively) who underwent ACB surgery without CPB. In the USA, Pfister and Corso[28] reported their experience with 220 patients. These studies demonstrate that the complications of CPB can be avoided during ACB surgery.

Despite the demonstration of statistically significant clinical benefits in those patients who were revascularized without CPB, the majority of ACB patients (80%) require revascularization to circumflex or posterior vessels or segmental disease, and thus were not candidates for this technique.[26–28] In these series, approximately 20% of ACB candidates were amenable to non-CPB ACB. In order to fully exploit the potential advantage of revascularization without CPB, it would be necessary to decompress the heart and support the circulation to facilitate access to circumflex and posterior vessels while avoiding the use of the pump oxygenator. Ventricular assist devices have been successfully adapted to this application. Extracorporeal non-oxygenator support with ventricular assist devices (VADs) has been used to support patients during ACB surgery. Use of VADs during ACB surgery avoids the risk of the artificial oxygenator, since the patient's own lungs are functioning, yet allows the surgeon to safely revascularize vessels that were inaccessible in the experiences of Buffolo, Benetti and Pfister.

The use of non-oxygenator extracorporeal support during ACB surgery has a number of theoretical advantages:

1. Ventricular decompression should decrease myocardial oxygen demand and increase coronary flow to ischaemic areas, thereby protecting the myocardium.
2. An artificial oxygenator and the associated circuit are not needed since the patient's own lungs oxygenate the blood.
3. Aortic cross-clamping and ischaemic arrest are not necessary.
4. The heparin dosage can be lowered and potentially there would be less blood loss.

Glenville and Ross[29] and Sweeney and Frazier[30] have demonstrated that a VAD may be used effectively for intraoperative haemodynamic support and ventricular decompression during ACB surgery. However, although the results with VAD-supported ACB surgery have been encouraging, the VADs currently available are not ideally suited to this application. VAD-supported ACB surgery currently adapts a centrifugal pump intended for use in a cardiopulmonary circuit as an extra-corporeal VAD with the use of large-bore cannulaes. There are several disadvantages to this approach.

The Hemopump system may avoid many of the limitations and potential problems inherent in extracorporeal VAD support. The small size of the pump assembly permits it to be placed intra-corporeally, without the need for a large-bore cannula. The pump could potentially be an ideal VAD for intraoperative support during ACB surgery. During the course of the phase I trial, five patients underwent ACB surgery during non-oxygenator Hemopump LV support, and all were successfully revascularized and survived. These results are very encouraging, particularly since these were high-risk patients with acute myocardial infarction and severe LV dysfunction.

The most serious complications related to CPB include severe bleeding secondary to CPB-induced abnormalities of the coagulation system that require reoperation or blood transfusion; pulmonary dysfunction or pneumonia secondary to haemodilution and cell-mediated toxic reactions from the oxygenator; and impairment of ventricular function requiring pharmacological support or intra-aortic balloon counterpulsation (IABC).

Recent experience with non-oxygenator bypass during ACB surgery, and ACB surgery on the unsupported heart, has demonstrated a significant potential to avoid many of the complications. Glenville and Ross[29] used non-oxygenator biventricular assist to perform ACB. In this study they demonstrated the absence of microbubbles, indicating less potential for neurological complications, and a reduction in sequestration of white cells in the lungs which would indicate the potential for fewer pulmonary complications. Benneti *et al.*[27] reported on the results of ACB surgery on the beating, unsupported heart; in this study 90% were free from transfusion and only 6% required inotropic support. In a similar series of patients, Buffolo *et al.*[26] reported pulmonary complications in 3.2% compared with a CPB control of 9.7%, and only 8 transfusions in a series of 593 patients. Pfister and Corso[28] reported freedom from blood transfusion in 72.7% of patients compared with 54.6% in a retrospectively matched CPB control

group. They also reported a requirement for pharmacological or mechanical ventricular support (IABC) in 5.5% of patients versus 12.7% in CPB control patients.

Protocol for the phase II trial

The phase II trial will evaluate the clinical utility of the sternotomy Hemopump for non-oxygenator support during aortocoronary bypass surgery. This trial will be a prospective, randomized study. A patient may be entered into the study if he or she meets all of the following criteria:

1. The patient is a candidate for isolated aorto-coronary bypass grafting using conventional CPB.
2. One to five grafts are planned.
3. The target vessels intended for bypass are among the following:
   Left coronary artery
   —left anterior descending artery
   —ramus medianus artery
   —diagonal artery
   —obtuse marginal artery 2 cm from the takeoff of the circumflex artery
   Right coronary artery
   —acute marginal artery
   —posterior descending artery
   —posterior left ventricular artery.

A patient will be *excluded* from the trial if he or she meets any one of the following criteria:

1. There is significant blood dyscrasia.
2. The patient has a prosthetic aortic valve or severe aortic stenosis or insufficiency.
3. He or she refuses to accept blood transfusions.
4. There is a left ventricular or atrial mural thrombus.
5. There is pulmonary hypertension.
6. The patient is a candidate for emergency surgery.
7. There is intravascular haemolysis greater than 25 mg/dl.

The clinical utility of non-oxygenator support with the Hemopump will be established by assessing freedom from serious complications and avoidance of heterogeneous blood transfusions. Serious complications will be taken to include:

1. Any reoperation due to bleeding.
2. Focal neurological deficit following surgery.

3. Pulmonary failure, defined as the need for ventilator support 24 hours after surgery.
4. A low-output state, defined as impaired haemodynamics requiring inotropic drug therapy for longer than 24 hours after surgery or the use of an IAB pump.
5. Disseminated intravascular coagulopathy (DIC).

An investigational device exemption, based on this protocol was approved by the United States FDA in 1993; these clinical trials are in progress.

What is the future of the Hemopump?

It is very clear that the Hemopump pumps blood effectively and safely, and has been life-saving. As the body of clinical experience grows, I must confess that there are still times when I, the inventor, am astonished that it works at all. How does the blood escape destruction as it passes through this high-speed 'Waring blender'? Companies, investors, engineers and clinicians have shared the vision of the Hemopump even when it did not work at all and, with their efforts, it was made to work. When one considers the instinctive reaction shared by many—that it shouldn't work—the clinical successes bear testimony to a substantial achievement. Many dramatic clinical cases serve as testimony to its potential. However, the pump has some rough ground to cover if it is to claim a prominent place in clinical practice. For it to be successful it must also get FDA approval.

It is my firm belief that this technology can revolutionize the management of cardiogenic shock and myocardial infarction, and shake up a few paradigms about the way we do heart surgery. It is gratifying to see that a large number of other groups are pursuing variations on the principle of axial flow and continuous-flow blood pumps, and I believe the Hemopump had some role in bringing about this shift. I could not close without acknowledging the substantial and essential contributions of all those that have helped to carry the Hemopump this far and for the faith, sacrifice and courage of the patients and their families.

At the time of writing, the sternotomy Hemopump is approaching the status of a mature technology, ready to be put to the test in rigorous trials. The percutaneous Hemopump has reached clinical readiness and will, it is hoped, find its proper place as an interventional tool by the cardiologist. This has been my hope all these years. I wait to see what will happen next.

References

1. Norman JC, Cooley DA, Igo SR, *et al.* Prognostic indices for survival during postcardiotomy intra-aortic balloon pumping. *J Thorac Cardiovasc Surg* 1977; **74**, 709–720.
2. Parmley W. Cardiac failure. In: Rosen MR, Hoffman BF (eds), *Cardiac Thérapy*. Boston: Martinus Nijhoff, 1983: 21–44.
3. Shoemaker WC, Bland RD, Appel PL. Therapy of critically ill postoperative patients based on outcome prediction and prospective clinical trials. *Surg Clin N Am* 1985; **65**, 811–833.
4. Schoen FJ, Palmer DC, Bernhard WF, *et al.* Clinical temporary ventricular assist. *J Thorac Cardiovasc Surg* 1986; **92**, 1071–1081.
5. Lass J, Campbell CD, Takanashi Y, Pick R, Replogle RL. Preservation of ischemic myocardium with TALVB using complete left ventricular decompression. *ASAIO Trans* 1979; **25**, 220–223.
6. Takanashi Y, Campbell CD, Laas J, Pick RL, Meus P, Replogle RL. Reduction of myocardial infarct size in swine: a comparative study of intra-aortic balloon pumping and transapical left ventricular bypass. *Ann Thorac Surg* 1981; **32**, 475–485.
7. Merhgie ME, Smalling RW, Cassidy D, Barrett R, Wise G, Short J, Wampler RK. Effect of the Hemopump left ventricular assist device on regional myocardial perfusion and function: reduction of ischemia during coronary occlusion. *Circulation* 1989; **80** (suppl. III), 158–166.
8. Magovern GJ, Park SB, Maher TD. Use of a centrifugal pump without anticoagulants for postoperative left ventricular assist. *World J Surg* 1985; **9**, 25–36.
9. Bernstein EF, Dorman FD, Blackshear PL, Scott DR. An efficient, compact blood pump for assisted circulation. *Surgery* 1970; **68**, 105–115.
10. Golding LR, Jacobs G, Groves LK, Gill CC, Nose Y, Loop FD. Clinical results of mechanical support of the failing left ventricle. *J Thorac Cardiovasc Surg* 1982; **83**, 597–601.
11. Pae WE, Pierce WS, Pennock JL, Campbell DB, Waldhausen JA. Long-term results of ventricular assist pumping in postcardiotomy cardiogenic shock. *J Thorac Cardiovasc Surg* 1987; **93**, 431–441.
12. Pennington DG, Samuels LD, Williams G, *et al.* Experience with the Pierce–Donachy ventricular assist device in postcardiotomy patients with cardiogenic shock. *World J Surg* 1985; **9**, 37–46.
13. Wampler RK, Moise JC, Frazier OH, Olsen DB. *In*

vivo evaluation of a peripheral vascular access axial flow blood pump. *ASAIO Trans* 1988; **34**, 450–454.

14. Wampler RK, Frazier OH, Lansing AM, *et al.* Treatment of cardiogenic shock with the Hemopump left ventricular assist device. *Ann Thorac Surg* 1991; **52**, 506–513.

15. Balley CP, May A, Lemon WM. Survival after coronary endarterectomy in men. *JAMA* 1957; **167**, 641.

16. Longmire WP, Cannon JA, Kattus AA. Direct-vision coronary endarterectomy for angina pectoris. *New Engl J Med* 1958; **259**, 993.

17. Murray G, Porcheron R, Hilario J, Rosemblau W. Anastomosis of a systemic artery to the coronary. *Can Med Assoc J* 1954; **594**, 71.

18. Favaloro RG. Saphenous vein autograft replacement of severe segmental coronary artery occlusion. *Ann Thorac Surg* 1968; **33**, 5.

19. Kolessov VI. Mammary artery–coronary artery anastomosis as method of treatment for angina pectoris. *J Thorac Cardiovasc Surg* 1967; **54**, 535–544.

20. Johnson WD, Lepley D. An aggressive surgical approach to coronary disease. *J Thorac Cardiovasc Surg* 1970; **128**, 59.

21. Garrett RE, Dennid EW, Debakey ME. Aortocoronary bypass with saphenous vein graft. *JAMA* 1973; **223**, 792.

22. Sabiston DC. The coronary circulation. *Johns Hopkins Med J* 1974; **314**, 134.

23. Miller DW, Ivey TD, Bailey WW, Johnson DD, Hessel EA. The practice of coronary artery bypass surgery in 1980. *J Thorac Cardiovasc Surg* 1981; **81**, 423–427.

24. Trapp WG, Bisarya R. Placement of coronary artery bypass graft without pump oxygenator. *Ann Thorac Surg* 1975; **19**, 1–9.

25. Ankeney JL. Coronary vein graft without cardiopulmonary bypass a surgical motion picture. *Ann Thorac Surg* 1975; **1**, 19.

26. Buffolo E, Andrade JCS, Branco JNR, Aguiar JNR, Aguiar LF, Ribeiro EE, Jatene AD. Myocardial revascularization without extracorporeal circulation: seven-year experience in 593 cases. *Eur J Cardiothorac Surg* 1990; **4**, 504–508.

27. Benetti FJ, Naselli G, Wood M, Geffner L. Direct myocardial revascularization without extracorporeal circulation. *Chest* 1991; **100**, 313–316.

28. Pfister AJ, Corso P. Coronary artery bypass without cardiopulmonary bypass. *Ann Thorac Surg* 1992; **54**, 1085–1092.

29. Glenville B, Ross D. Coronary artery surgery with patient's lungs as oxygenator. *Lancet* 1986; **333**, 1005–1006.

30. Sweeney MS, Frazier OH. Device-supported myocardial revascularization: safe help for sick hearts. *Ann Thorac Surg* 1992; **54**, 1065–1070.

14

Clinical use of the Hemopump®

OH Frazier and Michael P Macris

Introduction

Direct unloading of the left ventricle through peripheral vessels is not a new concept. In the 1950s, Dennis and colleagues[1] developed a technique for left heart bypass in which a cannula was advanced through the internal jugular vein, into the right atrium, and then into the left atrium by way of a puncture in the atrial septum. This was a remarkable achievement given that the cannula was advanced and the puncture was created without visual aid. During the late 1950s and the 1960s, the investigators used this technique in seven patients with severe heart failure, and the treatment was successful in six. Dennis, Spencer and others[2] later showed the inadequacy of attempting to allow for ventricular recovery by femoral–femoral bypass alone. The problem of this approach was and remains the inability to directly unload the left ventricle and the problems associated with increased resistance against a poorly functioning left ventricle.

In 1987, investigators at the Texas Heart Institute began testing a unique axial flow pump, invented by Richard Wampler, that could directly unload the left ventricle. The cannula assembly for the miniature Hemopump® (Johnson and Johnson Interventional Systems, Rancho Cordova, CA) is advanced through a peripheral artery into the aorta, and then across the aortic valve. Thus, unlike the earlier left heart bypass technique, circulatory support could now be imple-

mented without injuring the heart. The Hemopump also provides adequate circulation for end-organ function, which optimizes the potential for left ventricular recovery.[3,4] Extensive studies of the Hemopump in healthy calves showed that haemolysis was minimal, despite the high flow rates.[5] Thus, in 1988, we[6] began testing the Hemopump in patients with potentially reversible acute heart failure.

Device description

The Hemopump system comprises (1) a small rotating screw contained within a 21-F silicone cannula that serves as the pumping mechanism, (2) a drive cable contained within a 9-F polymeric sheath, and (3) a purge fluid system. The system is operated and monitored through an external console that contains an electric motor and a microprocessor.

Properly positioned, the silicone cannula crosses the aortic valve, so that its tip rests within the left ventricle and the pump within the aortic arch (Fig. 14.1). When the system is activated, the drive cable rotates the screw at up to 25 000 times per minute, drawing blood from the left ventricle into the cannula, then propelling the blood into the aorta. The pump can produce flows of up to 4 litres/min, depending on the resistance. When pump support is initiated, the pulse is usually absent, but blood pressure is maintained. In

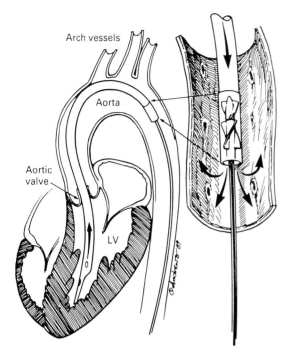

Fig. 14.1 Proper placement of the Hemopump. Reproduced with permission from reference 20.

addition, pulmonary capillary wedge pressure and left ventricular pressure are reduced.

The polymeric sheath containing the drive cable also contains the purge fluid system. An external roller pump on the console generates high-pressure flows to deliver the fluid (40% dextrose in water) to the bearings that support the rotating elements. The fluid lubricates the drive shaft and bearings and prevents thrombus formation.

Insertion techniques

A short (10 cm) and a long (26.2 cm) cannula have been used for the Hemopump, but because of FDA restrictions at the time of our initial studies, only one could be used. For technical and financial reasons, as well as its potential broader application to patients in nonoperative cardiogenic shock, the long cannula pump was utilized in the first large series of patients. Before that, the short cannula had been used successfully in two cases. Because this cannula can be inserted directly through the ascending aorta, it is suited for intraoperative treatment of postcardiotomy cardiogenic shock (Fig. 14.2).

Like the IABP, the long-cannula Hemopump is inserted through the femoral artery (Fig. 14.3), iliac artery, or distal abdominal aorta (Fig. 14.4). A 12-mm, low-porosity woven Dacron graft is sewn, end-to-side, to the arteriotomy, with continuous polypropylene sutures. The Hemopump cannula is introduced through the graft and advanced through the aorta, across the aortic valve, and into the left ventricle. Fluoroscopy is used to confirm the proper position of the cannula within the ventricle. Recently, a guide wire has been used during placement as an aid to fluoroscopy. To ensure that the pump functions properly, arterial pressure tracings are obtained at different pumping speeds. Finally, a silastic plug is placed in the distal opening of the graft and secured with a suture to prevent back bleeding and to protect the drive shaft. The skin incision is closed with monofilament suture.

Patient management

At initiation of support, the Hemopump is usually set to pump at full speed, producing nonpulsatile

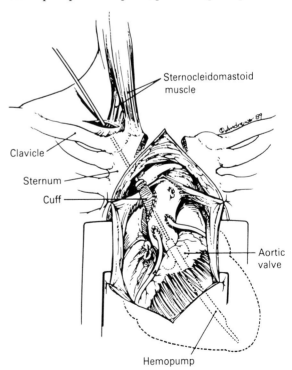

Fig. 14.2 Approach through the ascending aorta. Reproduced with permission from reference 20.

flow. Adequate function of the Hemopump depends on reducing mean aortic pressure, or afterload. Therefore, early after device insertion, a nitroprusside infusion may be used to maintain mean aortic pressure between 50 and 60 mmHg.[7] Reducing the afterload against which the device must pump increases its effectiveness. For example, at a mean pressure of 90 mmHg, flows at 2.6 litres/min are produced; at 55 mmHg, flows at 3.6 litres/min are produced. Inotropic agents should be avoided to decrease the heart rate and left ventricular end-diastolic pressure, further reducing myocardial oxygen requirements, afterload, and the risk of arrhythmia. Isoproterenol, prostaglandin E_1, or both, can be used to reduce pulmonary vascular resistance and improve right ventricular function. Finally, anticoagulative therapy usually consists of 1 mg/kg heparin.

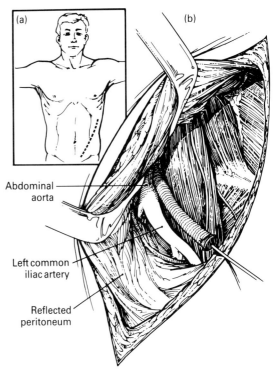

Fig. 14.4 Approach through the distal abdominal aorta. Reproduced with permission from reference 20.

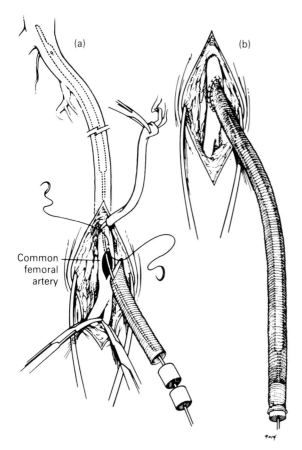

Fig. 14.3 Approach through the femoral artery by either (a) direct insertion through the arteriotomy, followed by graft anastomosis, or (b) insertion through the anastomosed graft. Reproduced with permission from reference 20.

As the heart recovers, pulse pressure returns and gradually increases, at which time weaning from LVAD support begins. If the pulse pressure fails to increase, support should be continued.

During Hemopump support, the patient must be monitored continually. Potential complications include dislodgement of the cannula due to restored ventricular function; drive cable breakage due to kinking; and obstruction of inflow due to mural thrombus, suction of the papillary muscle, or kinking of the cannula. The sudden onset of pulsatile flow and a decrease in cardiac output may indicate that the cannula has dislodged; the position of the cannula should be confirmed by chest X-ray.

Clinical experience

Originally, the Hemopump was intended for patients with cardiogenic shock occurring after cardiotomy or after acute myocardial infarction. In clinical trials, however, another group of suitable candidates for treatment emerged—heart transplant recipients (Table 14.1). In fact, the first

Table 14.1 Criteria for Hemopump treatment.

Indications
Severe cardiogenic shock
   Acute myocardial infarction
   Failure to wean from cardiopulmonary bypass
   Certain myocardial diseases
Heart transplantation
   Postoperative donor heart failure
   Acute myocardial rejection
Intraoperative circulatory support
   Coronary artery bypass
   Percutaneous transluminal coronary angioplasty

Contraindications
Aortic valve stenosis or insufficiency
Mechanical aortic valve
Dissecting aortic aneurysm
Intracardiac shunt (VSD, ASD, PFO)
Severe aortoiliac disease*
High peripheral vascular resistance*

* Relative contraindications.
ASD = atrial septal defect; PFO = patent foramen ovale;
VSD = ventricular septal defect.

patient ever treated with the Hemopump, a 62-year-old man, was experiencing severe allograft rejection.[6] Despite aggressive therapy with OKT3, the patient's haemodynamic status had failed to improve. After two days of Hemopump support, allograft function had gradually recovered, and we began to consider weaning the patient from support. Ultimately, the heart's pumping ejected the cannula, and the drive cable broke. The Hemopump was then removed without complications. The patient was eventually discharged from the hospital and became a long-term survivor of heart transplantation. Overall, this case proved that the Hemopump could support circulation and allow for full ventricular recovery in the transplant patient.

Our second patient was a 61-year-old man with chronic congestive heart failure who had suffered an acute myocardial infarction. He had severe hypotension, and treatment with the IABP had failed. Within 48 hours of instituting Hemopump support, pulmonary oedema, which had been evident on the chest X-ray at the time of admission, had completely cleared, and the patient remained alert. Despite adequate circulatory support, global cardiac dysfunction continued, so we considered bridging the patient to transplantation. Consent for this procedure could not be obtained, and the patient died shortly after treatment was discontinued.

The next patient, a small, 71-year-old woman, experienced cardiogenic shock after percutaneous transluminal coronary angioplasty. After emergency coronary artery bypass surgery, she could not be weaned from cardiopulmonary bypass. We decided to institute Hemopump support, and in this case, the intraoperative setting made it convenient to insert the device through the aorta, so that the pump exited directly from the chest. The pump worked well and was removed after 48 hours. This patient recovered and is alive and well.

These patients represent the various populations who can benefit from Hemopump treatment. In each case, the pump rapidly allowed improved function of the heart, reduced capillary wedge pressure, and improved end-organ function.

The small size of the Hemopump has allowed treatment of smaller patients, such as a woman with postpartum cardiomyopathy who required a bridge to transplantation (total duration of support, 13 days) and a young boy with severe allograft rejection. Owing to the small size of their femoral arteries, the pump was inserted by way of the distal abdominal aorta, which had been exposed through an extraperitoneal flank incision in one patient and an intraperitoneal incision in the other.

We do not believe that the Hemopump will ultimately play a large role in bridge-to-transplant procedures in the United States because transplant candidates face a potentially long wait for a donor heart. During this time, the candidate would have to remain bed-ridden. In addition, candidates with irreversible end-stage heart failure may require higher flows to maintain the body's circulatory requirements over a long-term period. Thus, in the bridge-to-transplant setting, a completely implantable left ventricular assist device that is capable of providing higher flows and that might allow outpatient treatment during the waiting period, such as the HeartMate, would be more practical than the Hemopump.[8,9]

Despite the variety of patients who can potentially benefit from Hemopump support, others have conditions that prevent insertion or exacerbate pre-existing conditions (Table 14.1). For example, a septal defect or patent foramen ovale can cause a severe right-to-left shunt; unrecognized, these shunts can cause death.[10] If a patent foramen ovale is found after support has been initiated, the Hemopump flow rate should be reduced in an attempt to increase left atrial pressure and, thus, reduce the shunt. If this manoeuvre is ineffective, the patent foramen ovale must be surgically repaired.[10]

In clinical trials at the Texas Heart Institute, a total of 10 patients were successfully weaned from Hemopump support and discharged from the hospital.[11] The protocol for the prospective study required that the following haemodynamic criteria be met before support could be initiated: cardiac index $< 2.0\,l/min/m^2$, pulmonary capillary wedge pressure > 18 mmHg, and systolic blood pressure < 90 mmHg or left ventricular work index < 1500 g-m/m^2/min. The average time of Hemopump support was 71 hours and the average postoperative hospital stay was 37 days. At a mean follow-up of 21 months, four patients each were in New York Heart Association functional classes I and II. Two patients had died: one at 2 months of ventricular fibrillation, and the other at 7 months of myocardial infarction.

Overall, 53 patients with refractory cardiogenic shock were included in the multicentre study of the Hemopump,[12] and the device was successfully inserted in 41 (77.3%) patients (Table 14.2). The mean duration of support was 52.8 hours (range, 1–94 hours) (Table 14.3). The Hemopump worked reliably and safely: haemodynamic indices

Table 14.2 Characteristics of 41 patients undergoing Hemopump support.[12]

Sex (%)	
Male	33 (80)
Female	8 (20)
Mean age (years)	54.7
Range	8.6–76.4
Prior IABP treatment (%)	31 (75.5)
Reason for Hemopump support (%)	
Acute myocardial infarction	17 (41.5)
Postcardiotomy	17 (41.5)
Other	7 (17)

Table 14.3 Results of Hemopump treatment in 41 patients.[12]

Mean duration of support (hours)	52 (range 1–94)
Weaned (%)	15 (36.5)
Alive at 30 days (%)	13 (31.7)
Acute myocardial infarction	7 (41.1)
Postcardiotomy	4 (23.5)
Other	2 (28.6)
Died* (%)	26 (63.4)

* During support or just after device removal.

improved, with a low incidence of complications, including thromboembolic events. Whereas 26 patients died during support or just after device removal, 13 patients (31.7%) were alive at 30 days. Of the total 53 patients, 12 (16.6%) (9 males, 3 females) had conditions that prohibited insertion (including atherosclerosis of the ileal system, small femoral arteries, and failure to cross the aortic valve); and ultimately, only two of these patients lived.

Based on this study, we were able to identify some factors as predictors of survival. A cardiac index of $>2.0\,l/min/m^2$ and a decrease in pulmonary capillary wedge pressure within the first 24 hours was associated with a high rate of weaning from support and of 30-day survival. In addition, preinsertion left ventricular work index (LVWI) appeared to be an important indicator of 30-day survival. LVWI was calculated as follows:

$$LVWI = CI(MAP - PCWP) \times 13.6$$

where CI = cardiac index, MAP = mean arterial pressure, and PCWP = pulmonary capillary wedge pressure. The calculated work index is normally about 3000 g-m/m^2/min. Only 1 of 7 (14%) patients with an initial LVWI of less than 500 g-m/m^2/min survived. Of 9 patients with an LVWI of 500 to 1000 g-m/m^2/min, 3 (33%) survived, and of 11 patients with an LVWI of 1000 to 1500 g-m/m^2/min, 7 (64%) survived. These findings provide good evidence of myocardial recovery. Improved methods for selecting patients may eventually increase survival in this high-risk population.

Complications

The main complications have been cannula ejection, drive cable fracture, and failure to insert. A few patients have had haemolysis and minimal ischaemia in the leg, which have resolved after support was stopped. Thromboembolic complications have also occurred in some patients due to mural thrombus, which typically forms after cardiogenic shock. The Hemopump can dislodge thrombi, which can block the cannula. This is a catastrophic, but rare, complication (2.4%).[12] No thromboembolic complications were related to the Hemopump.

Comment

The initial clinical trials proved that use of the Hemopump can potentially lead to reversal of acute left ventricular dysfunction. These findings may be particularly useful in the treatment of cardiogenic shock after acute myocardial infarction,[13] for which in-hospital mortality rates remain high (74–82%).[14,15] In the multicentre study of the Hemopump, 30-day survival for that group of patients was 41%.[12] Recent studies in a canine model of acute myocardial infarction have also shown that relieving the demand on myocardial oxygen consumption with the Hemopump can reduce the area of infarction.[16] Likewise, the chief cause of early death in transplant patients remains acute donor heart failure, and our studies showed that the Hemopump provides adequate circulatory support until the donor heart regains function.[6]

Another potential use for the Hemopump includes coronary artery bypass without an oxygenator.[17] Currently, we are studying the use of the short, 21-F Hemopump cannula for coronary artery bypass surgery. At a flow rate of 4 l/min, the device unloads the left ventricle, making it possible to bypass the left anterior descending, the right coronary, and obtuse marginal arteries. During operation, esmolol, a short-acting beta blocker, is administered to lower the heart rate, so that the heart is virtually asystolic. This circulatory support technique allows us to avoid cardiopulmonary bypass and operate under normothermic conditions, to reduce the dose of heparin to 1 mg/kg, and to completely avoid ischaemic arrest of the heart.

In Europe and elsewhere,[18] researchers are evaluating use of the 14-F Hemopump cannula in high-risk patients undergoing percutaneous transluminal coronary artery stenting. Eventually, the smaller 14-F cannula could make Hemopump treatment, with its advantage of direct myocardial unloading, as feasible as intra-aortic balloon pump treatment in patients needing circulatory support after cardiotomy. Since 1988, the overall survival in such patients undergoing intra-aortic balloon pump support has remained steady, at approximately 50%.[19] These results may improve with the Hemopump because it actively unloads the left ventricle, accentuating the potential for myocardial recovery, while at the same time supplying adequate systemic circulation.

Experimentally, this technology has also been used in the laboratory as early resuscitation in traumatic shock. Its use in the emergency room setting for such patients should be investigated.

We have found the Hemopump to be safe and reliable in animal studies and in clinical trials. Because of its small size, it can generally be easily inserted.[20] Our initial results show that it is very effective and safe in supporting the heart in severely compromised patients.

References

1. Dennis, C, Carlens, E, Senning A, *et al*. Clinical use of a cannula for left heart bypass without thoracotomy: 'experimental protection against fibrillation by left heart bypass. *Ann Surg* 1962; **156**, 623–637.
2. DeVries WC. The total artificial heart. In: Sabiston DC, Spencer FC (eds), *Gibbon's Surgery of the Chest*, 4th edn. Philadelphia: WB Saunders, 1983: 1629–1636.
3. Hoffman JIE, Buckberg, GD. Transmural variation in myocardial perfusion. In: Yu, PN, Goodwin JF (eds), *Progress in Cardiology*, vol 5. Philadelphia: Lea & Febiger, 1976: 37–89.
4. Brazier J, Cooper N, Buckberg GD. The adequacy of subendocardial oxygen delivery: the interaction of determinants of flow, arterial oxygen content and myocardial oxygen need. *Circulation* 1974; **49**, 968–967.
5. Wampler DG, Moise JC, Frazier OH, Olsen DB. *In vivo* evaluation of a peripheral vascular access axial flow blood pump. *ASAIO Trans* 1988; **34**, 450–454.
6. Frazier OH, Wampler R, Duncan JM, *et al*. First human use of the Hemopump, a catheter-mounted ventricular assist device. *Ann Thorac Surg* 1990; **49**, 299–304.
7. Baldwin RT, Radovancevic B, Duncan JM, Wampler RK, Frazier OH. Management of patients supported on the Hemopump cardiac assist system. *Tex Heart Inst J* 1992; **81**, 86.
8. Frazier OH, Rose EA, Macmanus Q, *et al*. Multicenter clinical evaluation of the HeartMate 1000 IP left ventricular assist device. *Ann Thorac Surg* 1992; **53**, 1080–1090.
9. Frazier OH. Chronic left ventricular support with a vented electric assist device. *Ann Thorac Surg* 1993; **55**, 273–275.
10. Baldin RT, Duncan JM, Frazier OH, Wilansky S. Patent foramen ovale: a cause of hypoxemia in patients on left ventricular support. *Ann Thorac Surg* 1991; **52**, 865–867.
11. Baldwin RT, Radovancevic B, Duncan JM, *et al*. Quality of life in long-term survivors of the Hemopump left ventricular assist device. *ASAIO Trans* 1991; **37**, M422–423.

12. Wampler RK, Frazier OH, Lansing AM, *et al.* Treatment of cardiogenic shock with the hemopump left ventricular assist device. *Ann Thorac Surg* 1991; **52**, 506–513.

13. Willerson JT, Frazier OH. Reducing mortality in patients with extensive myocardial infarction. *New Engl J Med* 1991; **325**, 1166–1168.

14. Goldberg RJ, Gore JM, Alpert JS, *et al.* Cardiogenic shock after acute myocardial infarction—incidence and mortality from a community-wide perspective, 1975 to 1988. *New Engl J Med* 1991; **325**, 1117–1122.

15. Gacioch GM, Ellis SG, Lee L, *et al.* Cardiogenic shock complicating acute myocardial infarction: the use of coronary angioplasty and the integration of the new support devices into patient management. *J Am Coll Cardiol* 1992; **19**, 654–656.

16. Smalling RW, Cassidy DB, Barrett R, Lachterman, B, Felli P, Amirian J. Improved regional myocardial blood flow, left ventricular unloading, and infarct salvage using an axial-flow, transvalvular left ventricular assist device: a comparison with intra-aortic balloon counterpulsation and reperfusion alone in a canine infarction model. *Circulation* 1992; **82**, 1152–1159.

17. Sweeney MS, Frazier OH. Device-supported myocardial revascularization: safe help for sick hearts. *Ann Thorac Surg* 1992; **54**, 1065–1070.

18. Loisance D, Deleuze P, Dubois-Rande JL, *et al.* Hemopump ventricular support for patients undergoing high risk coronary angioplasty. *ASAIO Trans* 1990; **36**, M623–626.

19. Baldwin RT, Slogoff S, Noon GP, Sekela M, Frazier OH. A model to predict survival at time of post-cardiotomy intraaortic balloon pump insertion. *Ann Thorac Surg* 1993; **55**, 908–913.

20. Duncan JM, Frazier OH, Radovancevic B, Velebit V. Implantation techniques for the Hemopump. *Ann Thorac Surg* 1989; **48**, 733–735.

15

The development and clinical use of centrifugal blood pumps

Leonard AR Golding

Development

The roller pump has been the basis of cardio-pulmonary bypass (CPB) for many years and, with appropriate adjustment of the occlusion, haemolysis can be minimized. Attempts to utilize the roller pump for cardiogenic shock and low cardiac output state began in 1957 when Stuckey and associates attempted to support patients with myocardial infarction by use of a pump oxygenator system.[1] In 1963, Spencer and coworkers had success with left-heart bypass in postcardiotomy cardiogenic shock patients.[2] Litwak and colleagues developed specific cannulae that were used in association with the roller pump and they reported good success.[3] It was found, however, that a roller pump could develop high afterload pressure or allow gas to come out of the fluid phase, with development of gaseous emboli.

Centrifugal pumps have been used in industry for many years because of their simplicity. The first description of their potential use to pump blood was by Saxton and Andrews in 1960.[4] They recognized that such a device would require less power and have fewer moving parts than would a pulsatile device of similar capability. They showed the pump output to be directly related to the input pressure and inversely related to the output pressure, but a major limitation to its use was the potential destruction of the red cell elements by the impeller. They actually undertook studies of short-term duration in anaesthetized dogs, but all

died owing to the development of pulmonary oedema.

A combined surgical and engineering effort at the University of Minnesota led to the development of a centrifugal-type blood pump that was ultimately aimed at prolonged intracorporeal left ventricular bypass with power being transmitted by magnetic coupling across the chest wall.[5] During that development, efforts at redesigning the impeller and pump housing resulted in pumps that had an index of haemolysis of less than 0.01 g per 100 litres of blood pumped. Over the next decade, studies with an extracorporeal version were undertaken in animals and demonstrated the capability of the system to be used as an LV assist device.[6] In 1978, the initial clinical use of this system was undertaken and resulted in the survival of some patients with postcardiotomy cardiogenic shock.[7] This Medtronic Hemadyne® pump saw only limited clinical use; it was discontinued in 1980 and its use since then has been limited to animal studies. Two other magnetically coupled centrifugal blood pumps have been developed and had clinical use. The Centrimed® pump has since been renamed the Sarns–Delphin® pump and has had some clinical use for postcardiotomy support since 1985.[8] Although it has proven effective, its use has been limited by its sometimes questionable durability. The Aries® centrifugal pump is produced by St Jude Medical and has seen even less clinical use.

In 1968, Rafferty and colleagues described the

development of a constrained force–vortex pump.[9] With modifications, they were soon able to demonstrate low haemolysis rates and these efforts resulted in the present-day Biomedicus® Biopump. It has been used clinically for temporary support since early efforts in 1980 by Magovern[10] and has become the most frequently used blood pump for postcardiotomy support. It has replaced the roller pump in almost 15% of CPB surgery. It is also used by some groups instead of the standard roller pump in CPB. The low haemolysis rate of the biopump has also encouraged its use in both extracorporeal membrane oxygenator (ECMO) systems and for emergency percutaneous CPB.

These various centrifugal blood pumps have required anticoagulation to prevent thrombus deposition with potential embolization. Without heparin, either the Medtronic pump by Pennington or the Biopump by Magovern resulted in a significant incidence of emboli.[11,12] Recent attempts to address this problem have resulted in the availability of pumpheads and inflow and outflow circuits in which the surface has been treated with a Carmeda heparin-bonding process.[13] Initial use of the Biopump treated in such a fashion has shown good clinical results. This has also encouraged the clinical use of percutaneous CPB for either emergency support[14] or in the catheterization room during high-risk cardiology procedures.

Table 15.1 summarizes the progress towards clinical use of centrifugal pumps since 1960.

Table 15.1 Progress towards the clinical use of centrifugal pumps.

1960	Saxton and Andrews[4]
	First report of use of a centrifugal blood pump
1963	Spencer *et al.*[2]
	First successful postcardiotomy LVAD
1966	Dorman[5]
	Description of impeller centrifugal pump
1968	Rafferty *et al.*[9]
	Description of vortex-shedding pump
1974	Bernstein *et al.*[6]
	Centrifugal pump for LV bypass in animals
1978	Golding *et al.*[7]
	Clinical use of Medtronic LVAD
1980	Magovern[10]
	Clinical use of Bio-medicus LVAD
1983	Phillips *et al.*[14]
	Percutaneous emergency cardiopulmonary bypass

Indications

Although roller pumps continue to be the mainstay of pumping systems in cardiopulmonary bypass, in 10–15% of cardiac procedures they have been replaced by the centrifugal type. It is, however, in the role of more prolonged short-term use that centrifugal pumps have found their niche. They have become the most frequently used blood pumps for postcardiotomy, low cardiac output state, unresponsive to standard supportive measures of vasoconstrictors, vasodilators, and intra-aortic balloon pumping. Most recently, with the development of percutaneous cannula systems, there has been an increasing use of these pumps as a part of emergency bypass systems in situations requiring acute resuscitation and/or diagnostic intervention.

In spite of improvements in preoperative and intraoperative management, a small number of patients develop a low cardiac output state during weaning from CPB in the early postoperative period. While many respond to pharmacological manipulation, in about 5% the use of intra-aortic balloon pumping is necessary. In spite of these additional measures, a few patients fail to respond, and at that point a mechanical blood pump is the only other therapeutic option available (in 0.5–1.0% of cardiac surgical patients). In general, the premise underlying the use of these devices is that there is a reversible myocardial injury that can recover with time provided there is a sufficient decrease in the workload of the failing ventricle while maintaining adequate blood flow to the systemic organs.[15] Less frequently, such as in bridging to cardiac transplantation, the major function is only to maintain blood flow to systemic organs and ensure their viability until a donor heart is found.

Historically, the earliest approach to a selection process was the set of haemodynamic criteria proposed by Norman *et al.*[16] for the abdominal LV assist device (ALVAD) (Table 15.2). At that

Table 15.2 Haemodynamic indications for temporary mechanical assistance.

Cardiac index <1.8
Systolic blood pressure <90 mmHg
Left atrial pressure >25 mmHg
Vascular resistance <1500 dyn/s/cm^{-5}

In spite of correction of metabolic abnormalities by:
   optimized pharmacology
   intra-aortic balloon pumping

Table 15.3 Short-term uses for a centrifugal blood pump.

Postcardiotomy low cardiac output state:
  Early in operating theatre to wean
  later in ICU
As part of cardiopulmonary bypass:
  ECMO
  Emergency percutaneous bypass
Acute cardiogenic shock (non-surgical):
  Acute myocardial infarction
  Acute myocardiopathy
Bridge to transplantation

Table 15.4 Contraindications to short-term cardiac support.

Incomplete correction of surgical problem
Uncontrolled bleeding
CNS damage
Intercurrent illness likely to limit patient's lifespan
Severe biventricular failure
Intercurrent infection

Table 15.5 Postcardiotomy VAD: negative prognostic indications.

For weaning	For discharge/survival
Bleeding	Perioperative myocardial infarction
DIC	Renal failure
Renal failure	Infection
Biventricular failure	Age >65 years
Poor systemic flow	

time, only postcardiotomy patients were considered as candidates. The clinical indications were later expanded as part of a NIH Cooperative Clinical Trial in the early 1980s to evaluate the short-term use of ventricular assist devices, and this has resulted in the presently accepted guidelines (Table 15.3).

The low cardiac output state was characterized as that situation in which, despite all other supportive measures, the cardiac index remained at less than $2\,1/min/m^2$, the mean arterial blood pressure at 60 mmHg or less, with a systemic vascular resistance of 1000–1500 $dyn/s/cm^{-5}$ and a left atrial pressure or capillary wedge pressure above 25 mmHg.

Importantly, however, these haemodynamic criteria did not allow any decision as to the presence of permanent as opposed to a reversible myocardial injury, and there have been many attempts to find a diagnostic procedure to allow this determination prior to instituting support. Many groups have analysed their experiences in an attempt to optimize patient selection and improve weaning and survival rates, and this has become even more important because of increasing economic cost and decreasing availability of resources.[17] Best results have been obtained in patients developing low cardiac output state, where the device is required as an aid to weaning from CPB; and inability to wean from CPB following an uneventful cardiac surgical procedure in a low-risk patient is an unexpected event. Perhaps consideration of absolute and relative contraindications to the use of temporary support devices is becoming more important than a list of indications (Tables 15.4 and 15.5).

Clinical uses

Critical to the successful use of short-term mechanical blood pumps is the recognition that the management of the pump is but one factor in the coordinated management of the whole patient. It is not sufficient to simply worry about the systemic blood pressure and the flow produced by the pump. An approach to the use of these devices in patients, therefore, involves consideration of all these factors; first in the operating room setting at the initiation of support and later in the intensive care unit.

In the operating room, two major problems to be addressed are achieving adequate flow through the device and control of any bleeding difficulty. For the latter problem good surgical haemostasis, the use of pledgetted tourniquets at any cannulation site, full reversal of heparin anticoagulation with protamine, and replacement of blood products are well established fundamentals. At my institution we now routinely aim to achieve a haematocrit of 30% with packed red cell replacement, and will give platelets and/or fresh frozen plasma cryoprecipitated after protamine administration. In spite of this, many groups report significant bleeding in up to 85% of patients in the first 24 hours after initiation of support.[10,18–21] Because of the high incidence of postoperative bleeding and some degree of pulmonary dysfunction, most groups no longer oppose the sternal edges and either close only the skin or place an occlusive dressing over the open sternotomy. In our own experience, leaving the chest open for 24 or 48 hours does not lead to an increased incidence of mediastinitis in those patients surviving.

Flow produced by a blood pump is measured through the associated flow probe in the circuit. More important, however, is the ability to monitor systemic blood flow through a thermodilution catheter and to be able to assist left and right heart function via atrial pressure monitoring lines. The use of these latter parameters will allow evaluation of the cause of the low flow state whether it is due to hypovolaemia, associated other ventricular failure, or a problem associated with the position of the inflow cannula. Inability to adequately oxygenate the patient supported with the blood pump makes exploration of the atrium mandatory to exclude the presence of a patent foramen ovale.[22] Associated RV failure can most frequently be managed with isoproteranol or the bipyridine compound Inocor. If the device is being inserted after prolonged attempts at resuscitation, frequently there has been significant fluid accumulation and a lowered haematocrit. In such circumstances, while the patient is supported on CPB, the early institution of ultrafiltration both to remove excessive fluid as well as to haemoconcentrate can be very beneficial.

Management in the intensive care unit involves support of all organ functions. Renal function is maximized by the use of renal doses of dopamine, and maintaining appropriate systemic flow and pressure. The patient is also best managed in the early phases with full ventilated support while sedated and paralysed to minimize the workload on the failing ventricle. Careful control of electrolyte administration will help minimize third-spacing of fluid, particularly into pulmonary tissues as well as the injured myocardium.

Heparin administration sufficient to maintain the activated clotting time (ACT) at approximately one and a half times normal is commenced as soon as bleeding is no longer an ongoing problem. More recently, with the advent of heparin-bonded systems, there is less need for this while good pump flows can be maintained through the circuit. Transfusions are given as required to maintain the haematocrit at a minimum of 30%, and particular care is given to monitoring platelet counts. This is done routinely twice a day while the patient is maintained on support, because a fall in platelet count can be very precipitous owing to the presence of the intra-aortic balloon pump and the centrifugal pump. With more prolonged use of the device, platelets can become affected by either Inocor or the development of antibodies to heparin itself.

An early sign of recovering ventricular function is the development of the pressure wave form on a previously non-pulsatile trace when balloon pumping is briefly discontinued. The development of a noise in the pumphead or of deteriorating pump function in the absence of any other haemodynamic changes necessitates rapid replacement of the pumphead. Finally, it is important to maintain adequate nutrition for the patient. After an initial stabilization period of 24 hours, we routinely initiate intravenous alimentation based on the belief that this will become necessary and may possibly aid in resisting infection in the long run.

A recent report by Pae analysed data from 965 patients undergoing postcardiotomy support with a variety of devices.[17] From that information it became apparent that there was no difference in survival rate whether the device was a centrifugal pump or a more sophisticated and expensive pulsatile pump. There was, however, a marked difference in the period of support: only 3 days for centrifugal devices, but 6 days for pulsatile pumps. Although unproven, it is possible that the continuous unloading with a centrifugal pump may promote more rapid recovery of the stunned myocardium, in contrast to pulsatile devices whose function necessitates filling by the damaged ventricle and so provides rest to the myocardium only through a part of the cardiac cycle. An overall survival rate of 24.6% was found, with the highest survival for LV assistance, and the worst results were obtained with biventricular support. We recently analysed our own series of patients who were supported for postcardiotomy low output state and found very similar results. We have also found that renal failure is associated with poor prognosis, but were unable to show that age is a significant prognostic indicator.[21]

Despite increasing experience by many groups, the overall survival rate has remained surprisingly unchanged. Analysis of results from eleven published series showed an overall survival rate of 28% for postcardiotomy support (Table 15.6).[8,10,18–21,23–27] For many years, it was our practice to have a perfusionist in constant attendance while a patient was supported with a centrifugal blood pump. It soon became apparent, however, that after the initial period of stabilization during the first 12 hours, intervention by the perfusionist

Table 15.6 Summary of survival rates with postcardiotomy centrifugal assist.

Series	Survival	
Golding et al.[21]	20/79	(25%)
Noon[20]	19/79	(24%)
Magovern[10]	27/77	(35%)
Curtis et al.[23]	11/54	(20%)
Moore et al.[24]	7/16	(44%)
Killen et al.[19]	8/41	(20%)
Wareing and Kouchoukos[25]	8/18	(44%)
Campbell et al.[18]	8/20	(40%)
Joyce et al.[8]	13/28	(46%)
Adamson et al.[26]	8/39	(21%)
Anstadt et al.[27]	1/17	(6%)
Total	130/468	(28%)

to change a pumphead was a rare event in postcardiotomy use. Additionally, there was a significant economic impact on the patient care. For the last two years, the perfusionist's role has become the supervision of pump management which is done by nursing staff who have undergone a training programme to familiarize themselves with the system. Nurses have successfully changed pumpheads with no detrimental effect to patient care.

The use of the Biomedicus centrifugal pump in association with percutaneous cannulae for acute resuscitation was originally described by Phillips et al.[14] The percutaneous cannulae were modified arterial intra-aortic balloon catheter sheaths and a Biomedicus pump was utilized for active venous drainage and pumping through the oxygenator. Since that time, specialized cannulae have been developed, and the addition of heparin bonding to coat the entire circuit has allowed the elimination of the use of heparin. Recently Dembitsky et al.[28] reported the results of resuscitation with a portable percutaneous CPB system.

A registry has collected information on 187 patients of which 40 (21%) ultimately survived. A total of 140 patients were able to have diagnostic and/or therapeutic interventions while supported on the system. It was recommended that these devices should be limited to use in patients with cardiac arrest following hypothermia or patients in whom the cardiac arrest episode has been witnessed.

The use of centrifugal devices in bridging to cardiac transplantation is becoming less frequent. We have had some success,[29] and a fourth patient was supported with biventricular assist and survived after transplantation 15 days later. Pae[17] recently reported that, although the results for pneumatic pulsatile, electric pulsatile and centrifugal pumps used as bridging devices were similar, there was a trend to worse results with the nonpulsatile devices.

References

1. Stuckey JH, Newman MM, Dennis C, et al. The use of the heart–lung machine in selected cases of acute myocardial infarction. *Surg Forum* 1957; **8**, 342–344.
2. Spencer FC, Eiseman NG, Trinkle JK, Rossi NP. Assisted circulation for cardiac failure following intracardiac surgery with cardiopulmonary bypass. *J Thorac Cardiovasc Surg* 1965; **49**, 56.
3. Litwak RS, Koffsky RM, Jurado RA, et al. Use of a left heart assist device after intracardiac surgery: technique and clinical experience. *Ann Thorac Surg* 1976; **21**, 191–202.
4. Saxton GA, Andrews, CB. An ideal heart pump with hydrodynamic characteristics analogous to the mammalian heart. *ASAIO Trans* 1960; **6**, 288.
5. National Research Council (Blockner TG, committee chair). Mechanical devices to assist the failing heart: Proceedings. Washington, DC: National Academy of Sciences, 1966, 107.
6. Bernstein EF, Dorman FD, Blackshear PL Jr, Scott DR. An efficient, compact blood pump for assisted circulation. *Surgery* 1970; **68**, 105–115.
7. Golding LR, Groves LK, Peter M, Jacobs G, Sukalac R, Nosé Y, Loop FD. Initial clinical experience with a new temporary left ventricular assist device. *Ann Thorac Surg* 1980; **29**, 66–69.
8. Joyce LD, Kiser JC, Eales F, King, RM, Toninato CJ, Hansen J. Experience with the Sarns centrifugal pump as a ventricular assist device. *ASAIO Trans* 1990; **36**, M619–623.
9. Rafferty EH, Kletschka HD, Wynyard M, Larkin JT, Smith LV, Cheathem B. Artificial heart. I. Application of nonpulsatile force—Vortex principle. *Minn Med* 1968; **51**, 11–16.
10. Magovern GJ Jr. The biopump and postoperative circulatory support. *Ann Thorac Surg* 1993; **55**, 245–249.
11. Magovern GJ, Park SB, Maher TD. Use of a centrifugal pump without anticoagulants for postoperative left ventricular assist. *World J Surg* 1985; **9**, 25–36.
12. Pennington DG, Merjavy JP, Swartz MT, Willman VL. Clinical experience with a centrifugal pump ventricular assist device. *Trans Am Soc Artif Intern Org* 1982; **28**, 93–99.
13. Arnander C, Olsson P, Larm O. Influence of blood flow and the effect of protamine on the thromboresistant properties of a covalently bonded heparin

surface. *J Biomed Mater Res* 1988; **22**, 859–868.

14. Phillips SJ, Ballentine B, Slonine D, *et al.* Percutaneous initiation of cardiopulmonary bypass. *Ann Thorac Surg* 1983; **36**, 223–225.

15. Braunwald E, Kloner RA. The stunned myocardium: prolonged, postischemic ventricular dysfunction. *Circulation* 1982; **66**, 1146–1149.

16. Norman JC, Cooley DA, Igo SR, *et al.* Prognostic indices for survival during postcardiotomy intraaortic balloon pumping. Methods of scoring and classification, with implications for left ventricular device utilization. *J Thorac Cardiovasc Surg* 1977; **74**, 709–720.

17. Pae WE Jr. Ventricular assist devices and total artificial hearts: a combined registry experience. *Ann Thorac Surg* 1993; **55**, 295–298.

18. Campbell CD, Tolitano DJ, Weber KT, Hines HH, Replogle RL. Mechanical support for postcardiotomy heart failure. In: Unger F (ed), *Assisted Circulation* 3rd edn. Berlin: Springer Verlag, 1989, pp. 167–180.

19. Killen DA, Piehler JM, Borkon AM, Reed WA. Biomedicus ventricular assist device for salvage of cardiac surgical patients. *Ann Thorac Surg* 1991; **52**, 230–235.

20. Noon GP. Bio-medicus ventricular assistance (editorial). *Ann Thorac Surg* 1991; **52**, 180–181.

21. Golding LAR, Crouch RD, Stewart RW, Novoa R, Lytle BW, McCarthy PM, Taylor PC, Loop FD, Cosgrove DM III. Postcardiotomy centrifugal mechanical ventricular support. *Ann Thorac Surg* 1992; **54**, 1059–1064.

22. Baldwin RT, Duncan JM, Frazier OH, Wilansky S. Patent foramen ovale: a cause of hypoxemia in patients on left ventricular support. *Ann Thorac Surg* 1991; **52**, 865–867.

23. Curtis JJ, Walls JT, Boley TM, Schmaltz RA, Demmy TL. Autopsy findings in patients on postcardiotomy centrifugal ventricular assist. *ASAIO J* 1992; **38**, M688–690.

24. Moore CH, Dailey JW, Canon DS, Rubin JMO. Non-pulsatile circulatory support in 90 cases. *ASAIO J* 1992; **38**, M627–630.

25. Wareing TH, Kouchoukos NT. Postcardiotomy mechanical support in the elderly. *Ann Thorac Surg* 1991; **51**, 443–447.

26. Adamson RM, Dembitsky WP, Reichman RT, Moreno-Cabral RJ, Daily PO. Mechanical support: assist or nemesis? *J Thorac Cardiovasc Surg* 1989; **98**, 915–921.

27. Anstadt MP, Tedder M, Hegde SS, Douglas JM Jr, Sperling RT, White WD, Van Trigt P, Lowe JE. Intraoperative timing may provide criteria for use of post-cardiotomy ventricular assist devices. *ASAIO J* 1992; **38**, M147–150.

28. Dembitsky WP, Moreno-Cabral RJ, Adamson RM, Daily PO. Emergency resuscitation using portable extracorporeal membrane oxygenation. *Ann Thorac Surg* 1993; **55**, 304–309.

29. Golding LA, Stewart RW, Sinkewich M, Smith W, Cosgrove DM. Nonpulsatile ventricular assist bridging to transplantation. *ASAIO Trans* 1988; **34**, 476–479.

16

Mechanical circulatory support: patient and device selection

D Glenn Pennington and Marc T Swartz

Introduction

Clinicians and researchers have long sought a mechanical device that could replace or supplement the functions of the heart. One potential device was described in 1928.[1] The clinical use of cardiopulmonary bypass (CPB) demonstrated the feasibility of mechanical circulatory support[2] in 1951, and Gibbon described the first successful intracardiac repair in 1954.[3] Subsequently, clinical application of CPB grew not only in the area of elective cardiac surgery, but also to support patients in cardiogenic shock following acute myocardial infarction.[4] By the mid-1960s, investigators had successfully supported a patient with postoperative cardiogenic shock with CPB.[5] In 1968 the introduction of the intra-aortic balloon pump[6] provided clinicians with an effective tool for treating cardiogenic shock. Progress in the field of mechanical circulatory support was accelerated by government funding, the development of more thromboresistant biomaterials, as well as the growing recognition of the clinical need.[7,8] During the decade of the 1970s, development continued on several new ventricular assist devices (VADs) and total artificial hearts.[9–12] By the end of the 1970s, results of the first clinical trials with ventricular assist devices were being reported.[13–18] The first use of a ventricular assist device as a bridge to transplantation was reported in 1978, as was the use of intra-aortic balloon pump for bridging.[19,20] These reports continued into the early 1980s in both myocardial recovery and bridge-to-transplant patients using mechanical devices such as centrifugal pumps and extracorporeal membrane oxygenation. In 1984 the first two successful ventricular assist device bridge-to-transplant procedures were performed.[21,22] Less than one year later, a total artificial heart was successfully used as a bridge to transplantation.[23]

Since that time, there has been increasing interest in the use of mechanical circulatory support devices for a variety of indications. The combined registry of clinical use of mechanical circulatory support devices, sponsored by the American Society for Artificial Internal Organs (ASAIO) and the International Society for Heart and Lung Transplantation (ISHLT), reports more than 1500 cases of mechanical circulatory support in patients awaiting either myocardial recovery or cardiac transplantation.[24,25] In reality, this number underestimates the total worldwide use of mechanical supports devices as many cases go unreported. Indications for mechanical circulatory support are varied, and a diverse selection of devices are available—either commercially, or for investigational use. Some devices have been designed specifically for a particular circumstance, whereas others are capable for a variety of applications. This review describes some guidelines that will be useful in selecting appropriate patients and attempts to classify devices by their best proven clinical use.

During the 1980s there was considerable progress in the field of mechanical circulatory support. Many advances were made in the areas of technology as well as patient management. Concurrently, there were improvements in patient selection. Some predictors of survival which can be evaluated prior to device placement have been identified, but these have usually been in small numbers of patients at a single institution. Investigational protocols, historical criteria and previous experience can also be used as guidelines. However, in many cases the decision the initiate mechanical circulatory support is based on limited objective criteria.

In this chapter, patient selection criteria will be discussed for each of the three major patient groups: postcardiotomy support, bridge-to-transplant, and acute deterioration. Information contained in this chapter is derived from our clinical experience, a literature review, device manufacturers, and data from the ASAIO/ISHLT registry.

Postcardiotomy support

Perioperative intra-aortic balloon pump support continues in 1–10% of patients undergoing cardiac surgical procedures, with survival rates in the range 45–60%.[26–30] Reports describe the incidence of postoperative patients requiring ventricular assistance to be 0.1–0.8%, with survival ranging from 29% to 50% in some of the larger series.[31–33] However, the overall survival rate of the postcardiotomy VAD population is 25%.[25] Survival rates for postoperative intra-aortic balloon pump and VAD patients have changed little over the last decade.[26–33]

The haemodynamic criteria generally used to evaluate a patient's candidacy for postcardiotomy VAD support are derived from the studies of Norman *et al.*[30] These criteria include a cardiac index of $<1.8\,\text{l/min/m}^2$, an elevated systemic vascular resistance, systolic arterial blood pressure <90 mm/Hg, left and/or right atrial pressures >20 mm/Hg, and urine output <20 ml/h. These parameters should be present despite maximal pharmacological and intra-aortic balloon pump support. These haemodynamics should be considered guidelines and not rigidly applied. Other factors such as previous medical history, the amount of pharmacological support necessary to wean from CPB, and other factors such as those

Table 16.1 Risk factors to evaluate before VAD insertion after CPB.

Unsuccessful operation
Preoperative or intraoperative myocardial infarction
Biventricular failure
Multiple previous infarctions or history of congestive heart failure
Physiological age
Uncontrollable bleeding while on CPB
Cardiac surgical procedure within 10 days

listed in Table 16.1, should be evaluated prior to VAD insertion. Some of the risk factors in the table have been shown to influence survival in retrospective studies, while others have been traditionally thought to be influential.

Pre-existing renal insufficiency is the single most important exclusion practised at the authors' institution. In our experience, a pre-existing serum creatinine of >2.5 mg/dl is highly predictive of post-VAD renal failure and death.[34] For this reason, we exclude patients who have an acute increase in creatinine above 2.5 mg/dl with a decrease in urine output and increased resistance to diuretic therapy from insertion of an assist device. Pre-existing ischaemia, CPB, bleeding and infectious complications can all influence the reversibility of renal insufficiency.

Patients with unsuccessful operations who cannot be weaned from CPB should be excluded from temporary mechanical circulatory support unless they are candidates for cardiac transplantation. Patients suffering acute perioperative myocardial infarctions have a reduced chance of cardiac recovery.[35] The development of biventricular failure decreases the likelihood of myocardial recovery.[36] In some cases it is possible to determine whether biventricular failure is present prior to placement of the assist device. This can be accomplished by evaluating left and right atrial pressures and by inspecting the heart visually. While off CPB, the atrium with the highest pressure usually indicates the ventricle with the worst failure. If both the left and right atrial pressures are elevated, biventricular failure is present.

Another important risk factor is advanced age, this being the most common reason why patients are excluded from advanced mechanical circulatory support. Data from the ASAIO/ISHLT registry show that the overall survival rate for patients under 59 years requiring postoperative VAD support is 34%, while patients over 70 have a survival rate of 13%.[25] It is important to evaluate physiological age rather than chronological age since some patients older than 65 years have a reasonable chance of survival. This factor was probably the reason why Wareing and Kouchoukos were able to report good results in postoperative support of older patients.[37] Physiological age is an extremely important factor to evaluate since the mean age of patients undergoing cardiac surgical procedures has increased over the last decade.[38]

Severe, diffuse intraoperative bleeding is considered a relative contraindication to advanced mechanical circulatory support. However, placement of devices in which heparin can be reversed leads to less bleeding. Some patients have died in the operating room from bleeding complications associated with coagulopathies or technical problems related to cannula placement. In Chapter 35 of this volume we describe our clinical experience with bleeding in patients receiving VADs. Severe postoperative bleeding complications are a predictor of mortality in the bridge-to-transplant patient population. However, in the myocardial recovery group, postoperative bleeding does not appear to independently affect survival.

Other factors have traditionally been thought to influence survival. Intraoperative ventricular arrhythmias are negative prognostic indicators if a stable rhythm cannot be maintained. However, intermittent episodes of ventricular tachycardia or fibrillation prior to device insertion do not predict survival.[39] Patients with controlled bacterial endocarditis (sterile blood cultures) preoperatively should be considered reasonable candidates for mechanical circulatory support once the infected valve has been removed. Patients in both the postcardiotomy and bridge-to-transplant populations have been successfully supported during and after episodes of bacteraemia.[33,40] Patients undergoing reoperations were once thought to have a decreased chance of survival, but our limited clinical experience with this group as well as the overall clinical experience from the Thoratec clinical trial does not prove this to be true.

Since most cardiac surgical procedures are performed electively, most VAD patients have not suffered major organ dysfunction preoperatively. However, patients undergoing emergency cardiac surgical procedures are more likely to develop renal or hepatic dysfunction, coagulopathy, or cerebral dysfunction which is made worse by the need for urgent cardiac surgical procedures. When such patients cannot be weaned from CPB

or deteriorate in the ICU, placement of a mechanical circulatory support device may reverse the acute haemodynamic deterioration. Unfortunately, major organ dysfunction is often irreversible and the survival rate is low.

Bridging to cardiac transplantation

The criteria used to determine whether a patient is a candidate for bridging to transplantation are quite different from the criteria used in post-cardiotomy and acute deterioration patients. Many bridge-to-transplant candidates are stable and do not require CPB at the time the decision to implant the circulatory support device is made. The adverse affects of CPB and resulting time constrains are not as great a problem and thus do not force a rapid decision, as is often the case in postcardiotomy patients. Many bridge-to-transplant patients can be effectively stabilized with pharmacological support and an intra-aortic balloon pump. While some may be acutely deteriorating, there is usually time for a thorough evaluation. In the early bridging experience the haemodynamics used to select a patient were similar to those used for postcardiotomy patients. Since the initial protocols were developed, a great deal has been learned concerning patient selection for bridging to transplantation, and the indications for support have recently changed for some clinical trials. Since myocardial recovery is usually not a concern, the question becomes how long the patient can be effectively maintained with conventional therapy prior to locating a donor heart. Owing to the success of cardiac transplantation, waiting lists continue to grow and the time necessary to locate a donor heart continues to increase. Waiting periods of weeks or months are now the rule even for patients in the most urgent category. Therefore, the decision of when to intervene in an unstable patient is crucial. Since the clinician is unable to predict when a compatible heart will be located, the decision to implant a mechanical circulatory support device needs to be made as soon as major organ function begins to be in jeopardy.

In our experience, some early patients initially rejected as candidates for bridging to transplantation because they were haemodynamically stable, later developed complications that excluded them from mechanical circulatory support and/

or cardiac transplantation.[41] Based on this experience, we concluded that haemodynamic stability alone should not exclude patients from mechanical assistance. The amount of pharmacological, respiratory and intra-aortic balloon pump support necessary to maintain stability must be considered. Patients suffering progressive renal, pulmonary or hepatic dysfunction should be considered for support prior to the development of irreversible major organ failure. Intra-aortic balloon pumps seem reasonable support mechanisms for up to 1–2 weeks. However, these patients often require inotropic support and have limited rehabilitative potential. It is our preference to insert a more sophisticated device which will provide adequate cardiac output without the need for associated inotropic support. Patients may then have all their intravenous lines removed, take oral medications and begin regular ambulation and exercises.

Some bridge-to-transplant candidates are unstable and require immediate implantation of an assist device. These patients may be at a higher risk of developing complications eliminating them from transplantation than the stabilized patient in whom device implantation can be performed under more controlled conditions. Criteria which should be rigidly applied to exclude patients from mechanical circulatory support prior to cardiac transplantation include:

1. Unresolved pulmonary emboli.
2. Renal failure requiring dialysis.
3. Recent unresolved cerebral vascular accident.
4. Unacceptable psychosocial history.
5. Severe bleeding.

This is not to say that at the time of device insertion all patients must meet all the transplantation criteria. Complications such as acute renal insufficiency, pulmonary oedema and minor infections can often be more effectively treated if the patient receives circulatory support. In this case, the patient can often be converted from a non-transplant candidate to a transplant candidate by the use of mechanical support.

Most of the patients in our experience who have been refused mechanical support prior to cardiac transplantation were rejected on the basis of infection and/or renal failure. Infection is a major concern since the device contains a large amount of prosthetic material which may worsen the infectious process. In addition, patients must be immunosuppressed after transplantation and

the infection may reappear or worsen. In our experience, 9 out of 44 bridge-to-transplant patients had pre-existing infectious complications. This included seven pneumonias and two cases of bacteraemia. The presence of bacteraemia was unknown in both these patients at the time of device implantation. None of these infections influenced the patient's outcome. For this reason, patients with superficial wound infections, urinary tract infections, or mild pneumonias with low-grade fever and minimal elevation in white blood cell count should be considered as reasonable candidates for mechanical circulatory support. Procedure-related risk factors such as the implantation of large amounts of prosthetic material, the potential need for invasive monitoring lines over a prolonged period, transcutaneous cannula or power cable sites also play a role in the development of infection. However, a recent review of 44 bridge-to-transplant patients at St Louis University showed that, when 54 risk factors for infection were analysed by multivariate analysis, no independent predictors for the development of infection could be identified.

Renal insufficiency or failure in any cardiogenic shock population is highly predictive of mortality. The factors aggravating renal insufficiency have been mentioned in the foregoing postcardiotomy section. It is often difficult or impossible to determine the reversibility of major organ dysfunction prior to device placement. However, patients with rising creatinine and blood urea nitrogen levels, decreasing response to diuretics and anuria should be carefully evaluated prior to device placement.

In our experience, a previous cardiac operation does not decrease a patient's chance of receiving a transplant during VAD support.[42] Pre-existing haemodynamic parameters such as cardiac index, right atrial pressure, and pulmonary capillary wedge pressure are not predictors of survival in our experience.[41] However, the presence of biventricular failure in the bridge-to-transplant patient population does appear to influence survival. In our experience, 78% of 26 patients receiving left ventricular assist devices were successfully transplanted and discharged, compared with only 22% of 18 patients who required biventricular support. In the Novacor, Thoratec and Thermo Cardiosystems clinical VAD trials the survival rates were lower in patients who received biventricular support.[43–45] However, this knowledge was only gained retrospectively and is made less useful as a selection criterion since the need for biventricular support is so difficult to predict preoperatively.

It is generally agreed that patients with coagulopathy should be excluded. Since coagulation, renal failure and infection can often be evaluated prior to device placement, some of these problems can be avoided in the post-implant period by limiting the entry criteria.

A growing number of patients have been successfully stabilized with mechanical circulatory support devices and successfully transplanted. Recent studies have documented that bridging to transplantation was at least as effective as routine cardiac transplantation.[46–48] The bridging experience has also greatly expanded clinical knowledge and experience, resulting in technological advancements and the identification of areas in which further work needs to be performed. Unfortunately, some patients initially improve after device placement and then deteriorate as a result of multiple complications which preclude transplantation. Owing to the scarcity of donor hearts and the amount of resources expended during each bridging procedure, it is imperative that only the best candidates for mechanical circulatory support be selected.

Acute deterioration

Some patients who develop acute cardiogenic shock or cardiac arrest qualify for circulatory support. These individuals may be already hospitalized or may arrive in the emergency department, ICU or catheterization room with acute massive injuries and cardiogenic shock. Some of them would not have had a previous evaluation of cardiac function, and many of them would be rapidly deteriorating or being actively resuscitated. In a significant percentage of such patients conventional resuscitative techniques such as pharmacological therapy and intra-aortic balloon pumps are ineffective. These patients may be successfully resuscitated with femoro-femoral extracorporeal membrane oxygenation (ECMO). After stabilization, their cardiac and major organ function can be evaluated and the plan of therapy formulated. Some of them may be best served by a percutaneous transluminal coronary angioplasty, corrective cardiac surgery or cardiac transplantation. Those who are candidates for angioplasty or cardiac surgery should be taken immediately to

the cardiac catheterization room or operating theatre. Patients who are candidates for cardiac transplantation should be stabilized and then switched to a more sophisticated device for long-term support.

Inpatients undergoing elective procedures such as coronary angioplasty or cardiac catheterization and who deteriorate should be supported, as should those who have undergone elective cardiac surgical repair and deteriorate in the ICU. Patients who have undergone emergency femoro-femoral CPB include those with postcardiotomy cardiogenic shock, failed coronary angioplasty, myocardial infarction with cardiogenic shock, massive pulmonary embolism, deterioration after cardiac transplantation, cardiomyopathy with acute shock, aortic stenosis, hypothermia, traumatic injury, and refractory ventricular fibrillation.[49–52] The survival rate has been seen to be best in those who had a failed coronary angioplasty and then underwent surgical revascularization after a brief period of stabilization with ECMO. Patients who have suffered large myocardial insults and are not cardiac transplant candidates, and patients who undergo conventional cardiopulmonary resuscitation for prolonged periods, have the least chance of survival.

Devices currently available

There are a variety of devices available that can be classified in several different ways. Some are investigational with limited availability while others can be purchased commercially. The position of a device can be described as extracorporeal, paracorporeal, heterotopic (internal or external) or orthotopic. Devices can also be classified according to their intended use; i.e. resuscitation or long-term support. There is no universal method of classification. In this chapter, five separate classes of devices will be discussed. These classes (see Table 16.2) include the devices currently being used clinically: resuscitative devices; external centrifugal and roller pumps; external pulsatile assist devices; implantable left ventricular assist systems; and total artificial hearts.

Resuscitative devices are systems that can be applied rapidly in the cardiac catheterization room, ICU or emergency room in patients suffering acute cardiogenic shock or haemodynamic

Table 16.2 Mechanical circulatory support devices.

Device	Position	Support	Anticoagulation required	Preferred application	Duration
BioMedicus	Extracorporeal	Rt,L,B	Moderate	P,B-Tx	Short–intermediate
Sarns/Centrimed	Extracorporeal	Rt,L,B	Moderate	P,B-Tx	Short–intermediate
ECMO	Extracorporeal	B	Full	R	Short
Abiomed BVS	Extracorporeal	Rt,L,B	Moderate	P,B-Tx	Short–intermediate
Pierce–Donachy VAD	Paracorporeal	Rt,L,B	Low	P,B-Tx	Intermediate–long
Hemopump	Internal	L	Moderate	P	Short–intermediate
Novacor LVAS	Internal	L	Low	B-Tx	Intermediate–long
Thermo Cardiosystems LVAS	Internal	L	Low	B-Tx	Intermediate–long

BVS = biventricular support system; ECMO = extracorporeal membrane oxygenation;LVAS = left ventricular assist system; VAD = ventricular assist device; AVAD = acute ventricular assist device; TAH = total artificial heart.
Rt = right; L = left; B = biventricular; R = resuscitative; P = postcardiotomy; B-Tx = bridge-to-transplantation.

deterioration that is unresponsive to pharmacological support and/or an intra-aortic balloon pump. The most commonly used and available of these systems are those that utilize femoro-femoral CPB or ECMO. Two methods of femoral cannulation are available, a percutaneous technique and a femoral cutdown technique.[50,53] This type of support uses a membrane oxygenator inline with a heat exchanger and a centrifugal pump. Femoro-femoral bypass systems are generally not recommended for periods of support longer than 24 hours, but they provide the option of rapid resuscitation and further patient evaluation. The chief disadvantages of these systems are that they require continuous heparin anticoagulation and provide incomplete biventricular support.

External centrifugal and roller pumps are commercially available and have been used extensively. Roller pumps have generally been used for postcardiotomy support, while centrifugal pumps have been used for both postcardiotomy (myocardial recovery) and for bridging to transplantation. There have been reported successes in both categories.[54,55] These devices are positioned extracorporeally and attached to cannulae that may be placed on any of the cardiac chambers to provide the desired type of support. Furthermore, insertion of these devices does not require complicated techniques and in many cases does not require CPB. Owing to the size, weight and extracorporeal nature of these devices, patient mobility is limited and patients are usually confined to bed or getting up in a chair. Results with these pumps are best if the duration of support is kept short (less than one week), but there have been cases of support for as long as 30 days.[54]

External pulsatile assist devices are now being used worldwide. The Pierce–Donachy ventricular assist device developed at Pennsylvania State University and manufactured by Thoratec Medical Corporation of Berkeley, California, has been used in more than 378 patients. Investigators have reported successful use of this VAD in both bridge-to-transplantation and postcardiotomy cardiogenic shock applications.[33,44] This device is positioned paracorporeally on the upper portion of the abdominal wall, allowing considerable patient mobility. It can be used to support either the right or the left side of the heart and atrial or left ventricular cannulation is available. The power source is compressed air. This device has been proven to be effective for intermediate term support. Many patients have been supported for more than 30 days and one patient was successfully transplanted after 225 days of support with this VAD.

The Symbion VAD, also known as the AVAD (acute ventricular assist device), is similar to one ventricle of the Symbion Jarvik 7 total artificial heart which will be discussed later. The power source is compressed air. Both right and left support can be provided, but the Symbion device can only be used with atrial cannulation. It is not currently available for clinical use in the USA.

The Abiomed (BVS 5000) or biventricular support system is different in configuration from other external pulsatile devices discussed in this section. It is located extracorporeally and significantly impairs patient mobility. It uses only atrial cannulae and can provide right, left or biventricular support. Filling of the devices is accomplished by gravity, so there is no need for diastolic vacuum. Patients have been supported with this device both in the USA and in Europe for both bridge-to-transplantation and myocardial recovery.

Implantable LV assist systems are important devices since they are prototypes of permanent, non-tethered systems which may provide an alternative to transplantation for patients with end-stage heart disease. Several manufacturers are developing permanent implantable systems. Two devices currently used clinically, the Novacor LV assist system and the ThermoCardiosystems LV assist device, are under investigation as bridges to transplantation.[43,45] These devices are not well-suited for postcardiotomy support since they are designed for LV cannulation only and require removal of a large portion of myocardium at the time of insertion. In addition, they can provide only LV support. The energy source for the Novacor LV assist system is electricity. An external power cable is the only element traversing the skin, allowing for excellent patient mobility. Patients have been successfully transplanted after as long as 370 days of support with this device. The ThermoCardiosystems device is similar, with two models presently available, one which uses compressed air, and one which uses electricity as its power source. A unique feature of the Thermo-Cardiosystems device is that it utilizes a textured rather than a smooth blood-contacting surface, so that a pseudo-neointimal layer develops which provides a decreased risk of thromboembolism and reduced requirements for anticoagulation.[45]

Orthotopic biventricular replacement devices or artificial hearts are perhaps the most publicized devices. The Jarvik 7 total artificial heart manufactured by Symbion has been used clinically in more than 180 cases worldwide but is not currently available for clinical use. Powered pneumatically, it requires removal of the patient's ventricles and can be used for bridging to transplantation or permanent applications. Two drivelines exit the abdomen so patient mobility is not severely restricted. A variety of other total artificial heart designs have been used clinically, but the numbers of patients are few and the survival has been minimal.

Selection of an appropriate device

Proper device selection is essential according to the circumstances leading to the patient's state of cardiogenic shock. Few facilities have all of the previously mentioned devices at their disposal.

In patients who suffer an acute haemodynamic deterioration outside the operating room, the immediate concern is the restoration of normal perfusion to the vital organs. With this patient population is it important to gain immediate access to the circulatory system. For this reason, resuscitative devices which can be inserted rapidly are the most appropriate devices. While these devices are not designed for long-term support, they do provide a period of stabilization in which further evaluation can be performed. After resuscitation with femoro-femoral ECMO, patients may be candidates for urgent cardiac repair or percutaneous transluminal coronary angioplasty. If the patient is determined to be inoperable, transplantation may be a consideration if the patient meets the transplant criteria. In this case, unless a donor organ is immediately available, the patient should be switched to another system which could provide more effective long-term support.

Patients requiring mechanical circulatory support for postcardiotomy cardiogenic shock remain the largest population, and survival in this group is just 25%. If this patient population has not suffered a large perioperative myocardial infarction or had previous extensive myocardial damage, the possibility for recovery should be assumed. For this reason, an artificial heart is not an appropriate device for this group. Resuscitative systems have little if any positive effect on myocardial recovery so these devices are usually not as effective for postcardiotomy cardiogenic shock.[56] In addition, resuscitative systems usually require high doses of intravenous heparin which would aggravate existing bleeding complications. External centrifugal pumps or external pulsatile assist devices are the most appropriate devices for this application. It is also important to determine whether the patient has right, left or biventricular failure. Since the incidence of biventricular failure is so high in the postcardiotomy group,[36] it is important to select a method of support which would optimize left and right ventricular recovery. If myocardial damage is so severe that recovery is unlikely, transplantation may be considered. The patient should be stabilized and meet all of the usual transplant guidelines prior to listing. Fortunately, the external pulsatile assist devices are effective for use as bridges to transplantation as well as postcardiotomy recovery. Centrifugal pumps may not be the best choice of device if it is thought that the patient may need a transplant, owing to the wait for a donor heart. However, few postcardiotomy patients requiring VAD support progress to the point that they would be candidates for cardiac transplantation. For this reason, centrifugal pumps are an appropriate choice and probably more than effective in the majority of postcardiotomy patients. In addition, data from the ASAIO/ISHLT registry show no difference in survival in postcardiotomy patients supported with external pneumatic versus centrifugal pumps.[25]

Another group often requiring mechanical circulatory support are patients awaiting cardiac transplantation or patients who have large irreversible cardiac injuries precluding recovery. Many of these patients have already been selected and listed for cardiac transplantation; therefore, short-term devices need not be considered. The waiting time for donor organs continues to increase annually. Therefore, it is important to support candidates with devices that are effective for periods of more than 30 days. At present all of the investigational pulsatile devices such as the Thoratec, Novacor and ThermoCardiosystems devices have proven to be very effective in this group. The overall survival rates and post-transplant survival rates with these three systems are similar.

Discussion

It is apparent that device selection criteria have evolved more rapidly than patient selection criteria. This is in part due to the fact that there are a small number of devices available whereas the variables involved in patient selection are infinite. While there have been dramatic improvements in patient selection criteria, especially in the bridge-to-transplant patient population over the last decade, several areas require further investigation. More objective determinations of major organ dysfunction and reversibility need to be identified. Very few hard criteria have been identified, and patients are often selected on the basis of study protocols and a clinician's impressions. Retrospective reviews have identified some risk factors in both the myocardial recovery and bridge-to-transplant patient populations. The improving survival rates after transplantation in patients bridged with VADs has sparked widespread interest and a significant amount of reporting in the literature. Patient selection for bridging to cardiac transplantations is expanding;

however, at the same time survival is increasing. Unfortunately, no single institution has enough patients to perform a reasonable multivariate analysis or identify predictors of survival. The survival rate in the postcardiotomy patient population has remained relatively constant for the past decade. Many centres now consider postcardiotomy VAD support as rescue therapy and shy away from its consistent use.

This technology currently benefits a small number of patients. However, in the future, it may significantly alter the morbidity associated with acute and chronic heart failure. It is unclear whether randomized trials are needed or if they would even be useful at this point in history. However, multicentre studies would be useful since so few patients are studied per year at any one institution.

References

1. Dale HH, Schuster EHJ. A double perfusion pump. *J Physiol* 1928; **64**, 356–365.
2. Dennis C, Spreng DS, Nelson GE, *et al.* Development of a pump–oxygenator to replace the heart and lungs: an apparatus applicable to human patients, and application to one case. *Ann Surg* 1951; **134**, 709–721.
3. Gibbons JH. Application of a mechanical heart and lung apparatus to cardiac surgery. *Minn Med* 1954; **37**, 171.
4. Stuckey JH, Newman MM, Dennis C, *et al.* The use of the heart–lung machine in selected cases of acute myocardial infarction. *Surg Forum* 1957; **8**, 342–344.
5. Spencer FC, Eiseman B, Trinkle JK, Rossi NP. Assisted circulation for cardiac failure following intracardiac surgery with cardiopulmonary bypass. *J Thorac Cardiovasc Surg* 1965; **49**, 56–73.
6. Kantrowitz A, Tjonneland S, Freed PS, *et al.* Initial clinical experience with intra-aortic balloon pumping in cardiogenic shock. *J Am Med Ass* 1968; **203**, 135–140.
7. Akutsu T, Kolff WJ. Permanent substitutes for valves and hearts. *ASAIO Trans* 1958; **4**, 230–234.
8. Boreto JW, Pierce WS. Segmented polyurethane: a new elastomer for biomedical applications. *Science* 1967; **158**, 1481–1482.
9. Bernhard WF, Poirier V, LaFarge CG, Carr JG. A new method for temporary left ventricular bypass: preclinical appraisal. *J Thorac Cardiovasc Surg* 1975; **70**, 800–885.
10. Donachy JH, Landis DL, Rosenberg G, *et al.* Design and evaluation of a left ventricular assist device: the angle port pump. In: Unger F (ed), *Assisted Circula-*

tion. Berlin: Springer Verlag, 1978: 138–146.

11. Portner PM, Oyer PE, Jassawalla JS, *et al.* An alternative in end-stage heart disease: long-term ventricular assistance. *J Heart Transplant* 1983; **3**, 47–59.

12. Cooley DA, Liotta D, Hallman GL, *et al.* Orthotopic cardiac prosthesis for two-staged cardiac replacement. *Am J Cardiol* 1969; **24**, 723–730.

13. Golding LR, Groves LK, Peter M, *et al.* Initial clinical experience with a new temporary left ventricular assist device. *Ann Thorac Surg* 1980; **29**, 66–69.

14. Holub DA, Hibbs CW, Sturm JT, *et al.* Clinical trials of the abdominal left ventricular assist device (ALVAD): progress report. *Cardiovasc Dis Bull Tex Heart Inst* 1979; **6**, 359–372.

15. Litwak RS, Koffsky RM, Jurado RA, *et al.* Use of a left heart assist device after intracardiac surgery: technique and clinical experience. *Ann Thorac Surg* 1976; **21**, 191–202.

16. Olsen EK, Pierce WS, Donachy JH, *et al.* A two and one-half year clinical experience with a mechanical left ventricular assist pump in the treatment of profound postoperative heart failure. *Int J Artif Organs* 1979; **2**, 197–206.

17. Pennington DG, Merjavy JP, Swartz MT, Willman VL. Clinical experience with a centrifugal pump ventricular assist device. *ASAIO Trans* 1982; **28**, 93–99.

18. Turina M, Bosio R, Sennig A. Clinical application of paracorporeal uni- and biventricular artificial heart. *ASAIO Trans* 1978; **24**, 625–631.

19. Norman JC, Cooley DA, Kahan BD, *et al.* Total support of the circulation of a patient with postcardiotomy stone heart syndrome by a partial artificial heart (ALVAD) for five days followed by heart and kidney transplantation. *Lancet* 1978; **i**, 1125–1127.

20. Reemstsma K, Drusin R, Edie R, *et al.* Cardiac transplantation for patients requiring mechanical circulatory support. *New Engl J Med* 1978; **298**, 670–671.

21. Hill JD, Farrar DJ, Hershon JJ, *et al.* Use of prosthetic ventricle as a bridge to cardiac transplantation for postinfarction cardiogenic shock. *New Engl Med* 1986; **314**, 626–628.

22. Starnes VA, Oyer PE, Portner PM, *et al.* Isolated left ventricular assist as a bridge to cardiac transplantation. *J Thorac Cardiovasc Surg* 1988; **96**, 62–71.

23. Copeland JG, Levinson MM, Smith R, *et al.* The total artificial heart as a bridge to transplantation: a report of two cases. *J Am Med Ass* 1986; **256**, 2991–2995.

24. Oaks TE, Pae WE, Miller CA, Pierce WS. Combined registry for the clinical use of mechanical ventricular assist pumps and the total artificial heart in conjunction with heart transplantation: fifth offi-cial report 1990. *J Heart Lung Transplant* 1991; **10**, 621–625.

25. Pae WE, Miller CA, Matthews Y, Pierce WS. Ventricular assist devices for postcardiotomy cardiogenic shock. *J Thorac Cardiovasc Surg* 1992; **104**, 541–553.

26. Bolooki H (ed.) *Clinical Application of Intra-aortic Balloon Pump*, 2nd edn. Mount Kisco, NY: Futura Publishing, 1984.

27. Creswell LL, Rosenbloom M, Cox JL, *et al.* Intra-aortic balloon counterpulsation: patterns of usage and outcome in cardiac surgery patients. *Ann Thorac Surg* 1992; **54**, 11–20.

28. DiLello F, Mullen DC, Flemma RJ, *et al.* Results of intra-aortic balloon pumping after cardiac surgery: experience with the Percor balloon catheter. *Ann Thorac Surg* 1988; **46**, 442–446.

29. Naunheim KS, Swartz MT, Pennington DG, *et al.* Intra-aortic balloon pumping in cardiac surgical patients: risk analysis and long-term follow-up. *J Thorac Cardiovasc Surg* 1992; **104**, 1654–1661.

30. Norman JC, Cooley DA, Igo SR, *et al.* Prognostic indices for survival during postcardiotomy intra-aortic balloon pumping. *J Thorac Cardiovasc Surg* 1977; **74**, 709–720.

31. Joyce LD, Kiser JC, Eales F, *et al.* Experience with the Sarns centrifugal pump as a ventricular assist device. *ASAIO Trans* 1990; **36**, 619–623.

32. Pennington DG, Joyce LD, Pae WE, Burkholder JA. Patient selection. *Ann Thorac Surg* 1989; **47**, 77–81.

33. Pennington DG, McBride LR, Swartz MT, *et al.* Use of the Pierce–Donachy ventricular assist device in patients with cardiogenic shock after cardiac operations. *Ann Thorac Surg* 1989; **47**, 130–135.

34. Kanter KR, Swartz MT, Pennington DG, *et al.* Renal failure in patients with ventricular assist devices. *ASAIO Trans* 1987; **43**, 426–428.

35. Pennington DG, McBride LR, Kanter KR, *et al.* The effect of perioperative myocardial infarction on survival of postcardiotomy patients supported with ventricular assist devices. *Circulation* 1988; **78** (suppl III), 111–115.

36. Pennington DG, Merjavy JP, Swartz MT, *et al.* The importance of biventricular failure in patients with postoperative cardiogenic shock. *Ann Thorac Surg* 1985; **39**, 16–26.

37. Wareing TH, Kouchoukos NT. Postcardiotomy mechanical circulatory support in the elderly. *Ann Thorac Surg* 1991; **51**, 443–447.

38. Naunheim KS, Fiore AC, Wadley JJ, *et al.* The changing mortality of myocardial revascularization: coronary artery bypass and angioplasty. *Ann Thorac Surg* 1988; **46**, 666–674.

39. Moroney D, Swartz MT, Reedy JE, *et al.* Importance of ventricular arrhythmias in recovery patients with ventricular assist devices. *ASAIO Trans* 1991; **37**, 516–517.

40. McBride LR, Swartz MT, Reedy JE, Miller LW, Pennington DG. Device related infections in patients supported with mechanical circulatory support devices greater than 30 days. *ASAIO Trans* 1991; **37**, 258–259.

41. Reedy JE, Swartz MT, Pennington DG, *et al.* Bridge to cardiac transplantation: importance of patient selection. *J Heart Transplant* 1990; **9**, 473–481.

42. McBride LR, Swartz MT, Reedy JE, *et al.* Bridging to transplantation in patients with previous cardiac operations (abstract). *J Heart Transplant* 1990; **9**, 57.

43. Portner PM, Oyer PE, Pennington DG, *et al.* Implantable electrical left ventricular assist system: bridge to transplantation and the future. *Ann Thorac Surg* 1989; **47**, 142–150.

44. Farrar DJ, Hill JD. Univentricular and biventricular thoratec VAD support as a bridge to transplantation. *Ann Thorac Surg* 1993; **55**, 276–282.

45. Frazier OH, Rose EA, MacManus Q, *et al.* Multi-centre clinical evaluation of the HeartMate 1000 IP left ventricular assist device. *Ann Thorac Surg* 1992; **53**, 1080–1090.

46. Reedy JE, Pennington DG, Miller LW, *et al.* Status I heart transplant patients—conventional *vs* ventricular assist device support. *J Heart Lung Transplant* 1992; **11**, 246–252.

47. Birovljev S, Radovancevic B, Burnett CM, *et al.* Heart transplantation after mechanical circulatory support: four years' experience. *J Heart Lung Transplant* 1992; **11**, 240–245.

48. Pifarre R, Sullivan H, Montoya A, *et al.* Comparison of results after heart transplantation: mechanically supported versus nonsupported patients. *J Heart Lung Transplant* 1992; **11**, 235–239.

49. Moore CH, Rubin JM, Shnitzler RN, Canon DS, Arpin A. Experience and direction using cardio-pulmonary support in fifty-three consecutive cases. *ASAIO Trans* 1991; **37**, 340–342.

50. Phillips SJ, Zeff RH, Kongatahworn C, *et al.* Percutaneous cardiopulmonary bypass: application and indications for use. *Ann Thorac Surg* 1989; **47**, 121–123.

51. Raithel SC, Swartz MT, Braun PR, *et al.* Experience with an emergency resuscitation system. *ASAIO Trans* 1989; **35**, 475–477.

52. Reichman RT, Joyo CI, Dembitsky WP, *et al.* Improved patient survival after cardiac arrest using a cariopulmonary support system. *Ann Thorac Surg* 1990; **49**, 101–105.

53. Pennington DG, Merjavy JP, Codd JE, *et al.* Extracorporeal membrane oxygenation for patients with cardiogenic shock. *Circulation* 1984; **70** (suppl I), 130–137.

54. Golding LAR, Stewart RW, Sinkewich M, *et al.* Nonpulsatile ventricular assist bridging to transplantation. *ASAIO Trans* 1988; **34**, 476–479.

55. Rose DM, Connolly M, Cunningham JN, Spencer FC. Technique and results with a roller pump left and right heart assist device. *Ann Thorac Surg* 1989; **47**, 124–129.

56. Bavaria JE, Ratcliffe MB, Gupta KB, *et al.* Changes in left ventricular systolic wall stress during biventricular circulatory assistance. *Ann Thorac Surg* 1988; **45**, 526–532.

17

The Thoratec® VAD system: patient selection and clinical results in bridging to transplantation

J Donald Hill and David J Farrar

Introduction

With increasing frequency, transplant centres around the world are relying on prosthetic devices to support the circulation of patients who are at imminent risk of dying before a donor heart becomes available.[1,2] The goal is to provide circulatory assistance until orthotopic cardiac transplantation can be performed. As in any new technology, a clearer picture of which patients can most benefit from the use of these devices comes with experience. In this chapter we report on 214 patients who have had circulatory support by means of a ventricular assist device for bridging to transplantation, since its first successful use in 1984.[3]

The Thoratec VAD system

The system consists of prosthetic ventricles with a 65 ml stroke volume (Fig. 17.1), appropriate cannulae for atrial or ventricular inflow and arterial outflow connections, and a pneumatic drive console. The blood pumping chamber and cannulae are fabricated from Thoratec's BPS-215M polyurethane elastomer, a blend of two polymers, one of which provides extensive flex life and strength, and the other thromboresistance.[4] The pneumatic drive console provides alternating positive and negative air pressure to empty and fill the blood pump and has three control modes depending on the needs of the patient: asynchronous (fixed rate), volume (full-to-empty variable rate), and synchronous.[5] The full-to-empty mode was used in most bridging cases, because it automatically adjusts beat rate and thus flow output in accordance with venous return and the needs of the body. These heterotopic prosthetic ventricles are placed in a paracorporeal position on the anterior abdominal wall and are connected to the heart and great vessels with cannulae crossing the chest wall (Fig. 17.2). The paracorporeal approach allows it to be used in a wide range of patient body sizes.

An advantage of the Thoratec VAD system is its versatility. For support of the left side of the heart, inflow cannulation can be achieved from the left atrial appendage, from the left atrium via the intra-atrial groove, or from the left ventricular apex, depending on the patient's anatomy or the surgeon's preference. VAD outflow is through a polyurethane cannula attached to a preclotted 14 mm polyester graft anastomosed to the ascending aorta. For support of the right side, cannulation is from the right atrium with return blood flow to the pulmonary artery. Detailed surgical techniques for these cannulation approaches have been published.[6] In addition to its use in bridging to transplantation, the device can be used for support pending recovery of the natural heart.[7,8]

Patient entry criteria

The decision to implant VADs in patients in this study was made when the clinical and haemodynamic status indicated that the patient would probably die or sustain permanent end-organ damage before a donor heart could be located. No patient was accepted for the study who had known contraindications to cardiac transplantation other than those considered to be reversible after restoration of adequate cardiac output. Patients who were found to have pre-existing contraindications to cardiac transplantation after device insertion (e.g. emergency insertion of VADs in patients subsequently found to be brain dead) were not transplanted. Likewise, patients in whom contraindications developed during the bridging period and whose condition could not

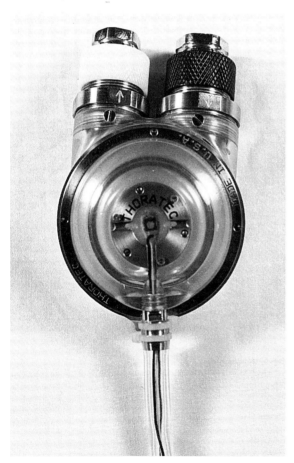

Fig. 17.1 The Thoratec ventricular assist device consists of a flexible polyurethane blood pumping chamber with a stroke volume of 65 ml encased in a rigid plastic housing.

be stabilized by circulatory support with ventricular assist devices did not receive a heart transplant and ultimately died.

At the time of device implant, patients must have been judged to be at imminent risk of death prior to obtaining a suitable donor heart, using haemodynamic guidelines of: a cardiac index $<1.8\,l/min/m^2$, a mean arterial pressure <70 mmHg, and a left atrial pressure >20 mmHg, despite appropriate use of conventional therapies such as inotropic agents, vasodilators and intra-aortic balloon pumps.

In the USA the studies were carried out under the investigational-device-exemption (IDE) regulations of the US Food and Drug Administration. Informed consent was obtained from either the patient or the next of kin.

The patient population

As of January 1993, 214 patients who were in imminent risk of dying prior to donor heart procurement received Thoratec VADs for left, right or biventricular support at 44 medical centres in ten countries. Excluded from this analysis are patients with mixed types of support such as Thoratec VADs used in combination with centrifugal pumps. Coronary artery disease was diagnosed in 85 patients (ischaemic cardiomyopathy in 63, acute myocardial infarction in 22) and cardiomyopathy in 98 (idiopathic in 75, postpartum in 11, viral in 9, hypertrophic in 3). An additional 31 'other' patients received devices for diagnoses such as graft failures following orthotopic cardiac transplantation, valvular disease, myocarditis, doxorubicin (Adriamycin) toxicity, and congenital heart disease. There were 165 males and 49 females with an average age of 43 years (range 11–63 years), an average body surface area of 1.84 m^2 (range 1.00–2.41 m^2) and an average weight of 72 kg (range 26–123 kg).

All patients undergoing implantation were receiving maximal inotropic support. In addition, 42% had experienced one or more cardiac arrests, 63% had received cardiac assistance with intra-aortic balloon pumps, and 57% were receiving mechanical ventilation. Despite this therapy, the average cardiac index in this patient population was $1.4 \pm 0.7\,l/min/m^2$ with a pulmonary capillary wedge pressure of 28 ± 8 mmHg and a mean arterial pressure of 65 ± 14 mmHg.

Clinical results

Of the 214 patients implanted with Thoratec VADs, three remain on support at the time of writing awaiting a suitable donor heart. Results are reported here on 211 patients in which the VAD had supported the circulation for up to 226 days until a donor heart could be located and transplantation performed.

One hundred and thirty-six of the 211 patients (64%) recovered sufficiently to undergo cardiac transplant. One hundred and thirteen of those patients undergoing transplantation were eventually discharged from the hospital. Early post-transplant survival was 83% and the overall survival from implant to patient discharge was 54% (Table 17.1).

One hundred and fifty-five patients (73%) were maintained on biventricular support. Ninety-nine of these patients (64%) went on to transplantation and 79 were eventually discharged for a post-transplant survival of 80% and an overall survival

of 51%. In 54 patients (26%) univentricular LVADs were sufficient to support the circulation. Their survival statistics (67% pre-transplant, 92% post-transplant, 61% overall) were slightly better than BVAD patients but the difference was not significant. Two patients were supported with univentricular RVADs following cardiac allograft failure; one patient survived to retransplant and was eventually discharged from the hospital (Table 17.1).

There was a significant difference in overall survival according to age, when divided into patients above and below 50 years. Of the 137 patients under this age, 94 (69%) went on to transplantation and 81 were eventually discharged (overall survival 59%) (Table 17.2). Of the 74 patients who were 50 years or older, 42 (57%) went on to transplantation and 32 were eventually discharged (overall survival 43%). The difference in overall survival between the groups was significant ($p = 0.03$). Young patients in general tended to do the best. Those under the age of

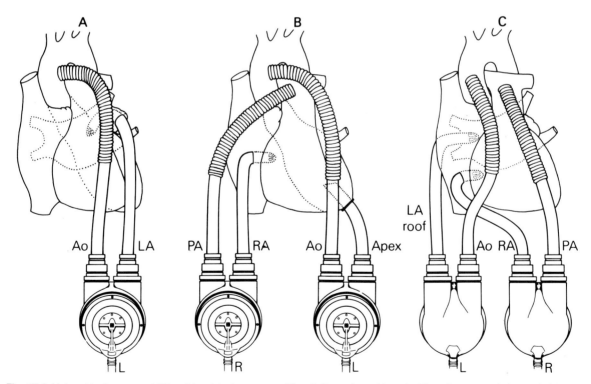

Fig. 17.2 Univentricular support (*A*) or biventricular support (*B* and *C*) can be achieved with various cannulation techniques. Inflow cannulation from the left side of the heart can be made from the left atrial appendage (*A*), the left ventricular apex (*B*) or the left atrial roof via the intra-atrial groove (*C*), with outflow to the aorta. On the right side, inflow cannulation is from the right atrium with outflow to the pulmonary artery (*B* and *C*). Reproduced with permission from reference 9.

Table 17.1 Overall* survival statistics for patients who received Thoratec biventricular (BVAD), left (LVAD) or right (RVAD) assist devices as a bridge to heart transplantation.

	Implanted	Transplanted (Tx)	Survival		
			Number	After implantation	After Tx
BVAD	155	99 (64%)	79	51%	80%
LVAD	54	36 (67%)	33	61%	92%
RVAD	2	1 (50%)	1	50%	100%
Totals	211	136 (64%)	113	54%	83%

* Does not include data on three patients waiting for a transplant at the time of writing.

40 had a 92% post-transplant survival.

There was no difference in survival according to duration of support (Table 17.2). One hundred and sixty-nine patients were supported for less than 30 days. One hundred and six of these patients went on to transplant and 91 were eventually discharged (86% post-transplant survival, 54% overall survival). The 42 patients who were supported for more than 30 days experienced similar post-transplant survival (73%) and overall survival (52%).

There was no significant difference in overall survival between patients with the preoperative diagnoses of dilated cardiomyopathy (56%), or ischaemic cardiomyopathy (47%). The group of patients required VAD support for an acute myocardial infarction had a non-significant higher overall survival rate of 68% (Table 17.3).

Complications

Complete data on complications for 185 patients are given in Table 17.4, and the causes of death in Table 17.5. Surgical bleeding and coagulopathies resulting in excessive chest tube drainage, tamponade, haemothorax or reoperation remain the most common complications during the bridge period and were reported in 44% of patients. Since our initial report on the use of Thoratec VADs for bridging to transplantation,[9] the proportion of patients undergoing reoperations for bleeding following device insertion has decreased from 38% to 23%, while the proportion of patients who died from this complication has increased slightly, from 14% to 18%. Infection was another major complication, occurring in 40% of patients and causing death in 28%. Hepatic dysfunction and renal failure requiring dialysis were both reported in 14% or patients during the bridging period, and 17 patients (28% of deaths) succumbed to multiorgan failure, mainly related to hepatic and renal dysfunction. Respiratory failure occurred in 13% of patients and was the pre-transplant cause of death in three patients. Non-thromboembolic neurologic events were reported in 12% of patients, including four patients who, prior to transplantation, had died from brain death (believed in retrospect to be present at the time of implant). Clinical haemolysis (defined as haemolysis requiring blood replacement) was seen in 9%, while elevations in plasma free haemoglobin (at least one measure-

Table 17.2 Survival statistics by age and by duration of support for patients who received Thoratec VADs as a bridge to heart transplantation (data on 211 patients).

	Implanted	Transplanted (Tx)	Survival		
			Number	After implantation	After Tx
Age (years)*					
<50	137	94 (69%)	81	59%	86%
≥50	74	42 (57%)	32	43%	76%
Duration (days)					
<30	169	106 (63%)	91	54%	86%
≥30	42	30 (71%)	22	52%	73%

* There was a significant difference ($p = 0.03$) in overall survival between age-groups.

Table 17.3 Comparison of survival by preoperative diagnosis (data on 178 patients).

Preoperative diagnosis	Implanted	Transplanted (Tx)	Survival Number	Survival After implantation	Survival After Tx
Dilated cardiomyopathy	94	64 (68%)	53	56%	83%
Ischaemic cardiomyopathy	62	40 (65%)	29	47%	73%
Acute myocardial infarction	22	15 (68%)	15	68%	100%
Totals	178	119 (67%)	97	54%	82%

ment greater than 3 times normal) were seen in 31%. Haemolysis tended to occur early in the support period and usually resolved with plasma free haemoglobin levels returning to normal. Nine per cent of patients experienced CVAs during the support period (significantly less for LV cannulation compared to LA cannulation[11]) and two patients died prior to transplantation following these embolic events. An additional 4% of patients suffered transient ischaemic attacks. Three patients died from what is described as 'peripheral shock'—that is, low systemic vascular resistance in the absence of sepsis. Three patients with unilateral LVADs died from right ventricular failure. Finally, one patient died when adequate inflow through the LVAD cannula could not be achieved.

Eight patients who underwent transplantation died from graft failure prior to discharge (Table 17.5). Additional deaths reported after transplantation but before discharge from hospital were infections in five patients, bleeding in three, multiorgan failure in two, rejection in one, and hepatitis in one (Table 17.5).

Discussion

Proper selection of patients and early initiation of support continue to be the principal factors affecting survival to transplant and ultimately overall survival. Patients who died prior to transplant, from multiorgan failure or from pre-VAD neurologic hypoxia, are examples of where the initiation of circulatory support and restoration of

Table 17.4 Complications reported on 185 patients while on Thoratec VADs for bridging to transplantation.

Complication	Patients (%)
Bleeding (Reoperations: 23%)	44
Infection	40
Hepatic dysfunction (Bilirubin >3× normal: 39%)	14
Renal dialysis (Creatinine >1.5× normal: 27%)	14
Respiratory failure	13
Non-TE neurologic events	12
Clinical haemolysis (Plasma free Hgb >3× normal: 31%)	9
Stroke	9
TIA	4

TE = thromboembolism; TIA = transient ischaemic attack.

Table 17.5 Causes of death in patients who died prior to transplant, and in transplanted patients who died prior to discharge from hospital (data on 185 patients).

Cause of death	Number	Deaths (%)
Patients not transplanted (61/185)		
Multiorgan failure	17	28
Sepsis	17	28
Bleeding	11	18
Pre-VAD hypotension	4	6
Peripheral shock	3	5
Respiratory failure	3	5
RV failure	3	5
Stroke	2	3
Inadequate LVAD filling	1	2
Transplanted patients (20/124)		
Graft failure	8	40
Infection	5	25
Bleeding	3	15
Multiorgan failure	2	10
Hepatitis	1	5
Rejection	1	5

blood flow occurred too late to reverse the effects of pre-VAD hypotension. Often it is only clear in retrospect that the window of opportunity has been missed.

The debate over the criteria for prosthetic support and the timing of VAD insertion continues. The ideal candidate is the patient in imminent risk of death from irreversible myocardial dysfunction but without end-organ involvement or contraindications to heart transplant. Specific haemodynamic criteria such as those adopted for the evaluation of the Thoratec VAD system (as cited above) are useful guidelines, but can be inappropriate indicators in patients who are deteriorating prior to satisfying these criteria.

In the absence of consistent prognostic indicators in selecting patients and the abundance of anecdotal case histories of patients *in extremis* who ultimately survived, it is more apparent that to implant devices when in doubt is the best course of action. This is especially true in the young, previously healthy patient or in the patient in cardiogenic shock following an acute myocardial infarction. While on support it will become apparent if they are suitable candidates for transplantation.

As our experience with prosthetic circulatory support grows, indicators for successful bridging to transplantation should emerge. As an example, in earlier analyses of Thoratec bridge-to-transplant patients, women tended to have a higher overall mortality than did men. Over time, as the total number of women receiving VADs has increased, this difference is no longer apparent. With this most recent analysis of the Thoratec data the difference in overall survival in patients younger than 50 years was significantly greater than in those older than 50 (59% and 43% respectively). Also of interest is that overall survival in patients with the pre-support diagnosis of acute MI is tending to be higher than in patients with chronic heart disease such as dilated or ischaemic cardiomyopathy. While the difference was not significant, and the majority of acute MI patients successfully bridged to transplant occurred at one centre, this finding certainly will be followed over time.

In addition to the data presented here, an analysis of preoperative predictors of survival in bridge-in-transplant patients with Thoratec VADs has recently been completed.[10] This study of pre-VAD variables identified two statistically significant risk factors for survival after VAD implantation: previous operations more than 30 days prior to a VAD implantation, and elevated pre-VAD measurements of blood urea nitrogen. In addition, preoperative measurements of total bilirubin were almost significant ($p = 0.07$). No other pre-VAD demographic, haemodynamic, or blood chemistry variable was found to be significantly related to survival. The results suggest that blood urea nitrogen is a marker of multiorgan pathophysiology that is useful in assessing bridge-to-transplant patients.

Obviously, proper patient selection and the timing of VAD insertion are not the only questions that require answers. For example, 13% of patients in this analysis experienced a thromboembolic event (stroke or TIA) while on support. Yet evaluating the individual embolic incidents is difficult. The data presented here are all-inclusive, regardless of aetiology. Because of changes in intrathoracic flow, haemodynamics and cardiac rhythms, all of which can effect the incidence of thromboembolism, we have come to consider the support circuit to begin at the vena cava and end in the aorta regardless of the type of support (BVAD, LVAD or RVAD). In this analysis there is no way to differentiate between emboli originating in the atria, ventricles or VADs, which are normally free of any evidence of thrombus when they are removed. The data is also uncorrected for anticoagulation regimens which are determined by the individual centres, for variations in VAD flow, and for the site of inflow cannulation, which was recently shown to be a significant factor in the risk for thromboembolism. In data not shown here, an analysis of 166 Thoratec bridge-to-transplant patients showed that the incidence of thromboembolism was significantly reduced with LV cannulation (2.8%) when compared with cannulation in the intra-atrial groove (10%) and in the left atrial appendage (13.8%).[11]

In conclusion it can be stated that univentricular or biventricular prosthetic circulatory support can provide an effective method of maintaining blood flow to vital organs until a donor heart becomes available for transplantation. Proper selection of patients and timing for initiation of support continue to be the principal factors affecting overall survival. It is hoped that as our knowledge of this technology increases, preoperative predictors of success will become more apparent.

Acknowledgement

We gratefully acknowledge the contributions of the principal investigators and cardiac surgical teams at the investigational centres that provided data reported here.

References

1. Hill JD. Bridging to cardiac transplantation. *Ann Thorac Surg* 1989; **47**, 167–171.
2. Pennington DG, Swartz MT. Assisted circulation and the mechanical heart. In: Branwald E, (ed), *Heart Disease: A Textbook of Cardiovascular Medicine*. Philadelphia: WB Saunders, 1991: 535–550.
3. Hill JD, Farrar DJ, Hershon JJ, *et al*. Use of a prosthetic ventricle as a bridge to cardiac transplantation for postinfarction cardiogenic shock. *New Engl J Med* 1986; **314**, 626–628.
4. Farrar DJ, Litwak P, Lawson JH, *et al*. In vivo evaluations of a new thromboresistant polyurethane for artificial heart blood pumps. *J Thorac Cardiovasc Surg* 1988; **95**, 191–200.
5. Farrar DJ, Compton PG, Lawson JH, Hershon JJ, Hill JD. Control modes of a clinical ventricular assist device. *IEEE Engr Med Biol* 1986; **5**, 19–25.
6. Ganzel BL, Gray LA, Slater AD, Mavroudis C. Surgical techniques for the implantation of heterotopic prosthetic ventricles. *Ann Thorac Surg* 1989; **47**, 113–120.
7. Holman WL, Bourge RC, Kirklin JK. Case report: circulatory support for seventy days with resolution of acute heart failure. *J Thorac Cardiovasc Surg* 1991; **102**, 932–934.
8. Pennington DG, McBride LR, Swartz MT, *et al*. Use of the Pierce–Donachy ventricular assist device in patients with cardiogenic shock after cardiac operations. *Ann Thorac Surg* 1989; **47**, 130–135.
9. Farrar DJ, Hill JD, Gray LA, *et al*. Heterotopic prosthetic ventricles as a bridge to cardiac transplantation: a multicentre study in 29 patients. *New Engl J Med* 1988; **318**, 333–340.
10. Farrar DJ. Preoperative predictors of survival in patients with Thoratec ventricular assist devices as a bridge to cardiac transplantation. *J Heart Lung Transplant* 1994; **13**, 93–101.
11. Farrar DJ. Atrial versus ventricular cannulation for bridge to transplantation with the Thoratec VAD system. *Thoratec's Heartbeat* 1993; **7**(1), 3–4.

Section V

Long-Term Support

18

End-organ function during mechanical left ventricular assistance

Howard R Levin, Jonathan M Chen, Kurt A Dasse and
Timothy R Graham

Introduction

Cardiac transplantation is an effective treatment for patients with end-stage heart disease. However, a lack of donor organs currently limits the number of transplants performed to approximately 5% of potential recipients in need.[1] Since they were first introduced by Cooley in 1969, temporary mechanical circulatory support devices have become critically useful tools in the therapeutic armamentarium available to patients awaiting transplantation.[2] Investigations with these devices have demonstrated encouraging results for the support of patients following cardiotomy, infarction and the development of end-stage cardiomyopathy.[3,4]

To ensure the future success of left ventricular assist devices (LVADs) in the community, it will ultimately be necessary to prove that these devices are safe, clinically useful and economically efficacious to society. In short, the devices must be demonstrated to exhibit minimal adverse effects such as right heart failure, haemolysis, bleeding, vital organ dysfunction, infection and thromboembolic complications. In addition, the devices must be shown to improve the health status, quality of life and overall survival of patients to a degree sufficient to justify the undertaking of these procedures, and their cost.

In this chapter we present a review of the available data on the effects of left ventricular mechanical assistance on end-organ function.

Without question, the frequency and severity of adverse effects caused by the use of these devices is dependent on numerous factors, including: (1) device design, (2) the team involved with the implantation and clinical management of device recipients, and (3) the overall health status of the recipient prior to, during and following implantation. Therefore, it is possible that the data presented may differ from the results ultimately obtained once these devices are out of the research stage.

Haemodynamics and exercise

In a recent study, eight of nine patients who preoperatively were New York Heart Association (NYHA) Class IV improved to Class I following mechanical circulatory support.[5] Resting cardiac output increased from 3.37 l/min preoperatively to 5.68 l/min at 2 months, a benefit that was documented to last as long as 10 months. Similarly, systolic blood pressure increased in these patients from 85 to 140 mmHg. Four of the patients underwent further exercise testing and achieved both a mean maximum oxygen consumption of approximately 15 ml/kg/min as well as a parallel increase in cardiac output with exercise. Such improvement in exercise capacity is comparable to that found by other investigators in studies evaluating patients with mechanical circulatory assistance.[6,7] However, there currently

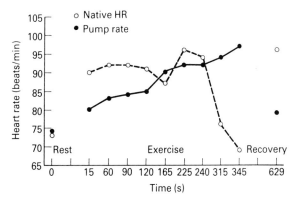

Fig. 18.1 Heart rate changes during exercise taken three weeks after device implantation.

are no conclusive data to determine if LVAD implantation improves exercise tolerance over time, and relatedly, no previous study has identified factors responsible for limited exercise tolerance in selected patients. In order for permanent LVAD implantation to be a practical therapeutic alternative, we must discover how to improve exercise capacity in recipients so that they may perform tasks that require moderate to vigorous of exercise.

Fig. 18.1 shows a typical response of native heart rate and LVAD rate in the 'pump-on-full' mode in a patient undergoing upright bike exercise 3 weeks after LVAD implantation. While the native heart rate increases monotonically (as expected during exercise), the LVAD rate falls abruptly at the end of exercise to maintain filling of the LVAD due to the decrease in venous return associated with the end of exercise. These changes in native heart and LVAD rates illustrate the proper functioning of the LVAD in the 'pump-on-full' mode and suggest that patients with LVADs can mount a normal autonomic response to exercise.

Right heart failure

Because the LVAD assists—but does not replace—the patient's own heart, the right side of the heart in the LVAD recipients is still responsible for moving enough blood through the lungs to provide adequate filling of the LVAD. The syndrome of right heart failure is seen in 20–40% of patients who have undergone LVAD placement.[8] In a

review of all implants performed at 12 centres, 49 of 213 (23%) LVAD patients either died or required the placement of an RV mechanical assist device for right heart failure.[9] Furthermore, other patients developed mild to moderate right heart failure requiring treatment with inotropic support and/or volume loading. This incidence of right heart failure suggests a poor understanding of the factors associated with proper patient selection.

Many factors have been suggested as the aetiology of right heart failure, including altered ventricular interdependence, increased pulmonary vascular resistance and changes in RV loading.[10–13] Fig. 18.2 is a diagram of the circulation showing the relationship of these factors during LVAD support. Performed mostly in animals, studies generally have provided conflicting results because they were performed either in animals with normal hearts, or in animals in which acute heart failure had been induced. This explains the opposing results from these studies, and their potentially limited applicability to the clinical arena may relate not only to interspecies differences, but also to differences in physiology between the normal, acute CHF and chronic CHF states. A better understanding of this complex situation will be required before we can develop proper selection criteria for LVAD candidates.

Haematology

Haemolysis

During the early phase of LVAD development, concern was expressed regarding the potential risk of haemolysis due to the presence of artificial valves, moving surfaces and high flow rates. However, in a recent study, haemoglobin and haematocrit levels were shown to be within the normal ranges following device insertion. The average plasma free haemoglobin level for these patients was 8 mg/dl which, while demonstrating slight haemolysis, was not considered to be clinically significant in the light of normal values for average haematocrit (34%) and platelet counts (249 000/ml).[14]

Bleeding

In the same trial,[14] bleeding occurred in all of the recipients, but non experienced device-related bleeding severe enough to require return to the

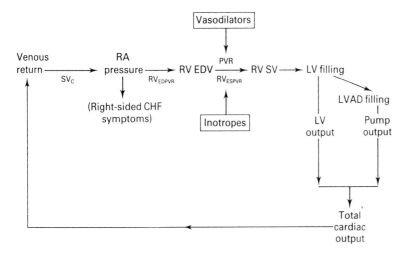

Fig. 18.2 The relationships of various factors during LVAD support. EDV = end-diastolic volume; SV = systolic volume; PVR = pulmonary vascular resistance; ESPVR = end-systolic PVR; EDPVR = end-diastolic PVR; SV_C = system venous compliance.

operating room. Thirty-nine per cent of the device recipients exhibited patient-related bleeding, of whom 64% later underwent transplantation, 71% of whom were long-term survivors. Of those patients who died, 50% required simultaneous support with a Biomedicus (Eden Prairie, MN) right ventricular assist device. No correlation was found between bleeding and overall outcome (as represented by successful transplantation and overall survival rates).

End-organ function

Hepatic dysfunction

Although hepatic dysfunction is commonly documented during the first month following device implantation, parameters of hepatic assessment usually return to normal within 2 months. In a recent study, average values of hepatic parameters prior to transplantation (total bilirubin = 0.7 mg/dl, SGOT = 35 U/L) were demonstrated to be significantly reduced when compared with average preoperative values (total bilirubin = 2.3 mg/dl, SGOT = 73 U/L).[15]

A second analysis was undertaken to evaluate the effect of hepatic dysfunction on the overall survival of device recipients. Values of total bilirubin both prior to device implantation as well as prior to transplantation (or at the time of death) were compared for survivors and non-survivors following device implantation. Interestingly, whereas total bilirubin values were significantly reduced after LVAD support in the case of survivors of LVAD implantation, these values either failed to decrease or actually increased in the case of non-survivors. For those patients ultimately receiving a heart transplant, hepatic function was not demonstrated to be significantly improved following transplantation when compared with function during previous mechanical circulatory assistance.[14]

In summary, although hepatic failure *per se* prior to implantation may be regarded as a potential contraindication to implantation, it demonstrates an excellent response following assistance with these devices. These data further support the notion that mechanical circulatory assistance may actually have led to improvement in hepatic function in the majority of patients who survived device implantation, and or whom the hepatic dysfunction was reversible. For those patients who did not survive implantation, it is reasonable to suggest that the total duration of circulatory support may have been insufficient to yield the presumptive benefit of improved hepatic perfusion.

Renal dysfunction

Renal failure has been associated with mortality rates of 70–100% in patients undergoing cardiac surgery,[16-18] and investigations with pneumatic ventricular assist devices have described the occurrence of renal failure to be highly predictive of mortality.[19] However, other investigators have shown that renal function actually may improve following prolonged mechanical circulatory assistance. In particular, comparisons of creatinine values prior to device insertion and prior to transplantation have revealed that creatinine significantly decreases during LVAD support.[14] A related study of renal function in recipients of assist devices revealed renal parameters to be significantly reduced from baseline (creatinine = 1.7 mg/dl, BUN = 37 mg/dl) at the time just prior to transplantation (creatinine = 1.2 mg/dl, BUN = 19 mg/dl).[15] These data indicate that mechanical circulatory assistance and subsequent improved renal perfusion may benefit renal function prior to transplantation. Following subsequent transplantation, creatinine values have been demonstrated to increase, a finding most likely due to the employment of nephrotoxic immunosuppressive therapy.

Pulmonary dysfunction

Improvement in pulmonary function during left ventricular assistance has been described in patients supported for more than 30 days.[20] For these patients, both the mean cardiac index and the pulmonary capillary wedge pressure were demonstrated to return to normal shortly following LVAD insertion in all patients studied. In addition, although mean pulmonary arterial pressure and pulmonary vascular resistance were demonstrated to decrease over time, neither parameter ultimately returned to normal. A related study described recovery of pulmonary function following device insertion on the basis of reductions in pulmonary capillary wedge pressure and clearing of pleural fluid during the initial days of left ventricular support.[21]

In general, recovery of pulmonary function may be expected to improve over the long-term in device recipients.

Gastrointestinal dysfunction

Upper GI bleeding following device implantation has been reported, but may in fact represent the stress response following a major operative procedure. It is possible that the LVAD exerts a degree of external irritation to the GI tract, but this appears to be an unlikely factor contributing to upper GI bleeding. Abdominal wound dehiscence and herniation of the small bowel though the drive line tunnel have also been noted. Both complications were successfully treated with operative intervention. Bowel adhesions to the drive lines have been noted to occur, and are most likely the result of contact between the bowel and textured drive line materials. However, these adhesions have not caused significant complications; rather, they have served to re-emphasize the need to reduce interactions between the bowel and drive lines.

Device recipients have also been noted to have a decreased appetite, a finding likely due to either external compression of the stomach by the device, or more generalized factors. Because of this potential complication, aggressive nutrition support should be considered early in the postoperative course.

Infection

The incidence of device-related infection has been reported to range from 20% to 75%. However, it is not entirely clear that these reported infections are all indeed device-related, owing to a lack of uniformity in the definition of infection. If infection is more strictly defined as a positive culture in association with an elevated white blood cell count, fever and the need for antimicrobial treatment, the incidence of infections documented is markedly lower.[14] In addition, infections may be considered device-related if the specific organism cultured was not detected prior to device implantation.

Several factors may contribute to a high rate of infection in patients with artificial implantable devices, including long and morbid pre-implant hospitalization, multiple sternotomies, chronic debilitation from heart failure and other factors.[22,23] In addition, contamination may result at the time of surgery from indwelling devices such as vascular cannulae, endotracheal tubes, intraaortic balloon pumps and urinary catheters. Infections may also occur at the site of skin insertion, but it remains unclear whether these infections are able to ascend via the drive line tunnel and infect the LVAD pocket, resulting in the haematologic spread of infection.

Other sources of potential infection specific to patients with implantable assist devices include potential spaces created around the device, adherence of certain bacteria to the internal device surfaces, sequestration of organisms from usual immunologic defences (e.g. in the pericardial space), empyemas resulting from aspiration or effusions, and chest drains into pericardial spaces.[22,23] It may also be postulated from previous studies that thrombi formed in the devices and device connections may themselves become colonized by bacteria and represent a further source of infection.[24]

In a study by Frazier and associates, 85% of the patients who had device-related infections went on to successful transplantation, and no infection precluded a transplantation.[14] Unlike the experience of documented mediastinal infections in patients receiving a total artificial heart as a bridge to transplant, few patients with left ventricular assist support have experienced mediastinitis.[22,25,26] A graft infection has been documented in the outflow conduit of a device in a bridge-to-transplant patient who ultimately was successfully treated. There appears, however, to be no difference in either the rate of transplants completed, or the rate of survival of patients with or without device-related infections.[14] Thus, while the rate of infectious complications in device recipients may be increased over standard cardiac surgery, the mortality from these complications is relatively low.

Thromboembolic complications

Although thromboembolic complications have historically represented a significant source of morbidity in recipients of implantable mechanical assist devices, only 3% of the patients in one study using the TCI HeartMate 1000 IP LVAD had a thromboembolic event.[14,27–30] Thrombosis within devices may be related to a number of factors, including the device flow pattern (turbulence, shear stress, areas of flow stasis), the device surface linings (texture and surface chemistry), and the inherent thrombogenicity of the blood.[23,26] As thrombi may themselves contribute to infection in the assisted host, so too may infections contribute to thromboembolism due to bacterial stimulation and activation of procoagulant pathways.[30] The asynchronous relationship of native heart to LVAD ejection may also have implications on the blood flow pattern through both the native heart and the device.

It should be noted that, although the rate of thromboembolic events in some LVADs (such as the TCI HeartMate) may be low, the native heart may still represent substantial sources of thromboembolism from artificial valves in the native heart, clots within the native ventricle, or pre-existing valvular disease. Indeed, thrombus within a heart with poor contractile function or in atrial fibrillation has been well documented as a source of embolic complications.[31] Thus, given the cohort of patients undergoing device implantation, thromboembolic complications still must be expected despite optimal device design.

Neurohumoral effects after device insertion

Implantation of ventricular assist devices has been shown to be associated with decreased plasma aldosterone activity, decreased plasma renin activity and decreased levels of atrial naturetic peptide.[5] During heart failure, all of these effectors are raised; indeed these changes during mechanical circulatory assistance may simply be indicative of the response due to an improvement in blood flow. The pathophysiological consequences of heart failure are complex, and such neurohumoral changes warrant further investigation as they may themselves have independent effects on renal, hepatic and gastrointestinal perfusion.

Conclusions

There is a growing body of knowledge regarding the benefits of LVAD support in patients with end-stage heart failure. While complications such as right heart failure, haemolysis, bleeding, infection and thromboembolism may occur, in most patients LVADs improve vital organ function and allow for successful bridging to transplantation.[14,15,32,33] Further controlled clinical studies must be undertaken to assess whether the LVAD improves both quality of life and mortality to a sufficient degree to justify the use of a permanent LVAD as an alternative to heart transplantation. Only in this way can the dream of freedom from the crippling effects of heart failure become a reality for the 80–90% of potential recipients who might otherwise die while awaiting transplantation.

References

1. United Network for Organ Sharing (UNOS). *UNOS Update* 1991; **7** (May), 2.
2. Cooley DA, Liotta D, Hallman GL, Bloodwell RD,

Leachman RD, Milam JP. Orthotopic cardiac prosthesis for two-staged cardiac replacement. *Am J Cardiol* 1969; **24**, 723–730.

3. McGee MG, Parnis SM, Nakatani T, *et al.* Extended clinical support with an implantable left ventricular assist device. *ASAIO Trans* 1989; **35**, 614–616.

4. Portner PM, Oyer PE, Pennington DG, Baumgartner WA, Griffith BP, Frist WR, Magilligan DJ, Noon GP, Ramasamy N, Miller PJ, Jassawalla JS. Implantable electrical left ventricular assist system: bridge to transplantation and the future. *Ann Thorac Surg* 1989; **47**, 142–150.

5. Levin HR, Oz MC, Burkhoff D, Catanese K, Krum H, Goldsmith RL, Packer M, Rose EA. Can left ventricular assist devices be used as outpatient therapy while awaiting transplant? Assessment of changes in long-term hemodynamics and functional capacity. *Ann Thorac Surg* 1994; **58**, 1515–1520.

6. Murali S, Uretsky BF, Quintero TE, *et al.* Metabolic and ventilatory responses to exercise in heart failure patients on left ventricular assist support. *Circulation* 1991; **84**, II-354.

7. Quintero TE, Uretsky BF, Murali S, *et al.* Amelioration of the heart failure state with left ventricular assist system support. *JACC* 1992; **19**, 254A.

8. Pae WE, Rosenberg G, Donachy JH, *et al.* Mechanical circulatory assistance for postoperative cardiogenic shock: a three-year experience. *ASAIO Trans* 1980; **26**, 256–260.

9. Farrar DJ, Compton PG, Herson JJ, *et al.* Right heart interaction with the mechanically assisted left heart. *World J Surg* 1985; **9** 89–102.

10. Elberry JR, Owen CH, Savitt MA, *et al.* Effects of the left ventricular device on right ventricular function. *J Thorac Cardiovasc Surg* 1990; **99**, 809–816.

11. Fischer EIC, Willshaw P, Armentano RL, *et al.* Experimental acute right ventricular failure and right ventricular assist in the dog. *J Thorac Cardiovasc Surg* 1985; **90**, 580–585.

12. Kormos RL, Borovetz HS, Pristas JM, *et al.* LVAS pump performance following initiation of left ventricular assistance. *ASAIO Trans* 1990; **36**, M703–705.

13. Farrar DJ, Chow E, Compton P, *et al.* Effect of acute right ventricular ischemia on ventricular interaction during prosthetic left ventricular support. *J Thorac Cardiovasc Surg* 1991; **102**, 588–595.

14. Frazier OH, Rose EA, Macmanus Q, Burton NA, Lefrak EA, Poirier V, Dasse KA. Multicentre clinical evaluation of HeartMate 1000 IP left ventricular assist device. *Ann Thorac Surg* 1992; **53**, 1080–1090.

15. Dasse KA, Frazier OH, Lesniak JM, Myers T, Burnett CM, Poirier VL. Clinical responses to ventricular assistance versus transplantation in a series of bridge-to-transplant patients. *ASAIO Trans* 1992; **38**, M622–626.

16. Yeboah ED, Petrie A, Pead JL. Acute renal failure and open heart surgery. *Br J Med* 1972; **1**, 415–418.

17. Bhat JG, Gluck MC, Lowenstein J, Baldwin DS. Renal failure after open heart surgery. *Ann Intern Med* 1976; **84**, 677–682.

18. Abel RM, Buckley MJ, Austen WG, Barnett GO, Beck CH, Fischer JE. Etiology, incidence and prognosis of renal failure following cardiac operations. *J Thorac Cardiovasc Surg* 1976; **71**, 323–333.

19. Kanter KR, Swartz MT, Pennington DG, Ruzevich SA, Madden M, McBride LR, Termuhlen DF. Renal failure in patients with ventricular assist devices. *ASAIO Trans* 1987; **33**, 426–428.

20. Baldwin RT, Duncan JM, Radovancevic B, Frazier OH, Abou-Awdi NL. Recovery of pulmonary function in patients undergoing extended left ventricular assistance. *Chest* 1992; **102**, 45–49.

21. Loisance DY. Mechanical circulatory support in the 1990s. *Eur J Cardiothorac Surg* 1992; **6** (suppl 1), S107–112.

22. Griffith BA, Kormos RL, Hardesty, Armitage JM, Dummer JS. The artificial heart: infection-related morbidity and its effect on transplantation. *Ann Thorac Surg* 1988; **45**, 409–414.

23. Didisheim P, Olsen DB, Farrar DJ, Portner PM, Griffith BP, Pennington DG, Joist JH, Schoen FJ, Gristina AG, Anderson JM. Infections and thromboembolism with implantable cardiovascular devices. *ASAIO Trans* 1989; **35**, 54–70.

24. Ward RA, Wellhausen SR, Dobbins JJ, Johnson GS, DeVries WC. Thromboembolic and infectious complications of total artificial heart implantation. *Ann NY Acad Sci* 1988; **516**, 638–650.

25. Rice LB, Karchmer AW. Artificial heart implantation: what limitations are imposed by infectious complications? *JAMA* 1988; **259**, 894–895.

26. Rooks JR, Burton NA, Lefrak EA, Macmanus Q. Mediastinitis complicating successful mechanical bridge to heart transplantation. *J Heart Lung Transplant* 1992; **11**, 261–264.

27. Levinson MM, Smith RG, Cork RC, *et al.* Thromboembolic complications of the Jarvik-7 total artificial heart: case report. *Artif Organs* 1986; **10**, 236–244.

28. DeVries WC, Anderson JL, Joyce LD, *et al.* Clinical use of the total artificial heart. *New Engl J Med* 1984; **310**, 273–278.

29. Termuhlen DF, Swartz MT, Pennington DG, *et al.* Thromboembolic complications with the Pierce–Donachy ventricular assist device. *ASAIO Trans* 1989; **35**, 616–618.

30. Icenogle TB, Smith RG, Cleavinger M, Vasu MA, Williams RJ, Sethi GK, Copeland JG. Thromboembolic complications of the symbion AVAD system. *Artif Organs* 1989; **13**, 532–538.

31. Maze SS, Kotler MJ, Parry WR. Flow characteristics in the dilated left ventricle with thrombus: qualitative and quantitative Doppler analysis. *JACC* 1989; **13**, 873–881.

32. Friedel N, Viazis P, Schissler A, Warnecke H, Hennig E, Trittin A, Böttner W, Hetzer R. Recovery of end-organ failure during mechanical circulatory support. *Eur J Cardiothorac Surg* 1992; **6**, 519–523.

33. Pantalos GM, Marks JD, Riebman JB, Everett SD, Burns GL, Burton NA, DePaulis R. Left ventricular oxygen consumption and organ blood flow distribution during pulsatile ventricular assist. *ASAIO Trans* 1988; **34**, 356–360.

19

Development and current status of the CardioWest C-70 ® (Jarvik-7) total artificial heart

Jack G Copeland, Richard G Smith and Marilyn R Cleavinger

Introduction

Since December 1982, when the first permanent total artificial heart (TAH) was implanted by a team led by DeVries,[1] approaching 200 Jarvik-7 total artificial hearts have been implanted in patients for durations that total nearly 13 years (Table 19.1).[2] Over 680 million beats have resulted in only one death from mechanical dysfunction. In the bridge-to-transplant experience, 57% of those transplanted lived at least one year, with major causes of death being sepsis (38%), multiple organ failure (25%), and post-transplant

Table 19.1 Experience of bridging to transplantation with the Jarvik-7.

Centres	Number of implants
Hospital La Pitié	63
University of Pittsburgh	20
Loyola University	19
Ottawa Heart Institute	12
University of Arizona	9
Minneapolis Heart Institute	9
Midwest Heart Institute	8
Milwaukee Mercy Medical Center	7
Others	
Two centres	4
Three centres	3
Ten centres	2
Five centres	1
DeVries (permanent TAH implants)	5

rejection (12%). Only nine strokes occurred in the bridging experience.[3] Individual institutional experiences have ranged from as little as one patient implanted for two days, to 63 patients implanted for over 1800 patient-days, with eight institutions having implanted seven or more devices, five having implanted three or four, and the remaining 15 two or less. Devices have been implanted for periods ranging from a few hours up to 620 days.[4] As one might expect, these experiences have been diverse. Selection of patients, surgical techniques, anticoagulation, antibiotic therapy, philosophies regarding the control of the device, management of complications, and timing of transplantation in the bridge-to-transplant setting have varied. Observations of the diversity of clinical experiences have been extremely variable and led to divergent opinions.

In the early 1980s, the world was exhaustively informed of the progress of the permanent artificial heart recipients' daily complications. The progression of strokes in William Schroeder, five in all, was interspersed with small human victories, a hero riding in the home town parade, going fishing with one good arm, and the asymmetric smile of a brave man. One cannot help feeling that a negative public opinion spread to the medical profession, among others. On the other hand, the investigators interpreted this initial experience as 'dramatically successful'.[4]

Diverse opinions have been evidence in the reports from nearly all investigators. In the long-term TAH experience, it was felt that the 'major limiting factor' was spread of infection from the drive lines to the mediastinal periprosthetic space.[5] In two patients, it was felt that biomaterials were susceptible to infection because they were 'not well integrated' with the host tissue on ultrastructural studies.[6] On the basis of this pioneering experience, further permanent implants were condemned as only serving to 'document further the magnitude of the complications, rather than to demonstrate an acceptable lifestyle of the recipient'. The idea that alterations in patient management could solve some of the problems was felt to be 'unlikely'.[7]

Mediastinitis in the bridge-to-transplant setting was felt by one group to be 'the current limiting factor' and to have a strikingly high incidence, but not to be related to ascending infection from the drive lines.[8] Another group with a similar number of implants did not experience mediastinitis in any patient, but were concerned with postimplant bleeding that was seen in more than 50% of their patients.[9] The La Pitié group, with an experience of over 60 implants, reported that significant factors in determining the outcome of TAH bridging were the size and age of the patient.[10,11] This agrees with our observation that the 'major problem' was fitting the device in the patient without causing systemic or pulmonary venous compression.[12] In spite of different views on what constituted the 'major problem' with the TAH, there was inter-observer agreement regarding the major complications: haemorrhage, thromboembolism, infection, and end-organ failure (often multiple organ failure). As time passed, a growing awareness of the importance of patient selection for implantation and for transplantation has been voiced.[8,9,12–17]

At present, thinking about the device is based upon careful observation and intuitive reasoning stemming from small series of patients in many institutions. Because of the diversity of baseline characteristics of the observed populations, as well as differences in techniques and management, these experiences and interpretations may not be comparable, even though they are valid. Experiences with this device extend from 1982 to the present, a time during which much has been learned. Looking back, we may not be so comfortable with the posture of pushing on to the fully implantable electrical devices of 'better design' before we have profited fully from what can be learned from this device, and our attempts to make it compatible with complex and incompletely understood biological systems of its host. It seems worthwhile to examine current results with this in mind.

The Jarvik-7, a product of nearly 30 years of development, is in jeopardy of being lost. Its use was banned in the USA in January 1990 by the Food and Drug Administration (FDA). Symbion Inc., producer of the device, discontinued production and dissolved, offering the production facility and patent rights to the University of Arizona Medical Center (UMC). UMC and Med Forte, a technology company associated with the University of Utah, now control manufacturing and distribution of the device under the name of CardioWest Technologies Inc., and have renamed the device the CardioWest C-70 (with the idea of producing only the 70 cm^3 ventricles). The reasons given for the FDA ban related primarily to manufacturing practices that failed to meet FDA standards. We believe that inadequate communication, primarily in the form of reporting the progress of investigations to the FDA, may have been an additional reason.

We believed that the preliminary investigations of the TAH were positive, and that tentatively the Jarvik-7 could be considered as beneficial in prolonging life in a select group of patients who decompensate while awaiting cardiac transplantation. We have, therefore, reapplied for and recently been granted an Investigational Device Exemption (IDE). A strictly controlled study will be undertaken with the hope of carefully defining the risks, benefits and recommended use of this technology.

Review of the development of the TAH

The first TAH was implanted in an animal laboratory in 1957 in dogs that survived about $1\frac{1}{2}$ hours.[18] Subsequently, pneumatically powered devices were developed at many centres.[19] Success was initially defined by length of animal survival. In the mid-1960s, calves were kept alive for a little longer than a day with sack-type hearts.[20] The first appropriation for targeted contracts by the National Heart Lung and Blood Institute (NHLB) was in 1964, and through fiscal year 1989 a total of $264.4 million had been spent (Fig. 19.1).[21] A diaphragm pumping mechanism[22] was introduced into the progression of heart models that reduced problems of breakage and haemolysis in

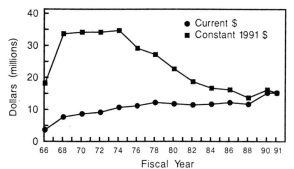

Fig. 19.1 Total expenditures of the US National Heart, Lung and Blood Institute for artificial heart development.[20]

the late 1960s, leading to 2-week survivals of calf implants by 1972. This was followed shortly by the design of a Jarvik-3 heart with a triple-layered diaphragm made of Biomer (Ethicon Inc., Somerville, NJ) and resulting survivals of up to 4 months. Another design iteration that followed was the Jarvik-7, specifically designed 'to fit the human anatomy'.[19]

Finally, the limits of the usefulness of the calf model were reached. Survivals exceeding 200 days were obtained in six centres worldwide.[18] Calves were not only outgrowing the devices by more than doubling their weight in 7 months, but were also failing to be a model sensitive enough with respect to neurological damage.[4] A huge experience with this model had accumulated and such things as the control, durability, thrombogenicity and infection had been addressed. The cardiac

output monitor and diagnostic unit (COMDU) was invented and perfected in monitoring the function of the Jarvik-7, based on measurements of the air outflow from the device.[23] Integration of the curve generated by plotting airflow measured by pneumotach with respect to time yielded the volume of air displaced by blood during diastole (Fig. 19.2). When averaged over a number of cycles, this is equal to the cardiac output. The COMDU unit plots airflow curves, integrates the curve, provides a calculated cardiac output every third beat, plots pressure waveforms, and plots a cardiac output trend, which includes the previous two hours. Using this information, it was shown in animals by Olsen and associates that actual failures of devices which included 13 valve failures and 11 diaphragm breaks could be diagnosed quickly enough to take corrective actions.[24]

An appreciation of the problem of thrombus formation within the TAH was documented by several investigators.[25] Much *in vitro* durability testing led to critical choices of appropriate valves and other components of the Jarvik-7.[26] Bjork–Shiley, Hall–Kaster and Medtronic–Hall valves were tested, with the latter found to be the most reliable. Diaphragms with four layers of Biomer separated by a tiny amount of graphite for lubrication and their attachments were perfected. The current form of this device, the CardioWest C-70, consists of two 70 cm³ ventricles that differ only in the spacing between the inflow and outflow valves (right ventricle valves are separated more to allow

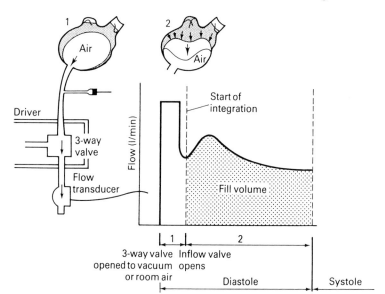

Fig. 19.2 Flow of air out of the pump is measured. The volume of air is obtained by integrating the area under the flow curve which is equal to the stroke volume (SV) under the condition of full ejection. This volume multiplied by heart rate equals pump output.[23]

a pathway for aortic outflow) (Fig. 19.3). The ventricle is controlled by a driver that provides air pressure pulses. Controls on the driver include left and right ventricular drive pressures, heart rate, and timing adjustment that allows for determination of the percentage of time the heart will be emptying (systole) or filling (diastole). The drive pressures are set just high enough to completely empty the ventricle with each beat as detected by a sharp peak on the end of the plateau of the pressure curve (left pressure usually about 160 mmHg with a dP/dT of less than 4500 mmHg per second; right ventricle usually about 60 mmHg with a dP/dT of less than 2000) (Fig. 19.4). Advantages of the pneumatic system, based on controlling the device so that it never completely fills, are that it automatically adjusts for the difference in volume pumped between the two ventricles (left pumps more because of bronchial collateral flow) and that, as venous pressure increases, the device pumps more blood up to the limit of its filling volume of 70 cm^3 (Starling mechanism). Thus, animal and *in vitro* work was considerable and had extended over a period of nearly 30 years when the first Jarvik-7 was implanted.

The first clinical use

Attempts to use a TAH as temporary support, or as a bridge to transplantation, had been made twice before December 1982,[27] when the Jarvik-7 was first placed in a human. At that moment, nothing was known about the human response to the device. Five permanent implants were attempted, four by DeVries and one by Semb (Table 19.2). What did we learn?

Observations of the initial experience sum up some of the most important points.[28,1] The device kept the patient alive for 112 days. He was not an excellent candidate for any surgical procedures,

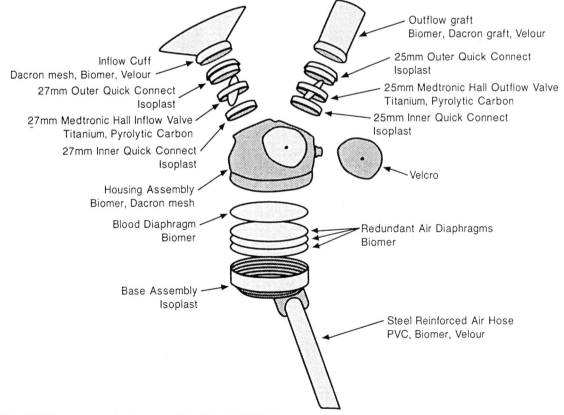

Fig. 19.3 Drawing showing the parts of the CardioWest C-70 pump.

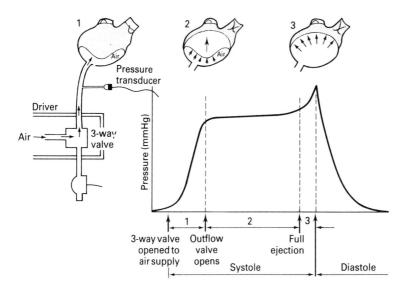

Fig. 19.4 Air pressure waveform during systole showing the typical morphology of a 'full eject' pattern. The sharp peak at the end of systole represents a slight rise in pressure occurring after maximal diaphragm excursion.

having been treated chronically with steroids for myocarditis. He was excessively anticoagulated, and consequently bled badly from his nose. He had no thromboembolic event, but he did have seizures, renal failure, and several infections, including a fatal episode of necrotizing enterocolitis. At autopsy, the observation was made that the fit of the device was tight.

All of DeVries' patients had renal failure during the first two postoperative weeks. Three of four had severe postoperative haemorrhage requiring reoperation. Two of four had thromboembolic strokes. All three survivors of more than 10 days had infections after 30 days. Notably, positive blood cultures seemed to be related temporally with thromboembolic events (Fig. 19.5).

Infections in this group were felt to be related to spread from the transcutaneous drive lines to the periprosthetic space[5] in one report. A second report on the two longest survivors revealed periprosthetic infections, but freedom from infection in the mid portion of the drive lines, and infection of the cutaneous portions. Thus there did

not appear to be a continuous spread from outside to inside via the drive lines,[29] suggesting another route of spread. Pseudomonas, Staphylococcus and Candida were the infecting species in both chronic patients. Both also had endoprosthetic infections.

In this setting—with renal failure, malnutrition, chronic infection, and chronic therapy with potent antibiotics—one wonders whether any meaningful observations of the immune systems could be made. Perhaps of significance are the observations of chronic lymphopenia[30] with depletion of both T helper and inducer cells. The lymphoid tissue in these patients revealed reduced numbers of germinal centres and a reticuloendothelial system engorged with degenerate erythrocytes, leading to the suggestion that this engorgement was the mechanism of the immunosuppression.[31] There is no doubt that these patients suffered from chronic haemolysis and were multiply transfused.

Two modifications of the Jarvik that stemmed directly from these initial experiences include

Table 19.2 The permanent implant experience with the Jarvik-7.

Patient	Age (years)	Duration (days)	Cause of death
1	61	112	Sepsis
2	54	620	Sepsis, endoprosthetic infection (SBE)
3	58	488	Sepsis, endoprosthetic infection (SBE)
4	53	228	Sepsis
5	62	10	Haemorrhage

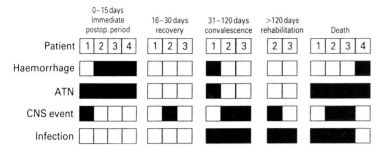

Fig. 19.5 The timing of complications with the Jarvik-7 in DeVries' series.

changing from Bjork–Shiley to Medtronic–Hall valves, and decreasing the dP/dT of air delivered from the driver-controller to the device from 6000–8000 to 4500 mmHg per second. The value change was made in response to a mitral valve strut fracture that occurred in the first patient on day 13, requiring reoperation and left ventricle replacement.[4] Testing in animals supported this change.[32] Thus, the permanent implant experience in many respects prepared us for bridging to transplantation.

One other investigation, before the beginning of bridging to transplantation, studied Jarvik-7 hearts implanted in brain-dead human subjects ranging in weight from 42 to 73 kg.[33] The investigators were able to implant the 100 cm³ ventricles in small patients using the standard technique[34] and also what they called the right and left heterotopic techniques. The right technique involved placement of the right ventricle in the right chest by attaching the right atrial quick-connect to the free wall of the right atrium. The left technique consisted of removing the left pericardium to near the level of the phrenic nerve and prolapsing the left ventricle into the left chest. The latter has been reported by several teams, including our own. I am not aware of clinical use of the right heterotopic technique thus far.

Statistics of bridging to transplantation

The bridge-to-transplant experience with the Jarvik-7 began on 26 August 1985 at the University of Arizona.[35] We were fortunate to have a patient of good size (height 185 cm, weight 84 kg, body surface area (BSA) 2.04 m²) who did not bleed (required one transfusion), had excellent renal function, had no significant haemolysis (free haemoglobin 4.7 mg/dl), no pre-transplant infection, and a reversible stroke characterized by expressive aphasia that persisted for 3 weeks.[10] After transplantation, he survived for 4.5 years before dying from lymphoma. The experience since then has been summarized in several registries,[3,36] as well as in reports of several series.[3,8–16,37–41] There are reported 175 Jarvik-7 hearts, 141 with 70 cm³ ventricles and 34 with 100 cm³ ventricles, implanted in 171 patients. Four patients received two hearts. There were 152 males and 19 females with a mean age of 42 years and weight of 74 kg. After the initial three implants in 1985, activity rose to a peak with 58 implants in 1988, falling to 20 in 1989 and 14 in 1990. Eighty-one per cent of the implants were done before 1989, a time that must be considered early on the device's learning curve. As can be seen in Fig. 19.6, the reported experiences of several of the centres cover different periods.

As one might expect, the registry results are a reflection of the entire experience from 1985 until 1990, while results from individual centres reflect not only the philosophy and technique of the centre, but also the time of the experience. As seen in Table 19.3, our experience at Arizona University and that at Pittsburgh University were characterized by transplanting a high percentage of those who were implanted (20/23), with results that yielded jointly a hospital discharge of 55% for those who received a transplant. We, in those days, felt a real pressure to 'get the patient off the device', even if this meant transplanting someone who might not have been an ideal candidate. Such a pressure may have been present in the La Pitié programme when they started, but it appears that for the majority they have not transplanted patients with implants unless they were good candidates (see Chapter 20). They, therefore, have only transplanted 39% of those with implants (11/28), but because of this have obtained an 82% post-transplant hospital discharge. Finally, the Loyola group has apparently been careful in selecting patients for bridging to

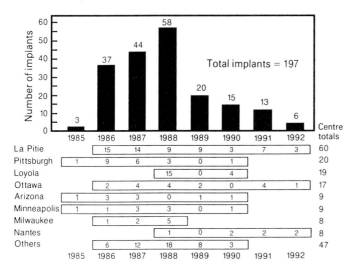

Fig. 19.6 Vertical bars show total number of implants by year. Horizontal bars show year-by-year experience of investigating centres.

transplantation from the beginning; thus they have obtained 89% transplantability of implanted patients (17/19) and then 88% survival to discharge and 76% one-year survival. Perhaps they have learned from other programmes, or perhaps their results are biased by the selection process. One must conclude, however, that their results with bridging to transplantation approximate international survival results with first-time transplants, and represent the best results to date. The combined results from La Pitié and Loyola, two programmes with the most recent experiences, give rise to hope that similar numbers (82–88% survival after transplant) could be generated in other institutions. The registry survival[3] after transplant of 70%, given our current better informed and more selective approach to bridging to transplantation, appears to be a standard that should be improved. As we review the results with Jarvik-7 bridging to transplantation, this

should be kept in mind. While it is tempting to compare the registry information with contemporary series using other devices, historically it would be appropriate only if one looked exclusively at the Loyola series, and then only with a matched series of candidates at the pre-implant interval.

Causes of death

Causes of death before and after transplantation from the Minneapolis registry[3] are shown in Fig. 19.7. Sepsis, multiple organ failure, and neurological death are the major causes, with the exception of 12% death from rejection post-transplant, for both groups. This coincides reasonably well with the experience at La Pitié, Loyola, Pittsburgh and Arizona with some notable exceptions (Table 19.4).

Table 19.3 Results of bridging to transplantation: comparison of the registry results with selected centres.

Source	Age (years)	Body surface area (m²)	Most common indication*	Number of patients	Number of transplants	Discharged	One-year survivors
Registry[3]	45 ± 12		Deterioration (36%) Cardiogenic shock (32%) Failure to wean (15%)	171	119(70%)	82	67
La Pitié[11]	39	1.8	Cardiogenic shock	28	11(39%)	9	8
Loyola[37]	46		Cardiogenic shock (58%) Failure to wean (42%)	19	17 (89%)	15	13
Pittsburgh[8]	47		Deterioration, chronic	16	14 (88%)	7	7
U. of Arizona[11]	31	1.8	Cardiogenic shock	7	6 (86%)	4	3

* Deterioration refers to haemodynamic deterioration of patients while on the waiting list for cardiac transplantation. Failure to wean refers to patients who could not be separated from CPB and, therefore, had a Jarvik-7 inserted.

First, haemorrhage was a major cause of death in three reported series. Fit problems in our programme[12] were found to be significant, causing two of the deaths. At La Pitié, in one study it was found that the only significant preoperative determinant of survival was the size of the patient; those who could be transplanted were larger.[10] In another report they cited age under 40 years as significant,[11] as does the registry[3] where a 15% greater mortality was seen in those over 40 years of age ($p < 0.04$). Also of interest was their finding that survival rates were significantly less in patients with implant times of less than 2 days, but not significantly different for other durations of implantation. Those transplanted at less than 2

days of Jarvik support had a 70% mortality at one month, compared with other groups which ranged from 2% to 45% for the same interval. Finally, mediastinitis, as a serious problem with the device,[8,39] was seen as a major factor only at Pittsburgh. In the Pittsburgh experience, those who developed mediastinitis had an average of 30 days pre-implant inotropic support compared with 12 days for mediastinitis-free patients; this is not statistically significant but is highly suggestive when one considers the increased risk of long-term intravenous and intra-arterial lines in these patients.[42]

Complications

Complications from Jarvik-7 bridging to transplantation, reported in the Minneapolis registry, included infection (37%), renal failure (20%), neurological abnormalities (9%), haemorrhage (26%), and device dysfunction (4%). Each of these merits some attention.

Infection

Clearly, some of the implanted patients had infections at the time of implantation (in the registry, 4% of patients). As other authors point out, heavily immunosuppressed patients, such as chronic transplant recipients,[41] do not make good bridging candidates. Nor are those who have been chronically decompensated (more than one

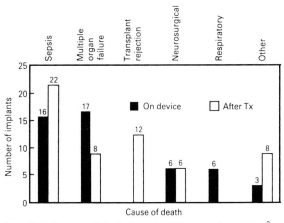

Fig. 19.7 Causes of death from the Minneapolis registry.[3]

Table 19.4 Causes of death in Jarvik-7 bridging to transplantation.

Source	Average number of days on device	Deaths	Causes of death on device	Deaths after transplant	Causes of death after transplant
La Pitié	15	17	Sepsis (8) Multiple organ failure (5)	3	Infection (2) Hepatitis (1)
Loyola	11	2	Neurologic (1) Haemorrhage (1)	4	Rejection (1) Neurologic (1) *Pneumocystis caranii* Pneumonia (1) Multiple organ failure (1)
Pittsburgh	9	2	Sepsis (1)	7	Mediastinitis (4) Infection (1) Sudden (1) Rejection (1)
U. of Arizona	53	3	Fit* (1) Fit*/haemorrhage (1) Graft failure (1)	0	None

* Failure of device to function optimally because of poor fit.

month) requiring inotropic support likely to benefit from Jarvik-7 bridging.[41] More stringent selection policies may help eliminate some of these problems, but it must be kept in mind that the patient with end-stage heart disease is, in many cases, a compromised host before he comes to the attention of the transplant/implant team. This group presents a great challenge to clinicians and basic scientists to improve current methods and technology. The stimulation of the coagulation system in the presence of infection and the complicity of infection and coagulation in the genesis of endoprosthetic infection is to be avoided.

From the clinician's point of view, a number of suggestions have been made and in some cases implemented. The Pittsburgh group has used gut sterilization. We, at the time of transplantation, have routinely used closed povidone-iodine (Betadine) irrigation for two days until intraoperative culture results are available. If negative, the irrigation is stopped. There has been at least one attempt to eliminate dead space around the Jarvik by mobilizing omentum; months later at transplant, an infection was found between the omentum and the device (DG Pennington, personal communication). Other simpler approaches that we have used have included avoidance of central and arterial lines except when absolutely necessary, and continued use of oral prophylactic antibiotics while the device is in place. We have used dicloxacillin (anti-staphylococcal) and trimethoprim-sulfa. We have tried to avoid the use of broad-spectrum intravenous antibiotics and nephrotoxins, using them only for short courses as necessary. Finally, it is obvious that the course of the patient in this process is extremely important. If every patient develops renal failure as was the case for DeVries, then they will all be fluid overloaded, immune compromised, chronically intubated, subject to pneumonia, and likely to develop a variety of infections. The art of 'getting in and getting out' is one that can never be overemphasized. Minimal bleeding and short runs on cardiopulmonary bypass minimize the need for blood transfusion and the chance of major haemolysis, as well as the chance for excessive clot formation in the pericardial space. Renal failure is commonly seen in longer cases, with massive bleeding and transfusions. Reoperation has been used successfully in this setting by the Loyola group to minimize the potential for clot becoming a culture medium[37] and to control haemorrhage.

As Didisheim *et al.*[43] have pointed out, there are also many problems that await a more basic solution in the form of improved materials, because biomaterial centred infections result from the ability of relatively primitive cells (bacteria and fungi) to colonize 'inert' materials. They suggest that if there were complete and successful integration of the foreign material (outer surface of the device) with the tissues of the host and the host tissues won the 'race to the surface' of the device, becoming integrated before bacterial colonization, a more satisfactory and permanent solution will have been reached.

Renal failure

Renal failure is currently a contraindication to cardiac transplantation, and from a review of the reported experiences should be a contraindication to bridging to transplantation with the Jarvik-7. The La Pitié experience shows us that patients with renal failure can be supported, but do not qualify as transplant candidates.[10] We have observed return of renal function in patients on Jarvik support, but have the impression that renal failure then subjects the patient to other risks and one is likely to find the number of complications rising exponentially. The obligatory time of device support is obviously increased by renal failure, making the likelihood of some interim complication increase. Essentially the same arguments can be made about hepatic failure.

Haemorrhage and thromboembolism

The most amazing part of the Minneapolis registry is the finding of only 16 neurologic events, being nine strokes (5.3%) and seven transient ischaemic attacks (4.1%). When one considers the number of patient-days of exposure to the Jarvik-7, our relatively crude management of anticoagulation, that most participating institutions were at the beginning of their own learning curves, and the time at which most of these implants were done (early in the experience with bridge-to-transplant), and especially in view of the strokes in the permanent implants, this statistic gives considerable optimism about the ultimate usefulness of such a device. It appears that bleeding has been a more significant problem. The salient facts are that bleeding, besides causing tamponade, leads to transfusion, which in turn leads to haemolysis of the more fragile stored red blood cells by the Jarvik device, which in turn can cause renal failure and perhaps immunosuppression (Fig. 19.8). Transfusion risks immunization by donor white cells and the formation of cytotoxic antibodies that may preclude transplantation. Thus, bleeding must be avoided.

On the other hand, the risks of thromboembolism are well known and are to be avoided. Attention is given in Chapter 36 to the equilibrium that must be attained to avoid these two major complications. In brief, it is suggested that the current diagnostic and therapeutic efforts are inadequate. It is not enough to simply follow one test and use one or two agents and expect to have control of the haemostatic system that is being continuously stimulated by the Jarvik-7. Aprotonin can be of great benefit at the end of CPB by controlling the plasminogen plasmin system. It is also extremely helpful during the subsequent course while the device is in place. Dipyridamole has been used, but in general the doses have been too small to result in the desired effect. Heparin is the most efficacious of anticoagulant drugs but is generally given in massive doses that predispose to bleeding. This and other information can be found in the experience of La Pitié[44] that is remarkable for having very few problems with bleeding and almost no evidence of thrombosis and no documented neurological thromboembolic events. Their favourable experiences strongly suggest that multi-institutional trials are not only indicated, but may lead to the conclusion that 'the device is not so bad'.

The device: fit and dysfunction

It was appreciated early in the experience with the Jarvik-7 that fit, or surgical positioning, was of great importance. Compression of left-sided pulmonary veins and/or the inferior vena cava may have catastrophic consequences.[12,45] Attempted closure of the chest that is too small results in obstruction. Obstruction of either venous systems, or both, drastically limits cardiac output from the device and is a fatal complication. Guidelines for the safe positioning of the device have never been strict. A cooperative study attempted to set some guidelines, but may have been too liberal,[46] concluding that the device could in its smaller form (70 cm^3 ventricles, now the only size produced) be used successfully in patients of 50 kg or greater. Our own experience suggests that patients in the 80 kg region with large hearts are the best candidates. The measurements suggested by the Jarvik[46] using CAT scan to define the distance from the sternum to the spine and one half the diameter from left to right at the level of the tenth thoracic vertebra may be helpful in considering whether the device will fit. It appears that a depth of 12–15 cm and a half-width of 12–15 cm are reasonable and that 'leftward positioning' is likely to be necessary if these are smaller.

Device malfunction, a problem that must be constantly suspected, has occurred several times, with one fatal right diaphragm rupture. All other occurrences were not fatal, and four of the total of seven consisted only of a momentarily stuck diaphragm. The potential for value dysfunction and

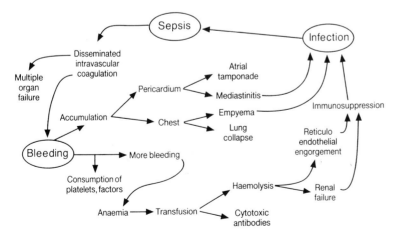

Fig. 19.8 The relationship of bleeding to other complications in Jarvik-7 implants.

diaphragm rupture are ever present but, thanks to the good work of the Utah group, extremely unlikely.

Conclusions

The Jarvik-7, now CardioWest C-70, is a product of years of careful research and development by one of the leading groups in the field. It is simple in design and function. It has been tested extensively in animals to a point of diminishing return of information. The entrance of this device into clinical use has been less than graceful. From our perspective, much was learned, but the image of this device suffered. The bridge-to-transplant experience with this device has done much to re-establish the worth of the technology. Contemporary experiences have been about as good as one could expect in such a critically ill group of patients. New approaches to the monitoring and treatment and treatment of the haemostatic system have, in one series, eliminated thromboembolic stroke, while at the same time caused minimal bleeding. The continuing threat of infection in what is already a compromised host has resulted in infection being the major complication. It has not, however, resulted in the pattern seen with the permanent implant patients, that of chronic endoprosthetic infections associated temporally with strokes; nor has infection taken the form of fatal mediastinitis.

Experience has shown that the device is most successfully used in patients under the age of 40 years who are of good size (at least 70–80 kg). The results seem to be best if use is limited to those patients who meet the selection criteria for heart transplantation not only before device implantation but also before subsequent transplantation. The optimal time for transplantation of implanted patients is after the first two days when the patient is completely stable. It also appears that waiting more than 30 days to proceed with transplantation may decrease the chance of success. This may be related to longer exposure to the potential complications of the device or to increasing technical difficulties encountered at reoperation.

An international study is envisaged to evaluate the risks and benefits of the CardioWest C-70 device. It is expected that such a study might result in the device being made more widely available for bridging to transplantation.

Acknowledgement

The work upon which this chapter is based was supported by the University Medical Center, the Marshall Foundation and the University Heart Center, Arizona.

References

1. DeVries WC, Anderson JH, Joyce LD, Anderson FL, Hammond EH, Jarvik RK, Kolff WJ. Clinical use of the total artificial heart. *New Engl J Med* 1984; **310**, 273–278.
2. CardioWest Investigational Device Exemption (G920101). Submitted to the Food and Drug Administration, September 1992.
3. Johnson KE, Prieto M, Joyce LD, Pritzker M, Emery RW. Summary of the clinical use of the Symbion total artificial heart: a registry report. *J Heart Lung Transplant* 1992; **11**, 103–116.
4. DeVries WC. The permanent artificial heart: four case reports. *JAMA* 1988; **259**, 849–859.
5. Kunin CM, Dobbins JJ, Melo JC, Levinson MM, Love K, Joyce LD, DeVries WC. Infectious complications in four long-term recipients of the Jarvik-7 artificial heart. *JAMA* 1988; **259**, 860–864.
6. Gristina AG, Dobbins JJ, Giammara B, Lewis JC, DeVries WC. Biomaterial-centered sepsis and the total artificial heart. *JAMA* 1988; **259**, 870–874.
7. Pierce WS. Permanent heart substitution, better solutions lie ahead (editorial). *JAMA* 1988; **259**, 891.
8. Griffith BG. Interim use of the Jarvik-7 artificial heart: lessons learned at Presbyterian University Hospital of Pittsburgh. *Ann Thorac Surg* 1989; **47**, 158–166.
9. Pifarre R, Sullivan HJ, Montoya A, Bakhos M, Grieco J, Foy BK, Blakeman B, Constanzo-Nordin MR, Altergott, R, Lonchyna V. The use of the Jarvik-7 total artificial heart and the Symbion ventricular assist device as a bridge to transplantation. *Surgery* 1990; **108**, 681–685.
10. Kawaguchi AT, Gandjbakhch I, Pavie A, Muneretto C, Solis E, Leger P, Bors V, Szefner J, Vaissier E, Levasseur JP, Cabrol A, Cabrol C. Liver and kidney function in patients undergoing mechanical circulatory support with Jarvik-7 artificial heart as a bridge to transplantation. *J Heart Transplant* 1990; **9**, 631–637.
11. Muneretto C, Pavie A, Solis E, Kawaguchi A, Leger P, Bors V, Gandjbakhch I, Desreunnes M, Vaissier E, Szefner J, Cabrol C. Special problems in use of the total artificial heart as a bridge to transplantation. *Transplant Proc* 1989; **21**, 2551–2552.
12. Copeland JG, Smith R, Icenogle T, Vasu A, Rhenman B, Williams R, Cleavinger M. Orthotopic artifi-

cial total artificial heart bridge to transplantation: preliminary results. *J Heart Transplant* 1989; **8**, 124–138.

13. Cabrol C, Gandjbakhch I, Pavie A, Bors V, Szefner J, Kawaguchi A, Cabrol A, Leger P, Vaissier E, Levasseur JP, Petrie J, Simmonneau F. Assistance circulatoire: resultats actuel et indications. In: Cabrol C, Gandjbakhch I, Pavie A (eds), *Transplantation Cardiaque et Pulmonaire*. Paris: Laboratoires Sandoz, 1992: 130–134.

14. Leger P. LeMoment de la greffe. In: Cabrol C, Gandjbakhch I, Pavie A (eds), *Transplantation Cardiaque et Pulmonaire*. Paris: Laboratoires Sandoz, 1992: 79–81.

15. Copeland JG, Smith RG, Cleavinger MR, Icenogle TB, Sethi GK, Rosado LJ. Bridge to transplantation indications for Symbion TAH, Symbion AVAD and Novacor LVAS. In: Akutsu T, Koyanagi H (eds), *Artificial Heart—Proceedings of the Third International Symposium on Artificial Heart and Assist Devices*. Tokyo: Springer Verlag, 1991: 303–308.

16. Loisance D, Dubois Rande JL, Deluze P, Benvenuti C, Dervanian P, Brunet S, Hillion ML, Castiagne A, Cachera JP. Improved patient selection for total artificial heart implantation. *ASAIO Trans* 1989; **35**, 242–244.

17. Reedy JE, Swartz MT, Termuhlen DF, Pennington DG, McBride LR, Miller LW, Ruzevich SA. Bridge to heart transplantation: importance of patient selection. *J Heart Transplant* 1990; **9**, 473–481.

18. Akutsu T, Kolff WJ. Permanent substitute for hearts and valves. *ASAIO Trans* 1958; **4**, 230–235.

19. Pierce W. The artificial heart 1986: partial fulfilment of a promise. *ASAIO Trans* 1986; **22**, 5–10.

20. Jarvik RK. The total artificial heart. *Sci Am* 1981; **244**, 74–80.

21. Institute of Medicine: Committee to Evaluate the Artificial Heart Program of the National Heart, Lung and Blood Institute (NHLBI). Hognes JR, VanAntwerp M (eds), *The Artificial Heart: Prototypes, Policies and Patients*. Washington, DC: National Academy Press, 1991: 298.

22. Kwan-Gett CS, Wu Y, Collan R, Jacobsen S, Kolff WJ. Total replacement artificial heart and driving system with inherent regulation of cardiac output. *ASAIO Trans* 1969; **15**, 245–251.

23. Willshaw P, Nielsen SD, Nanas J, Pichel RH, Olsen DB. A cardiac output monitor and diagnostic unit for pneumatically driven artificial hearts. *Artif Organs* 1984; **8**, 215–219.

24. Taenaka Y, Olsen DB, Nielsen SD, Dew PA, Holmberg DL, Chiang BY. Diagnosis of mechanical failures of artificial hearts. *ASAIO Trans* 1985; **21**, 79–83.

25. Olsen DB, Unger F, Oster H, Lawson J, Kessler T, Kolff J, Kolff WJ. Thrombus generation within the artificial heart. *J Thorac Cardiovasc Surg* 1975; **70**, 248–255.

26. Dew PA, Olsen DB, Kessler TR, Coleman DL, Kolff WJ. Mechanical failures in *in vivo* and *in vitro* studies of pneumatic total artificial hearts. *Trans ASAIO* 1984; **30**, 112–116.

27. Cooley DA. Staged cardiac transplantation: a report of three cases. *J Heart Transplant* 1982; **1**, 145–153.

28. Kolff WJ, DeVries WC, Joyce LD, Olsen DB, Jarvik RK, Nielsen S, Hastings I, Anderson J, Anderson F, Menlove R. Lessons learned from Dr Barney Clark, the first patient with an artificial heart. *Int J Artif Organs* 1983; **1**, 165–174.

29. Dobbins JJ, Johnson S, Kunin CM, DeVries WC. Postmortem microbiological findings of two total artificial heart recipients. *JAMA* 1988; **259**, 865–869.

30. Stelzer GT, Ward RA, Wellhausen SR, McLeish KR, Johnson GS, DeVries WC. Alterations in select immunologic parameters following total artificial heart implantation. *Artif Organs* 1987; **11**, 52–62.

31. Wellhausen SR, Ward RA, Johnson GS, DeVries WC. Immunologic complications of longterm implantation of a total artificial heart. *J Clin Immunol* 1988; **8**, 307–318.

32. Levinson MM, Copeland JG, Smith R, Cork RC, Devries WC, Mays JB, Griffith BP, Kormos R, Joyce LD, Pritzker MR, Semb BKH, Koul B, Menkis AH, Keon WJ. Indexes in hemolysis in human recipients of the Jarvik-7 total artificial heart: a cooperative report of fifteen patients. *J Heart Transplant* 1986; **5**, 236–248.

33. Kolff J, Deeb M, Cavarocchi NC, Riebman JB, Olsen DB, Robbins PS. The artificial heart in human subjects. *J Thorac Cardiovas Surg* 1984; **87**, 825–831.

34. Levinson MM, Copeland JG. Technical aspects of total artificial heart implantation for temporary applications. *J Card Surg* 1987; **2**, 3–19.

35. Copeland JG, Levinson MM, Smith R, Icenogle TB, Vaughn C, Cheng K, Ott R, Emery RW. The total artificial heart as a bridge to transplantation. *JAMA* 1986; **256**, 2991–2995.

36. Oaks TE, Pae WE, Miller CA, Pierce WS. Combined registry for the clinical use of mechanical ventricular assist pumps and the total artificial heart in conjunction with heart transplantation: fifth official report 1990. *J Heart Lung Transplant* 1991; **10**, 621–625.

37. Lonchyna VA, Piffare R, Sullivan H, Montoya A, Mamdouh B, Grieco J, Foy B, Blakeman B, Altergott R, Calandra D, Hinkamp T, Istanbouli M, Sinno J, Bartlett L. Successful use of the total artificial heart as a bridge to transplantation with no mediastinitis. *J Heart Lung Transplant* 1992; **11**, 803–811.

38. Griffith BP, Hardesty RL, Kormos RL, Trento A, Borovetz HS, Thompson ME, Bahnson HT. Temporary use of the Jarvik-7 total artificial heart

before transplantation. *New Engl J Med* 1987; **316**, 130–134.

39. Griffith BP, Kormos RL, Hardesty RL, Armitage JM, Dummer S. The artificial heart: infection related morbidity and its effect on transplantation. *Ann Thorac Surg* 1988; **45**, 409–414.
40. Kormos RL, Borovetz HS, Griffith BP, Hung TC. Rheological abnormalities in patients with the Jarvik-7 total artificial heart. *ASAIO Trans* 1897; **37**, 413–417.
41. Cabrol C, Solis E, Muneretto C, Pavie A, Gandjbakhch I, Bors V, Szefner J, Leger P, Cabrol A. Orthotopic transplantation after implantation of a Jarvik-7 total artificial heart. *J Thorac Cardiovasc Surg* 1989; **97**, 342–350.
42. Tsao MM, Katz D. Central venous catheter induced endocarditis: human correlate of the animal experimental model of endocarditis. *Rev Infect Dis* 1984; **6**, 783–790.
43. Didisheim P, Olsen DB, Farrar DJ, Portner PM, Griffith BP, Pennington DG, Joist H, Schoen FJ, Gristina AG, Anderson JM. Infections and thrombolism with implantable cardiovascular devices. *ASAIO Trans* 1989; **35**, 54–70.
44. Bellon JL, Szefner J, Cabrol C. *Coagulation et Coeur Artificial.* Masson: Paris, 1989.
45. Cabrol C, Gandjbakhch I, Pavie A, Bors V, Mestiri T, Cabrol A, Leger P, Levasseur JP, Vaissier E, Szefner J, Auriol A, Aupetit B, Solis E. Total artificial heart as a bridge for transplantation: La Pitié 1986 to 1978. *J Heart Transplant* 1988; **7**, 12–17.
46. Jarvik RK, Devries WC, Semb BKH, Koul B, Copeland JG, Levinson MM, Griffith BP, Joyce LD, Cooley DA, Frazier OH, Carrol C, Keon WJ. Surgical positioning of the Jarvik-7 artificial heart. *J Heart Transplant* 1986; **5**, 184–195.

20

European clinical experience with total artificial hearts

A Pavie, Ph Leger, G Rabago, G Tedy, C Cabrol and J Gandjbakhch

Introduction

In the 1930s, Demikhov was the first surgeon to remove a dog's heart and replace it with a mechanical device,[1] but it was not until the 1960s that Cooley and others attempted the first clinical use of a total artificial heart (TAH) as a bridge to transplantation.[2] Fourteen years of human effort and technological development made the first permanent implantation of a Jarvik-7 possible (Symbion, Salt Lake City) by DeVries on his patient, Barney Clark, who lived for 112 days.[3] The first five implantations were performed as permanent circulatory support. Thereafter, due to complications, the US Food and Drug Administration (FDA) only allowed testing as a bridge to heart transplantation. In August 1985, three years later, Copeland and others achieved the first successful use of a Jarvik-7 TAH as a bridge procedure. After this success, many implantations were performed all around the world.

In April 1986, the first European case was performed in La Pitié hospital with a Symbion TAH.[5] Other European teams in England, France, Spain, Sweden and Turkey developed a Symbion TAH programme. During the same period, a few European teams developed their own devices and performed some human implantations (Berlin Heart, Brno, Ellipsoid Heart).[6,7] Recently the FDA banned the use of the Symbion TAH in the United States and consequently the number of implantations decreased, but in Europe this device is still used by some teams. More recently, Copeland and the University of Arizona have restarted the FDA approval procedure with a new company, CardioWest, and are able to deliver some devices in Europe.

This chapter summarizes the overall European experience of TAH use, but with an emphasis on the Symbion TAH as a bridge to heart transplantation because of the large number of implantations of this device for this purpose.

The extent of the European experience

European experience with the Symbion TAH up to the end of 1990 was analysed by Johnson et al.[8] These data have been compared with the preliminary data from the European registry of the Concerted Action 'Heart' proceedings.[9] The more recent implantations in France since October 1992, have also been considered.

Johnson and associates reported 171 patients having received 175 Symbion TAHs as a bridge to heart transplantation; 65 of these implantations were performed in Europe (37%). Owing to the withdrawal of the Symbion TAH in the USA, only 20 other implantations were performed, two in Canada and 18 in Europe.

Between April 1986 and November 1992, 83 patients received 83 Symbion TAHs in Europe. Bridging implantations were performed in nine centres (Table 20.1). Nineteen implants were

Table 20.1 The European centres considered in this review.

Centre	Number of implants	Died on device	Transplanted
La Pitié, Paris	63	37	26
Hospital of Nantes	7	2	5
Henri Mondor Hospital, Paris	4	2	2
Karolinska Institute, Stockholm	3		3
Hospices Civils, Lyon	2	2	
Clinica puerta de Hierro, Madrid	1		1
H. Santa Creu i Sant Pau, Barcelona	1		1
Papworth Hospital, Cambridge	1		1
University of Ankara	1	1	
Totals	83	44	39

performed with the 100 cm³ model and the others with the 70 cm³ model. There were 72 male recipients and 10 females. Since 1986, the number of implantations per year has decreased; but available ventricles through the new manufacturer explain the slight increase since 1991 (Fig. 20.1).

Age ranged from 15 to 57 years (Fig. 20.2). The durations of support ranged from less than one day up to 603 days (Fig. 20.3). This longest duration was due to the presence of antibodies not allowing transplantation.

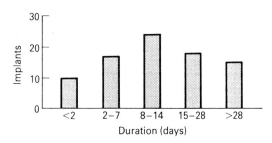

Fig. 20.3 Duration of support with a TAH.

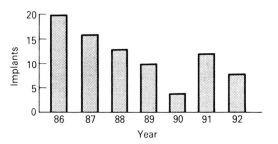

Fig. 20.1 Number of Jarvik-7 implantations per year in Europe.

Fig. 20.4 gives an idea of the aetiologies of the heart disease leading to implantation. Ischaemic disease accounted for 46% of cases.

Fig. 20.5 summarizes the indications for implantation. Here, deterioration on the waiting list was most often implicated (45%), followed by acute shock (43%), acute rejection of a transplanted heart (9%) and those not weanable from CPB (4%).

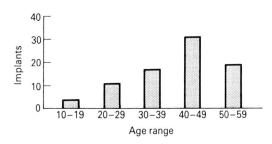

Fig. 20.2 Ages of patients.

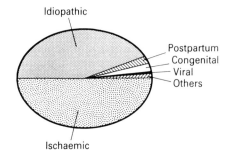

Fig. 20.4 The aetiologies of implantations.

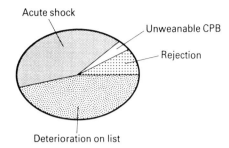

Fig. 20.5 Indications for implantations.

Device description

The Symbion ventricle has an air-driven intra-corporeal diaphragm coated with polyurethane urea. Medtronic–Hall valves are situated in the outflow and inflow orifices. Two different sizes are available, as mentioned above.

The Utah-drive controller works in an asynchronous mode with an internal fixed rate. Three parameters have to be preset before starting the support: heart rate (available range 0–199 beats/min), delay (from 0 to 99 ms) and systole duration (from 0 to 99%). Each unit is delivered with one active drive system and a second backup drive.

The activation pressure can be varied between 0 and 300 mmHg, and a negative pressure can be used if there is poor ventricular filling (0–20 mmHg).

A COMDU computer is connected to the Utah-drive system allowing continuous monitoring of cardiac output from each ventricle, on the basis of the air coming out from the ventricle at each diastole. Trend curves are displayed on a monitor.[10]

Indications for use of TAHs

The use of temporary mechanical cardiac support has increased rapidly, so that today many aspects of patient and device selection are clearer. Some problems remain unsolved.

The haemodynamic criteria are widely accepted. There should be a cardiac index $<2\,l/min/m^2$, with an arterial pressure <80 mmHg and a very high left or right atrial pressure (>20 mmHg). This very low cardiac output is associated with decreased urine output

(<30 ml/h) and sometimes anuria. All these conditions should be occurring with 'maximal' inotropic support. The definition of 'maximal' remains unclear, but in fact the real doses are not that important. The evolution of the drug support appears to be the best index.[11] The need for adrenaline is a particularly adverse factor.

In some instances, the use of a bolus test of enoximone allows one to select patients for bridging to transplantation. About two-thirds of the patients improve and can then wait for a suitable donor.[12] They require careful follow-up since the initial improvement is sometimes very short. In such cases, it is very important to implant an assist device before the onset of multiple organ failure (MOF). We consider the presence of a low vascular resistance as a strict contraindication for the test and probably for implantation.[13]

Contraindications

Few contraindications are absolute, but some clearly defined circumstances decrease the chance of success and require careful evaluation.[11–14]

Age is generally the first matter for discussion. In the La Pitié TAH series,[15] the patients successfully transplanted were younger than those who died under TAH; but this difference was not statistically significant. Patients under 40 years of age had 56% chance of being transplanted, compared with older patients of whom only 23% were transplanted ($p = 0.001$). This finding was also reported by Johnson *et al.*[8] On the other hand, survival was not influenced by sex and device model.[8–16]

Body surface area was a preoperative variable for which there was a significant difference between the patients with and without subsequent transplantation.[16] This seems to implicate a poor fit, with a small patient's thorax causing obstruction in the systemic or pulmonary venous return. This can be a theoretical explanation of organ dysfunction secondary to increased pressure in the inferior vena cava.[17]

However, the major contraindications are related to the status of other organs. Evaluation of reversible damage to organ function is essential, but unfortunately it is often impossible to be completely sure during the preoperative period. All teams specify a 'severe' dysfunction, but this non-quantitative assessment varies from one surgical group to another.

In cases of severe renal insufficiency, a creatinine level >2 mg/dl seems to be an important risk factor.[18,19] On the other hand, whereas dialysis is a strict contraindication for US teams, numerous European groups have reported success in such circumstances.[6–11] Liver dysfunction with a considerable increase in bilirubin level is another adverse factor.[11]

To evaluate multiple organ failure, the evolution of the cardiac decompensation is important. The type of decompensation could be deemed as a risk factor if we consider that chronic patients could have greater organ dysfunction due to the chronicity of their disease.[19]

The issue of infection requires careful analysis. Three groups can be distinguished:[11]

1. Pulmonary infection is very common, especially where there is pulmonary oedema. Most teams do not consider this as a contraindication.
2. With septicaemia, which is often the result of prolonged intensive-care hospitalization, we have to be more circumspect. The decision depends on the bacterium: only Candida and germs not open to antibiotic therapy are a contraindication.
3. Septic shock is an absolute contraindication, since it is impossible to obtain a high flow owing to the collapse of vascular tone.[13]

A focal neurological problem is a strict contraindication, as is gastrointestinal bleeding. With an obtundent patient the decision is more difficult to take because it can be due to a low cardiac output.

Candidate scoring

Analysis of the foregoing indications and contraindications leads to the idea of giving candidates for implantation a preoperative score.

The La Pitié team has selected some preoperative factors from their Jarvik-7 patients, including high-risk contraindications: rejection, postoperative failure, mode of decompensation, patient size, biliburin above 24 µmol/l and dialysis. The successful bridge cases had an average score of 1.3, compared with the failed cases with a score of 6.6 (Fig. 20.6). The European Concerted Action 'Heart' groups have also proposed a score which

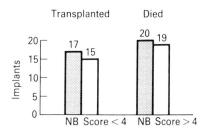

Fig. 20.6 A preoperative risk analysis of the La Pitié experience with 37 patients (sensitivity 94%, specificity 90%).

considers some other parameters. In the future, patient scoring will be very helpful and can lead to an improvement of results.

Surgical technique

The implantation of a Jarvik-7 TAH requires a special technique. Through a median sternotomy,[20] the pericardium is opened from the ascending aorta to the diaphragm. The ventricle drive-lines are placed through two separate skin incisions in the upper left quadrant of the abdomen, and a tunnel is created from the skin incision to the pericardial cavity. Once the drive-lines are perfectly in place, both ventricles are carefully checked (Fig. 20.7).

Cardiopulmonary bypass is established using two right-angled caval cannulae inserted anteriorly, and an arterial cannula is placed into the ascending aorta.

The heart excision should be performed carefully so as to ease subsequent cardiac transplantation. The pulmonary artery and the aorta are transected just above their respective valves. Right and left ventricles are transected on a 2–3 cm length distally from the atrioventricular groove. The coronary sinus ostium and the venous coronary sinus are closed to avoid bleeding.

The anastomosis between the atrial cuffs and the atrioventricular remnants is started at the cephalic portion of the septum, a double anastomosis with a simple running suture joining both cuffs to the remnant septum. Then each cuff is sutured to its respective right and left free ventricular wall. The aortic and pulmonary grafts (7 cm long) are sutured end-to-end to their respective bessels. In Europe, before testing the suture line, it is possible to supplement all anastomoses with fibrin glue or gelatine–resorcin–

formal adhesive (GRF). This technique allows one to avoid many postoperative bleeding complications as described by the US teams. The artificial ventricles are attached to their respective cuffs and, after air-purging, support is started. The left ventricle is activated first.

Coagulation control

Anticoagulation regimens vary. The complex device/blood interface (the presence of mechanical valves, large exposure between foreign materials and blood, localized blood turbulences) requires a systemic and personalized approach to avoid thromboembolic complications.[21] All

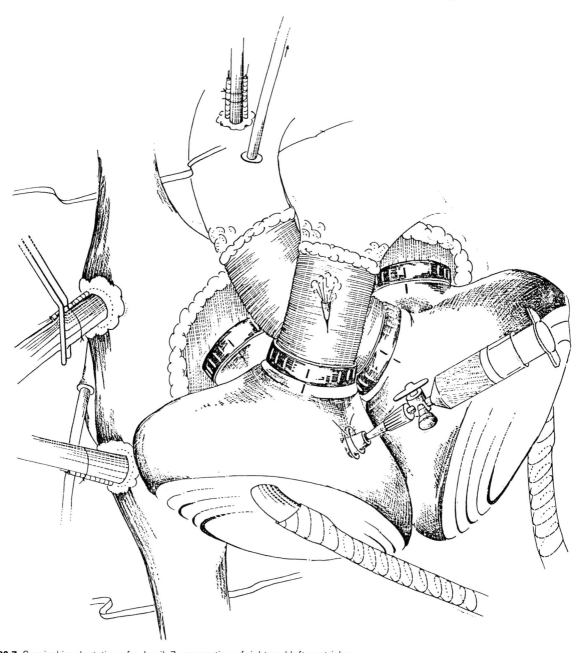

Fig. 20.7 Surgical implantation of a Jarvik-7: connection of right and left ventricles.

Table 20.2 Coagulation monitoring checklist.

Platelet functions
Platelet aggregation to ADP, epinephrine, collagen and
    arachidonic acid by Born method
Platelet count, haematocrit
Platelet aggregate evaluation by Wu–Hoak method
Ivy–Borchgrevink bleeding time
Platelet factor 4 (PF-4)
Beta-thromboglobulin (BTG)

Thrombin formation and its regulatory pathways
Prothrombin time
Activated partial thromboplastin time (APTT)
Fibrinogen titration
Thromboelastography (TEG) recalcified whole blood
Plasma and serum antithrombin III titration
Calculation of antithrombinic potential index (API)
Plasma and serum factor Xa titration
Raby's transfer test on plasma by thromboelastography
    (TEG)
Protein C—protein S—heparine cofactor II

Fibrinolytic system
Reptilase time
Fibrinogen degradation products (FDP)
Alpha-2-antiplasmin (A-2-AP)
Plasminogen

API = plasma AT-III minus serum AT-III.

patients at La Pitié were surveyed in terms of platelet functions, thrombin formation pathways and fibrinolytic status at least once a day (Table 20.2). Individualized treatments were established according to the test results. (Table 20.3). Dipyridamole was given to stabilize platelet activity and aspirin to lower aggregation. If a pathological fibrinolytic state was found, aprotinin was given until normalization of the laboratory and clinical status. All the systems involved in haemostasis were controlled in order to adapt the treatment to each individual.

Table 20.3 Anticoagulation regimen.

Heparin 1000–5000 IU/day (IV)
Dipyridamole 150–300 mg every 6 hours (IV)
Aspirin 50 mg/day
Aprotinin 12 500 kIU/bolus (IV), then 500 kIU/min in
    continuous drip
Pentoxyphylline 400 mg/day

Only when indicated:
Ticlopidine 250 mg every 2–3 days
Fresh frozen plasma
Antithrombin-III concentrates
Blood cell concentrates
Fibrogen concentrates

Results

Of the 83 patients who received a Symbion TAH in Europe between April 1986 and November 1992, 44 died while on the device. Mechanical dysfunction of the device was exceptional: it occurred once, in a case of a ruptured right ventricle diaphragm. The diagnosis was easily made by echography, and the ventricle was changed during a short reoperation. Unfortunately the patient died later of MOF, but death was not device-related. The ventricle and the Utah-drive console seem very safe, even for very long-term support (603 days).

There were two main causes of death in this group. The first was progressive deterioration of haemodynamic function associated with MOF, with the impossibility of maintaining a stable blood pressure despite vasoactive drugs.[13,15,16] The second main cause was untreatable sepsis.

Kidney failure was one of the most common complications after implantation. The prognosis depends on the evolution of the renal function, the need for dialysis being an adverse sign.[8] On the other hand, pre-implantation anuria had no influence on survival. Among MOF patients, alteration of the liver function had a bad prognosis.

Untreatable sepsis is often associated with MOF. In many cases it is difficult to know which is the cause and which is the consequence. It is hard to be completely sure that the patient is free of infection before implantation. Frequently, the systematic culture of the native heart comes back positive,[8,18] especially in cases of long stays in the intensive care unit before implantation.

On the other hand, mediastinitis is a very rare complication in the European experience when compared with some US reports.[22] Only a few infections of the drive-lines were reported but were generally without severe consequences.

Bleeding complications have decreased and are still rare owing to the use of glue during surgery, and to the special management of coagulation carried out by several teams in Europe.[12–21]

Thirty-nine patients (47%) could be transplanted. Owing to the shortage of donors, the transplant could be made only in cases of haemodynamic stability, on an extubated patient with normal renal and liver functions, without coagulation problems or infection. With such strict criteria for transplantation, the rate was low, but all ethical problems were avoided with the other patients on the waiting list. These results from Europe are largely influenced by the team with the most experience (Table 20.1).

Conclusions

It is clear today that some indications had a bad prognosis: patients not weanable from cardiopulmonary bypass, cardiac arrest and acute rejection.[8-15,16,18] These can now be considered as contraindications.

It is not very helpful to make comparisons with other international registries of mechanical support[23] or transplantation[24] which have only voluntary participation. For this reason, their results are probably very optimistic and perhaps misleading.

It seems that, despite relatively high overall morbidity and mortality, use of the Jarvik-7 has saved the lives of some patients. Continued use of the device in Europe has permitted the indications and contraindications to be more clearly defined.

References

1. Demikhov VP. *Experimental Transplantation of Vital Organs* (translated by Basil Haig). New York: Consultans Bureau, 1947: 212.
2. Cooley DA, Liotta D, Hallman Gl, *et al.* Orthotopic cardiac prosthesis for two-staged cardiac replacement. *Am J Cardiol* 1969; **24**, 723–730.
3. Jarvik RK, DeVries WC, *et al.* Clinical use of total artificial heart. *J Heart Transplant* 1986; **5**, 184–195.
4. Copeland JG, Emery WR, Levinson MM, *et al.* The role of mechanical support and transplantation in treatment of patients with end-stage cardiomyopathy. *Circulation* 1985; **72** (suppl II), 7–12.
5. Cabrol C, Gandjbakhch I, Pavie A, *et al.* Total artificial heart as a bridge for transplantation: La Pitié 1986 to 1987. *J Heart Transplant* 1988; **7**, 12–17.
6. Viazis P. The Berlin pneumatic device. In: Pavie A (ed), *European Concerted Action 'Heart' Proceedings: Medical Indications and System Choice*. The Netherlands, University of Twente, 1990: 35–36.
7. Unger F, Genelin A, Hager J, *et al.* Functional heart replacement with non-pulsatile assist devices. In: Reichart B, Fasol R, Odell J, *et al.* (eds), *Assisted Circulation*, vol 2. New York: Springer Verlag, 1984: 163.
8. Johnson KE, Prieto M, Joyce L, *et al.* Summary of the clinical use of the Symbion total artificial heart: a registry report. *J Heart Lung Transplant* 1992; **11**, 104–116.
9. Del Canizo JF. Clinical registry of mechanical circulatory support system applications in Europe. In: Del Canizo JF (ed), *European Concerted Action 'Heart' Proceedings*. The Netherlands, University of Twente, 1992: 5–24.
10. Leger Ph. Control of the Jarvik artificial heart. In: Arts T (ed), *European Concerted Action 'Heart' Proceedings: Physiological Interaction Between Circulatory Support System and Circulation*. The Netherlands, University of Twente, 1992: 117–120.
11. Meli M. Protocols in clinical applications. In: Mambrito B (ed), *European Concerted Action 'Heart' Proceedings: General Meeting*. The Netherlands, University of Twente, 1990: 95–97.
12. Heinz U. Clinical protocol for evaluation of the preoperative status of patients. In: Meli M, Pavie A (eds), *European Concerted Action 'Heart' Proceedings: Clinical Protocols for the Use of Assist Devices*. The Netherlands, University of Twente, 1992: 55–60.
13. Deleuze P, Loisance D, Shiiya N, *et al.* Irreversible drop of systemic vascular resistance in patients implanted with a Jarvik total artificial heart. *Int J Artif Organs* 1991; **14**, 286–289.
14. Leger Ph. Clinical indications and contraindications. In: Pavie A (ed), *European Concerted Action 'Heart' Proceedings: Medical Indications and System Choice*. The Netherlands, University of Twente, 1990: 43–50.
15. Kawaguchi AT, Gandjbakhch I, Pavie A, Muneretto C, Solis E, Bors V, Leger Ph, Vaissier E, Levasseur JP, Szefner J, Sasako Y, Cabrol A, Cabrol C. Factors affecting survival in total artificial heart recipients before transplantation. *Circulation* 1990; **80** (suppl IV), 322–327.
16. Pavie A, Muneretto C, Aupart M, Rabago G, Leger Ph, Tedy G, Bors V, Gandjbakhch I, Cabrol C. Prognostic indices of survival in patients supported with temporary devices (TAH, VAD). *Int J Artif Organs* 1991; **14**, 280–285.
17. Kawaguchi AT, Muneretto C, Pavie A, Solis E, Leger Ph, Gandjbakhch I, Bors V, Desruennes M, Cabrol A, Cabrol C. Hemodynamic characteristics of the Jarvik-7 total artificial heart. *Circulation* 1989; **79** (suppl III), 152–157.
18. Meli M. Definition and limits of the clinical protocols and their necessity. In: Meli M, Pavie A (eds), *European Concerted Action 'Heart' Proceedings: Clinical Protocols for the Use of Assist Devices*. The Netherlands, University of Twente, 1992: 45–53.
19. Kawaguchi, AT, Cabrol C, Gandjbakhch I, Pavie A, Bors V, Muneretto C. Preoperative risk analysis in patients receiving Jarvik-7 artificial heart as bridge to transplantation. *Eur J Cardiothorac Surg* 1991; **5**, 509–514.
20. Solis E, Muneretto C, Cabrol C. Total artificial heart. In: Cooper DK, Novitzky D (eds), *The Transplantation and Replacement of Thoracic Organs*. Boston: Kluwer Academic, 1988; 431–444.

21. Szefner J, Bellon JL, Cabrol C. *Coagulation et Coeur Artificiel.* Paris: Masson, 1988.
22. Griffith BP, Kormos RL, Hardesty RL, Armitage JM, Dummer JS. The artificial heart: infection-related morbidity and its effect on transplantation. *Ann Thorac Surg* 1988; **45**, 409–414.
23. Oaks TE, Pae WE, Miller MA, Pierce WS. Combined registry for the clinical use of mechanical ventricular assist pump and the total artificial heart in conjunction with heart transplantation: fifth official report. *J Heart Transplant* 1990; **10**, 621–625.
24. Kriett JM, Kaye MP. The registry of the International Society for Heart Transplantation: seventh official report, 1990. *J Heart Transplant* 1990; **9**, 323–330.

21

The future of artificial hearts

George M Pantalos

Heart disease causes more than 700,000 deaths each year in the United States alone. Decades of research have led to drugs, medical devices, and procedures that provide effective treatment for many forms of heart disease, yet even today an individual suffering from end-stage heart disease faces a bleak outlook and has few treatment options.

US Institute of Medicine,
The Artificial Heart, 1991[1]

The scary part of living on the edge of the next century is that sometimes we no longer have to accept life as a lottery. We have been given the power, in some cases, to refuse the orders of Fate and rewrite our lives.

Bill Hall, syndicated columnist, 1993

Our task is not to fix the blame for the past, but to fix the course for the future.

John F Kennedy

My philosophy is very simple and has never changed. If we can reasonably expect that the patient can be restored to a happy existence for him or her, then the patient should be treated with an artificial kidney or an artificial organ, and if it is unlikely or impossible that he will be restored, then the patient should not be treated.

Willem J Kolff, 'Father of Artificial Organs'

As in the past, the future goal of the mechanical circulatory support community is to develop devices and techniques which restore cardiac and circulatory function, so that patients may be rehabilitated to the point where they may once again become productive members of society. As we

look to the future, we envision a spectrum of circulatory support devices and techniques that are not only safe and effective, but also affordable and forgettable, so as to minimize the associated anxiety to the recipient, their attending surgeon, and indeed, the anxiety to society as a whole.

The intra-aortic balloon pump (IABP) will remain the primary device for mechanical circulatory support, but it will become more user-friendly, fully automatic[2] and easily portable, permitting patient ambulation and exercise as the myocardium recovers. Variations on the IABP will include balloon pumping of the ventricles and pulmonary artery, and even combining a balloon and an axial flow pump on the same catheter to maximize the amount of ventricular unloading and blood flow generated. Until undisputable evidence to the contrary comes forth, it appears that when IABP support is inadequate, the 'depulsed' flow from rotary blood pumps will continue to be effective for the short-term ventricular support required by most patients when the recovery of ventricular function is anticipated. Advances in the pharmaceutical modification of both pump and circuit components will eliminate the need for systemic anticoagulation. Automatic controllers will eliminate the need for constant staff attention in the intensive care unit, and refinements in pump design will extend the duration of reliable function, thus eliminating the need to change pump heads during circulatory support. Smaller, implantable centrifugal pumps are being re-examined as a means of providing long-term circulatory support. All this will be accomplished while continuing to keep the cost of these continuous flow systems notably lower than their pulsatile counterparts.

Despite advances in medical therapy and the growing use of the 'presumed consent' policy for increasing the number of donor organs, it is unlikely that these approaches will sufficiently restore cardiac function or increase donor organ supply to match the need of end-stage heart disease patients in the near future. Consequently, there will still be the need for artificial hearts and other circulatory support devices in the bridge-to-transplantation setting. The early experience with implanted left ventricular assist systems, utilizing a wearable controller, is already charting the course for eventual patient discharge and outpatient management protocols, as well as the return to a productive life style. However, this left ventricular assist system experience, coupled with the current total artificial heart experience, continues to reiterate the challenges of thromboembolism, foreign-body response and infection, as well as recipient quality of life and psychological well-being.

Many new and innovative ways of providing mechanical circulatory support are being explored. Among other approaches considered for artificial hearts are small, intraventricular or intravascular axial flow pumps. These devices are emerging as potential alternatives to the larger, pulsatile systems. A scaled-up version of the Hemopump that is actually smaller than a scalpel handle is being developed jointly at Nimbus Inc. and the University of Pittsburgh.[3] The pump inlet is connected to an uptake cannula and the pump outlet is connected to a vascular graft anastomosed to the corresponding great vessel. It is envisioned that this device could either be a left ventricular assist device, or be used as a biventricular, long-term circulatory support device. Taking this approach one step further, Dr Robert Jarvik is developing what he refers to as an intraventricular artificial heart. Called the Jarvik-2000, the pump housing acts as its own uptake cannula as well, and is inserted into the apex of the left ventricle with the outlet then being connected to a vascular graft that is anastomosed to the descending, thoracic aorta. One can appreciate the amazing size, weight and space savings of this device compared with a current pulsatile left

ventricular assist system if this approach proves to be successful.

Exploring the versatility of axial flow pumps even one step further are Dr Mitamura and colleagues working at the Hokkaido Tokai University in Japan.[4] These developers have actually built into a mechanical valve ring an axial flow pump capable of pumping 6–8 litres per minute. They envision implanting this device in the aortic valve position using the surgical technique identical to an aortic valve replacement.

While the devices considered so far are for adults, we should also expect that there will be paediatric devices to address the heretofore unmet needs of the paediatric population as recently reviewed by Pennington and Swartz.[5] The registry from the International Society for Heart and Lung Transplantation indicates that the number of paediatric cardiac transplants has increased in recent years, and that the greatest increases occurred in patients less than one year old.[6] At the University of Utah in Salt Lake City, we have worked on a 6 cc stroke volume neonatal artificial heart to bridge newborn patients to transplantation, particularly patients with hypoplastic left heart syndrome.[7] At the moment, we are limited by the unavailability of an appropriate valve, so the device has been scaled-up to a 10 cc ventricular assist device that is currently in animal evaluation prior to submission of an application to initiate clinical trials. Significant effort to develop paediatric ventricular assist devices is also being undertaken at the Pennsylvania State University Hershey Medical Center and by the Berlin Heart company; the latter has already developed a larger paediatric ventricular assist device and initiated clinical trials.

> It was silver, shaped like a flattened egg, a trifle smaller than the laboring human pump. To it was attached a pair of long, flexible silver pipes. Electricity worked the air pumps, which in turn supplied the little silver egg implanted in the patient with both pressure and vacuum. The regulating device kept the blood circulating at the proper rate. The surgeon seemed satisfied with it all.
>
> HE Flint, *The Devolutionist*, 1921[8]

What do we look for in artificial hearts of the future, both in the near-term and the far-term? First of all, if they are going to be considered 'safe and effective', they have to match the current record with biological transplants, which means nearly 70% survival for five years.[6] Given the fact that, to date, there has never been a completely implantable artificial heart system that has even pumped for five years, one is only left with the anticipation that there is still a long and trying developmental path ahead. These systems are envisioned to have an orthotopically positioned blood pump coupled to a physiological controller and batteries that will be implanted in the abdomen, along with a subcutaneous coil of varying design to receive transcutaneously transmitted energy from a primary source coil on top of the skin. Criteria for these artificial hearts require that they be completely implantable with compact components and minimal dead space for ease of implantation and removal.[9] Initial requirements for the entire system must have a high two-year electromechanical and biocompatible reliability (e.g. 80% reliability at a 95% confidence level) and must be physiologically responsive to the needs of the recipient. The patient should be able to resume an acceptable quality of life, with infrequent medical intervention, creating an autonomous livelihood out of the hospital. The devices need to have autodiagnostic capabilities that can be easily interpreted by the recipient and attendee with a minimum of training as well as the possibility of remote transmission of data to the attending surgeon. Soft failures of the device should not endanger the life of the recipient and autodiagnostic alarms should alert the recipient to the nature of the problem.

There are three programmes currently being funded in the United States under contract by the National Heart, Lung and Blood Institute to develop completely implantable cardiac replacement devices. The device being developed by Abiomed, in collaboration with the Texas Heart Institute, uses an electrohydraulic energy converter and trileaflet, polymer valves. The Division of Artificial Organs at the Pennsylvania State University Hershey Medical Center, in collaboration with Sarns 3M, is developing a roller-screw pusher plate bloodpump with tilting disc valves. The Cleveland Clinic Foundation, in collaboration with Nimbus Inc., is developing an electrohydraulic, magnetically coupled pusher plate device using bioprosthetic valves and a biolized blood-contacting surface. Substantial progress in the development of completely implantable total artificial hearts has also been made at the Baylor College of Medicine, the University of Utah, the Milwaukee Heart Institute and several other

organizations. All of these implanted systems require not only the blood pump and energy converter mechanism, but also a physiological controller, implanted battery pack, transcutaneous energy transmission system and, in some cases, an implanted volume compliance chamber. Indeed, these systems represent a substantial amount of hardware, reiterating the requirements for good fit, high reliability and patient acceptance. In spite of this major surgical and biomedical engineering challenge, our colleagues at the Hershey Medical Center have already demonstrated tether-free animal survival in excess of 150 days with their system completely implanted.[10]

For the future development of implantable artificial hearts, further examination of some of the previously mentioned criteria is merited. It is hoped that devices in the future will not only be haemodynamically sound, but also metabolically smart, immunologically improved and 'user friendly' compared with present devices. Paramount to the appropriate physiological control of these devices is maintaining an appropriate balance between the left and right ventricular output and keeping the inflow and outflow pressures in an acceptable range. Yet, as can be demonstrated on a mock circulation, these haemodynamic criteria can be met without addressing the metabolic adequacy of the cardiac output. Consider an experiment conducted at the University of Utah Institute for Biomedical Engineering in which the perfusion of animals with pneumatically driven artificial hearts was varied from a baseline condition to hyperperfusion, followed by graded hypoperfusion to extreme cardiogenic shock, and then recovery.[11] The following observations were made during the different perfusion states. In an attempt to make up for the reduced oxygen delivery with a lower cardiac output, greater levels of oxygen extraction as indicated by reduced mixed venous oxygen saturation were measured. Ultimately, however, there was a limitation as to how much oxygen can be extracted, so that as the experiment progressed to even lower levels of cardiac output, the transition from aerobic to anaerobic metabolism occurred as indicated by increasing levels of serum lactate. While devices have already been made that can keep the haemodynamic parameters at the proper level, for the future we can also envision artificial hearts being metabolically smart so that the anaerobic threshold could be avoided by incorporating oxygen saturation sensors in the right and left ventricles. From the oxygen saturation data of these sensors, an index of metabolic adequacy can be calculated to be used as a physiological modifier to the haemodynamic algorithms of the physiological controller.[11]

An elusive developmental criterion for artificial hearts to date has been to make these devices more biologically compatible in terms of being infection-resistant. In the past, Dacron Velour® has been used on drivelines and around devices to promote tissue ingrowth for device anchoring and to form a percutaneous external barrier. The tissue ingrowth stimulated by the Dacron Velour is a tough, fibrous tissue with little vascularity, making surgical explanation of the device difficult and providing a limited vascular access for immune mechanisms to respond to localized infection when and where it occurs. An alternative approach, evolving from plastic and reconstructive surgical research, is the special texturing of implant external surfaces with a spatially specific, porous, silicone material.[12] This material can be made to cover the entire implant. Evaluated both in clinical plastic surgery cases and in animal artificial heart and assist device implantation experiments, unlike materials that stimulate a fibrous encapsulation, this material stimulates a biointegration with soft tissue and a true neovascularity. Based on the nearly two years of cumulative implantation experience in animals, including quantitative bacterial analysis, this textured silicone material holds promise as a relatively infection-free implant interface that may be appropriate for future implantable artificial hearts.

Quality of fit is another critical issue for artificial hearts in the future; if the device does not fit so that it can function properly, the patient cannot be helped. Fundamentally, a good device design and a good surgical positioning of the device would be defined as a good fit. Either an inadequate design or poor device positioning results in a poor fit. When recalling the amount of hardware that will go into a completely implantable artificial heart system, and the desire to accommodate a range of patient sizes, the challenge is formidable. With adequate studies of the three-dimensional anatomy of the cardiac space and remnant attachment tissues, better designed blood pumps will be developed. Using computer-generated, three-dimensional images of the devices coupled with preoperative images of the

thoracic anatomy of the recipient candidate, a preoperative fit assessment can be made by taking the computer image of the artificial heart, placing it in the native cardiac cavity, and check for regions of impingement. Such computer graphic imaging opportunities will aid the patient evaluation and surgical implantation processes as well as lead to the evolution of devices of superior fit.

> 'Well I must go to Oz and get my heart,' said the Woodman. So he walked to the throne room and knocked at the door.
> 'Come in,' called Oz, and the Woodman entered and said, 'I have come for my heart.'
> 'Very well,' said the little man,' but I shall have to cut a hole in your breast so I can put your heart in the right place.' And Oz brought a pair of tinner's shears and cut a small, square hole in the left side of the Tin Woodman's breast. Then he showed the Woodman a pretty heart, made entirely of silk and stuffed with sawdust. 'Isn't it a beauty?' he asked.
> 'Oh, indeed!' replied the Tin Woodman. 'But is it a kind heart?'
> 'Oh, very!' answered Oz. He put the heart in the Woodman's breast, and replaced the square of tin, soldering it neatly.
> The Woodman exclaimed his gratitude and returned to his friends.
> L Frank Baum, *The Wizard of Oz*[13]

There is something else to be said about these hearts; they must be 'user friendly', 'recipient acceptable', or in the words of the Tin Woodman, 'kind'. The image of the Tin Woodman seeking a new heart in the *Wizard of Oz* portrays the perspective of the end-stage heart disease patient simply and clearly. The Wizard, being the 'device developer', is quite pleased with himself, because he has made a heart that looks very nice. The Tin Woodman, however, taking the perspective of the recipient of such a high-risk device, is not so much concerned with how it looks, but if it is 'kind'. What is it that makes a heart kind? It is very simple, as shown in Fig. 21.1—an unkind heart makes you frown, and a kind heart makes you smile. Possibly the issue is not quite that easy, but it gives some insight into the notion of future artificial hearts being 'user friendly' or 'recipient acceptable'.

Current artificial hearts, both pneumatic and electric, generate a great deal of vibration and sound. Therefore, one of the qualities that makes for a 'kind heart' is a device that produces a minimum of noise so that it does not disturb the patient and those around. Although quantitative measurements have demonstrated the dramatic difference between the sound and vibration production of the natural heart and artificial hearts,[14-16] the qualitative experience of visiting with a recipient with one of these devices is sufficient evidence that these devices are much more intrusive than the natural heart. Is it any wonder that more than one artificial heart recipient from farming regions has likened the sound of their artificial heart to that of a tractor or threshing machine? Admittedly, artificial heart and left ventricular assist system recipients report that they learn to accommodate the continuous noise and vibration made by their implant. However, if given the opportunity to choose a quieter device, they would probably select it. Clearly, we have a way to go before we have a 'kind heart' based on noise and vibration production criteria. Improvements in valve closure and energy

converter mechanics may also be able to reduce the sound and vibration production to a more acceptable level.

In the next 25 years, carefully designed and controlled clinical trials will ultimately demonstrate that implanted mechanical pumps will be as safe, reliable, patient compatible, and cost effective as the biological donor heart. This clinical trial result will bring about the reclassification of selected, end-stage heart disease patients as candidates for 'cardiac replacement', instead of 'cardiac transplant'. In the current bridge-to-transplant scheme (Fig. 21.2), the patient with irreversible cardiac dysfunction has failed to be sustained with conventional and experimental medical and surgical therapy or primary mechanical circulatory support (e.g. IABP) before requiring an artificial heart or ventricular assist device(s) to sustain him or her prior to receiving a donor heart. In the future scheme (Fig. 21.3),

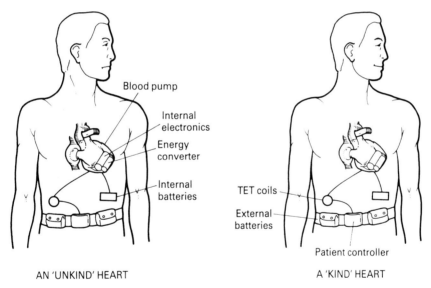

Blood pump
Internal electronics
Energy converter
Internal batteries

TET coils
External batteries
Patient controller

AN 'UNKIND' HEART   A 'KIND' HEART

Fig. 21.1 A 'kind' artificial heart of the future will be completely implantable with compact components for ease of implantation and removal. The entire system must have a high two-year electromechanical and biocompatible reliability and must be physiologically responsive to the needs of the recipient. The devices need to have autodiagnostic capabilities that can be easily interpreted by the recipient and attendee with a minimum of training as well as the possibility of remote transmission of data to the attending surgeon. Of prime importance is that the artificial heart recipient should be able to resume an acceptable quality of life. The recipient should expect normal mobility and freedom from irritating noise and vibration with infrequent medical intervention creating an autonomous livelihood out of the hospital. Soft failures of the device should not endanger the life of the recipient and autodiagnostic alarms should alert the recipient to the nature of the problem. In other words, a 'kind' artificial heart of the future will bring a smile, not a frown, to the face of the recipient and to those people around them.

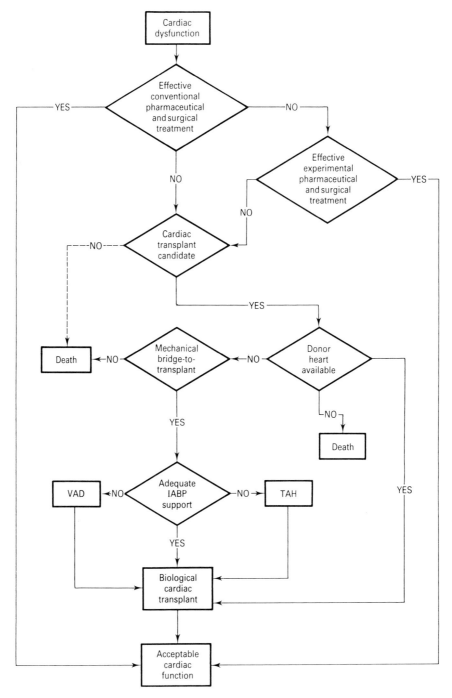

Fig. 21.2 The decision-making chart for the current bridge-to-transplantation scheme. The patient with irreversible cardiac dysfunction has failed to be sustained with conventional or experimental medical and surgical therapy or primary mechanical circulatory support (IABP) before requiring an artificial heart or ventricular assist device(s) to sustain him or her prior to receiving a donor heart.

patients who are accepted as 'cardiac replacement' candidates following the failure of conventional and experimental medical and surgical therapy to reverse their cardiac dysfunction will either receive a biological transplant or mechanical implant, but not have the chance of a staged procedure; bridging to cardiac transplantation will no longer be an option. In the new scheme, the candidate may choose to wait a period of time for a donor heart which will result in a biological

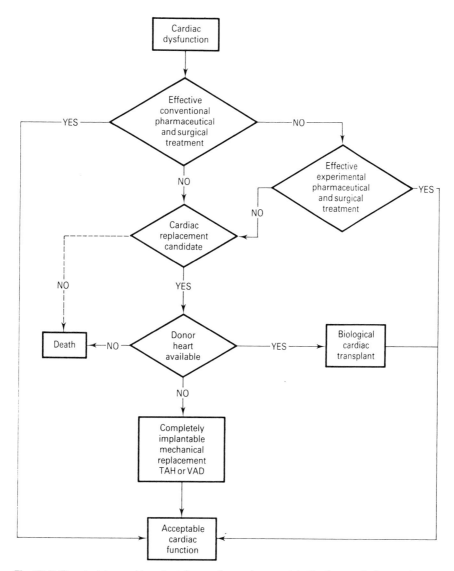

Fig. 21.3 The decision-making chart for cardiac replacement in the future. Patients who are accepted as 'cardiac replacement' candidates following the failure of conventional and experimental medical and surgical therapy to reverse their cardiac dysfunction will receive either a biological transplant or a mechanical implant, but not have the chance of a staged procedure; bridging to cardiac transplantation will no longer be an option. In the cardiac replacement scheme, the candidate may choose to wait for a donor heart which will result in a biological transplant, and the anticipated restoration of health. If a donor heart is not available, the candidate may opt for a mechanical implant, and the anticipated restoration of health, or face the prospect of death.

transplant and the anticipated restoration of health. If a donor heart is not available, the candidate may opt for a mechanical implant and the anticipated restoration of health, or face the prospect of death.

Somewhere in this discussion of the future, we must consider the question, 'How shall we pay the bill?' The economic analysis for the future use of these devices has been expertly presented elsewhere in this book (see Chapter 43). Clearly, these devices must be proven to be cost-effective and quality-effective when compared with conventional therapy if they are to be accepted into standard clinical practice. Complementary to that finding is that health care systems must become even more creative in the identification and mobilization of resources to continue to provide the highest quality and most realistic level of diagnosis-appropriate health care services possible. In the not-too-distant future, it is possible to anticipate that cardiac replacement will take place only at specified regional centres as a cost containment and skills consolidation measure. Cardiogenic shock patients will be stabilized at tertiary care centres with inexpensive, temporary circulatory support devices (e.g. IABP, continuous flow blood pumps) creating time to evaluate the patient's condition and the appropriate course of action. Patients meeting the selection criteria for cardiac replacement will then be transferred to specified regional centres for their surgical procedure, postoperative care, instruction and rehabilitation. The cardiac mobile intensive care unit (MOBI™) developed at the University of Arizona[17] and SWAT team programme developed by the Institut de Recherches Cardio-Vasculaires (Sion, Switzerland)[18] have already demonstrated the feasibility of this approach to treating cardiogenic shock patients not responsive to other therapy.

Regardless of the availability of reliable cardiac replacement devices, in the future there will remain a place for portable, pneumatic or rotary, paracorporeal assist devices. For a yet to be characterized group of cardiac dysfunction patients previously considered only for cardiac transplantation, these temporary pumps will be used for extended, temporary circulatory support until ventricular recovery is achieved.[19] One recent anecdotal case report was for a patient who, after being sustained with a left ventricular assist device as a bridging-to-transplantation for 70 days, ultimately experienced recovery of cardiac function.

The device was removed and the patient was discharged with his own heart, avoiding the lifetime expense and detrimental aspects of cardiac transplantation.

Within the next 50 years, *in vitro* or transgenically bred, genetically engineered biological hearts designed in a manner that will not provoke a rejection response from the immune system will be available for cardiac replacement.[20–22] That prospect may really not be so far-fetched when one considers that it was only 40 years ago that Watson and Crick first identified the sequence of the DNA molecule and all that has been accomplished with genetic engineering in the brief period since their discovery.[23] The advent of these propagated organs will eliminate the need for the bulkier, less efficient mechanical devices if the biological organs can be produced in a great enough quantity.

Within the next 100 years, the collaboration between molecular biologists, genetic engineers, and nanomachinery engineers[24] will develop a therapeutic hybrid device that will be injected into the coronary arteries. These nanomachines will be programmed to support and direct the creation of new, intramyocardial channels for blood flow and the repair of injured or infected myocytes at the cellular level, leading to eventual full recovery of myocardial function, except in the sickest of patients who will still require cardiac replacement. And within the next 500 years, well, perhaps we should save that projection for another edition of *Mechanical Circulatory Support*. In the meantime, it can be anticipated that artificial hearts still represent real hope to patients in end-stage heart disease.

Final thoughts

> The quality of life is at best a relative concept, especially in the context of the artificial-heart project.
>
> Reasonable quality may mean that the patient's level of function is consistent with that of a 'typical' person of the same age. On the other hand, some would argue that for patients eligible for an artificial heart, life at any functional level above coma should be considered of adequate quality.
>
> F Ross Woolley, 1984[25]

I would like to conclude by recognizing the immense amount of inspiration I have received from the mechanical circulatory support patients and their families who have allowed me to become acquainted with them through the course of my career. Particularly, I would like to pay tribute to Michael Templeton, who was a patient implanted with the Thermo Cardiosystems Heart-Mate® left ventricular assist system for 16 months at the Texas Heart Institute. My cardiac function experiments with NASA took me to Houston several times in 1992. During these trips, I always stopped to visit with colleagues at the Texas Heart Institute, at which time Mike and I became acquainted. The last time we visited was in November of 1992. That evening, like any group of colleagues or friends, a few of us, including Mike, hopped into the car and drove to a local pub where we had a couple of pints of beer together before returning Mike to the hospital for the evening. We must have visited for over two hours. The amazing thing about the evening is that other than the four of us in the group, nobody in the pub knew that Mike had an artificial heart. This is exactly the vision that we want for our patients in the future.

I will close with an excerpt from a story about an artificial-heart patient support group:

> Abe began, 'Something happened the other day that helped me. I went to the cardiac ward where I had Lub, my artificial heart, installed.'
>
> 'Why?' asked Colleen.
>
> 'I don't know. There was a little boy there, Colleen, and the intern told me he was in there for an implant. Internal drive. No hose and box stuff. He'll hardly be different from other kids.'
>
> Her eyes widened. 'I didn't know the internal drive had gotten past the experimental stage.' She glanced at him, cautiously. 'Anything like that in the works for us?'
>
> 'The intern said, there is research into the idea. That means, we probably won't be linked to these drives much longer.'
>
> 'We'd be so much happier,' she breathed.
>
> Abe nodded. 'In the future, there will be thousands of kids like that boy, Colleen. They'll all be happier because of us.'
>
> Paula Robinson, *Hearts and Dandelions*, 1989[26]

Thank you, Mike Templeton, and all of the patients who have been willing to be pioneers so that in the future, there will be many happy people that had formerly suffered from end-stage heart disease.

Acknowledgements

Many friends and colleagues in the mechanical circulatory support community generously provided resource material to augment the preparation of this futuristic view, including Jean Kantrowitz (L·VAD Technology Inc.), Ken Butler (Nimbus Inc.), Steve Parnis (Texas Heart Institute), Robert Jarvik (Jarvik Research Inc.), Yoshinori Mitamura (Hokkaido Tokai University, Japan), Erik Koppert (University of Utah), Gus Rosenberg (Pennsylvania State University), William Seare (University of Utah), Rich Smith (University of Arizona Medical Center), Center for Engineering Design (University of Utah), and Harvey Borovetz (University of Pittsburgh). Assistance in the preparation of this chapter was kindly received from Carol Rice and Scott Everett at the Artificial Heart Research Laboratory of the Institute for Biomedical Engineering at the University of Utah. To all of these people, I would like to express my grateful thanks and appreciation for their contributions.

References

1. Hogness JR. Preface. In: Hogness JR, VanAntwerp M (eds), *The Artificial Heart: Prototypes, Policies and Patients*. Washington, DC: National Academic Press, 1991: vii–ix.
2. Kantrowitz A, Freed PS, Cardona RR, Gage K, Marinescu GH, Westveld AH, Litch BA, Hayakawa H, Takano T, Rios CE, Rubenfire M. Initial clinical trial of a closed loop, fully automatic intra-aortic balloon pump. *ASAIO J* 1992; **38**, M617–621.
3. Butler KC, Maher TR, Borovetz HS, Kormos RL, Antaki JF, Kameneva M, Griffith BP, Zerbe T, Schaffer FD. Development of an axial flow blood pump LVAS. *ASAIO J* 1992; **38**, M296–300.
4. Mitamura Y, Yozu R, Tanaka T, Yamazaki K. The Valvo-Pump: an axial, nonpulsatile blood pump. *ASAIO Trans* 1991; **37**, M510–512.
5. Pennington DG, Swartz MT. Circulatory support in infants and children. *Ann Thorac Surg* 1993; **55**, 233–237.
6. Kaye MP. The registry of the International Society for Heart and Lung Transplantation. *J Heart Lung Transplant* 1993; **12**, 541–548.
7. Koppert E, Holfert JW, Dew PA, Pauley J, Pantalos G, Crump K, Burns G. A total artificial heart for neonates allowing bridging to transplantation. *ASAIO Trans* 1990; **36**, M226–230.
8. Flint HE. The devolutionist. *Argosy*, July 1921.
9. White RK, Pantalos GM, Olsen DB. Total artificial heart development at the University of Utah; the

Utah-100 and electrohydraulic cardiac replacement devices. In: Quaal SJ (ed), *Cardiac Mechanical Assistance Beyond Balloon Pumping*. St Louis: Mosby–YearBook Inc., 1993: 181–193.

10. Snyder AJ, Rosenberg G, Weiss WJ, Ford SK, Nazarian RA, Hicks DL, Marlotte JA, Kawaguchi O, Prophet GA, Sapirstein JS, Schwartz M, Pierce WS. *In vivo* testing of a completely implanted total artificial heart system. *ASAIO J* 1993; **39**, M177–184.

11. Robinson P, Pantalos G, Long J, Bliss R, Price D, Everett S, Goldman P, Goldenberg I, Olsen D. Toward development of a physiologic control system modifier based on continuous measurement of oxygen consumption and arterial–venous oxygen saturation following total artificial heart implantation. *Int J Artif Organs* 1993; **16**, 135–140.

12. Seare WJ, Pantalos GM, Burns GL, Burt WR, Olsen DB. Quantitative bacterial analysis of porous, fabric, and smooth non-blood contacting implant surfaces and their tissue interfaces in a 169–day pneumatic total artificial heart animal recipient. *ASAIO J* 1993; **39**, M668–674.

13. Baum LF. *The Wizard of Oz*. New York: Jelly Bean Press, 1991: 79.

14. Pantalos G, Kim C, Robison P, Everett S, Olsen D. Characterization of natural heart and total artificial heart acceleration. *ASAIO Trans* 1989; **35**, 235–238.

15. Reul H, Taguchi K, Herold M, Lo HB, Reck H, Muckter H, Messmer BJ, Rau G. Comparative evaluation of disk and trileaflet valves in left-ventricular assist devices (LVAD). *Int J Artif Organs* 1988; **11**, 127–130.

16. Pantalos G, Kim C, Flatau A. Variation in artificial heart acceleration and sound production with prosthetic valve selection *in vitro*. *Int J Artif Organs*. In press.

17. Icenogle TB, Sato DJ, Smith RG, Cleavinger M, Loffing D, Mikitish SA. Transport of the critically ill cardiac patient. In: Ott RA, Gutfinger DE, Gazzaniga AB (eds), *Cardiac Surgery: State of the Art Reviews (Mechanical Cardiac Assit)*, vol 7, no 2. Philadelphia: Hanley & Belfus, 1993: 241–248.

18. Meli M, Odermatt R, Brugger J-P, Hahn C. Organization and experience of a mobile team to support European cardiac centers. In: Quaal SJ (ed), *Cardiac Mechanical Assistance Beyond Balloon Pumping*. St Louis: Mosby–YearBook, 1993: 355–369.

19. Holman WL, Bourge RC, Kirklin JK. Case report: circulatory support for seventy days with resolution of acute heart failure. *J Thorac Cardiovas Surg* 1991; **102**, 932–934.

20. Michler RE, Chen JM. Cardiac xenotransplantation: a therapy whose time has come. *Xeno* 1994; **2**(4): 55–57.

21. Gundry S. Is it time for clinical xenotransplantation (again)? *Xeno* 1994; **2**(4): 60–61.

22. Smith JA, Rosengard BR, Wallwork J. Cardiopulmonary xenotransplantation: the past, the present, and future prospects. In press.

23. Watson JW, Crick FHC. A structure for deoxyribose nucleic acid. *Nature* 1953; **171**, 737–738.

24. Jacobsen SC, Wood JE, Price RH. Micromotors split hairs: mechanical systems join electronics in the microscopic world. *IEEE Potentials*, Feb 1991, 12–15.

25. Woolley FR. Ethical issues in the implantation of the total artificial heart. *New Engl J Med* 1984; **310**, 292–296.

26. Robinson P. Hearts and dandelions. *Analog*, Oct 1989, 94–112.

22

The Novacor® left ventricular assist system

Peer M Portner, Jal S Jassawalla and Philip E Oyer

Introduction

Cardiac transplantation is the only therapy currently available for terminal heart failure. After a period of clinical development in the 1970s, the introduction of cyclosporine resulted in the proliferation of transplant centres and a rapid growth in cardiac transplants in the early 1980s.[1] However, the supply of donor organs has not kept pace with the demand, and both the waiting period for a cardiac allograft and the number of patients who die while waiting have increased substantially.[2,3] The potential for heart replacement in the United States has been estimated to be greater, by an order of magnitude or more, than the donor supply.[4]

Implantable, electrically powered left ventricular assist and biventricular replacement systems have been under development for more than a decade. Intended for chronic, untethered circulatory support in patients with end-stage heart failure, these systems will provide the first therapeutic alternative to transplantation. The Novacor® left ventricular assist system (LVAS) was the first integrated electrically powered system designed for long-term human use[5,6] and the first such technology to be used clinically.[7,8]

The shortage of donor hearts has prompted the increasing investigational use of circulatory assist and replacement devices to prolong survival while waiting for a suitable organ. The first successful bridge-to-transplant (BTT) was performed in 1984 at the Stanford University Medical Center with a Novacor assist system.[7] The 51-year-old patient with end-stage ischaemic disease, first in a multicentre clinical trial, remained alive and well as he approached nine years post-transplantation.

Design considerations

The Novacor LVAS was designed, from first principles, for long-term circulatory support—electrically powered, self-regulating, physiologically responsive and, ultimately, totally implantable. Performance specifications included low filling pressures, full support of the systemic circulation and efficient operation. Blood compatibility imposed design constraints on the blood pump and its actuating mechanism. The need for high reliability and durability dictated mechanical simplicity and electronic functional redundancy. The overriding design consideration was for quality of life with primary attention to recipient safety, comfort and confidence.

System configuration

System configuration[9] and anatomic placement of the totally implantable LVAS are illustrated in Fig. 22.1. The pump/drive unit is implanted within the abdominal wall, in the left upper

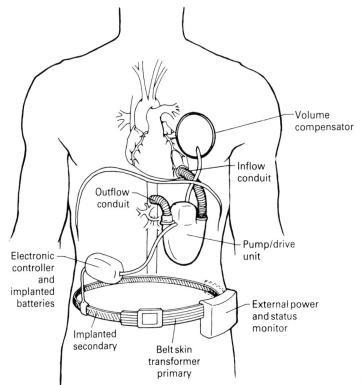

Fig. 22.1 Anatomic placement of the totally implantable Novacor assist system.

quadrant, anterior to the posterior rectus sheath and between the costal margin and iliac crest. Externally reinforced inflow and outflow conduits, of low-porosity woven Dacron (Meadox Medical Inc., New Jersey), penetrate the diaphragm at the costal margin and connect the pump between the left ventricular apex and the ascending aorta. The variable volume compensator (VVC) is placed in the left pleural space and communicates with the space enclosed by the pump/drive unit encapsulation through a flexible, wire-reinforced tube that traverses the diaphragm. The electronic controller is implanted in the right subcostal region and connected by flexible leads to the pump/drive unit and belt skin transformer (BST) secondary.

The BST consists of a pair of flexible concentric coils positioned around the waist with a five-turn external primary overlying the subcutaneously implanted, single-turn, compliant secondary. This geometry, unlike that of more traditional pancake coils, is insensitive to axial alignment of the primary and secondary, thus greatly facilitating stable magnetic coupling.[10] Other externally worn components include the external power and sta-

tus monitor (EPSM) and rechargeable batteries. The EPSM provides visual and audible system status indicators and alarms. A hospital monitor (not shown) allows for periodic monitoring of system performance and adjustment of LVAS operating parameters. A home monitor with power supply (also not shown) enables periodic interrogation of LVAS data, and serves as an alternative night-time (or stationary) power source.

In the first, developmental, configuration, LVAS power and control electronics were externalized within an extracorporeal console (Fig. 22.2). This configuration was used during the early evaluation in experimental animals and in the initial phase of clinical studies. Modular in design, console circuits are redundant. Uninterruptible power supplies protect against power failure and enable patient transport or ambulation. A percutaneous vent tube, containing power and control leads, is tunnelled from the pump pocket inferior to the umbilicus to exit near the right anterior superior iliac spine. A Dacron–velour covering, to encourage tissue ingrowth, and a long subcutaneous path minimize the risk

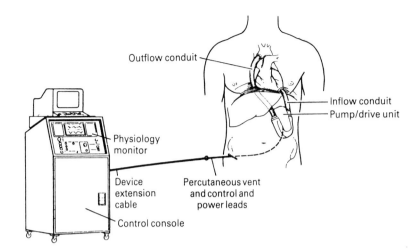

Fig. 22.2 Console-based bridge-to-transplant system.

of infection. A 7 m extension cable from the percutaneous lead to the console allows considerable patient mobility. The console incorporates a physiology monitor that continuously displays electrocardiogram, left ventricular pressure, systemic pressure and instantaneous pump volume.

A 'wearable LVAS' configuration, representing a hybrid of the totally implantable and console-based systems, was recently introduced. Offering considerably improved mobility and freedom from a tether, the wearable system utilizes the controller/EPSM circuitry and batteries of the totally implantable design and the pump/drive unit and percutanous lead of the console-based configuration. The wearable, ergonomically designed, controller can be worn within the recipient's clothing. It obtains power from redundant sources: the wearable primary and reserve battery packs (Fig. 22.3) for an ambulating recipient, or a single battery pack and the hospital or home monitor during stationary periods such as during sleep.

Pump/drive unit

The pump/drive unit consists of a dual pusher-plate sac-type blood pump (Fig. 22.4) integrally coupled to a unique spring-decoupled pulsed-solenoid energy converter and encapsulated in a fibreglass-reinforced polyester shell (Fig. 22.5). The blood pump has a one-piece seamless sac with a smooth polyether–urethane (Biomer, Ethicon Inc., New Jersey) blood contacting surface. The sac is bonded to a pair of symmetrically opposed pusher plates and to a lightweight aramid/epoxy housing that incorporates fittings for 21 mm, silicone-flanged, custom bovine pericardial valves (Edwards CVS Division, Baxter Healthcare Corp., Irvine, California).

The balanced energy converter (drive) has only two moving parts: identical armature/spring assemblies pivoting symmetrically within a skeletal aluminium frame. This simple and reliable design provides efficient and physiological transformation of electrical to mechanical energy. With a nominal maximum stroke volume of 70 ml, pump outputs in excess of 10 litres/min and synchronous operation at cardiac rates as high as 240 beats/min have been achieved.

The pump/drive unit utilized in the initial evaluation of the totally implantable system had a trilaminate sac of Biomer/butyl rubber/Biomer to limit moisture diffusion, 25 mm silicone-flanged custom porcine xenograft valves and a 90 ml stroke volume.

Electronic controller

Power conditioning circuits and all LVAS control functions, including solenoid energization and timing, are incorporated within the microprocessor-based controller. Optimal solenoid closure is achieved with real-time servo-control.[11] LVAS operation is programmed for synchronous counterpulsation and utilizes a 'Frank–Starling' control algorithm responsive to pump fill, without the need for physiological sensors. All control information is derived from internal proximity displacement transducers, which provide a continuous measure of solenoid

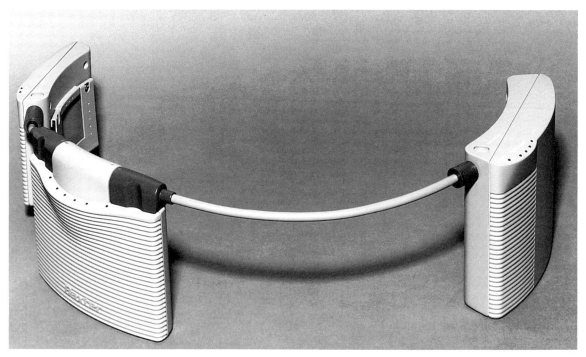

Fig. 22.3 Wearable controller (left foreground) connected to primary (right) and reserve battery packs.

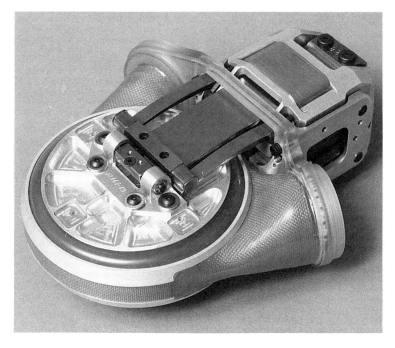

Fig. 22.4 Unencapsulated, dual-pusher-plate blood pump coupled to spring-decoupled solenoid energy converter.

armature gap, pump volume and pump fill and ejection rates. Asynchronous, fixed-rate or fill-to-empty modes may also be selected.

While the console-based controller employed discrete circuits, the miniaturized implantable and wearable controllers incorporate custom-hybrid power and surface-mount control circuits utilizing large-scale CMOS application-specific integrated circuits. The implantable controller contains a rechargeable NiCd battery that provides approximately one half hour of independent LVAS operation and freedom from external components to facilitate bathing and general hygiene.

Preclinical testing

Extensive *in vitro* testing was conducted to characterize performance and to demonstrate reliability and durability. Characterization over a wide range of preloads, afterloads and rates was performed on customized NIH mock circulatory loops. Synchronous counterpulsation with substantial left ventricular decompression was demonstrated over the physiological range of haemodynamics.[9] The LVAS has been shown to be instantaneously responsive to changes in haemodynamic variables.

Long-term durability testing has been carried out at the system, subsystem and component levels. More than 130 years of pump testing has been accumulated on multi-station pump testers and in pump/drive *in vitro* testing. Four pumps continue on test after 8 years. Energy converters have accumulated more than 60 years of endurance testing in pump/drive units, without failure. Accelerated testing of the most highly stressed system components (decoupling springs, energy storage capacitors) has also been carried out.

Reliability testing, under formal refereed conditions, of twelve totally implantable systems was

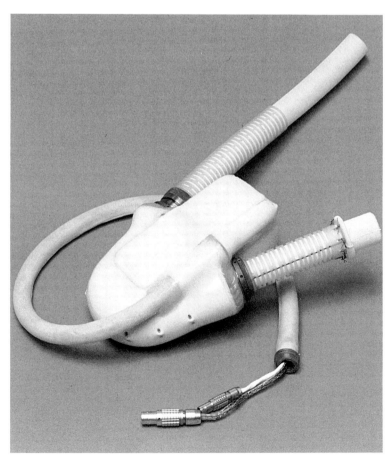

Fig. 22.5 Encapsulated unit, with inflow (right) and outflow conduits and percutaneous vent tube containing power and control leads.

conducted as part of an NIH-sponsored pre-clinical device readiness testing (DRT) pro-gramme.[12] Systems were placed on test in individual, instrumented, mock circulatory loops under conditions simulating a physiological envi-ronment (implantable components immersed in saline at body temperature). Pump flows were cycled, on a diurnal basis, between 6 and 9 litres/min to simulate sleeping and waking periods, while maintaining a physiological preload and afterload. Each system was switched to its internal battery for 20 minutes each day. More than 26 years of life testing were accumulated (average 2.2 years) without failure. All systems completed the two-year mission (two systems were run for nearly three years) before elective termination (Fig. 22.6). The resulting demonstrated reliability of 89% at an 80% confidence level significantly exceeded the NIH objective (80% reliability at 60% confidence). In addition, five complete wear-able systems continued on life test without failure after more than two years.

Since the initiation of animal testing in 1972, more than 250 experiments have been conducted to characterize system performance. Until early 1984, young bovines were used in pump/drive experiments and dogs were used for BST studies. The adult ovine has been used since then, obviat-ing the problems of growth, pannus and accel-erated valve mineralization observed in the immature bovine model.[13] Anticoagulation and platelet anti-aggregating agents were not used. Experimental animals were instrumented for chronic measurement of pressures and flows, and data acquisition/analysis was carried out in real-time.

In vivo experiments have demonstrated support of the entire systemic circulation under condi-tions of severe myocardial failure and ventricular fibrillation. Chronic studies have demonstrated system safety and efficacy. More than 18 years of pump/drive implant experience have been accu-mulated with 30 experiments exceeding 3 months, 12 exceeding 5 months and the longest extending to 10 months. Haematology, coagula-tion and blood chemistry values remained within the normal range. Device-related complications, including haemolysis, infection and thromboem-bolism, were infrequent. Implant duration was limited by valve calcification and, in the bovine, by pseudoneointimal proliferation in the inflow con-duit, resulting in progressive stenosis, declining flow and elective termination.

Normal VVC function was documented, both in total system (to 9 months) and subsystem (to 2 years) studies, with stable compliance and no gross or histologic evidence of fibrous encapsula-tion. More than 40 years of BST experience has been accumulated in experiments extending to 3 years. The subcutaneous belt was well tolerated

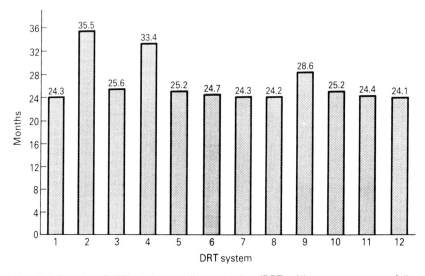

Fig. 22.6 Results of NIH device readiness testing (DRT). All systems successfully completed a two-year test with no failures. Total test time = 26.6 years; mean test time = 26.6 months.

with minimal evidence of inflammatory response and no fibrous encapsulation.

Clinical evaluation

A multicentre BTT clinical trial, utilizing the console-based Novacor system, was initiated in 1984 at Stanford and subsequently expanded to more than 25 centres in the USA and Europe. The results of this clinical evaluation are presented in Chapter 24.

More recently, the BTT study has been extended to include the wearable Novacor system. The first wearable implant was successfully carried out at the Henri Mondor Hospital of the University of Paris (D Loisance *et al.*, personal communication). Two additional patients have since been successfully bridged at other European centres (Universities of Munich and Münster). The duration of support in these three patients ranged from 44 to 57 days. All were fully rehabilitated prior to transplantation and each demonstrated the freedom provided by the wearable configuration.

Discussion

An implantable assist system specifically designed for definitive treatment of patients with terminal heart failure, the Novacor LVAS, is at an advanced stage of development. A considerable body of *in vitro* testing, animal studies and clinical evaluation has demonstrated safe and effective long-term performance.

The design of the Novacor LVAS offers some unique advantages over systems with motor-driven diaphragm pumps. The simplicity of the solenoid energy converter, with only two moving parts, has resulted in high reliability and durability. Its symmetric design ensures balanced closure and obviates the transfer of reaction forces or motion to adjacent tissues. Symmetric displacement of the pump's two pusher plates substantially reduces deformation and stress on the polyurethane sac while, at the same time, maintaining optimal flow characteristics throughout the pumping cycle. The increased area provided by two pusher plates minimizes pump filling pressures. Controller independence from physiological sensors ensures stable LVAS operation. The controller can be readily programmed to vary the

load on the left ventricle—a unique capability of the system design. During the early postoperative period, ventricular unloading may facilitate improved myocardial function while, at a later time, increased loading may prevent myocardial decompensation secondary to chronic unloading.

The BTT clinical experience has clearly demonstrated the ability to fully rehabilitate severely incapacitated patients with terminal congestive heart failure. It has, therefore, provided a unique opportunity to demonstrate feasibility in the intended long-term application.

References

1. Kaye MP. The Registry of the International Society for Heart and Lung Transplantation: Ninth Official Report. *J Heart Lung Transplant* 1992; **11**, 599–606.
2. Evans RW, Mannion DL, Garrison LP, Maier AM. Donor availability as the primary determinant of the future of heart transplantation. *JAMA* 1986; **225**, 1892–1898.
3. Copeland JG, Emery RW, Levinson MM, Copeland J, McAleer MJ, Riley JE. The role of mechanical support and transplantation in treatment of patients with end-stage cardiomyopathy. *Circulation* 1985; **72** (Suppl 2), 7–12.
4. Hogness JR, Antwerp MV. *The Artificial Heart: Prototypes, Policies and Patients*. Washington, DC: National Academy Press, 1991.
5. Portner PM, Oyer PE, Jassawalla JS, Miller PJ, Chen H, LaForge DH, Skytte KW. An implantable permanent left ventricular assist system for man. *ASAIO Trans* 1978; **24**, 98–102.
6. Portner PM, Oyer PE, Jassawalla JS, Miller PJ, Chen H, LaForge DH, Green GP, Shumway NE. An alternative in end-stage heart disease: long-term ventricular assist. *Heart Transplant* 1983; **3**, 47–59.
7. Portner PM, Oyer PE, McGregor CGA, Baldwin JC, Ream AK, Wyner J, Zusman DR, Shumway NE. First human use of an electrically powered implantable ventricular assist system. *Artif Organs* 1985; **9**(a), 36.
8. Portner PM, Oyer PE, Pennington DG, Baumgartner WA, Griffith BP, Frist WR, Magilligan DJ, Noon GP, Ramasamy N, Miller PJ, Jassawalla JS. Implantable electrical left ventricular assist system: bridge to transplantation and the future. *Ann Thorac Surg* 1989; **41**, 142–150.
9. Portner PM, Jassawalla JS, Oyer PE, Chen H, Miller PJ, LaForge DH, Ramasamy N, Lee J, Billich J, Beering FK, Conley MG, Sohrab B, Ryan M, Daniel MA, Strauss LR, Brugler JS, Ream AK, Shumway NE. A totally implantable ventricular assist system

for terminal heart failure. In: Kantrowitz A (ed), *Primers in Artificial Organs: Left Ventricular Assist Devices.* JB Lippincott, Philadelphia: JB Lippincott, 1988: 57–76.

10. LaForge DH, Lee J, Beering FK, Portner PM. The belt skin transformer for energy transmission to implanted circulatory support devices. In: Andrade JD (ed), *Artificial Organs.* New York: VCH Publishers, 1987: 95–107.

11. Brugler JS, LaForge DH, Lee J, Rising DL, Billich J, Miller PJ, Jassawalla JS, Portner PM. Implanted control and power electronics for a left ventricular assist system. *Proc Intersoc Energy Conv Eng Conf* 1985; **20**, 1613–1627.

12. Jassawalla JS, Daniel MA, Chen H, Lee J, LaForge DH, Billich J, Ramasamy N, Miller PJ, Oyer PE, Portner PM. *In vitro* and *in vivo* testing of a totally implantable left ventricular assist system. *ASAIO Trans* 1988; **34**, 470–475.

13. Ramasamy N, Miller PJ, Green GF, Oyer PE, Baldwin JC, Ream AK, Wyner J, Portner PM. Long-term studies with an electromechanical ventricular assist system in the calf and sheep. In: Nose Y, Kjellstrand C, Ivanovich P (eds), *Progress in Artificial Organs—1985.* Cleveland: ISAO Press, 1986: 456–463.

23

Clinical experience with the Novacor® left ventricular assist system

D Glenn Pennington, Peer M Portner and Marc T Swartz

Introduction

The Novacor® left ventricular assist system (LVAS) was the first integrated system designed for long-term use in humans. It was also the first electrically powered implantable circulatory support device to be used clinically.

The first attempt to bridge a patient to cardiac transplantation was performed in 1969 using an orthotopic pneumatic total artificial heart.[1] In 1978, the first patient was bridged to cardiac transplantation using a ventricular assist device (VAD);[2] unfortunately this patient died of infection soon after transplantation. The first successful bridge to transplant using a VAD was performed at Stanford University Medical Center in 1984 using the Novacor LVAS.[3] The first successful bridge with a total artificial heart was achieved early in 1985 at the University of Arizona.[4]

In the Novacor bridge-to-transplant trials described here, the LVAS power and control electronics were contained in a free-standing console. This console is modular in design, with redundant control circuits and uninterruptible power supplies. It has a monitor that displays an electrocardiogram and left ventricular and systemic pressure waveforms in addition to the pump volume trace.

Clinical evaluation

After extensive preclinical evaluation, including *in vitro* and *in vivo* testing (see Chapter 22) a clinical protocol for temporary application using the console-based system was approved by the US Food and Drug Administration. The clinical trial was initiated at Stanford University Medical Center and subsequently expanded to 17 centres in the USA and five in Europe.

Patients selected for the bridge-to-transplant clinical trial had to be in terminal heart failure either as a result of chronic cardiomyopathy or a massive acute myocardial infarction. Appropriate candidates all demonstrated deteriorating end-organ function despite maximal pharmacological and/or IABP support. Inclusion criteria for the Novacor bridge-to-transplant clinical trial are shown in Table 23.1. Exclusion criteria are shown

Table 23.1 Patient inclusion criteria.

- Accepted/acceptable transplant candidate
- Age between 15 and 65 years
- Body surface area between 1.5 and 2.5 m^2
- Haemodynamic deterioration as evidenced by one of the following:
  - ■ Cardiac index <2.0 litres/min/m^2 *and* mean arterial pressure <65 mmHg or left atrial pressure (pulmonary capillary wedge pressure) >18 mmHg

OR

  - ■ Increasing inotropic support and/or need for IABP (to include two inotropes at a predetermined high dose, or IABP and one inotrope)

Table 23.2 Exclusion criteria.

- Pulmonary parenchymal disease and/or fixed pulmonary hypertension (pulmonary vascular resistance >6 wood units, pulmonary artery systolic >65 mmHg)
- Renal or hepatic dysfunction not explained by underlying heart failure and deemed irreversible
- Systemic infection unresponsive to treatment
- Documented cerebrovascular or peripheral vascular disease
- Cancer with metastases
- Blood dyscrasia that would predispose to uncontrollable bleeding
- Prosthetic aortic valve

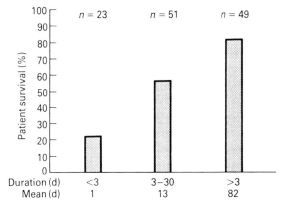

Fig. 23.1 Survival to transplant *versus* duration of support.

in Table 23.2 and are very similar to those routinely followed for cardiac transplantation.

Prophylactic antibiotics were administered during the perioperative period. Postoperatively, clinically significant infections were treated on an individual basis. Anticoagulation, usually with heparin (partial thromboplastin time 1.5 times control), was started when chest tube drainage decreased to acceptable levels. Most patients were converted to an oral anticoagulant regimen of warfarin (prothrombin time 1.5 times control) within one to two weeks. Platelet deaggregating drugs, initially intravenous low-molecular-weight dextran and then aspirin and/or dipyridamole for the duration of support, were also administered. In patients with postoperative bleeding complications, the initiation of anticoagulation was often delayed.

After a donor heart was located and at the time of cardiac transplantation, cardiopulmonary bypass was instituted, LVAS pumping discontinued and the inflow and outflow conduits cross-clamped and divided. The vent tube was isolated from the sterile field and transected near the pump. The pump/drive unit and the percutaneous vent tube were removed from the sterile field and cardiac transplantation performed in the usual manner.

Clinical results

At the time of writing, 129 patients (116 male, 13 female) had been bridged to transplant using the Novacor LVAS. Ages ranged from 15 to 67 years (mean 45) with 60% of the patients in their 40s and 50s. Patient weight ranged from 49 to 142 kg (mean 78) and body surface area was 1.54–2.78 m^2 (mean 1.91). The aetiology of heart

failure was cardiomyopathy (mainly idiopathic) in 60 patients (47%), end-stage ischaemic disease in 39 patients (30%), acute myocardial infarction in 27 patients (21%), acute viral myocarditis in two patients and acute allograft rejection in one patient.

Duration of LVAS support ranged from hours to 370 days (mean 42 days). Twenty-three patients (19%) were supported for less than three days, 51 patients (41%) were supported for 3–30 days and 49 patients (40%) were supported for greater than 30 days. As shown in Fig. 23.1, survival to transplant improves significantly with duration of support. Excluding ongoing implants, 60% of patients were transplanted and 89% of those transplanted were discharged. The overall survival for patients supported greater than 30 days has been 82%.

Forty-nine patients died while on LVAS support, nine intraoperatively and 40 in the postoperative period. The primary cause of death in patients supported less than three days was bleeding, respiratory failure and multiorgan failure. In patients supported 3–30 days, the primary cause of death was multiorgan failure. No primary cause of death could be identified in the patients supported longer than 30 days. In all of these cases, however, the complications and cause of death had developed early in the period of support.

Pre-LVAS haemodynamics improved significantly after placement of the device. Pre-implant cardiac index increased from 1.89 ± 0.47 to $3.02 \pm 0.62 \, 1/m^2/min$ ($p < 0.0005$) within 24 hours, while during the same period the pulmonary artery diastolic pressure decreased from 28.0 ± 8.4 to 19.3 ± 6.1 mmHg ($p < 0.0005$).

Adequate right ventricular function was maintained in most patients in the early postoperative period with low to moderate amounts of inotropic or pulmonary vasodilator support. In 25 patients (19%), it was necessary to insert a right ventricular assist device (RVAD) using an extra-corporeal centrifugal pump. Eighteen of these patients did not survive to transplantation. Seven patients were weaned off RVAD support after an average of 6.4 days, and were then maintained on univentricular support. Three were successfully transplanted.

At the time of LVAS implantation, most patients exhibited moderate to severe major organ dysfunction. Pre-implant blood chemistries were not useful in predicting reversibility of organ dysfunction. For example, there was no statistically significant difference in pre-LVAS creatinine between transplanted and non-transplanted patients. However, creatinine continued to rise despite adequate perfusion in many of those who died during the period of support.

Once stabilized after LVAS implantation, most haematological values remained within normal limits. There was little or no haemolysis, with plasma-free haemoglobin levels usually below 5 mg/dl.

The most common complications during LVAS support were bleeding/coagulopathy and infection. There have been some minor technical problems, but there have been no mechanical failures. The incidence of device-related complications including infection and thromboembolism was low—the same for patients successfully transplanted as for those who died while supported—and, therefore, did not significantly affect outcome.

Sixty-six (89%) of the 74 patients transplanted were discharged and 61 (82%) are long-term survivors. Post-transplant actuarial survival compares favourably with that for routine, non-staged cardiac transplantation (Fig. 23.2). Early post-transplant mortality (less than 30 days) was due to allograft failure, sepsis or presumed sepsis, and acute rejection. Late mortality was due to rejection, infection, presumed arrhythmia, and colon cancer.

Discussion

The Novacor LVAS was specifically designed for chronic support in patients with end-stage heart

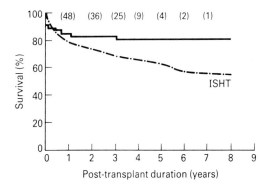

Fig. 23.2 Post-transplant actuarial survival of Novacor LVAS bridge-to-transplant patients *versus* conventional cardiac transplant recipients (International Society of Heart and Lung Transplantation).

disease. Pre-clinical and clinical (bridge application) evaluations have shown that the Novacor LVAS is capable of long-term, safe and effective performance. Reliability and durability have been documented in all phases of the programme to date.

The Novacor design offers a number of significant advantages when compared with other systems in development. The presence of dual pusher plates substantially reduces stress on the blood sac and ensures optimal flow throughout the pumping cycle. Solenoid drive is simple with only two moving parts, resulting in a high level of reliability. The control modes allow physiological control of pump function throughout a wide range of patient activity levels.

Patient selection criteria and better methods to detect irreversible organ dysfunction need to be developed. Post-implant right ventricular failure, bleeding, thromboembolism and infection remain significant problems to overcome, although there has been dramatic improvement in all of these areas within the past five years. Further advances are expected as experience is gained and technology continues to evolve.

The clinical experience with bridging to transplantation has gone a long way toward demonstrating the rehabilitative potential of mechanical circulatory support in patients with end-stage heart disease. The positive correlation between the duration of support and survival demonstrates the ultimate benefits of this technology. The bridge-to-transplant clinical trials have provided clinicians with a unique opportunity to explore the potential of chronic mechanical circulatory support and have provided a glimpse of what the future has to offer.

References

1. Cooley DA, Liotta D, Hall GL, Bloodwell RD, Leachman RD, Milam JD. Orthotopic cardiac prosthesis for two-staged cardiac replacement. *Am J Cardiol* 1969; **24**, 723–730.
2. Norman JC, Cooley DA, Kahan BD, Keats AS, Massin EK, Solis RT, Luper WE, Brook MI, Klima T, Frazier OH, Hacker J, Duncan JM, Dasco CC, Winston DS, Reul GJ. Total support of the circulation of a patient with postcardiotomy stone-heart syndrome by a partial artificial heart (ALVAD) for five days followed by heart and kidney transplantation. *Lancet* 1978; **i**, 1125–1127.
3. Portner PM, Oyer PE, McGregore CGA, Baldwin JC, Ream AK, Wyner J, Zusman DR, Shumway NE. First human use of an electrically-powered implantable ventricular assist system. *Artif Organs* 1985; **9(a)**, 36.
4. Copeland JG, Levinson MM, Smith R, Icenogle TB, Vaughn C, Cheng K, Ott R, Emery RW. The total artificial heart as a bridge to transplantation: a report of two cases. *JAMA* 1986; **256**, 2991–2995.

24

The TCI HeartMate® blood pump

Victor L Poirier

Introduction

Thermo Cardiosystems Inc. (TCI) developed the HeartMate® blood pump that can be driven by either air or electrical energy. This device is designed for long-term use and is therefore configured to be fully implantable.[1] The pump and driver are positioned in the abdominal cavity, just inferior to the left hemidiaphragm (Fig. 24.1). The inlet conduit is inserted into the left ventricular cavity, while the outlet conduit is attached to the ascending aorta. With this arrangement, blood from the ventricle simply drains into the blood pump chamber, whence it can be expelled through the outlet conduit into the arterial system.

System description

The HeartMate blood pump is a pusher-plate type of device as shown in Fig. 24.2. It has a discoid shape and is fabricated from titanium with 6% aluminium and 4% vanadium. The pump body is 11.2 cm in diameter and 4 cm thick. The inlet conduit consists of a 19 mm-diameter inlet tube connected to a 25 mm porcine xenograft valve. The pump body has a stroke volume of 83 cm^3 and the pump can produce flows in excess of 10 l/min. The pumping chamber consists of a polyether polyurethane diaphragm bonded to a rigid piston. The outlet conduit consists of a

25 mm diameter porcine xenograft valve attached to a 20 mm Dacron conduit.

All blood-contacting surfaces are textured.[2,3] Metal components are textured with titanium spheres bonded to the substrate, while the polyurethane surface is textured by extruding filaments from the base membrane. Fig. 24.3 illustrates these surfaces.

The electric HeartMate system[4] consists of an implantable blood pump and driver coupled with electrical and vent lines to an external console and battery pack. Support hardware consists of a bedside battery charger and power unit, as well as an auxiliary digital display unit that can be used in the operating theatre or ICU, or under other non-ambulatory conditions.

Diagnostic evaluation of the system is obtained through a software program developed by TCI. A personal computer can be linked to the power unit to document motor performance as a function of time, and to reprogram the portable patient controller. All data are kept on disk for evaluation.

As shown in Fig. 24.4, the electromechanical driver[5] consists of an electronically commutated low-speed torque motor that drives the pusher plate through a pair of nested helical cams. The torque motor itself consists of a stationary copper wave-wound stator, a rotating magnet assembly and an electronic commutator. The electronic commutator uses solid-state Hall-effect devices to sense rotor position and, through electronic logic, switches the power transistors that control power distribution to the windings. This starts from any position when power is applied. No startup sequence is required.

The motor operates at physiological speeds, with one motor revolution corresponding to one pump ejection cycle. As the magnet assembly of the torque motor rotates, two diametrically opposed ball-bearing cam followers bear against nested helical face cams. These face cams are fixed to the pusher plate and serve to convert the rotary motion of the pump to the linear motion of the pusher plate.

The control system reacts to each ejection cycle as an individual event. When the commutator receives a start signal, it rotates one revolution and stops. The motor then sits in the standby configuration until another start signal is received. There is no need to predict future events based on past history. The stop position is determined by a Hall sensor on the commutator ring and a small magnet buried in the titanium hub of the rotor.

The weight of the combined pump, torque motor and energy converter is 908 g and the displacement is 460 cm^3. The conduits weigh an additional 161 g and the displacement is 174 cm^3. This includes all protective housing, cables, tubes and connectors.

The blood pump driver assembly is connected to the external environment by two lines: one to carry electrical energy and the other to allow air to transfer in and out of the motor chamber. Air transfer is required to maintain the pressure in this cavity at atmospheric conditions. For every beat, a volume of air equivalent to the volume of blood pumped must be accommodated.

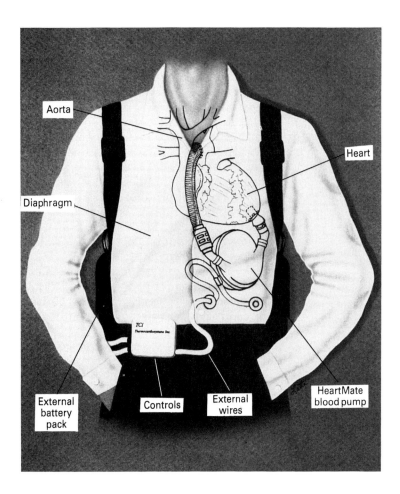

Fig. 24.1 Implant position for the vented electric model of the HeartMate blood pump.

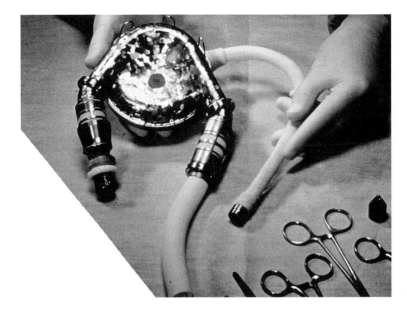

Fig. 24.2 The HeartMate blood pump.

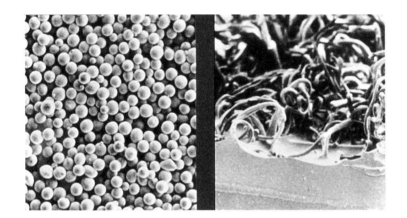

Fig. 24.3 Magnified views of rigid and flexible textured surfaces. On the left is a sintered titanium microsphere (STM) surface (×40). On the right is an integrally textured polyurethane (ITP) surface (×80).

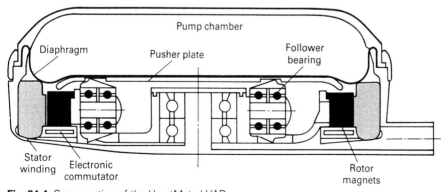

Fig. 24.4 Cross-section of the HeartMate LVAD.

The vented electric system is operated by a portable control system (Fig. 24.5) which is worn by the patient. It is designed to be as small as possible so that it can be conveniently clipped on to a belt. Its dimensions are $6.2 \times 7.6 \times 1.9$ cm with a total weight with attached cables and connectors of 275 g. Permanently mounted to the housings are two leads that connect to a pair of batteries via a positive acting, push-type sealed connector. Power is derived from either one or two batteries to provide redundancy. The preferred orientation to maximize battery life is to use the system coupled in parallel to two batteries. When one battery is used, battery life will be reduced to approximately one half the expected time that two batteries would provide.

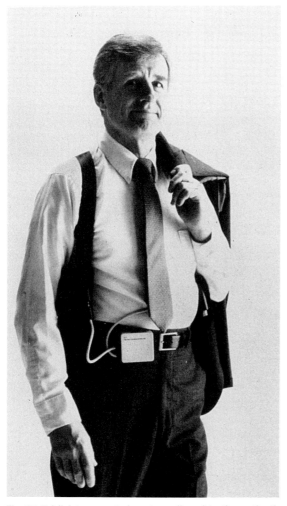

Fig. 24.5 Miniature control system clipped to the patient's belt.

The control system is designed to provide power conditioning to the motor, rate control, documentation of operating parameters, diagnostic information, basal level default capability as well as a sophisticated alarm system to provide the patient with a warning on malfunction.

Motor rate control is optional and can be modified by either the patient or by the attending physician. The control system incorporates a two-position membrane switch that can be controlled by the patient. The primary position establishes a predetermined fixed rate that can be varied between 50 and 120 beats/min in increments of 1 beat/min. When the switch is depressed by the patient, the control function will be changed to either a fixed-rate augmentation by a step difference between 1 and 20 beats/min or to an 'auto-mode'. The auto-mode automatically varies the rate as a function of the volume of blood entering the pump chamber to maintain the pump stroke volume at 75 cm^3 per beat. The rate of change can be adjusted between 1 and 5 beats/min.

The control system digitizes the analogue signals of motor current and voltage. These waveforms (Fig. 24.6) are used to calculate stroke volume as well as to determine motor operating voltage. In addition, the waveforms can be accessed through a software system for display on a personal computer for permanent storage on disk. System performance can then be documented on a real-time basis to establish wear trends over time.

This system utilizes two commercially available gel cell type lead–acid batteries. These standard six-cell packs are $18 \times 6 \times 2$ cm and weigh 636 g each.

A power unit (Fig. 24.7) provides the patient with an isolated 12 V source to energize the electrical system during periods when the batteries are not appropriate. In addition, this unit recharges up to six batteries at a time. A digital display can also be attached to this power unit to continuously display stroke volume, rate and flow.

Two emergency systems are provided to the patients. First, because the pump can be driven pneumatically, a portable hand-pump is provided to every patient in the event of a malfunction. The hand-pump can be attached quickly to the vent line exiting the patient. Pumping can then be restored with pneumatic energy to nearly equivalent flows as with electrical acutation. The operation of the hand-pump can be carried out for

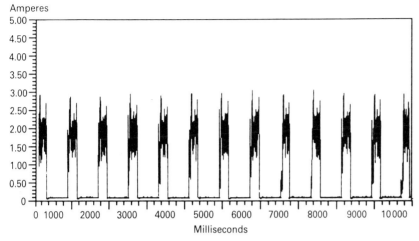

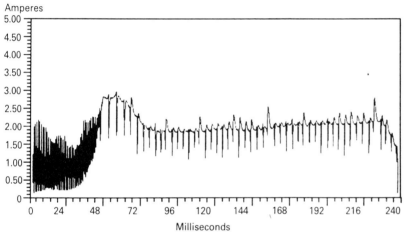

Fig. 24.6 The top trace shows a series of current waveforms obtained from the miniature control system; an expanded view of one cycle is shown in the bottom trace. Average power = 6.05 W; average current = 1.41 A; no load = 29 ms; stroke volume = 78 ml.

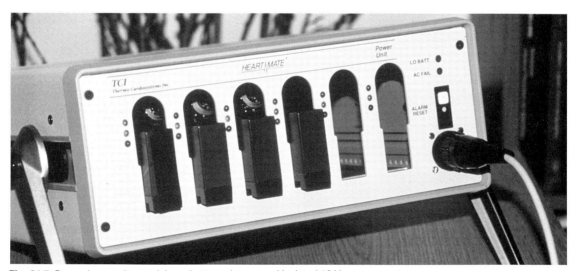

Fig. 24.7 Power base unit containing a battery charger and isolated 12 V power supply.

extended durations without undue strain on the operator. Pneumatic operation can also be carried out by attaching the patient's vent line to the standard pneumatic clinical console.

Patients who are discharged from the hospital are also supplied with two independent 24-hour battery packs. These packs can provide up to 48 hours of uninterrupted power in the event of power failure due to storms or other environmental factors.

The protocol for patient release

The portable HeartMate electrical system is designed to be operated by the patient. The system is simple to operate and lends itself to home use, and to this end a three-phase programme has been designed to release patients to a home environment. The programme is structured for a controlled release under the following conditions:

Phase I

1. A minimum of 30 days has elapsed since the implant.
2. The patient has NYHC I status.
3. There is echocardiographic evidence of aortic valve function with the HeartMate operating at its lowest level;
   or
   Arterial pressure is maintained at >60 mmHg while the HeartMate blood pump is off for 60 seconds.
4. Release is for 16 hours per day.
5. The patient has a trained companion.
6. The home is within one hour or 30 miles from hospital.
7. The physician's consent has been obtained.

Phase II

1. The patient has successfully carried out five day trips during phase I.
2. The patient is now released for weekends or three consecutive days.
3. Conditions 5–7 of phase I must still apply.

Phase III

1. The patient has successfully completed five weekend or multiple trips during phase II.
2. There can now be permanent discharge.
3. Conditions 5–7 of phase I must still apply.

This programme has been conditionally approved by the Food and Drug Administration (FDA) and has been operating successfully since August 1992. Patients are free to do whatever they wish and to go wherever they would like. With continued success of this programme, patients will be released with a portable, battery-operated pneumatic power source.

Clinical results

At the time of writing, 88 bridge-to-transplant patients had been supported with a *pneumatic* blood pump (Table 24.1).[6–11] The average implant duration was 89 days (range 1–324 days). The cumulative duration of support was 15 years.

Of the 88 patients, five were ongoing at the time of writing, leaving 83 in the study. Of these, 30 died, leaving 53 patients (64%) being supported to transplantation. Eight patients died after transplantation, leaving 45 patients (85%) either discharged or awaiting discharge.

An additional five bridge-to-transplant patients were supported with the portable *electrical* system (Table 24.1).[12] The average implant duration was 144 days (range 1–450 days, ongoing). The cumulative duration of support was two years. Of these five patients, two were ongoing, leaving three in the study. Of these, two have died, leaving one patient to transplant and subsequent discharge.

Of these patients, the pre-implant baseline cardiac index was 1.9 ± 0.6 l/min/m^2. Average pump index on the LVAD was 2.7 ± 0.4 l/min/m^2, resulting in a 42% increase in index.

Table 24.1 HeartMate® clinical summary.

	Pneumatic	Electric
Total number of patients	88	5
Cumulative duration of support (years)	15	2
Longest support to date (days)	324	450
Pump index (l/min/m^2)	2.7	2.7
Average flow (l/min)	4.8	5.8
Maximum flow (l/min)	10.1	9.6
Mean arterial pressure (mmHg)	90	97
Haematocrit (%)	33	37
Haemoglobin (g/dl)	11	12
Plasma-free haemoglobin (mg/dl)	8	8
Platelet count (×10^3/ml)	256	228

Summary

Ventricular assist devices can be used to support patients suffering from cardiac insufficiency. Our emphasis in the design and testing of the Heart-Mate system has always been oriented toward long-term support. It is now clear that patients supported on the device can return to a NYHC I status and can go back into society as normal individuals.

The simple design of this system, coupled with its safety in terms of freedom from thromboembolic complications, makes it ideally suited for long-term use as an alternative to transplant. Patients are ambulatory, feel well, look well and are confident in operating the system themselves with very limited supervision.

We have taken a stepwise path in developing the ultimate system. The concept that we have been following is to develop a blood pump which can be operated by either a simple air system or by electrical energy. Having an electrical system that can be operated by air is a major advantage in terms of safety. For this reason, a vented system is very attractive as opposed to a sealed system. With a sealed system, in the event of an electrical or mechanical malfunction, nothing can be done to maintain cardiac function. Under the same conditions with a vented system, a pneumatic driver or portable air pump can be attached to the vent tube and pumping can immediately be resumed.

A unique characteristic of this blood pump is its textured blood contacting surfaces. These surfaces have, after 17 patient-years of experience, proven to be beneficial to the patient. The only anticoagulant therapy is the use of aspirin and dipyridamole. Heparin or a coumarin are not required to prevent thrombotic complications.

The blood-derived biologic surface that is developed on the textured biomaterials is smooth, continuous, thin, well-adhered and rich in collagen. Of the 93 patients reported here, only three thromboembolic complications have been experienced even though the patients are not anticoagulated. One complication is believed to be secondary to a Candida infection with vegetative growth in the inlet conduit, another is believed to be due to thrombus accumulation on a mechanical valve in the native heart, and the third is believed to be due to be the result of thrombus accumulation in the dilated native ventricle.

Portability is the key for long-term systems. The HeartMate air and electrical systems are portable so that patients can be discharged to lead an active life.

References

1. Macoviak J, Dasse K, Poirier V. Mechanical cardiac assistance and replacement. *Cardiol Clin* 1990; **8**, 39–53.
2. Dasse K, Frazier O, Macoviak J, Menconi M, Clay W, Poirier V. Textured blood contacting surfaces for heart assist systems: current clinical experience. In: *Transactions of the Society of Biomaterials*, Lake Buena Vista, Florida, 1989: p. 36.
3. Dasse K, Menconi M, Lian J, Stein G, McGee M, Poirier V, Frazier O. Characterization of TCI's textured blood contacting materials following long-term clinical LVAD support. In: *Cardiovascular Science and Technology: Basic and Applied*, Louisville, KY, 1990, vol 2: 218–220.
4. Poirier V, Frazier OH. Portable electric systems for long-term use. In: Akutsu T, Koyanagi H (eds), *Artificial Heart*, vol 4. New York: Springer Verlag, 1992: 103–114.
5. Poirier V, Sherman C, Clay W, Graham T, Withington P, Marrinan M, Lewis C. An ambulatory intermiate-term left ventricular assist system. *ASAIO Trans* 1989; **35**, 452–455.
6. Nakatani T, Frazier OH, McGee M, Parnis S, Dasse K, Duncan M, Poirier V. Extended support prior to cardiac transplant using a left ventricular assist device with textured blood contacting surfaces. *ISAIO (Japan)* 1990; **14** (suppl 1), 154–157.
7. McGee M, Parnis S, Nakatani T, Myers T, Dasse K, Hare W, Duncan M, Poirier V, Frazier OH. Extended clinical support with an implantable left ventricular assist device. *ASAIO Trans* 1989; **35**, 614–616.
8. McGee M, Myers T, Dasse K, Hare W, Gernes D, Sherman C, Poirier V, Frazier OH. The HeartMate Assist Device: Recent clinical experience and evolving concepts in design. In: *Transactions of the American Society of Mechanical Engineers*, Dallas, Texas, 1990.
9. Poirier V, Dasse K, Frazier OH. TCI HeartMate assist device: clinical experience with first and second generation systems. *ISIAO (Japan)* 1991; **15**, 315.
10. Frazier OH, Rose E, Macmanus Q, Burton N, Lefrak E, Poirier V, Dasse K. Multicenter clinical evaluation of the HeartMate 1000 IP left ventricular assist device. *Ann Thorac Surg* 1992; **53**, 1080–1090.
11. Dasse K, Frazier OH, Lesniak J, Myers T, Burnett C, Poirier V. Clinical response to ventricular assistance versus transplantation in a series of bridge to transplant patients. *ASAIO J* 1992; **38**, M622–626.
12. Poirier V, Sherman C, Dasse K, Graham T, Withington D, Marrinan M, Lewis CT. The next step in cardiac assist. In: *Cardiovascular Science and Technology: Basic and Applied*, Louisville, KY, 1989, vol 1: 210–211.

25

Clinical experience with the TCI HeartMate® left ventricular assist device

OH Frazier and Michael P Macris

Introduction

In the early 1970s, the National Heart and Lung Institute (NHLI) instituted a programme aimed at treatment of acute and chronic heart failure with left ventricular assist devices.[1] This programme was based upon earlier experience from the 1960s, which had shown that ventricular function could recover in patients who could not be weaned from cardiopulmonary bypass if the ventricle was given time to rest.[2] In 1966, DeBakey[3] first successfully used a left ventricular assist device in a patient who could not be weaned from CPB, but who was subsequently weaned from the assist device. Dennis and associates[4] had developed a temporary device for use in acute heart failure before DeBakey, although none of their patients survived. They were, however, able to demonstrate the feasibility of left ventricular unloading by cannulating the left atrium through the atrial septum and effectively supporting the systemic circulation.

The NHLI programme was the first government-supported research in the field of left ventricular assistance. This research culminated in clinical use of a left ventricular assist device (LVAD) in the 1970s, when Norman and associates[5] implanted an abdominal left ventricular assist device (ALVAD), designed by Thermo Electron Corporation, in patients with postcardiotomy cardiogenic shock as part of a structured clinical trial. Unfortunately, survival in Norman's early series of 22 patients was poor,[6] as the device was used only in moribund patients who had already sustained multisystem end-organ failure before device implantation. The ALVAD was, however, successful in supporting the circulation in all patients. In 1978, this assist device was used as a bridge to transplant.[7] The patient had developed 'stone heart' following emergency surgery to repair an aortic valve. Although his heart function never recovered, the device supported this patient's entire circulation for five days prior to transplant. Unfortunately, he died of infection and rejection soon after his transplant operation.

With the introduction of cyclosporine in the early 1980s, infectious complications after transplant decreased. Because of better results with this immune suppressant, assist devices could finally be used successfully in patients infected prior to device implantation. Oyer first successfully used the Novacor left ventricular assist device as a bridge to transplant in such a patient.[8] This device was powered externally by a large console and monitoring system.

The next major breakthrough in our clinical research came in 1986, when we began testing the pneumatic version of the HeartMate LVAD (Thermo Cardiosystems, Inc.). During the first phase of testing, the pump was powered by a portable pneumatic console. Because the pump has proved to be extremely successful as a bridge-to-transplant,[9] we have recently begun clinical trials with a vented electric version of the pump, which is powered by an external battery pack (see Fig. 24.1). The device is vented because, to date, an internal compliance chamber suitable for long-term human use has not been developed. The vented electrical model provides substantially improved freedom of movement and allows patients with end-stage heart disease to participate in normal activities as they wait for their heart transplant. This chapter describes our experience with the HeartMate LVAD.

Characteristics of the HeartMate

The blood pump housing is made of a rigid titanium alloy and measures 11.2 cm in diameter × 4.0 cm in thickness. A flexible diaphragm separates the blood chamber from the air chamber in the pneumatic pump and separates the blood chamber from the motor in the electric device. Within the pump, blood flows in one direction. The inlet and outlet tubes contain 25-mm porcine valves (Medtronic Blood Systems, Irvine, CA).

A safe blood–biomaterial interface has proved to be one of the greatest challenges in development of mechanical circulatory support devices. In an effort to prevent thrombus from forming, most investigators have used smooth linings to prevent cellular elements from adhering to blood-contacting surfaces. Patients in whom these devices were implanted, however, still experienced thromboembolic complications.

Instead of preventing cellular elements from adhering to the blood-contacting surfaces of the pump, developers of the HeartMate promoted this natural process.[10] During the 1960s, Jordan and associates[11] proved that endothelial cells could be carried in the bloodstream. They suspended Dacron patches in thoracic aortic grafts in pigs. After 20 days, microscopic studies showed endothelium covering the patches. In 1969, Cooley implanted the first total artificial heart in man.[12] The heart he implanted, which was developed by Domingo Liotta, had pumping chambers lined with reticulated Dacron. Liotta also believed that the textured surface would trap formed elements from the blood and form a biological lining. Although this pump was implanted for only 72 hours, haemolysis *was* minimal.

Within the HeartMate's pumping chamber are two types of textured surfaces. Integrally textured polyurethane covers the moveable diaphragm,

and sintered titanium microspheres cover the metallic surface. Within 5 days of initiation of support, a smooth, adherent lining composed of biologic elements begins to form on these surfaces.

Immunochemical analyses have been performed to determine the components of the pseudointimal lining.[13] Samples were taken from two explanted pumps; one had supported a patient for 132 days, the other for 189 days. The samples were cultured to detect factor VIII-related antigen (von Willebrand factor), acetyl low-density lipoprotein receptors, smooth-muscle-cell actin, and surface adhesion molecules specific for monocytes and macrophages. Macrophage cells were predominant in both pumps, but in the second pump, cultures from the centre of the diaphragm were positive for acetyl low-density lipoprotein receptor and von Willebrand factor, indicating the presence of endothelial cells (Fig. 25.1). We believe that blood-borne endothelial cells or endothelial cell precursors were deposited on the blood-contacting surfaces. This finding is important, as it may explain the decreased incidence of thromboembolic complications seen in our patients, which may reduce the need for systemic anticoagulation in patients who need long-term support.

Device implantation

The HeartMate was initially implanted clinically (in two patients) in the extraperitoneal space. Both of these patients, however, developed haematomas, a result of severe coagulopathy present at the time of implant. We, therefore, decided to implant the next pump intra-abdominally, and, in general, we have continued to implant the pump in the abdomen.[14] Although there have been reports of patients with intestinal obstruction and other problems related to intra-abdominal implantation, these complications have been minimal in our experience. With the development of the vented electric device, however, pump exchange in patients who are undergoing long-term (>5 years) assistance may become a possibility. As a result, we have again used the extraperitoneal approach and have not encountered the complications seen in the earlier implantations. After implantation, a capsule forms around the pump (Figs 25.2 and 25.3, which may help guard against infection.

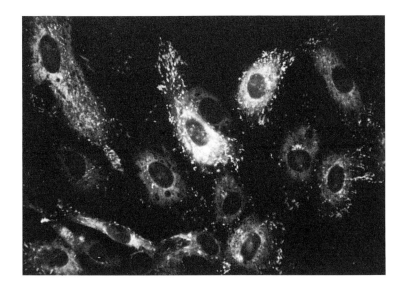

Fig. 25.1 Cell culture obtained from the lining at the centre of the LVAD diaphragm. In immunofluorescent studies, the cells stained positively for factor VIII-related antigen as shown (×240). The cells were also bound by acetyl low-density lipoprotein receptors, which identified them as endothelial cells.

Implanting the device requires total cardiopulmonary bypass. Blood inflow to the pump is obtained by cannulating the left ventricular apex. Blood first drains passively from the left ventricle into the pump, after which it is propelled through an outflow conduit into a graft that has been anastomosed to the ascending aorta. Unidirectional, pulsatile flow is ensured by using two porcine bioprosthetic valves. Best results are achieved in patients with a preconditioned right ventricle, one that can pump against the higher pulmonary artery pressure caused by chronic left ventricular failure. A dilated left ventricle facilitates implantation of the pump. Patients with

acute heart failure have not done as well if their right ventricle is functioning normally. In our series, only 1 of 6 patients with acute myocardial infarction survived. Treating patients with subacute infarctions, however, may be performed successfully.

The pneumatic console is actuated directly, which eliminates the need for tanks of compressed air. The console sits on a steerable, wheeled base and can be easily manoeuvred by the patient or an assistant. It can be operated synchronously or asynchronously, in either automatic rate-responsive or set-rate mode. Programmed pulses of air are delivered to the air

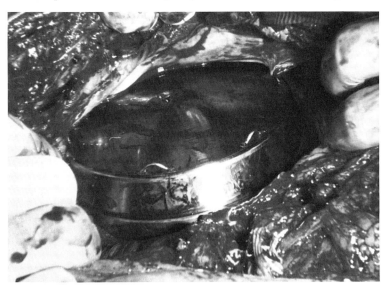

Fig. 25.2 LVAD encapsulated after implantation.

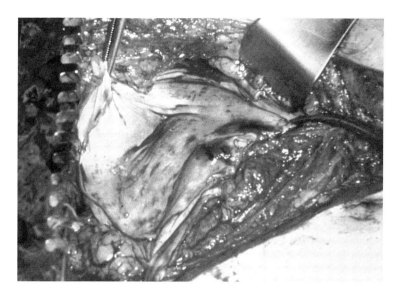

Fig. 25.3 Capsule, shown after pump removal.

chamber, actuating the pusher-plate diaphragm to eject blood from the device chamber.

Clinical results

Indications for use

To be enrolled in clinical trials of the HeartMate, each patient had to be an approved transplant candidate, receiving inotropic drugs, and on an intra-aortic balloon pump (if possible). In addition, the following haemodynamic criteria had to be met: pulmonary capillary wedge pressure ≥ 20 mmHg, with either a cardiac index ≤ 2.0 l/min/m^2 or a systolic blood pressure ≤ 80 mmHg. Moreover, the patient must not have met a lengthy list of exclusion criteria, including severe right heart failure or pulmonary, neurologic, renal, and/or hepatic dysfunction (Table 25.1).

Patient demographics

Since 1988, 36 patients have been supported with the HeartMate, 35 men and one woman (average age 47 years; range 17–64 years). Admission diagnoses included ischaemic cardiomyopathy in 18 of the patients and idiopathic cardiomyopathy in 18 patients.

Results

Haemodynamic and haematological responses to LVAD support

The patients were supported for an average implant duration of 78 days (range 0–504 days). The average pump flow was 5.0 ± 1.0 l/min, and the mean blood pressure was 93 ± 12 mmHg. The average haemoglobin, plasma free haemoglobin, haematocrit, and platelet count during support were 11 g/dl, 7 mg/dl, 32%, and 240 000/ml, respectively. The HeartMate 1000 LVAD provided adequate circulatory support. In 16 patients sup-

Table 25.1 Patient exclusion criteria.

Age greater than 70
BSA less than 1.5 m^2
Chronic renal failure
Severe emphysema
Severe chronic obstructive pulmonary disease
Severe chronic pulmonary hypertension
Unresolved pulmonary infarction
Severely depressed right heart function
Intractable ventricular tachycardia
Severe hepatic disease
Severe gastrointestinal malabsorption
Severe blood dyscrasia
Active systemic infection
Diffuse peripheral vascular disease
Cancer/metastases
Refractory anuria
BUN greater than 100 mg%
Creatinine greater than 5.0 mg%
Positive HIV test
Long-term, high-dose steroid treatment

ported greater than 30 days who subsequently underwent transplantation, long-term survival was 100% at two years.

Heart function

We have seen native heart function gradually improve in these patients. Cardiac index increased 50% in our patients. During ventricular fibrillation, the pump can maintain a reasonable cardiac output, although *output* is better when the heart is beating (Fig. 25.4). Right ventricular function, however, usually remains depressed (as

shown by echocardiography) in the early post-operative period.

Improvement in the condition of the heart has also been shown by histological examination. We compared tissue specimens from the core of the left ventricular apex, which is removed at the time of LVAD implantation, to specimens from the explanted hearts at the time of cardiac transplantation.[15] Apical core specimens from all patients showed extensive areas of attenuated myocardial fibres, combined with wavy patterns in some areas. In these regions, the nuclei of the cardiac myocytes from idiopathic cardiomyopathy

Ventricular
tachycardia

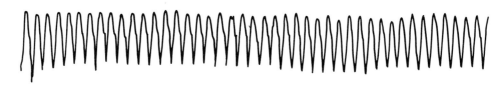

Radial arterial
pressure: 100/50

Pump flow:
3 l/min at 80 bpm

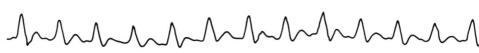

Ventricular
fibrillation

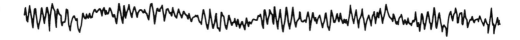

Radial arterial
pressure: 90/50

Pump flow
3 l/min at 80 bpm

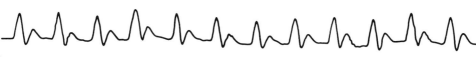

Cardioversion
(after sedation)
sinus tachycardia

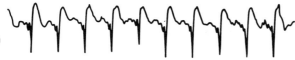

Radial arterial
pressure: 140/70

Pump flow
4 l/min at 80 bpm

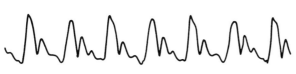

Fig. 25.4 Electrocardiographic tracings, showing pump flow during episodes of ventricular tachycardia (top) and ventricular fibrillation (middle), and after conversion to sinus rhythm (bottom). The LVAD was able to support the circulation successfully throughout periods of tachycardia and fibrillation.

specimens were neither pyknotic nor disappearing, as was noted in an infarcted area of a specimen from one patient with ischaemic cardiomyopathy. At the time of heart transplantation, myocardial tissue specimens from the explanted hearts had a significant decrease or disappearance of stretched fibres, as well as an increase in the diameter of the myocardial fibres. These findings appear to correlate with the clinical impression of improved native ventricular function and with radiographic findings of decreased chamber size during prolonged ventricular support (Fig. 25.5).

Effect on end-organ function

Renal function improved, as levels of blood urea nitrogen and serum creatinine progressively decreased (Fig. 25.6).[16] Liver function also improved, although total bilirubin did increase in the first 48 hours (Fig. 25.7). The pump did not cause haemolysis; plasma haemoglobin levels actually decreased slightly overall and remained within acceptable levels in all patients.

Complications

Thromboembolic complications

We have seen only one possible device-related thromboembolic episode. In this patient, the device implantation was his third cardiac operation, and the posterior aspect of the heart was dissected. This resulted in angulation of the inlet cannula which, coupled with the diastolic flow, contributed to pannus formation and resulting thromboembolism. We view this as more of a complication of device implantation than of the device.

In the postoperative period, we give low-molecular-weight dextran followed by dipyridamole (Persantine) and aspirin. We have occasionally given heparin or Coumadin when LVAD support is diminished by recovery of native heart function. We also give Coumadin when the native heart is known to contain left atrial or ventricular thrombus prior to implantation.

Infections

Although some patients have developed infections around the drive-line, no lasting complica-

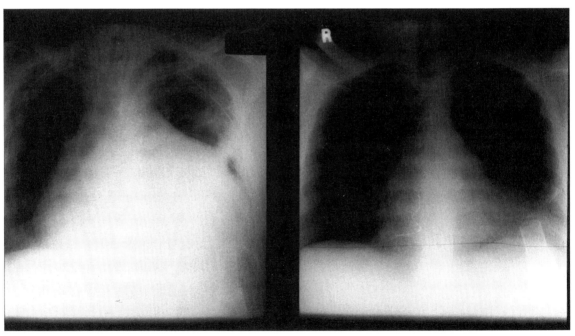

Fig. 25.5 Chest X-ray prior to LVAD implantation (left) and 30 days later, with the LVAD in place (right). Heart size decreased markedly following LVAD implantation.

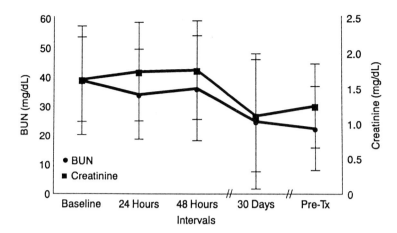

Fig. 25.6 Improved renal function in patients who underwent extended (>30 days) LVAD support. Reproduced from reference 16.

tions have occurred. In no instance has removal of the pump been necessitated by infection. In no instance has heart transplantation been delayed or denied due to infection. Cultures of all pump surfaces have been negative.[17]

Bleeding

Bleeding is frequently a problem in these patients. Episodes of bleeding are usually secondary to coagulopathy, which is related to hepatic dysfunction and correlates with right heart failure, which is most likely due to increased pulmonary vascular resistance secondary to microemboli.

Comment

In the early days of this research, controversy centred on whether the condition of the heart would improve after implantation of an assist device. Thus far, we have been pleased with the clinical results.

We have also found that patients who undergo extended support with the LVAD (until end-organ function recovers) fare better than patients who are supported for short periods of time.[16] Patients supported by the LVAD feel well, begin to exercise, and grow stronger. Thus, we believe that early use of the LVAD as an extended bridge will ultimately make the patient a better transplant candidate.[18] In addition, earlier use of the device would also decrease the costs of treating severely ill patients waiting for a transplant. Rather than spending $3000 per day or more on ICU care, patients could be supported in minimal care units (at about $100 per day) or, even, at home.[19] (See also Chapter 24.)

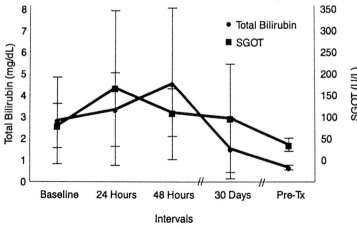

Fig. 25.7 Improved liver function in patients who underwent extended (>30 days) LVAD support. Reproduced with permission from reference 16.

Addendum

The HeartMate has recently been approved by the US Food and Drug Administration for use as a bridge to transplantation.

References

1. The left ventricular assist device: assistance to the failing circulation. DHEW Publication (NIH) 75-626, 11 Jan 1974.
2. National Heart Institute. *Cardiac Replacement: A Report by the Ad Hoc Task Force on Cardiac Replacement.* National Heart Institute, Oct 1969.
3. DeBakey ME. Left ventricular bypass pump for cardiac assistance: clinical experience. *Am J Cardiol* 1971; **27**, 3.
4. Dennis C, Carlens E, Senning A, Hall DP, Moreno JR, Cappelletti RR, Wesolowski SA. Clinical use of a cannula for left heart bypass without thoracotomy: experimental protection against fibrillation by left heart bypass. *Ann Thorac Surg* 1962; **156**, 623–637.
5. Norman JC, Fuqua JM, Hibbs CW, Edmonds CH, Igo SR, Cooley DA. Intracorporeal (abdominal) left ventricular assist device: initial clinical trials. *Arch Surg* 1977; **112**, 1442–1451.
6. Norman JC, Duncan JM, Frazier OH, Hallman GL, Ott DA, Reul GJ, Cooley DA. Intracorporeal (abdominal) left ventricular assist devices or partial artificial hearts: a five-year clinical experience. *Arch Surg* 1981; **116**, 1441–1445.
7. Norman JC, Cooley DA, Kahan BD, Keats AS, Massin EK, Solis RT, Luper WE, Brook MI, Klima T, Frazier OH, Hacker J, Duncan JM, Dasco CC, Winston DS, Reul GJ. Total support of the circulation of a patient with post-cardiotomy stone-heart syndrome by a partial artificial heart (ALVAD) for 5 days followed by heart and kidney transplantation. *Lancet* 1978; **i**, 1125.
8. Portner PM, Oyer PE, McGregor CGA, *et al.* First human use of an electrically powered implantable ventricular assist system. *Artif Organs* 1985; **9**(A), 36.
9. Frazier OH, Duncan JM, Radovancevic B, Vega JD, Baldwin RT, Burnett CM, Lonquist JL. Successful bridge to heart transplantation with a new left ventricular assist device. *J Heart Lung Transplant* 1992; **11**, 530–537.
10. Graham TR, Dasse K, Coumbe A, Salih V, Marrinan MT, Frazier OH, Lewis CT. Neointimal development on textured biomaterial surfaces during clinical use of an implantable left ventricular assist device. *Eur J Cardiothorac Surg* 1990; **4**, 182–190.
11. Jordan GL, Stump MM, DeBakey ME, Halpert B. Endothelial lining of Dacron prostheses of porcine thoracic aortas. *Proc Soc Exp Biol Med* 1962; **110**, 340–343.
12. Cooley DA, Liotta D, Hallman GL, Bloodwell RD, Leachman RD, Milam JD. Orthotopic cardiac prosthesis for two-staged cardiac replacement. *Am J Cardiol* 1969; **24**, 723–730.
13. Frazier OH, Baldwin RT, Eskin SG, Duncan JM. Immunochemical identification of human endothelial cells on the lining of a ventricular assist device. *Tex Heart Inst J* 1993; **20**, 78–82.
14. Radovancevic B, Frazier OH, Duncan JM. Implantation technique for the HeartMate® left ventricular assist device. *J Card Surg* 1992; **7**, 203.
15. Scheinin SA, Capek P, Radovancevic B, Duncan JM, McAllister HA, Frazier OH. The effect of prolonged left ventricular support on myocardial histopathology in patients with end-stage cardiomyopathy. *ASAIO J* 1992; **38**, M271–274.
16. Frazier OH, Macris MP, Myers TJ, Duncan JM, Radovancevic B, Parnis SM, Cooley DA. Improved survival after extended bridge to cardiac transplantation. *Ann Thorac Surg* 1994; **57**, 1416–1422.
17. Myers TJ, McGee MG, Zeluff BJ, Radovancevic B, Frazier OH. Frequency and significance of infections in patients receiving prolonged LVAD support. *ASAIO Trans* 1991; **37**, M283–285.
18. Dasse KA, Frazier OH, Lesniak JM, Myers T, Burnett CM, Poirier VL. Clinical responses to ventricular assistance *versus* transplantation in a series of bridge to transplantation patients. *ASAIO J* 1992; **38**, M622–626.
19. Myers TJ, Dasse KA, Macris MP, Poirier VL, Cloy MJ, Frazier OH, Use of a left ventricular assist device in an outpatient setting. *ASAIO J* 1994; **40**, M471–475.

Section VI _____

Biological Assistance

26

Current indications for, and results of, cardiac transplantation

JR Anderson and DJ Parker

Introduction

The true number of patients suffering from congestive heart failure is unknown as most clinical data are from large studies of patients who have already been identified with incipient heart failure or risk factors for developing heart failure. Large epidemiological studies show that 1% of patients have heart failure by their fifth decade and this figure rises to 10% by the 8th decade. The incidence of heart failure in men exceeds that in women in nearly all age groups.[1] Congestive cardiac failure is the final common pathway for a wide variety of cardiac disorders. The death rate from ischaemic heart disease has fallen in the last few decades but, despite this, the incidence of congestive cardiac failure has risen. This may be due, in part, to improved management of ischaemic heart disease and better control of hypertension. The treatment of advanced cardiac failure has improved but the prognosis remains poor in those with very advanced disease.

The changing pattern of cardiac failure

Two decades ago, cardiac transplantation was the only available treatment option for patients with unrelenting heart failure despite the then optimal medical management. However, the natural history of congestive cardiac failure has changed since the introduction of angiotensin converting enzyme (ACE) inhibitors. Large studies have shown that the prognosis in NYHA stage 3 and 4 heart failure is significantly improved in patients receiving ACE inhibitors compared with those taking a placebo.[2–4] The clinical picture of congestive heart failure has also changed. Evidence from recent trials shows that patients with heart failure, even if asymptomatic, are more likely to suffer sudden cardiac death than progression of heart failure. Some patients die suddenly without preceding clinical deterioration, others gradually deteriorate but die suddenly whilst in reasonably good health, and still others die with severe symptoms that respond poorly to therapy.

The CONSENSUS and SAVE trials have demonstrated that ACE inhibitors reduce the mortality and morbidity of heart failure in a number of ways. The delay in or prevention of the progression of heart failure is the major factor underlying the improved prognosis with ACE inhibitors. In 1987 the CONCENSUS investigators reported a 31% decrease in mortality at one year in patients with NYHA class IV symptoms. The multiple effects of ACE inhibitors may reduce the risk of arrhythmias and therefore sudden cardiac death.[5] It is now clear that ACE inhibitors should be given to all patients with significant impairment of systolic left ventricular function in the absence of contraindications.[6] For patients with advanced dysfunction, prevention of sudden death by using an implantable defibrillator could allow more patients to defer or avoid transplantation until haemodynamic symptoms made daily life intolerable.[7]

Indications for heart transplantation

The major indication for heart transplantation is end-stage cardiac disease including heart failure, refractory ischaemia and arrhythmias, which have lead to unacceptable prognosis for survival and unacceptable disability even after careful consideration of all other medical and surgical therapies. The ideal candidate for transplantation is one who has severe irreversible cardiac dysfunction despite optimal medication but no requirement for intravenous or circulatory support and no evidence of end-organ damage. There are a very small minority of patients who have inoperable coronary artery disease where angina is the dominant symptom.

The changing clinical picture of heart failure has lead to a more critical and objective appraisal of patients referred for heart transplantation. This treatment mode obviously benefits a selected group of patients in terms of symptomatic improvement and survival. The results of transplantation will be discussed later.

It is difficult to identify those patients who would benefit the most from transplantation in terms of survival and quality of life. Only a minority of patients with end-stage disease will be offered alternatives to medical treatment, such as revascularization, transplantation or cardiomyoplasty. With increased understanding of conditions that may be helped by transplantation, many patients are often referred early on in the natural history of their disease, whilst there is no secondary end-organ damage, and there may not be a requirement for transplantation at that time.

Regardless of the aetiology of disease, identification of who needs transplantation must focus on the relative survival compared with other alternative therapies. The NYHA classification for the assessment of the severity of the functional impairment is limited by the subjectivity of its criteria. In contrast, determination of peak oxygen consumption ($\dot{V}_{O_2}$ max) has not only been shown to be a more objective but also a useful tool in determining the optimum timing of transplantation.[8] Once maximal therapy has been instituted and maintained, $\dot{V}_{O_2 max}$ measured during maximal exercise testing provides an objective assessment of functional capacity in patients with heart failure and gives an indication of cardiac reserve. Patients with a peak $\dot{V}_{O_2}$ of greater than 14 ml/kg/min have a survival rate of 94% at one year with medical treatment, and this confirms that transplantation could be deferred in these patients. However, they still remain at risk for sudden death. The worst survival rates are in those with $\dot{V}_{O_2 max}$ of less than 10 ml/kg/min. The importance of this test is that it can be measured accurately and not estimated by exercise duration or metabolic equivalents. Peak $\dot{V}_{O_2}$ on exercise testing has been shown to be a strong predictor of death in patients with congestive heart failure and can be used to select patients with heart failure for transplantation.[9] It should also be used to evaluate other strategies in this group of patients (such as cardiomyoplasty). Patients with a lower (14 ml/min/kg) peak $\dot{V}_{O_2}$ have a higher risk of sudden death rather than progression of heart failure irrespective of the aetiology of heart failure.[10]

Ischaemic heart disease or cardiomyopathy are the most frequent indications for transplantation (Table 26.1), but patients with congenital or valvular heart disease may be suitable candidates. Other indications include HOCM, sarcoid, myocarditis, amyloid and other miscellaneous conditions. A number of relative and absolute contraindications to transplantation are listed in Table 26.2.

Experience in some centres has challenged the presence of some exclusion criteria (i.e. transplanting patients with active endocarditis, those with renal impairment and those with diabetes) with good results. Advanced age is a relative contraindication for transplantation. There is no agreed cut-off point, but a figure of 60 years is a common limit in many transplant units. There is evidence to suggest that selected patients over the age of 60 have results similar to those below this age, but transplant centres are now required to

Table 26.1 Indications for heart transplantation: International Society for Heart and Lung Transplantation registry data.[11]

Cardiomyopathy	49%
Coronary artery disease	41%
Rejection	3%
Valvular	4%
Congenital	1%
Other	2%

Table 26.2 Contraindications to heart transplantation.

Absolute
Active infection
Malignancy (untreated)
Severe systemic disease with independent poor prognosis
Irreversible, severe organ dysfunction
Raised PVR that cannot be reversed with vasodilators
   (>4 Wood units)

Relative
Age >60 years
Recent pulmonary embolism
Insulin-dependent diabetes with end-organ damage
Active peptic ulceration
Severe peripheral vascular disease
Drug or alcohol dependency or psychological problems

make the best use of an increasingly scarce resource and, in general, younger patients are selected for transplantation.[12] Patients with a pulmonary vascular resistance of greater than 4 Wood units (after vasodilators) are at risk of right ventricular failure in the early postoperative period and may be offered an alternative treatment such as heterotopic heart transplantation or heart–lung transplantation.[13] For patients with an ischaemic aetiology to their heart failure, the option of CABG despite poor left ventricular function may be a reasonable option as the mortality rate is around 10% and many patients derive significant early and long-term benefits.[14] Long-term survivors of CABG and cardiomyoplasty usually require medication for heart failure despite functional improvement.

The overall success of heart transplantation has lead to a severe shortage of donor organs and this has a number of effects on current practice. Data from large centres show an 8% mortality for patients who were referred for transplantation but never reached the stage of evaluation, and a 22% mortality for those on the waiting list. Patients who are rejected for being too well usually have a good survival rate on medication.[15] Only about 60% of potential heart transplant recipients ever undergo transplantation.[16]

Results of heart transplantation

Analyses of benefits after transplantation have focused almost exclusively on survival with little reference to quality of life. Assessment of quality of life variables are important when comparing patients who have had transplantation with those whose functional capacity is improved by modern aggressive medical management. The National Transplantation Study in the USA has shown that 80–85% of patients are physically active and over 30% return to gainful employment (a figure comparable with the employment rates for other solid-organ transplants).[17] Transplant patients must tolerate the inconvenience of repeated endomyocardial biopsies, problems of immuno-suppression, the constant fear of rejection and other complications.

There has been an alarming increase in the cost of heart transplantation over a four-year period coinciding with a shift in the recipient population towards more severely ill patients. In the United States, the waiting lists have become top heavy with ill patients. If this trend continues there is the feeling that all heart transplants in the United States will soon be emergencies. In the past, morbidity and mortality were considered parameters of success, but with rising health care costs, the quality of life of patients and cost–benefit analyses of procedures is much more carefully scrutinized. Length of pre-transplant stay rose from 8.9 days to 17.5 days between 1989 and 1991. Total length of stay rose from 29.5 days in 1988 to 44.9 days in 1991 and 34% were transplanted from ITU in 1988 compared with 62% in 1991.[18] As the number of donor organs available for transplantation remains limited, the mean length of time a potential recipient is on the waiting list increases. Data from the ISHLT Registry[11] show that one-year survival following transplantation approaches 80% with a steady decline in subsequent years, with a 5-year survival of 70% and 10-year survival of around 53%. The 30-day mortality following heart transplantation in the UK in 1991 was 14%. Thereafter there was a further 10% mortality for the following year. From the second year on there was a 3% annual mortality. The 1-, 5- and 10-year survival currently stands at 75, 65 and 50% respectively for transplants carried out in the British Isles.[19]

Donor shortages

This is the critical issue in all aspects of organ transplantation. The criteria for accepting a donor for heart transplantation is becoming increasingly liberalized to accommodate the increasing number of potential recipients that are placed on transplant lists.[20] The decision to use a

Table 26.3 Contraindications to accepting a donor heart for transplantation.

Absolute
HIV positivity
Intractable ventricular arrhythmia
Poor oxygenation with Po_2 of <60 mmHg despite 100% O_2
  on PEEP
Documented previous MI
Significant heart disease or poor ejection fraction (<20%)
Severe occlusive coronary artery disease on arteriogram or
  detected at time of harvesting

Relative
Hepatitis B sAg positive
Bacterial sepsis
Hepatitis C positivity
History of metastatic cancer
Extensive chest wall trauma with evidence of contusion on
  ECG or echo
Prolonged hypotension, i.e. <60 mmHg systolic pressure for
  more than 6 hours
Recurrent atrial arrhythmia
Prolonged need for inotropic support
Severe left ventricular hypertrophy on echocardiography
Hypokinesia on echocardiogram (ejection fraction >20%)
Non-critical coronary artery disease on arteriogram
History of intravenous drug abuse

donor depends on the recipient's clinical state and the relative contraindications (Table 26.3).

The main goal of donor management is to maintain donor haemodynamic stability. Constant monitoring of arterial pressure, central venous pressure and urinary output is essential. The ideal circumstances are a donor with an arterial pressure of >100 mmHg with a CVP of less than 12 mmHg. Large volumes of fluid may be required to maintain adequate filling pressures. Brain death is often associated with low-pressure pulmonary oedema and frequent endotracheal suction is required with the addition of PEEP. There are a number of preoperative factors that are predictive of a poor outcome. These are young recipient age, old recipient age, ventilator support at the time of transplantation, higher pulmonary vascular resistance, older donor age, small donor body surface area and donor diabetes mellitus.[21]

Transplantation for salvage situations

A number of patients on the waiting list deteriorate to the point where they can no longer generate a sufficient cardiac output to survive without medical intervention. Supporting the poorly functioning myocardium takes a number of forms, from inotropic support to intra-aortic balloon counterpulsation and ventricular assist devices. With the lack of available donors, it has become common for patients to wait over one year for transplantation. It is likely that a number of these patients will deteriorate to the point where they will require some form of circulatory support as a bridge to transplantation until a suitable donor organ is found.[22] Such patients may have good survival and quality of life.[23]

Complications of heart transplantation

Rejection

Rejection of the allograft is a natural response to a foreign antigen if the immune system is not suppressed. Many improvements have been made in the field of immunosuppression, especially with an increased understanding of the immune system and principally since the introduction of cyclosporin A. However, acute allograft rejection accounts for up to 30% of all deaths in the first year after transplant.

Acute cellular rejection

The mean number of rejection episodes in the first year is 1.3 ± 0.7 per patient. In the first year, 37% of patients have no rejection episodes, 40% have only one episode and the remaining 23% have more than one episode. The majority are asymptomatic and are detected by routine endomyocardial biopsy. Numerous attempts have been made to screen for rejection using noninvasive means but none is reliable enough, at present, to replace endomyocardial biopsy. The risk factors for developing acute cellular rejection despite seemingly adequate immunosuppression are: HLA mismatch, female gender, young age, female and younger donor hearts, panel reactive antibody screen >10%, and CMV infection. The therapy for acute cellular rejection remains varied but in all cases the immunosuppression is increased and the response monitored by endomyocardial biopsy.[24]

Humoral rejection

Unlike cellular rejection which can be diagnosed by light microscopy, the diagnosis of humoral rejection requires immunofluorescent staining. Evidence of immunoglobulin and complement deposition on the endothelium together with endothelial swelling is sought. The antibodies are against class II donor HLA antigens on the endothelium. It may actually occur in 20% of patients receiving antilymphocyte immunosuppression and is a likely cause of fatal rejection, transplant coronary vascular disease and decreased late survival. The consensus view is that treatment is required if there is graft dysfunction in which case treatment is with high-dose steroids, antithymocyte globulin, cyclophosphamide and plasmapheresis.[25]

Rejection prophylaxis

Most immunosuppression regimens are triple therapy with steroids, azathioprine and cyclosporin A. Induction therapy with antilymphocyte globulins increases the time to first rejection but does not decrease the number of rejection episodes. Steroids are generally stopped at 3 months but this decision is dictated by biopsy findings. Cyclosporin A has a number of undesirable side effects, particularly renal impairment, hypertension, osteoporosis and, in the long term, lymphoproliferative disorders. Despite these side effects, cyclosporin has been largely responsible for the increased survival in heart transplantation since the early 1980s.

Bacterial infection

The use of immunosuppressants predisposes patients to infection. The introduction of cyclosporin has led to decreased numbers of all infections and their severity. However, infection is still a major cause of death in the first year after transplant. Early infections (those in the first 4 weeks after transplantation) are usually the result of line-borne infections whereas later ones are due to opportunistic infection. The lung is the most common site, followed by blood, urine, gastrointestine and the sternal wound.[24]

Viral infection

Patients are susceptible to all viral infections but particularly to cytomegalovirus (CMV). This may occur as a primary infection in individuals not previously exposed to the virus, as a result of blood-borne or organ transmission from seroposi-

tive donors. More commonly the disease is a reactivation of a previously acquired infection in immunosuppressed individuals. CMV viraemia is associated with malaise and pyrexia, but the disease can affect certain organs with devastating results. One of the most serious manifestations is CMV pneumonitis which, if not treated early, can be rapidly fatal. Symptomatic patients may be treated with a gancyclovir which is successful in controlling the symptoms although does not necessarily eradicate the organism. Quite apart from the acute illness caused by CMV, there is considerable evidence that it is responsible in part for the development of acute rejection and accelerated graft coronary artery disease.[26]

Allograft coronary disease

An accelerated form of coronary disease is a major cause of death after the first year post-transplant.[27] Despite all the improvements in immunosuppression, the incidence of this complication has not decreased over 20 years. It is detectable in 30–50% of patients 5 years after transplantation. The only reliable way to detect and monitor the progression of the disease is by routine surveillance coronary angiography. Because of denervation of the transplanted organ, there is usually no anginal like syndrome to herald the onset of myocardial ischaemia, although there is increasing evidence of late, partial re-innervation. The angiographic appearances are those of a diffuse concentric narrowing of the epicardial arteries particularly in the distal branches. This arrangement makes effective treatment virtually impossible. The histological appearances show that there is hyperplasia of the smooth muscle cells and macrophages that migrate into the intima. These changes occur in a concentric fashion and there is little calcification and almost no thrombus formation or ulceration. The process is probably immune-mediated and risk factors include HLA mismatch at the DR locus, hyperlipidaemia and CMV infection.[28] No treatment has been shown to influence the course of the disease. Angioplasty has been undertaken in some patients and some have been offered re-transplantation, although the results in general are poor.

Malignancy

This is a well recognized side effect of chronic immunosuppression for solid-organ transplants.

An almost unique malignancy is the post-transplant lymphoproliferative disease that occurs in a small number of patients and is more common in those who have had induction therapy with OKT3 or antilymphocyte globulin.[29] Up to 40% respond to a reduction in immunosuppression and treatment of an Epstein–Barr viral infection. Those who do not respond to this may respond to chemotherapy regimens.

Summary

Heart transplantation is not the easy option in the treatment of end-stage cardiac failure. Careful selection using objective assessment of the severity of the heart failure by $\dot{V}_{O_2\,max}$ is now appropriate. Whilst a selected group do very well following transplantation, there is considerable inconvenience and the constant threat of complications. The current donor shortage remains the limiting factor for cardiac transplantation, and until xenografting becomes practical, the search for a suitable alternative therapy must be ongoing.

References

1. McKee PA, Castelli WP, McNamara PM, Kannell WB. The natural history of congestive heart failure: the Frammingham study. *New Engl J Med* 1971; **285**, 1441–1446.
2. The SOLVD Investigators. Effect of enalapril on survival in patients with reduced left ventricular ejection fractions and congestive heart failure. *New Engl J Med* 1991; **327**, 685–691.
3. The SOLVD Investigators. Effect of enalapril on mortality and the development of heart failure in asymptomatic patients with reduced left ventricular ejection fractions. *New Engl J Med* 1992; **327**, 685–691.
4. Cleland JGF. The clinical course of heart failure and its modification by ACE inhibitors: insights from recent clinical trials. *Eur Heart J* 1994; **15**, 125–130.
5. Armstrong PW, Moe GW. Medical advances in the treatment of congestive heart failure. *Circulation* 1993; **88**, 2941–2952.
6. Stevenson WG, Stevenson LW, Middlekauff HR, Saxon LA. Sudden death prevention in patients with advanced ventricular dysfunction. *Circulation* 1993; **88**, 2953–2959.
7. Kubo SH, Ormaza SM, Francis GS, Holmer SC, Olivari MT, Bolman RM, Shumway SJ. Trends in patient selection for heart transplantation. *JACC* 1993; **21**, 975–981.
8. Dunselman PHJM, Kunzem EE, Van Bruggen A, *et al.* Value of NYHA classification, radio nucleotide ventriculography, and cardiopulmonary exercise tests for selection of patients for congestive heart failure studies. *Am Heart J* 1988; **116**, 1475–1482.
9. Mancini DM, Eisen H, Kussmaul W, Mull R, Edmunds LH, Wilson J. Value of peak exercise oxygen consumption for optimal timing of cardiac transplantation in ambulatory patients with heart failure. *Circulation* 1991; **83**, 778–786.
10. Mudge GH, Goldstein S, Addonizio LJ, Caplan A, Levine BT, Ritsch ME, Stevenson LW. Task Force 3: Recipient guidelines/prioritization (from 24th Bethesda Conference: Cardiac Transplantation). *JACC* 1994; **22**, 21–32.
11. The Registry of the International Society for Heart and Lung Transplantation: Tenth Official Report, 1993. *J Heart Lung Transplant* 1993; **12**, 541–548.
12. Olivari MT, Antolick, Kaye MP, Jamieson SW, Ring WS. Heart transplantation in elderly patients. *J Heart Transplant* 1988; **7**, 258–264.
13. Costard-Jackle A, Fowler MB. Influence of pre-operative pulmonary artery pressure on mortality after heart transplantation: testing of potential reversibility of pulmonary hypertension with nitroprusside is useful in defining a high risk group. *J Am Coll Cardiol* 1992; **19**, 48–54.
14. McGovern JA, Magovern GJ, Maher TD, Benckart DH, Park SB, Christlieb IY, Magovern GJ. Operation for congestive cardiac failure: transplantation, coronary artery bypass, and cardiomyoplasty. *Ann Thorac Surg* 1993; **56**, 418–425
15. McManus RP, O'Hair DP, Beitzinger JM, Schweiger J, Seigel R, Breen TJ, Olinger GN. Patients who die awaiting cardiac transplantation. *J Heart Lung Transplant* 1993; **12**, 159–172.
16. Campana C, Gavazzi A, Berzuini C, Larizza C, Marioni R, D'Armini A, Pederzolli N, Martinelli L, Vigano M. Predictors of prognosis in patients awaiting heart transplantation. *J Heart Lung Transplant* 1993; **12**, 756–765.
17. Young JB, Winters WL, Bourge R, Uretesky BF. Task Force 4: Function of the heart transplant patient. *J Am Coll Cardiol* 1993; **22**, 31–41.
18. Reetsma K, Berland G, Merrill J, Arons PH, Evans C, Drusin R, Smith CR, Rose EA. Evaluation of surgical procedures: changing patterns of patient selection and costs in heart transplantation. *J Thorac Cardiovasc Surg* 1992; **104**, 1308–1313.
19. UKTSSA. *Thoracic Organ Transplant Audit 1985–92.* UKTSSA, 1994.
20. Baldwin JC, Anderson JL, Boucek MM, Bristow MR, Jennings B, Ritsch ME, Silverman NA. Task Force 2: Donor considerations. *J Am Coll Cardiol* 1993; **22**, 15–20.
21. Young JB, Naftel DC, Bourge RC, *et al.* Matching

the heart donor and heart transplant recipient. Clues for successful expansion of the donor pool: a multivariable, multi-institutional report. *J Heart Lung Transplant* 1994; **13**, 353–365.

22. Mulcahy D, Fitzgerald M, Wright C, Sparrow J, Pepper J, Yacoub M, Fox KM. Long term follow up of severely ill patients who underwent urgent cardiac transplantation. *Br Med J* 1993; **306**, 98–101.

23. Reedy JE, Pennington G, Miller LW, McBride LR, Lohmann DP, Noedel NR, Swartz MT. Status I heart transplant patients: conventional versus ventricular assist device support. *J Heart Lung Transplant* 1992; **11**, 246–252.

24. Miller LW, Schlant RC, Kobashigawa J, Kubo S, Renlund DG. Task Force 5: Complications. *J Am Coll Cardiol* 1993; **22**, 41–54.

25. Olsen SL, Wagoner LE, Taylor DO, *et al.* Treatment of vascular rejection in the 1990s: the Utah experience. *Circulation* 1992; **86**, 2500–2506.

26. Kirklin JK, Naftel DC, Levine TB, *et al.* Cytomegalovirus infection after heart transplantation. Risk factors for infection and death: a multi-institutional study. *J Heart Lung Transplant* 1994; **13**, 394–404.

27. Miller LW. Transplant coronary artery disease (editorial). *J Heart Lung Transplant* 1993; **11**, S1–4.

28. Hosenpud JD, Shipley GD, Wagner CR. Cardiac allograft vasculopathy: current concepts, recent developments and future directions. *J Heart Lung Transplant* 1992; **11**, 9–23.

29. Chen JM, Barr ML, Chadburn A, *et al.* Management of lymphoproliferative disorders after cardiac transplantation. *Ann Thorac Surg* 1993; **56**, 527–538.

27

Xenotransplantation: current status and future prospects

J Dunning and J Wallwork

Introduction

The field of organ transplantation has grown dramatically over the last 35 years and a few key advances stand out. Undoubtedly one of the most significant has been the introduction of cyclosporin as an effective immunosuppressive agent. As a result of this the success of allotransplantation—that is the transplantation of organs within a species—has led to an ever greater number of patients being referred by the physicians for consideration of transplantation. Unfortunately this has led to a relative shortage of donor organs and in no area is this more marked than in the field of cardiopulmonary transplantation. In the year ending 31 December 1992, 454 patients received thoracic organ transplants while the waiting list for transplantation grew to 706 patients[1] and the number of patients assessed is estimated to be five times that number.

Better education of the public has ensured that fewer potentially transplantable organs are lost through ignorance and prejudice, but even so the shortfall of donor organs relative to the number of potential recipients remains, and even worsens. Artificial organs such as the dialysis machine provide partial answers, but progress in the field of total artificial organs has perhaps been disappointing, particularly in view of the immense resources directed towards finding a solution. The artificial heart is perhaps the closest to a mechanical replacement organ, and although it is a simple pump with no metabolic function there remain problems with biocompatibility, thrombosis, infection and power source. It seems likely, however, that this concept may be developed to a state of clinical usefulness, but there is currently no prospect of an artificial alternative to the more complex metabolic organs such as the liver or kidney.

It is our belief that the field of xenotransplantation—that is transplantation of organs between species—provides the only true solution to the shortage of transplantable organs. The use of animals such as pigs that breed rapidly and in large numbers ensures a ready supply of organs, while the use of domestic animals already slaughtered in large numbers for food also poses fewer moral problems than those posed using closely related species such as primates as donors.

The use of such animal organs has largely been prevented to date by the phenomenon of hyperacute xenograft rejection (HXR) which occurs almost immediately. Debate centres on the mechanism of this violent reaction, with groups investigating the relative roles of preformed natural antibodies and the complement system. It is true that the use of non-human primate organs may partially overcome this problem since HXR is not seen in the same way, but first-set rejection still occurs. In addition it is unlikely that these animals can provide the organs in the quantity required and there are ethical and moral objections to the use of closely related animals.

It is clear that if xenotransplantation is to move from dream to reality the areas of antibody-mediated and cell-mediated rejection must be addressed and overcome. After this has been achieved there remain many other questions such as whether the graft will be more susceptible to chronic rejection than an allograft, although transplantation across ABO blood barriers[2] and in the presence of initially high HLA antibodies[3] suggest that this will not be so.

Another area which needs exploration is the function of one species organ within another. Observations have been made of non-human primate kidneys and a liver over relatively long periods, and of a few non-primate livers in man for short periods, but our detailed knowledge of their behaviour is still extremely limited. However, there is optimism that a pig liver, for example, will be able to function satisfactorily in man.[4]

An historical perspective

It has been observed that the first successful cross-species transplant was performed by Daedelus when he grafted bird feathers to his arms to escape to mainland Greece from his island prison of Crete. His son Icarus was perhaps less successful when he tried to repeat the experiment.[5] Perhaps this early failure discouraged experimenters for it was not until 1905 that the first report of cross-species grafting appeared in the scientific literature.[6] Slices of rabbit kidney were inserted into a nephrotomy in a child with renal insufficiency. The immediate effects were astonishing, with an increase in the volume of urine produced and cessation of vomiting, but the child died 16 days later with 'pulmonary congestion'.

Over the next five years several other attempts were made at xenografting with vascular anastamoses but all failed due to thromboses.[7,8] The next real attempt at treating a patient with renal failure secondary to poisoning by mercury bichloride was made in 1923 when Neuhof[9] attempted renal transplantation using a lamb's kidney. The patient died 9 days later but encouragement was obtained from the experience since thrombosis did not occur at the anastamotic sites.

Some interest was lost in transplantation once the immunological basis of rejection had been established, but as the immunosuppressive agents were demonstrated to be successful there was renewed interest in the field. As programmes gathered pace so the problems of organ procurement began to be apparent, and ethical considerations posed difficult problems. Organs harvested from human cadavers required rapid transfer and preservation to ensure a good result. This posed many logistical problems when planning transplants and the cumbersome results militated against the growth of this therapy.

So it was that Reemtsma and his colleagues at Tulane University in New Orleans turned to animal sources for organs for clinical renal transplantation. Their hypothesis was that kidneys from non-human primates (i.e. animals phylogenetically closely related to man) would respond similarly to human kidneys when transplanted into man. Six patients in the terminal phase of renal failure received chimpanzee renal grafts in 1963/64.[10] The results were encouraging, with good graft function and survival of one patient to 9 months after transplant. Subsequently Hardy *et al.*[11] reported the first case of heart transplantation in man using a chimpanzee heart, and Hume[12] attempted a renal transplant again using a chimpanzee as the donor. Both of these enterprises were unsuccessful. Meanwhile Starzl began a series of baboon-to-man renal transplants.[13–15]

Soon the concept of brain-stem death became acceptable and this led to a more ready supply of human donor organs, and many institutions also acquired chronic renal dialysis programmes. The combination of these two factors removed the main justification for the use of animal organs and led to reduced interest in the field of xenotransplantation, although there had by this stage been adequate proof of its potential. One problem remained and that was the limited number of donor organs available. In turn this led to a restricted waiting list, and as the indications for transplantation have widened, this restriction has become more apparent.

Following the early clinical efforts in xenografting there was increased scientific interest in the area, but the lack of need for animal donors and the apparent lack of answers to the problems of rejection of animal organs led to a decline in this effort after ten years or so. The number of organ transplants performed every year continued to rise as it became a more successful modality of treatment for end-stage organ disease, and once more the donor organ shortage became a problem. Today this is underlined by the number of kidneys required for transplantation in the

United Kingdom which is estimated at between 2500 and 4000 per year,[16] while a recent audit of intensive care units suggested an annual maximum of 1700 potential organ donors.[17] As a result of such a wide discrepancy in donor and potential recipient numbers, attention was turned again to the potential of xenotransplantation and led to the 'Baby Fae' transplant in 1984.[18] Although this clinical effort was unsuccessful it further boosted scientific research in the area of xenotransplantation.

Xenogenic relationships

Two types of xenogenic relationship were defined by Calne in 1969.[19] He differentiated between species combinations in which a rapid rejection process resembling second-set allograft rejection occurred (a discordant combination) and those in which a delayed reaction occurred resembling first-set rejection (a concordant relationship).

The difference between the two relationships has been underlined both clinically and in the research laboratory. Clinical experience of xenografting has been limited to around 30 cases and these attempts have been predominantly with concordant combinations. Although none of these grafts has survived beyond 9 months, and indeed most have survived for much shorter periods, they have helped to demonstrate that one species' organs can function usefully in another species body. At present the most likely organ to function usefully is the heart, and comparative physiological studies of human and porcine hearts have shown similar haemodynamic function suggesting that they may function successfully in man.[20,21]

While clinical experience has been limited to concordant combinations, the results have not as yet shown themselves to be a successful long-term strategy for the treatment of end-stage organ failure. However, with more modern research into concordant rejection and its modification and the more recent immunosuppressive regimens, programmes could well be established. The use of non-human primate donors, while desirable from the immunologist's viewpoint, poses many ethical and logistic problems and is unlikely to be adopted in large numbers. In view of this, and despite the difficulties associated with discordant transplantation, it is this object which has

become the aim of most xenotransplantation research programmes.

The rejection process

Much has been written about the discordant xenograft rejection process. Preformed antispecies (heterophile) IgM antibodies bind to donor endothelium and activate complement via the classical pathway.[22] It seems likely that the antigenic determinants are glycoproteins although this remains unproven. Tissue factor and plasminogen activator inhibitor are synthesized and heparan sulphate is lost.[23] These processes promote the accumulation of fibrin and in addition platelet activating factor is released stimulating the adhesion of platelets.[24,25] Polymorphs and neutrophils are retained in the organ by their cell surface complement receptors and play an intravascular role, generating further inflammatory mediators and disrupting the endothelial barriers to blood cells and proteins. Platelet thrombus results in ischaemia and failure of the transplanted organ.

If hyperacute rejection could be completely prevented it is not clear what would be the fate of the discordant xenograft, although studies of concordant grafts suggest that there would be many features in common with allograft rejection. Cellular rejection and destruction by newly generated antibody both occur and both these processes may be controlled by existing immunosuppressive techniques.

Experimental techniques such as plasmapheresis to remove heterophile antibody and xenoabsorption prolong xenograft survival from minutes to hours. Complement depletion with cobra venom factor has a similar effect. Cell depletion also prolongs graft survival, but none of these techniques has produced a xenograft which functions for more than a few hours and none can be envisaged in clinical use to provide long-term maintenance of xenografted organs.

The role of heterophile antibody in HXR is clear, but another area which is becoming more clearly defined is the role of complement, through both the classical and the alternative pathways. It appears that down-regulatory proteins in the donor organ fail to inhibit complement activity in the recipient. Clearly the control proteins are species-specific, and it may be that expression of the appropriate control proteins on donor organ cell surface may provide control.

This approach to cell protection is in use in nature already. *Schistosoma mansoni* does not activate the human complement cascade after it has been in the human blood stream. The failure to activate complement is blocked by antibody against DAF (Decay Accelerating Factor—a complement control protein) suggesting that the parasites insert host DAF into their surfaces.[26] Similarly, Vaccinia virus is able to encode for secretory proteins which find host C3 and C4 products to protect against attack by complement.[27]

Experimental evidence suggests that the manipulation of complement-controlling proteins does indeed protect against the action of xenogenic complement. Transfection of cell lines with gene constructs coding for human DAF and MCP (membrane cofactor protein) have provided almost complete protection against human complement but not rabbit complement.[28]

It may be that incorporation of human MCP or DAF into the genome of a transgenic animal could protect transplanted donor organs from hyperacute complement-mediated rejection. Attempts to produce such transgenic animals are already being made with cDNA constructs injected into mouse ova, but at present expression is variable.[29,30]

Clearly there is a long way to go before expression of human control proteins is reliably consistent throughout organ systems and on the vascular endothelium, and there will need to be detailed assessment before clinical transplantation can be made between discordant species. However, this approach is now seen as a likely strategy for clinical transplantation,[31,29] and attempts are already under way to produce larger transgenic animals.

Conclusions

There have been dramatic improvements in the survival of patients receiving allografts over the last 30 years, and these have mainly been due to the improvements which have taken place in immunosuppressive agents. Several new drugs which have novel modes of action may provide further improvements in graft and patient survival. However, allotransplantation remains limited by organ shortage and xenotransplantation is probably the only way to provide an adequate number of organs for the treatment of end-stage organ failure. Currently available drugs have not been shown to confer any advantage in preventing the rejection of xenografts, and many other physiological and ethical obstacles remain before xenotransplantation is widely accepted. However, there is growing impetus in this direction and it may only be a matter of years before clinical xenotransplantation programmes become established.

References

1. United Kingdom Transplant Support Service Authority. *Transplant Update,* January 1993.
2. Alexandre GPJ, Squifflet JP, De Bruyere M, *et al.* Present experience in a series of 26 ABO-incompatible living donor renal allografts. *Transplant Proc* 1987; **19**, 4538–4542.
3. Palmer A, Welsh K, Gjorstrup P, Taube D, Bewick M, Thick M. Removal of anti-HLA antibodies by extracorporeal immunoadsorption to enable renal transplantation. *Lancet* 1989; **1**, 10–12.
4. Auchincloss HJ. Xenogeneic transplantation. *Transplantation* 1988; **46**, 1–20.
5. Reemtsma K. Xenotransplantation—a brief history of clinical experiences 1900–1965. In: Cooper DKC, Kemp E, Reemtsma K, White DJG (eds), *Xenotransplantation: The Transplantation of Organs and Tissues Between Species.* Berlin: Springer Verlag, 1991: 9.
6. Princeteau M. Greffe renale. *J Med Bordeaux* 1905; **26**, 549.
7. Jaboulay M. Greffe de reins au pli du coude par soudures arterielles et veineuses. *Lyon Med* 1906; **107**, 575.
8. Unger E. Nierentransplantationen. *Klin Wschr* 1910; **47**, 573.
9. Neuhof H. *The Transplantation of Tissues.* New York: Appleton and Co., 1923: 260.
10. Reemtsma K, McCracken BH, Schlegel JU, *et al.* Renal heterotransplantation in man. *Ann Surg* 1964; **160**, 384–408.
11. Hardy JD, Chavez CM, Kurrus FD, *et al.* Heart transplantation in man: developmental studies and report of a case. *JAMA* 1964; **188**, 1132–1140.
12. Hume DM. Discussion of paper by Reemtsma *et al. Ann Surg* 1964; **160**, 409.
13. Starzl TE. Discussion of paper by Reemtsma *et al. Ann Surg* 1964; **160**, 409.
14. Starzl T. *Experiences in Renal Transplantation.* Philadelphia: WB Saunders, 1964.
15. Starzl TE, Marchioro TL, Peters GN, *et al.* Renal heterotransplantation from baboon to man:

experience with six cases. *Transplantation* 1964; **2**, 752–776.

16. Hoffenberg R. *Report of a Working Party on the Supply of Donor Organs for Transplantation.* London: HMSO, 1987.

17. Gore SM, Hinds CJ, Rutherford AJ. Organ donation from intensive care units in England. *Br Med J* 1989; **299**, 1193–1197.

18. Bailey LL, Nahlsen-Cannarella SL, Concepcion W, Jolley WB. Baboon-to-human cardiac xenotransplantation in a neonate. *J Am Med Ass* 1985; **254**, 3321–3329.

19. Calne RY. Organ transplantation between widely disparate species. *Transplant Proc* 1969; **2**, 550–556.

20. Hannon JP. Haemodynamic characteristics of the conscious resting pig. In: Tumbleson ME (ed). *Swine in Biomedical Research.* London: Plenum, 1985: 1341–1352.

21. Erickson HH, Faraci FM, Olsen SC. Effect of exercise on cardiopulmonary function in domestic pigs. In: Tumbleson ME (ed), *Swine in Biomedical Research.* London: Plenum, 1985: 709–717.

22. Fischel RJ, Bolman RM, Platt JL, Najarian JS, Bach FH, Matas AJ. Removal of IgM anti-endothelial antibodies results in prolonged cardiac xenograft survival. *Transplant Proc* 1990; **22**, 1077–1078.

23. Platt JL, Vercolotti GM, Lindman BJ, Oegema TR, Bach FH, Dalmaso AP. Release of heparan sulfate from endothelial cells. *J Exp Med* 1990; **71**, 1363–1368.

24. Otte KE, Jorgensen KA, Bonnevie V, *et al.* Xenoperfusion of rabbit kidney and the impact of

BN52021: a specific antagonist of platelet activating factor. *Transplant Proc* 1990; **22**, 1089–1090.

25. Reding R, Maldague P, Massion P, Lambotte L, Otte JB. Differential effect of plasma exchange and platelet activating factor antagonist WEB2170 on hyperacute vascular rejection of discordant xenografts in rodents: preliminary results. *Min Chir* 1991; **46**, 167–168.

26. Pearce EJ, Hall BF, Sher A. Host-specific invasion of the alternative complement pathway by schistosomes correlates with the presence of a phospholipase C-sensitive surface molecule resembling human decay accelerating factor. *J Immunol* 1990; **144**, 2751–2756.

27. Kotwaj GJ, Moss B. Vaccinia virus encodes a secretory polypeptide structurally related to complement control proteins. *Nature* 1988; **335**, 176–178.

28. Oglesby TJ, White D, Tedja I, *et al.* Protection of mammalian cells from complement-mediated lysis by transfection of human membrane cofactor protein and decay accelerating factor. *Trans Ass Am Phys* 1991; **104**, 164–172.

29. White D, Oglesby TJ, Liszewski K, *et al.* Expression of human decay accelerating factor or membrane cofactor protein genes on mouse cells inhibits lysis by human complement. *Transplant Proc* 1992; **24**, 474–476.

30. White DJG. Transplantation of organs between species. *Int Arch All Immunol* 1992; **98**, 1–5.

31. Platt JL, Bach FH. The barrier to xenotransplantation. *Transplantation* 1991; **52**, 937–947.

28

Educating skeletal muscle to do cardiac work

Stanley Salmons and Jonathan C Jarvis

Skeletal muscle as a functional autograft

Moving skeletal muscles around is not new: it is the daily routine of many plastic surgeons. There is a difference, however, between using muscles for physical reconstruction and using them to generate useful mechanical work. For example, we have to be sure that both the blood supply and the nerve supply are adequate. The muscle should be stimulated in such a way that all parts of it are used. It must operate under appropriate conditions of stretch and load. It must not fatigue progressively under the working conditions it encounters in the new application. In short, our use of skeletal muscle as a surgical biomaterial should be guided by a detailed understanding of its structure and capabilities. Much of the necessary information comes from an examination of the properties of its constituent fibres.

These properties are not uniform. At one extreme are fibres that contain many mitochondria and get their energy largely from aerobic oxidation, particularly of fats and fatty acids. These fibres are served by numerous capillaries, which maintain the necessary supply of oxygen and nutrients. They are well suited to functions such as standing, which call for steady forces to be exerted over long periods. At the other extreme are fibres with few mitochondria, which derive their immediate energy requirements largely from anaerobic glycolysis. Such fibres engage in intermittent bursts of intense activity, separated by relatively long quiescent periods during which glycogen and other reserves are replenished. This pattern of use can be supported by a much less extensive capillary network.

Fibres may also be distinguished on the basis of cytochemical techniques that are sensitive to differences in molecular isoforms of myosin. The so-called fast (types 2A and 2B) and slow (type 1) classes of skeletal muscle fibre synthesize distinct myosin isoforms that confer different contractile speeds. Combining this classification with metabolic differences yields the following simplified scheme:

> Type 2B fibres are fast-contracting and susceptible to fatigue.
> Type 2A fibres are fast-contracting and fatigue-resistant.
> Type 1 fibres are slow-contracting and fatigue-resistant.

The motor system employs these elements in an elegant way. Motor units that are active for much of the time are composed of slow, type 1 fibres—the type that is best suited for sustaining tension for long periods. Motor units that are active only infrequently are composed of fast, type 2B fibres—the type that is best suited to generating powerful contractions on an intermittent basis. Between these extremes, the type 2A motor units cope with routine activity against a background of more continuous postural tension provided by the type 1 motor units.

This organization minimizes the possibility of muscle fatigue. The units that are recruited most frequently have the metabolic capability for sustained use. The units that are recruited only infrequently have time to replenish their anaerobic reserves between bouts of activity. Fatigue can also be deferred if the muscle is activated in an economical way. The calcium ion fluxes that are triggered each time an impulse reaches a muscle fibre are energy-consuming, so the demand is less if the required force can be developed and maintained with fewer impulses. In practice this happens in three ways. First, motor units discharge at a rate that correlates closely with the contractile speed of the muscle fibres: thus, motoneurones innervating slow muscle fibres fire at lower frequencies than those innervating fast fibres. Second, motor units discharge asynchronously, and as a consequence tension at the whole muscle level can develop smoothly at lower average impulse frequencies. Third, individual motor units do not fire at a constant frequency. Fast motor units, in particular, tend to commence firing at a high frequency, usually in the form of a double pulse that produces a rapid rise of tension. The impulse frequency then declines, but tension is sustained, a phenomenon sometimes referred to as the 'catch' property of skeletal muscle.

Unfortunately all these benefits are lost when a muscle is activated by stimulating the nerve electrically in the conventional way. First, the normal order of recruitment is inverted, and as a result the largest motor units—those least resistant to fatigue—are the most heavily used. Second, electrical stimulation excites all motor units synchronously at the same frequency, resulting in a contraction that is grossly oscillatory unless the frequency of stimulation is raised. Finally, although commercial stimulators usually accommodate some adjustment of frequency, few are designed to cope with variation within individual bursts of activity. This is why skeletal muscle is potentially much more susceptible to fatigue under conditions of electrical stimulation than it would be if it performed the same amount of work in a physiological way. Whether or not this is a problem depends crucially on the rate of working, or power, that is demanded of the muscle.

Power requirements for cardiac assistance

The object of cardiac assistance is to restore the patient to a reasonable quality of life while improving, or at least preventing further deterioration in, the condition of the heart. How hard must a skeletal muscle pump be able to work to achieve this goal? For a normal 70 kg subject with a body surface area of $1.7 \, \text{m}^2$, the mean cardiac output is about 6 l/min at rest.[1] For an average systemic pressure of 100 mmHg, the corresponding power is about 1.3 W. The flow would rise to at least 14 l/min during walking or climbing stairs, corresponding to 3 W. In practice, part of this power would be provided by the patient's own heart, but these figures provide sensible targets to strive for.

In single contractions, skeletal muscle can perform more work per unit mass than cardiac muscle and it can generate a force per unit cross-sectional area that is between two and five times higher. Faced, however, with unrelenting power levels of 1.3–3 W, candidate muscles—such as diaphragm, rectus abdominis, pectoralis major or latissimus dorsi—would rapidly lose most of their capacity for work because of fatigue. For this reason, early attempts to use skeletal muscle in a cardiac assist role were thwarted. The situation changed only with the realization that skeletal muscles could actually adapt to the more demanding pattern of use if they were allowed to respond over a longer time-scale.

Stimulation-induced transformation

This property was discovered by Salmons and Vrbová in the course of experiments in which rabbit muscles of the fast-twitch, fatiguable type were subjected to a chronic increase in their pattern of use by electrical stimulation.[2] It turned out that if these conditions were maintained for a number of weeks, the fast muscle acquired a completely new set of physiological, biochemical and morphological characteristics. A considerable literature has now accumulated on the morphological and biochemical changes that underlie this adaptive response (see reference 3 for a recent review). The metabolism of the muscle switches to the oxidation of fats and fatty acids, increasing its capacity for the generation of energy substrates through oxidative phosphorylation.[4,5] These changes are supported by an enhanced blood supply to the muscle. Energy-consuming processes related to changes in intracellular calcium transport and binding, and the rate of recycling of cross-bridges between actin and myosin, are altered in a way that enables the muscle to generate and to sustain contractions with reduced energy expenditure. An important long-term consequence of these changes is a substantial slowing of muscle contraction and relaxation. Whereas some of the early features of this response are seen in the muscles of athletes undergoing prolonged endurance training, chronic electrical stimulation can accomplish the complete spectrum of adaptive change in a matter of weeks. These changes, referred to collectively as 'conditioning', make the muscle fibres much more resistant to fatigue than even the type 1 fibres used to maintain posture.[6] The phenomenon makes it possible to utilize skeletal muscle for cardiac assistance.

The changes take place within individual fibres, rather than by the degeneration of some fibre types and proliferation of others.[7] Moreover, the transformation is completely reversible. Thus if stimulation is discontinued at any stage, the muscle goes through a sequence of changes in a mirror-image of the transformation process until its original properties are restored in every detail.[8-10] Stimulation-induced transformation involves qualitative as well as quantitative changes in dozens of muscle proteins, and many of these changes have now been traced back to the messenger RNA level. Nonetheless, elucidation of the sequence of intracellular events that links depolarization of the surface membrane with re-expression of the muscle genome remains a major challenge for researchers in the field.

The adaptive hypothesis

The phenomena just described may be interpreted as evidence of a natural adaptive capacity of skeletal muscle. According to this hypothesis,[11] muscles subjected to sustained high levels of use tend to develop properties at the slow, fatigue-resistant end of the spectrum. Muscles that are less active revert to a native fast state. The concept emerges of a tissue that is interacting continuously with its environment, optimizing its properties according to demands. Thus the functional matching of the neural and muscular elements of

a motor unit should be seen not as a masterpiece of specific connectivity but as a simple consequence of the plasticity of the muscle fibres. And conditioning is a mere extension of this natural ability to adapt to a change in working requirements.

Conditioning protocols

Now that we have this knowledge it is no longer difficult to make a muscle fatigue-resistant. Unfortunately it is only too easy to make it slow as well, and this is almost always undesirable. In cardiomyoplasty, for example, if the skeletal muscle wrap contracts and relaxes more slowly than the myocardium, then it cannot follow wall movements precisely. This results in incomplete reinforcement during systole and the possibility that filling may be restricted during diastole. Slowness is equally disadvantageous in other approaches to skeletal muscle assist, for it produces a substantial loss of power-generating capacity and poses difficulties of synchronization with the cardiac cycle.[12]

The main reason for slowness is that long-term stimulation induces the synthesis of type 1 isoforms of myosin. Recent work from the authors' laboratory shows that this is not a prerequisite for fatigue resistance[13] and could, furthermore, be avoided by an appropriate choice of stimulation pattern.[14] Existing protocols should therefore be re-examined and optimized by systematic experimental work. There are additional benefits to be gained from timing the onset and progressive escalation of the conditioning regime more precisely. If conditioning is started too soon or too vigorously, the grafted muscle may suffer ischaemic damage; if, on the other hand, the onset is too gradual, the muscle begins to atrophy, revascularization is less rapid than it could be, and the assist is delayed unnecessarily. Improved methods for monitoring non-invasively the changes in the grafted muscle would enable the clinical protocol to be matched more closely to individual patients. Basic studies of this type will be helpful in developing any form of skeletal muscle assistance.

It should be clear by now that the light-hearted title of this chapter needs to be approached with a certain humility. Skeletal muscle is already 'smart': in reality, it is we who have been educating ourselves over the last 30 years or so about what it can actually do. But it is not enough to 'educate muscle': we must learn to teach it to do the right things.

Acknowledgements

The authors gratefully acknowledge grant support from the British Heart Foundation, Medical Research Council, Engineering and Physical Sciences Research Council, and Wellcome Trust.

References

1. Hurst JW (ed), *The Heart, Arteries and Veins*, 4th edn. New York: McGraw-Hill, 1978: 76.
2. Salmons S, Vrbová G. The influence of activity on some contractile characteristics of mammalian fast and slow muscles. *J Physiol* 1969; **201**, 535–549.
3. Pette D, Vrbová G. Adaptation of mammalian skeletal muscle fibers to chronic electrical stimulation. *Rev Physiol Biochem Pharm* 1992; **120**, 115–202.
4. Clark BJ, Acker MA, McCully K, Subramanian HV, Hammond RL, Salmons S, Chance B, Stephenson LW. *In vivo* ^{31}P–NMR spectroscopy of chronically stimulated canine skeletal muscle. *Am J Physiol* 1988; **254**, C258–266.
5. Mayne C, Anderson WA, Hammond RL, Eisenberg BR, Stephenson LW, Salmons S. Correlates of fatigue resistance in canine skeletal muscle stimulated electrically for up to one year. *Am J Physiol* 1991; **261**, C259–270.
6. Salmons S, Sréter, FA. Significance of impulse activity in the transformation of skeletal muscle type. *Nature* 1976; **263**, 30–34.
7. Lexell J, Jarvis JC, Downham DY, Salmons S. Quantitative morphology of stimulation-induced damage in rabbit fast-twitch muscles. *Cell Tiss Res* 1992; **269**, 195–204.
8. Brown JMC, Henriksson J, Salmons S. Restoration of fast muscle characteristics following cessation of chronic stimulation: physiological, histochemical and metabolic changes during slow-to-fast transformation. *Proc Roy Soc Lond* 1989; **235B**, 321–346.
9. Salmons S. On the reversibility of stimulation-induced muscle transformation. In: Pette D (ed), *The Dynamic State of Muscle Fibres*. Berlin: Walter de Gruyter, 1990: 401–414.
10. Brownson C, Little P, Jarvis JC, Salmons S. Reciprocal changes in myosin isoform mRNAs of rabbit skeletal muscle in response to the initiation and cessation of chronic electrical stimulation. *Muscle Nerve* 1992; **15**, 694–700.
11. Salmons S, Henriksson J. The adaptive response of skeletal muscle to increased use. *Muscle Nerve* 1981; **4**, 94–105.
12. Salmons S, Jarvis JC. Cardiac assistance from skeletal muscle: a critical appraisal of the various approaches. *Br Heart J* 1992; **68**, 333–338.
13. Jarvis JC. Power production and working capacity of rabbit tibialis anterior muscles after chronic electrical stimulation at 10 Hz. *J Physiol* 1993; **470**, 157–169.
14. Salmons S. Exercise, stimulation and type transformation of skeletal muscle. *Int J Sports Med* 1994; **15**, 136–141.

29

Circulatory assistance with skeletal muscle ventricles

Timothy L Hooper and Larry W Stephenson

Introduction

In the last few years skeletal muscle has emerged as a potential power source for supporting cardiac function in patients with severe heart failure. The latissimus dorsi muscle has attracted particular interest since, anatomically, its size, location and mobility are well-suited to a cardiac assist role; and, functionally, it is capable of sustaining a continuous level of work comparable with that of the resting heart.[1] Various approaches to muscle-powered cardiac assistance have been proposed, including cardiomyoplasty, aortomyoplasty and muscle-driven biomechanical devices. However, the use of skeletal muscle ventricles (SMVs) as auxiliary blood pumps in the circulation offers a particularly attractive and potentially more versatile option. Either left or right heart assistance is possible, for either congenital or acquired cardiac abnormalities, and SMV size and geometry can be tailored to provide the most favourable loading conditions for the muscular wall, so that the pumping capabilities of the muscle are utilized maximally. Much progress has been made in SMV research over the last few years, and this review will outline some of the major developments.

Historical perspective

Several workers have previously proposed the concept of creating a neoventricle from skeletal muscle, but they found that sustained function was not possible owing to early muscle fatigue. An important development at this time was the discovery by Salmons and Vrbová that skeletal muscle could be transformed by chronic electrical stimulation to a form more resistant to fatigue.[2] In Stephenson's laboratory, Mannion constructed multilayered, thick-walled SMVs from the latissimus dorsi muscle, rested the muscle for three weeks to allow recovery of vascularity, and then transformed the muscle with continuous electrical stimulation over several weeks. He then demonstrated that such a pump was capable of generating systemic levels of pressure in a hydraulic system over several hours.[3] Subsequently, Acker connected an SMV to an implantable mock-circulation device, and showed that meaningful systemic workloads could be sustained over several weeks.[4] SMVs were then connected in circulation with the thoracic aorta, where they were able to achieve a level of stroke work intermediate between that of the right and left ventricles over several hours.[5]

Functional characteristics of SMVs

In 1974, when Spotnitz et al.[6] evaluated skeletal muscle pouches constructed from canine rectus abdominis muscle, they demonstrated functional characteristics similar to those which Frank[7] and

Starling[8] had previously shown for cardiac ventricles. An important difference, however, was that SMVs were considerably less compliant than cardiac ventricles, requiring much higher preloads to generate high pressures. The question of poor compliance has since been addressed by a better understanding of the geometric aspects of SMV design, and this has resulted in improved performance at more physiological filling pressures.[9,10]

A more comprehensive evaluation of systolic and diastolic SMV function has recently been carried out. Using data derived from continuous pressure–volume measurements during variable SMV stimulation protocols, the end-diastolic pressure–volume relationship of SMVs has been found to be comparable to that of cardiac ventricles, although SMVs are relatively less compliant. Interestingly, whilst higher burst stimulation frequencies result in a greater force of muscle contraction, and therefore enhanced systolic function, they also increase SMV compliance. It is unclear why this should be the case, but it has been suggested that greater muscle contraction might be matched by more intense activation of those processes which allow the muscle to relax. Varying the rate of SMV contractions up to 97 per minute did not appear to have a detrimental effect on compliance, though one would anticipate diastolic filling to be impaired by still higher contraction rates as a consequence of the inherent slowness of transformed muscle. Although higher burst stimulation frequencies result in a greater force of contraction, end-systolic elastance, a reflection of contractility, does not appear to be influenced by the pattern of stimulation, and this constancy of SMV contractility differs importantly from the properties of a cardiac ventricle.

Right heart assist

Attempts to use SMVs to achieve partial or total right heart bypass have met with some success in short-term experiments, though at the expense of relatively high systemic venous pressures necessary to provide effective SMV preload.[11,12] An alternative way to provide effective SMV preload is to use a right ventricle to pulmonary artery SMV configuration which exploits right ventricular systolic pressure for SMV filling. In short-term studies this arrangement achieved an augmentation in

pulmonary blood flow of around 25% over several hours.[13] In subsequent experiments dogs were supported in this way for up to 16 weeks without thromboembolic complications, demonstrating that SMVs may have a potential role in certain congenital cardiac abnormalities.[14] However, an interesting problem encountered during this study was a progressive 'shrinkage' of SMV cavity size, to the extent that pump function eventually deteriorated. This phenomenon has not been observed when SMVs are connected to the systemic circulation, suggesting that lower right-sided pressures may inadequately support and sustain skeletal muscle fibre length in the long term.

Left heart assist

In theory, for effective left heart support, SMVs could be used to pump blood from the left atrial or left ventricular chamber to the systemic circulation, in a similar way to a true assist device, or alternatively may pump blood within the systemic circulation, synchronous with diastole, so as to generate arterial counterpulsation. In practice, all these forms of assist have been applied experimentally, and the findings have been encouraging. Moreover, whereas SMVs have previously been placed extrathoracically, an intrathoracic position has recently been evaluated,[15] since this may prove a more convenient location for long-term clinical use. Intrathoracic placement has not led to respiratory problems, albeit in healthy animals, but importantly has been associated with better SMV diastolic function.[16] This has led to SMVs being used to pump blood successfully between the left atrium and thoracic aorta for several hours, achieving flows of around 20% of the resting cardiac output at physiological left atrial preloads.[17] This configuration has yet to be assessed long-term, particularly in relation to thromboembolic phenomena.

As diastolic counterpulsators, SMVs have proved particularly effective in short- and long-term experiments. Connected 'in series' with the thoracic aorta using a bifurcated vascular graft, SMV function benefits not only from the high preload supplied by arterial pressure, but also because the 'washing' effect of the aortic circulation through the SMV appears to reduce the likelihood of thromboembolic complications. Diastolic pressure augmentation, in association with improved subendocardial viability and tension time indices, has been achieved in animals for periods of up to two years, demonstrating their capacity for long-term function in the circulation.[18–21] Thromboembolism, a serious complication in the early experience, has not been a significant problem in recent years even without formal anticoagulation. This may in part relate to the use of autogenous linings[18] or more rheologically favourable SMV geometry.[19] Non-valved SMV configurations in series with aorta theoretically allow reflux of blood from the distal aorta back into the SMV during its relaxation, which might prejudice the degree of LV off-loading achieved. It has been suggested that the introduction of a valve into the efferent vascular conduit may improve efficiency of the system, and a homograft valve in this position has functioned well for up to 4 months in dogs.[22] In terms of left heart assistance, such a valved configuration has been investigated in short-term experiments, demonstrating improved coronary blood flow in association with a reduction in LV stroke work of around 25% during SMV counterpulsation,[23] thus establishing a more favourable myocardial oxygen supply/demand relationship.

A potential concern of using SMVs to generate counterpulsation is that of adequacy of intramural blood supply, since the pouch wall is continuously exposed to systemic pressures which mirror those within the nutrient arteries. This may help to explain why SMVs have sometimes been observed to rupture in the early postoperative phase, or to dilate after long-term function. Recent work has focused on a valved LV apex to aorta configuration, which provides a low-pressure phase for the SMV during the cardiac cycle, while still providing high preloads to optimize SMV function. Acute experiments have provided encouraging results, with SMVs pumping in excess of 40% of the native cardiac output through the assist circuit during 1:2 synchrony with the heart.[24] This form of assist appears particularly promising, and long-term studies are currently under way.

In summary, SMVs have been shown to be effective blood pumps both short- and long-term, in various configurations. It is likely that they will ultimately be used to treat patients with various left and right-sided cardiac diseases.

References

1. Salmons S, Jarvis JC. Cardiac assistance from skeletal muscle: a critical appraisal of the various approaches. *Br Heart J* 1992; **68**, 333–338.
2. Salmons S, Vrbová G. The influence of activity on some contractile characteristics of mammalian fast and slow muscles. *J Physiol* 1969; **201**, 535–549.
3. Mannion JD, Hammond R, Stephenson LW. Hydraulic pouches of canine latissimus dorsi: potential for left ventricular assistance. *J Thorac Cardiovasc Surg* 1986; **91**, 534–544.
4. Acker MA, Hammond RL, Mannion JD, Salmons S, Stephenson LW. An autologous biologic pump motor. *J Thorac Cardiovasc Surg* 1986; **92**, 733–746.
5. Mannion JD, Acker MA, Hammond RL, Faltemeyer BS, Duckett S, Stephenson LW. Power output of skeletal muscle ventricles in circulation: short-term studies. *Circulation* 1987; **76**, 155–162.
6. Spotnitz HM, Merker C, Malm JR. Applied physiology of the canine rectus abdominis: force–length curves correlated with functional characteristics of a rectus powered ventricle; potential for cardiac assistance. *ASAIO Trans* 1974; **20**, 747–756.
7. Frank O. Zur dynamik des herzmuskels. *Am Heart J* 1959; **58**, 282–317.
8. Chapman CF, Mitchell JH (eds). *Starling on the Heart.* London: Dowsons, 1965: 121–147.
9. Bridges CR, Brown WE, Hammond RL, et al. Skeletal muscle ventricles: improved performance at physiologic preloads. *Surgery* 1989; **106**, 275–282.
10. Hammond RL, Bridges CR, Dimeo F, Stephenson LW. Performance of skeletal muscle ventricles: effects of ventricular chamber size. *J Heart Transplant* 1990; **9**, 252–257.
11. Bridges CR, Hammond RL, Dimeo F, Anderson WA, Stephenson LW. Functional right heart replacement with skeletal muscle ventricles. *Circulation* 1989; **80**, 183–189.
12. Bridges CR, Woodford E, Mora G, Anderson DR, Stephenson LW, Norwood WI. Use of skeletal muscle power to augment the pulmonary circulation. *Surg Forum* 1990; **41**, 267–270.
13. Niinami H, Hooper TL, Hammond RL, et al. A new configuration for right ventricular assist with a skeletal muscle ventricle: short-term studies. *Circulation* 1991; **84**, 2470–2475.
14. Niinami H, Hooper TL, Hammond RL, et al. Skeletal muscle ventricles in the pulmonary circulation: up to 16 weeks experience. *Ann Thorac Surg* 1992; **53**, 750–757.
15. Hooper TL, Niinami H, Hammond RL, et al. Intrathoracic skeletal muscle ventricles: a feasibility study. *J Cardiac Surg* 1991; **6**, 387–395.
16. Niinami H, Hooper TL, Hammond RL, et al. Functional evaluation of intrathoracic versus extrathoracic skeletal muscle ventricles. *J Surg Res* 1993; **54**, 230–236.

17. Hooper TL, Niinami H, Hammond RL, *et al.* Skeletal muscle ventricles as left atrial-aortic pumps: short-term studies. *Ann Thorac Surg* 1992; **54**, 316–322.

18. Anderson DR, Pochettino A, Hammond RL, *et al.* Autogenously-lined skeletal muscle ventricles in circulation. *J Thorac Cardiovasc Surg* 1991; **101**, 661–670.

19. Pochettino A, Mocek FW, Lu H, *et al.* Skeletal muscle ventricles in circulation with improved thromboresistance: up to 28 weeks experience. *Ann Thorac Surg* 1992; **53**, 1025–1032.

20. Ruggiero R, Anderson DR, Niinami H, *et al.* Skeletal muscle ventricles in circulation: 24-month update. In: Carraro U (ed), *Muscle Driven Devices for Cardiac Assistance*. Padova, Italy: Unipress, 1991: 81–89.

21. Mocek FW, Anderson DR, Pochettino A, *et al.* Skeletal muscle ventricles in circulation long-term: from 191 to 836 days. *J Heart Lung Transplant* 1992; **11**, S334–340.

22. Fietsam R, Lu H, Hammond RL, *et al.* Skeletal muscle ventricles with efferent valved homograft: up to four months in circulation. *J Cardiac Surg* 1993; **8**(2), 184–194.

23. Hooper TL, Niinami H, Hammond RL, *et al.* Aortic counterpulsation with a valved skeletal muscle ventricle: short-term studies of coronary flow and left ventricular function. *Basic Appl Myol* 1992; **2**(3), 159–168.

24. Lu H, Fietsam R, Hammond RL, *et al.* Skeletal muscle ventricles: left ventricular apex to aorta configuration. *Ann Thorac Surg* 1993; **55**, 78–85.

30

Aortic counterpulsation with skeletal muscle

Magdi H Yacoub and John R Pepper

Introduction

Appropriately trained skeletal muscle can be used to augment the systolic function of the heart, as in cardiomyoplasty, or to produce counterpulsation. The early work on skeletal muscle counterpulsation was carried out in 1959 by Kantrowitz and McKinnon,[1] who used the muscular portion of the left hemidiaphragm to wrap around the thoracic aorta. The muscle was stimulated repeatedly via the phrenic nerve and timed to contract in diastole. A transitory rise in mean arterial pressure of up to 26.5% of the baseline value was achieved before muscle fatigue occurred.

The fundamental observations of Buller *et al.*[2] and the work of Salmons,[3] Pette[4] and associates on muscle transformation and fatigue resistance led to a renewed interest in the feasibility of using skeletal muscle to augment the failing heart. The development of pulse train stimulators appropriate for skeletal muscle contraction and the use of conditioning protocols have contributed to the improved performance of assist devices. After transformation into a fatigue-resistant state, canine latissimus dorsi configured into auxiliary ventricles have subsequently demonstated adequate work performance for long-term cardiac assistance.[5,6]

Methods

Two broad approaches to the use of skeletal muscle for counterpulsation have emerged. They are skeletal muscle ventricles, which have been extensively studied by Stephenson's group,[5] and extra-aortic counterpulsation, involving either the ascending aorta[7] or the descending thoracic aorta.[8]

Skeletal-muscle counterpulsation devices have been constructed from various body-wall muscles, including pectoralis major and rectus abdominis, but latissimus dorsi (LD) has been the most widely used. It is readily mobilized on a neurovascular pedicle, is of a suitable size, is able to contract in two directions, and leaves minimal residual deformity.

We have developed a method of extra-aortic counterpulsation based on the descending aorta.[8] The left LD is mobilized on an intact neurovascular pedicle and two stimulating leads are attached proximally for neuromuscular stimulation. The thoracic cavity is approached through a 3rd rib resection and approximately 8 cm of the proximal descending aorta is mobilized, at least two pairs of intercostal arteries being divided in the process. The mobilized LD is wrapped twice around the aorta in a spiral fashion. A right ventricular epicardial sensing lead is placed (Fig. 30.1). Our standard regimen is as follows: 3 V, pulse width 240 μs, burst width 240 ms, 35 Hz. Stimulation of the LD wrap is begun after

4 hours and is most commonly delivered in our studies in a 1:4 mode. We have tested these wraps after a 6-month period on a mock circulation apparatus and demonstrated resistance to fatigue.

Assessment of the performance of skeletal muscle counterpulsation devices has included a range of physiological and biochemical approaches.

Echocardiography

Rates of contraction and relaxation may be calculated from M-mode images obtained from transthoracic echocardiography. In addition, the percentage of aortic occlusion produced by the LD wrap can be assessed (Fig. 30.2). This allows us to assess the physiological characteristics of the muscle as it is transformed from a fast fatiguable muscle towards a slow fatigue-resistant muscle with altered power characteristics.

Mock circulation

We have developed a mock circulation model (Fig. 30.3).[9] The model consists of two fluid-filled compliance chambers representing the elastic component of the ascending aorta, aortic arch and the major vessels arising from it. The second chamber represents the elastic component of the remainder of the systemic vasculature. The two chambers are connected by a length of rubber tubing which represents the descending thoracic aorta.

Table 30.1 illustrates the haemodynamic performance of the skeletal muscle wrap at different lengths: 5 cm and 8 cm. The results indicate that in this model the LD wrap is capable of conferring definite haemodynamic benefit.

Mock circulation models have been used by others to assess the potential power of skeletal muscle ventricles[10] and to investigate performance at different preloads and afterloads. The effect of stretch and burst frequency has also been examined.

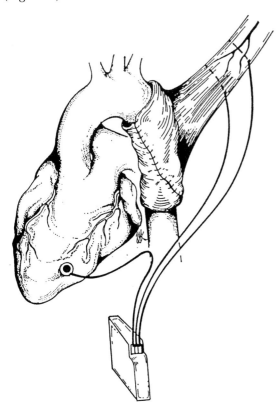

Fig. 30.1 Extra-aortic counterpulsation.

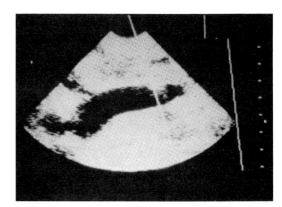

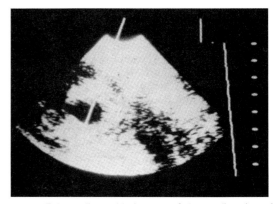

Fig. 30.2 Echocardiographic images of descending thoracic aorta. The two images are of a longitudinal section, showing the muscle wrap (*top*) relaxed and (*bottom*) contracted.

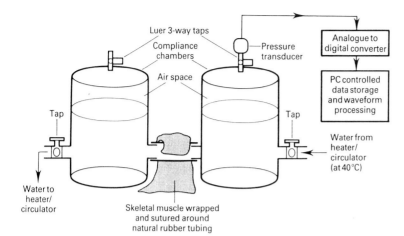

Luer 3-way taps
Compliance chambers
Air space
Pressure transducer
Analogue to digital converter
PC controlled data storage and waveform processing
Tap
Tap
Water from heater/ circulator (at 40°C)
Water to heater/ circulator
Skeletal muscle wrapped and sutured around natural rubber tubing

Fig. 30.3 Mock circulation apparatus for *in vivo* assessment of muscle wrap performance.

Biochemistry

Optimal muscle transformation to a particular fibre type composition has not yet been defined. The observation that a complete transformation to a homogeneous slow fibre composition is associated with an 8–10-fold loss of power[11] has led to the suggestion that a mixed fibre type population may be a more desirable goal. A broad spectrum of techniques, including molecular biology, enzymology, electrophoresis and magnetic resonance spectroscopy, are currently used to determine the degree of transformation achieved in any particular study.

Discussion

The precise application and indications for the use of conditioned skeletal muscle in humans remains controversial, although the exclusive use of one technique would appear restrictive. In the counterpulsation mode the skeletal muscle in the wrap is relaxed during the systolic phase of systemic blood flow and this may be important in limiting fatigue in the long term. Furthermore, immediately prior to contraction the muscle wrap is at maximum end-systolic distension of the aorta. The effect which this may have on the loading of this muscle is a difficult problem to study and to our knowledge is at present largely unknown. The increased pressure that may be generated by multiple layers of muscle around a tube in comparison with a single layer around the larger diameter heart, may be an important advantage.

Skeletal muscle used for counterpulsation remains at the research stage. Cardiomyoplasty and skeletal muscle counterpulsation, although different in approach, both depend upon the concept of muscle plasticity, and the fundamental molecular architecture of myofibrils. This includes myosin isoforms, calcium handling apparatus and the metabolic handling of glucose. All these mechanisms are ultimately influenced by the stimulation regime which is adopted.

References

1. Kantrowitz A, McKinnon WMP. The experimental use of the diaphragm as an auxiliary myocardium. *Surg Forum* 1959; **9**, 266–268.
2. Buller A, Eccles JC, Eccles RM. Interaction between motor neurones and muscles in respect of the characteristic speeds of their responses. *J Physiol (Lond.)* 1960; **150**, 417–439.
3. Salmons S, Sréter FA. Significance of impulse activity in the transformation of skeletal muscle type. *Nature* 1976; **263**, 30–34.
4. Pette D, Staron PS. Cellular and molecular diversities of mammalian skeletal muscle fibres. *Rev Physiol Biochem Phar* 1990; **116**, 1–76.

Table 30.1 Haemodynamic benefit of skeletal muscle counterpulsation. Period of conditioning: 2 weeks at standard regime.

	5 cm wrap	8 cm wrap
Volume displacement (cm^3)	14.1 (±1.8)	18.36 (±0.5)
Pressure augmentation (mmHg)	14.9 (±2.1)	17.54 (±0.8)
Work done (J)	0.18 (±0.07)	0.24 (±0.07)
Power generated (W)	0.80 (±0.1)	0.92 (±0.04)

5. Acker MA, Anderson WA, Hammond RL, *et al.* Skeletal muscle ventricles in circulation: one to eleven weeks' experience. *J Thorac Cardiovasc Surg* 1987; **94**, 163–174.

6. Acker MA, Mannion JD, Brown WE, *et al.* Canine diaphragm muscle after 1 year of continuous electrical stimulation: its potential as a myocardial substitute. *J Appl Physiol* 1987; **62**, 1264–1270.

7. Chachques JC, Grandjean PA, Fischer EIC, Latremouille C, Jebara VA, Bourgeois I, Carpentier A. Dynamic aortomyoplasty to assist left ventricular failure. *Ann Thorac Surg* 1990; **49**, 225–230.

8. Pattison CW, Cumming DVE, Williamson A, Clayton-Jones DG, Dunn MJ, Goldspink G, Yacoub M. Aortic counterpulsation for up to 28 days using autologous latissimus dorsi in sheep. *J Thorac Cardiovasc Surg* 1991; **102**, 766–773.

9. Bowles CT, Shah SS, Nishimura K, Clark C, Cumming DVE, Pattison CW, Pepper JR, Yacoub M. Development of mock circulation models for the assessment of counterpulsation systems. *Cardiovasc Res* 1991; **25**, 901–908.

10. Pochettino A, Anderson DR, Hammond RL, Salmons S, Stephenson LW. Skeletal muscle ventricles. *Sem Thorac Cardiovasc Surg* 1991; **3**, 154–159.

11. Salmons S, Jarvis JC. *Cardiomyoplasty*: a look at the fundamentals. In: Carpentier A, Chachques JC, Grandjean P (eds), *Cardiomyoplasty*. Mount Kisco, NY: Futura, 1991: 3–17.

31

The experimental evidence for skeletal muscle support in cardiomyoplasty

Russell Millner

Introduction

The concept of biomechanical support (e.g. dynamic cardiomyoplasty) utilizing the patient's own muscle as the mechanical element, and normal or modified muscle metabolism as the power source, is very attractive. Many patients who are not of a high enough priority to be offered a transplant could benefit from cardiac augmentation with their own muscle, a procedure that though still experimental has the potential to be relatively simple. In addition, cardiomyoplasty can be planned and performed electively and avoids the immunological hazards that surround organ transplantation. It would also avoid the use of external energy sources as used in total artificial hearts and ventricular assist devices.

Clinical assessment of dynamic cardiomyoplasty has been limited by logistical, cost and consent difficulties and has mostly been confined to non-invasive methods.[1-4] Whilst evidence of success with dynamic cardiomyoplasty has been presented on clinical grounds[3-7] and in the treatment of acute cardiac failure in animal models,[8-11] there has been until recently very little evidence that it is effective in experimental chronic heart failure.

Models of cardiac failure

A major difficulty with animal models has been the production of a reliable model of chronic heart failure that is appropriate to the study of dynamic cardiomyoplasty. One result of the lack of effective and reliable models of chronic heart failure is that, until recently, the majority of experimental studies published have been either acute studies using muscle that has not been previously transformed, or studies using muscle that has been transformed *in situ* and moved at the time of the operation with the animals studied acutely at that time. A further group of studies are those where the operation has been performed and the animals allowed to recover and undergo a muscle transformation protocol with an acute type of study after the muscle transformation period.

Agents such as doxorubicin or beta-blocking drugs have been used to induce experimental chronic LV failure,[12-17] as have manoeuvres such as rapid ventricular placing[18-22] and global cardiac ischaemia. These techniques have been used in attempts to create animal models that mimic the human pathologies. In spite of this, these studies are criticized either on the grounds that the acutely operated muscle will produce more power with a much faster twitch than the transformed muscle,[23] before it very rapidly fatigues, or that the acutely failing ventricle after propranolol or similar agents is not representative of the clinical situation.

Although doxorubicin produces an effect similar to a dilated cardiomyopathy, the toxicity and narrow 'therapeutic' window have resulted in very high mortality rates. In a recent experimental study of cardiomyoplasty, of 12 animals treated with doxorubicin, only five eventually survived the experimental protocol to provide usable haemodynamic data.[24] The cost of these agents and the haematological monitoring that they need also inhibits their use. Theoretical worries about the effects of long-term beta adrenoceptor blockade on skeletal muscle have also been raised in relation to dynamic cardiomyoplasty. There is experimental evidence that the training adaptations of skeletal muscle are impaired by long-term beta adrenoceptor blockade and that the effects depend on both the fibre type studied and the type of beta adrenoceptor antagonist used.[25]

A model of LV aneurysm in sheep has recently been reported.[26] The model comprises ligation of the homonymous coronary artery (equivalent to the left anterior descending in humans) and its second diagonal branch in open-chested sheep. It has since been confirmed that this is a usable model of moderate chronic LV failure.[27] The coronary anatomy of the sheep is similar to that in humans, without pre-existing coronary collaterals,[26] unlike the dog,[28] and probably for this reason produces a reliable model of aneurysm and LV failure. The relatively normal heart rate, as opposed to the tachycardia of pacing-induced heart failure, and the absence of implanted electronics, makes this model of more practical use in large-animal experimental studies both of skeletal muscle support and mechanical support in heart failure.

Haemodynamic evidence of benefit in cardiomyoplasty

The haemodynamic evidence for benefit comes from four major combinations of experimental procedures in cardiomyoplasty. These are acute heart failure studies in non-transformed muscle, acute heart failure studies in transformed muscle, chronic heart failure studies in non-transformed muscle, and finally chronic heart failure studies in transformed muscle.

Acute heart failure studies in non-transformed muscle

Some of the pioneering work here comes from Termet and coworkers, who used the latissimus dorsi muscle, based on its neurovascular pedicle,

to wrap around the heart.[29] They showed that it was possible with two latissimus dorsi muscle flaps, one wrapped in front and the other behind, to maintain a mean blood pressure of up to 60 mmHg in acute experiments in which the muscles were stimulated together whilst the heart was in induced ventricular fibrillation. Like all the other experimental work at that time, this failed to produce chronic support as the muscles rapidly fatigued.

Acute heart failure studies in transformed muscle

Evidence for haemodynamic benefit has been presented under these conditions for both right ventricular[30] and left ventricular[10] cardiomyoplasty.

After an RV cardiomyoplasty and the standard transformation protocol in 40 kg sheep, acute heart failure was induced with a high dosage of intravenous propranolol (1 mg/min for one hour). Multiple invasive measurements of haemodynamic parameters, including arterial blood pressure, cardiac output, pulmonary artery capillary wedge pressure, right ventricular dP/dT and end-diastolic pressures were performed before induction of heart failure, after induction of heart failure, and with pacing of the cardiomyoplasty flap in established heart failure.[30]

Data from seven animals were presented (Table 31.1). The heart rate fell after propranolol administration and then rose slightly after the cardiomyostimulator was switched on. Systolic aortic pressure fell and then rose slightly. Cardiac output fell markedly and then returned almost to its initial levels. Right ventricular dP/dT fell moderately and increased to above its initial level. RV systolic pressure fell slightly and then increased. There was an increase in RV end-diastolic pressure and a decrease after the cardiomyostimulator was turned on.

Similar data have been provided from LV cardiomyoplasty by Chagas *et al.*[10] (Table 31.2), who showed haemodynamic benefit after acute heart failure had been induced with intravenous propranolol, the benefit being demonstrated by invasive haemodynamic monitoring. In this study six dogs underwent cardiomyoplasty after a muscle transformation protocol. One week after the cardiomyoplasty, acute heart failure was induced with propranolol using an infusion of 2.0 mg/kg. Cardiac output fell markedly after propranolol,

Table 31.1 Results of an RV cardiomyoplasty study in acute heart failure.[30]

	Before propranolol	After propranolol	Cardiomyostimulator on
Heart rate (beats/min)	123 ± 8	91 ± 4	95 ± 6
Systolic aortic pressure (mmHg)	95.6 ± 7.5	86 ± 6.2	87.4 ± 5.8
Cardiac output (l/min)	4.35 ± 0.3	3.74 ± 0.18	4.26 ± 0.17
RV dP/dT (mmHg/s)	275 ± 25	230 ± 25	300 ± 25*
RV systolic pressure (mmHg)	28.5 ± 2.0	27.8 ± 0.9	35.0 ± 0.5†
RV end-diastolic pressure (mmHg)	4.8 ± 1.5	8.0 ± 1.0‡	6.31.0*

* $p < 0.01$; † $p < 0.05$; ‡ $p < 0.001$.

but returned towards the original level after the cardiomyostimulator was turned on. LV systolic pressures behaved similarly. LV end-diastolic pressures rose, as would be expected, after propranolol and then fell after the cardiomyostimulator was turned on, though none of these measures returned completely to their original level.

Chronic heart failure studies in non-transformed muscle

Lee *et al.*[31] used rapid ventricular pacing at a rate of 240–260 beats/min to create chronic heart failure in seven 20 kg dogs. At a second operation, the animals were instrumented and a dynamic cardiomyoplasty with the left latissimus dorsi muscle was performed. As the muscle had not been transformed, brief periods only of muscle stimulation could be used, with muscle fatigue becoming apparent by the end of the 20-second data-acquisition period. Their data (Table 31.3) showed that muscle flap stimulation increased both cardiac output and peak systolic LV pressure

significantly. LV end-diastolic pressure fell with muscle stimulation, and peak left ventricular dP/dT increased.

Using piezoelectric crystals to assess LV dimensions in a number of these animals, they also showed increased fractional shortening across the minor axis of the ventricle and therefore a decreased LV wall stress. As they pointed out, this combination of increased cardiac output and decreased wall stress suggests the possibility of a beneficial effect on myocardial oxygen utilization, together with an increase in 'contractility' of the heart–muscle complex.

Chronic heart failure studies in transformed muscle

Data have been presented from two different models of chronic heart failure to suggest that cardiomyoplasty produces mechanical benefit in experimental animals that have undergone a muscle transformation protocol. Firstly, data from

Table 31.2 Results of an LV cardiomyoplasty study in acute heart failure.[10]

	Before propranolol	After propranolol	Cardiomyostimulator on
Cardiac output (l/min)	2.42 ± 0.25	1.46 ± 0.13	2.01 ± 0.16
LV systolic pressure (mmHg)	140 ± 10	127 ± 10	131 ± 8
LV end-diastolic pressure (mmHg)	7.2 ± 1.2	18 ± 2.2	12.1 ± 1.47

Table 31.3 Results of a study of chronic heart failure in dogs using non-transformed muscle.[31]

	Stimulator off	Stimulator on
Cardiac output (ml/min)	966 ± 124	1166 ± 112*
LV systolic pressure (mmHg)	94 ± 4	104 ± 4*
LV end-diastolic pressure (mmHg)	18 ± 1	15 ± 1*
Peak LV dP/dT (mmHg/s)	867 ± 38	1254 ± 96*

* $p < 0.001$, from paired *t* tests.

Sink's laboratory[24] in dogs pretreated with doxorubicin have shown improvement in both radionuclide angiocardiography and LV pressures measured at cardiac catheterization. They showed that there were improvements in global ejection fractions as measured by MUGA scan, and in the regional ejection fractions of the low lateral, apical and low septal regions. There were significant falls in LV end-diastolic pressures from 11.2 ± 1.48 mmHg without stimulation to 9.6 ± 1.52 mmHg with 10 V stimulation (mean $\pm$ SD, $p < 0.05$). Although there were trends towards improved left ventricular dP/dT and LV systolic pressures in this study, they did not reach statistical significance.

Data have recently been presented from a study of cardiomyoplasty in 40 kg sheep using the LV aneurysm model of chronic LV failure,[32] in which the sheep underwent a muscle transformation protocol prior to haemodynamic studies. Three groups of animals were studied, one with LV aneurysms alone, a second with unpaced muscle wraps over their LV aneurysms, and a third group with a conventional paced dynamic cardiomyoplasty over their LV aneurysms. Haemodynamic studies included cardiac output, invasive measures of systemic arterial and pulmonary artery pressures, together with intracavity LV pressures with a catheter-tipped pressure transducer.

Analysis of the haemodynamic data showed little benefit at baseline on/off studies, either between the three groups or within on/off studies in the paced cardiomyoplasty group. Nonetheless, significant improvements in cardiac output and indices of LV function were seen when the animals were volume-loaded to worsen their heart failure (Table 31.4). These improvements were most apparent when the animals had received 1000–1500 ml of plasma expander, which increased their LV end-diastolic pressures to around 32.4 mmHg with the cardiomyostimulator off, falling to 26.4 mmHg with the cardiomyosti-

mulator on in the paced cardiomyoplasty group. At the same point on the curves, after 1000 ml of plasma expander, cardiac output in this group increased from 3.09 l/min with the cardiomyostimulator off to 3.59 l/min with the cardiomyostimulator on; after 1500 ml of plasma expander, cardiac output in this group increased from 3.47 l/min to 3.96 l/min. Left ventricular dP/dT and stroke volume were also improved when the cardiomyostimulator was turned on.

Benefits were also seen in this study when comparison was made between the animals with unpaced cardiomyoplasty and those with paced cardiomyoplasty. In particular, when function curves were drawn of volume transfused against pulmonary artery capillary wedge pressure and against stroke volume, there were statistically significant improvements in the paced cardiomyoplasty group, with their cardiomyostimulators switched on, compared with the animals with unpaced cardiomyoplasty. These benefits were abolished when the cardiomyostimulators were switched off.

The improved ventricular performance seen in this study cannot be solely due to a 'splinting' of the heart by the latissimus dorsi muscle: if this were so then there would not be any improvement in cardiac output when the cardiomyostimulator was switched *on* in the paced cardiomyoplasty group, nor would there be a difference between the paced and unpaced cardiomyoplasty groups.

It has also been shown in acute experiments[30] that the orientation of the wrap used in this particular study is mechanically inefficient in transferring energy from muscle contraction to mass transport of blood. The usual explanation for the clinical improvement seen after cardiomyoplasty is that the heart is 'squeezed' by the muscle wrap as it contracts, which implies that the improvements seen in cardiac performance in this model underestimate those that could be

Table 31.4 Results of a study of chronic heart failure in sheep using transformed muscle.[32]

	Stimulator off	Stimulator on
LV end-diastolic pressure (mmHg)	32.4 ± 2.43	26.4 ± 2.43*
Cardiac output (l/min)	3.09 ± 0.25	3.59 ± 0.35†
Cardiac output (+1500 ml)	3.47 ± 0.41	3.96 ± 0.37‡
LV dP/dT (mmHg/s)	650 ± 55	875 ± 50§
Stroke volume (ml/beat)	34.02 ± 3.19	39.14 ± 3.67

$p = 0.009$; †$p = 0.057$; ‡$p = 0.018$; §$p = 0.039$; from paired t tests.
The infusion was 1000 ml unless indicated otherwise.

seen if the wrap were more mechanically efficient.

There is an alternative suggestion that part, at least, of the transfer of energy from the muscle to the blood stream comes about as a result of forceful displacement of the heart within the mediastinum. It is harder to visualize the exact mechanism by which this might occur, although in the model used here it was obvious that there was significant potential for cardiac displacement to occur (R. Millner, unpublished observation).

Conclusions

There has emerged a considerable body of evidence for haemodynamic benefit in cardiomyoplasty. We are beginning to be able to resolve the dichotomy between the symptomatic benefit reported by patients and the difficulty in quantifying in the same patients a measurable haemodynamic benefit from the procedure of cardiomyoplasty. It is becoming clearer that we should be focusing our attention on the responses to stress in the experimental studies, and that in the assessment of patients we should be looking for correlations between their symptomatic benefit and their haemodynamics during exercise or other forms of stress.

References

1. Magovern GJ, Park SB, Kao RL, Christlieb IY, Liebler GA, Magovern GJ. Dynamic cardiomyoplasty in patients. *J Heart Transplant* 1990; **9**, 258–263.
2. Molteni L, Almada H, Ferreira R. Synchronously stimulated skeletal muscle graft for left ventricular assistance. *J Thorac Cardiovasc Surg* 1989; **97**, 439–446.
3. Moreira LFP, Stolf NAG, Bocchi EA, Pereira-Barretto AC, Meneghetti JC, Giorgi MCP, Moraes AV, Leite JJ, Da Luz LP, Jatene AD. Latissimus dorsi cardiomyoplasty in the treatment of patients with dilated cardiomyopathy. *Circulation* 1990; **82**(suppl 4), 257–263.
4. Moreira LFP, Stolf NAG, Jatene A. Benefits of cardiomyoplasty for dilated cardiomyopathy. *Sem Thorac Cardiovasc Surg* 1991; **3**, 140–144.
5. Carpentier A, Chachques JC. Latissimus dorsi cardiomyoplasty to increase cardiac output. In: Rabago G, Cooley DA (eds), *Heart Valve Replacement: Current Status and Future Trends*. London, Futura, 1987: 473–486.
6. Molteni L, Almada H. Clinical cardiac assist with synchronously stimulated skeletal muscle. *J Thorac Cardiovasc Surg* 1988; **95**, 940–941.
7. Chachques JC, Grandjean PA, Pfeffer TA, Perier P, Dreyfus G, Jebara VA, Acar C, Levy M, Bourgeois I, Fabiani J-N, Deloche A, Carpentier A. Cardiac assistance by atrial or ventricular cardiomyoplasty. *J Heart Transplant* 1990; **9**, 239–251.
8. Soberman MS, Wornom IL, Justicz AG, Coleman JJ, Austin GE, Alazraki NP, Sink JD. Latissimus dorsi dynamic cardiomyoplasty of the right ventricle. *J Thorac Cardiovasc Surg* 1990; **99**, 817–827.
9. Chachques JC, Grandjean PA, Schwartz K, Mihaileanu S, Fardeau M, Swynghedauw B, Fontaliran F, Romero N, Wisnewsky C, Perier P, Chauvaud S, Bourgeois I, Carpentier A. Effects of latissimus dorsi dynamic cardiomyoplasty on ventricular function. *Circulation* 1988; **78**(suppl 3), 203–216.
10. Chagas ACP, Moreira LFP, da Luz PL, Camarano GP, Leirner A, Stolf NAG, Jatene AD. Stimulated preconditioned skeletal muscle cardiomyoplasty: an effective means of cardiac assist. *Circulation* 1989; **80**(suppl 3), 202–208.
11. Chachques, Grandjean PA, Serraf A, Latremouille C, Jebara VA, Ponzio O, Mihaileanu S, Chauvaud S, Bourgeois I, Carpentier A. Atrial cardiomyoplasty after Fontan type procedures. *Circulation* 1990; **82**(suppl 4), 183–189.
12. Arnolda L, McGrath BP, Cocks M, Johnston CI, 1986. Vasoconstrictor role for vasopressin in experimental heart failure in the rabbit. *J Clin Invest* 1986; **783**, 674–679.
13. Tomlinson CW. Left ventricular geometry and function in experimental heart failure. *Can J Cardiol* 1987; **36**, 305–310.
14. Jones SM, Kirby MS, Harding SE, Vescova G, Wanless RB, Dalla Libera L, Poole-Wilson PA. Adriamycin cardiomyopathy in the rabbit: alterations in contractile proteins and myocyte function. *Cardiovasc Res* 1990; **24**, 834–842.
15. Kao RL, Christlieb IY, Magovern GJ, Park SB, Magovern GJ. The importance of skeletal muscle fiber orientation for dynamic cardiomyoplasty. *J Thorac Cardiovasc Surg* 1990; **99**, 134–140.
16. Doherty JD, Cobbe SM. Electrophysiological changes in an animal model of chronic cardiac failure. *Cardiovasc Res* 1990; **24**, 309–316.
17. Shenasa H, Calderone A, Vermuelen M, Paradis P, Stephens H, Cardinal R, de Champlain J, Rouleau JL. Chronic doxorubicin induced cardiomyopathy in rabbits: mechanical, intracellular action potential, and beta adrenergic characteristics of the failing myocardium. *Cardiovasc Res* 1990; **24**, 591–604.
18. Wilson JR, Lanoce V, Frey M, Ferraro N. Arterial baroreceptor control of peripheral resistance in experimental heart failure. *Am Heart J* 1990; **119**, 1122–1130.

19. Holtz J, Munzel T, Sommer O, Dassenge C. 1990. Converting enzyme inhibition by enalapril in experimental heart failure. *Nephron* 1990; **55**(suppl 1), 73–76.
20. Wang W, Chen JC, Zucker IH. Carotid sinus baroceptor activity in experimental heart failure. *Circulation* 1990; **81**, 1957–1966.
21. Spinale FG, Hendrick DA, Crawford FA, Carabello BA. Relationship between bioimpedance, thermodilution, and ventriculographic measurements in experimental heart failure. *Cardiovasc Res* 1990; **24**, 423–429.
22. Moe GW, Angus C, Howard RJ, De Bold AJ, Armstrong PW. Pathophysiological role of changing atrial size and pressure in modulation of atrial naturetic factor during evolving experimental heart failure. *Cardiovasc Res* 1990; **24**, 570–577.
23. Salmons S, Jarvis JC. Cardiomyoplasty: the basic issues. *Cardiac Chron* 1990; **4**, 1–7.
24. Cheng W, Justicz AG, Soberman MS, Alazraki NP, Santamore WP, Sink JD. Effects of dynamic cardiomyoplasty on indices of left ventricular systolic and diastolic function in a canine model of chronic heart failure. *J Thorac Cardiovasc Surg* 1992; **103**, 1207–1213.
25. Thomas DP, Jenkins RJ. Effects of beta 1 *vs* beta 1–beta 2 blockade on training adaptations in rat skeletal muscle. *J Appl Physiol* 1986; **60**, 1722–1726.
26. Markowitz LJ, Savage EB, Ratcliffe MB, Bavaria JE, Kreiner G, Iozzo RV, Hargrove WC, Bogen DK, Edmunds LH. Large animal model of ventricular aneurysm. *Ann Thorac Surg* 1989; **206**, 211–219.
27. Millner RWJ, Mann JM, Pearson I, Pepper JR. An experimental model of left ventricular failure. *Ann Thorac Surg* 1991; **52**, 78–83.
28. Flameng W, Vanhaecke J, Vandeplassche G. Studies on experimental myocardial infarction: dogs or baboons? *Cardiovasc Res* 1986; **20**, 241–247.
29. Termet H, Chaleneon JL, Estourm E, Gaillard P, Favre JP. Transplantation sur le myocard d'un muscle strie excite par pacemaker. *Ann Chir Thor Cardio* 1966; **5**, 270.
30. Millner RWJ, Guvendik L, Clarke T, Hynd J, Pepper JR. Right ventricular dynamic cardiomyoplasty: an experimental model. *Eur J Cardiothorac Surg* 1991; **5**, 311–314.
31. Lee KF, Dignan RJ, Parmar JM, Dyke CM, Benton G, Yeh T, Abd-Elfattah AS, Wechsler AS. Effects of dynamic cardiomyoplasty on left ventricular performance and myocardial mechanics in dilated cardiomyopathy. *J Thorac Cardiovasc Surg* 1991; **102**, 124–131.
32. Millner RWJ, Burroughs M, Pearson I, Pepper JR. Dynamic cardiomyoplasty in chronic left ventricular failure: an experimental model. *Ann Thorac Surg* 1993; **55**, 493–501.

32

Dynamic cardiomyoplasty at nine years

Alain F Carpentier, Juan-Carlos Chachques and Pierre A Grandjean

Introduction

End-stage heart failure is a major concern in cardiology because of the severity of its prognosis and its prevalence in western countries. About twelve years ago, actuarial survival at 3 years was reported to be only 20%.[1] Recent advances in medical treatment have improved and prolonged the survival, but progression remains inexorable and fatal outcome only delayed. Heart transplantation is a reasonable alternative to medical treatment but is limited by shortage of donors, contraindications and complications.

Cardiomyoplasty, a technique that we first introduced clinically in 1985, has the advantage of using the patient's own living tissues, thus avoiding rejection and related problems.[2] The haemodynamic effect of this technique has been demonstrated in short-term experiments. Skeletal muscle wrapped around the heart and electrically stimulated was able to enhance heart performance.[3-7] Normal cardiac output was restored when right or left ventricular walls were partially replaced by the latissimus dorsi muscle.[6] Haemodynamic improvement has also been documented in the presence of acutely induced myocardial dysfunction.[5-7] However, muscle fatigue was thought to be an insurmountable barrier whenever long-term stimulation was used. The introduction by our group of the concept of progressive sequential stimulation[2] was able to

overcome this difficulty, as shown by long-term experiments.[3]

Since the first clinical application in 1985,[8] cardiomyoplasty has been used clinically in the treatment of various cardiac diseases: tumour, aneurysm, ischaemic cardiomyopathy, dilated cardiomyopathy and Chagas disease, by others[9-16] and ourselves.[17,18] Results have been encouraging so far, although extreme variations have been found due to the heterogenicity of the patient population and of the techniques used. Our own experience, the longest and the largest so far, permits us to summarize the techniques, indications, and results.

Surgical technique

The surgical technique has evolved through the years with the aim of reducing pre-assist mortality and increasing the efficiency of the procedure. In the past four years, use of the 'non-cardiac suture' technique[19] and the 'flap sliding manoeuvre'[20] effectively reduced the operative mortality to 12%. There are, however, still controversial technical points which must be discussed.

Muscle orientation

Recent experimental studies have shown that an anterior positioning with a counterclockwise wrapping of the flap can be more efficient than posterior positioning,[21] but in patients with enlarged hearts, anterior positioning of the muscle flap does not allow the left ventricle to be completely covered. A pragmatic approach must be preferred in clinical practice taking into consideration the type of ventricular failure, the size of the heart and the size of the flap (Figs 32.1 and 32.2).

In *predominant left heart failure*, the flap must be positioned posteriorly in contact with the left ventricle. In *predominant right heart failure* the flap is positioned anteriorly. Enlarged heart size is a serious limitation to muscle wrapping particularly when the size of the muscle flap is small. Partial excision of the ventricle in order to reduce its size has not been associated with good results in our experience. Poor results were also observed whenever trying to reduce the size of the heart by excess tension on the muscle flap. It seems that severely dilated ventricles have adapted themselves to a given wall tension which cannot be reduced without impairing the residual contractility.

It is unfortunate that, owing to the short neurovascular pedicle, only the distal half of the flap, the less efficient, can be used for the wrapping. The use of a free flap with revascularization by the internal mammary vessels would be an ideal solution to this problem, but experimental section of the nerve has always led to progressive dystrophy of the muscle.

Muscle stimulation and ventricular compliance

Although some haemodynamic benefits have been obtained with single-pulse muscle stimulation,[9,16] it is now widely accepted that the protocol of progressive sequential stimulation and trains of pulses are preferable for muscle transformation and cardiac assistance.[2,3] The interval between the sensed QRS complex and each pulse train is of paramount importance. Both experimental and clinical data have shown that muscle contraction may affect ventricular filling when no delay is present between the QRS complex and the pulse

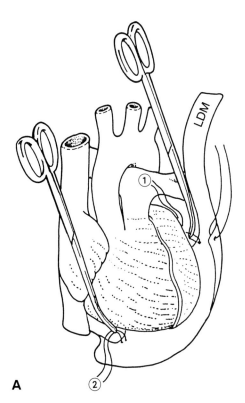

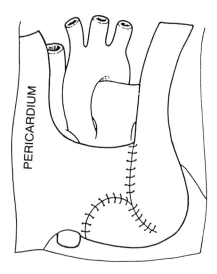

Fig. 32.1 (A) Extracardiac suture technique of cardiomyoplasty (posterior-anterior wrapping). The latissimus dorsi muscle (LDM) flap is positioned behind the heart using two long forceps, then is fixed to the pericardium, at the vicinity of pulmonary artery (suture 1) and inferior vena cava (suture 2). (B) The wrapping is completed by fixing the anterior part of the LDM to itself and to a pericardial flap tailored from the right edge of pericardiotomy.

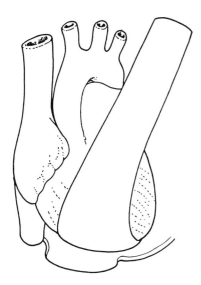

Fig. 32.2 Anterior-posterior wrapping of the heart for cases of preponderant right ventricular failure.

train.[22] Echocardiography must be used to adjust this delay in order to provide optimal synchronization between muscle contraction, ventricular systole and mitral valve closure.

Tachycardia is another factor which may impair ventricular filling, since in the current model of cardiomyostimulator (SP 1005) the pulse train has a fixed duration (185 milliseconds). For this reason, the stimulator automatically increases the heart muscle contraction ratio (2/1, 3/1, 4/1) with increasing heart rates, which results in assisting only one systole over two, three or four during exercise. The heart muscle contraction ratio must be adapted to each individual patient according to functional improvement. Most of the time the optimal ratio is 2/1. Whenever synchronization between heart and muscle contraction is adequate, the muscle does not impair the ventricular compliance because of the greater wall tension of the dilated ventricles.

Clinical results

From January 1985 to November 1993, 65 patients suffering from severe heart failure were operated on at Hôpital Broussais in Paris (Table 32.1). Their ages ranged from 15 to 69 years (mean 50.8 years). There were 54 males and 11 females.

Table 32.1 Surgical modalities.

Reinforcement technique	51 (78%)
Substitution technique	14 (22%)
Anterior wrap	6 (9%)
Posterior wrap	58 (89%)
Atrial wrap	1 (2%)
Extracorporeal circulation	23 (35%)
Intra-aortic balloon counterpulsation	27 (42%)

Aetiology

The two main causes of heart failure were chronic myocardial ischaemia and dilated cardiomyopathy.

Myocardial ischaemia

The 39 patients with myocardial ischaemia had suffered several myocardial infarctions and four had had previous coronary artery revascularization. All were considered to be beyond the possibility of efficient myocardial revascularization at the time of cardiomyoplasty. Ten patients, however, had one severely obstructed coronary artery suitable for bypass which, in the absence of pain, raised the question of the need for revascularization. Thirty-four patients had a global dilatation of the heart and 11 had an extensive anteroapical left ventricular aneurysm.

Dilated cardiomyopathy

Twenty-one patients presented with a dilated cardiomyopathy. Nineteen were idiopathic and two had a valvular origin. Among the 21 patients with a dilated cardiomyopathy, 18 had a predominant left ventricular cardiomyopathy and three (mean age 22) had an isolated right ventricular cardiomyopathy.

Cardiac tumour

Four patients suffered from a cardiac tumour. The first patient had an extensive fibroma involving the posterior wall of both ventricles and the diaphragm. The second had a lymphoma of the right heart involving the right atrium, the tricuspid valve and the aterior wall of the right ventricle. The third patient had a fibroma involving the anterior wall and the infundibulum of the right ventricle, a portion of the tricuspid valve and one cusp of the pulmonary valve. The fourth patient had an angioma localized in the ventricular septum. After the resection of the tumour, he needed an RV cardiomyoplasty.

Congenital malformation

One patient, aged 27, had elevated pulmonary resistances and severe venous and liver congestion developed 6 years after a Fontan operation made to correct a single ventricle with pulmonary artery stenosis.

Clinical status

All patients but one were in New York Heart Association functional class III or IV before operation (mean 3.3) (Table 32.2). Most of the patients had been hospitalized repeatedly for congestive heart failure with an average of 2.5 episodes/patient/year. Twenty-three of these patients had one or several episodes of pulmonary oedema, reversible with maximal medical therapy, in the year preceding the operation. Sixty patients were in sinus rhythm and the remaining five were in atrial fibrillation. Ventricular extrasystoles were present in 37 patients, among whom seven had several episodes of ventricular tachycardia. Other clinical or functional data are listed in Table 32.2.

Mitral valve incompetence (MVI) was present in six patients, severe in two and mild to moderate in four. The functional mechanism was MVI with normal leaflet motion (Type I) in one patient, leaflet prolapse (Type II) in two patients and restricted leaflet motion (Type III) in three. Tricuspid valve insufficiency was present in five patients. The functional mechanism involved was normal leaflet motion (Type I) in one patient and restricted leaflet motion (Type III) in two patients. In the remaining two patients, tricuspid

Table 32.3 Associated pathology (contraindications to heart transplantation).

Insulin-dependent diabetes	11
Pulmonary artery hypertension	11
Respiratory insufficiency	9
Gastric ulcer	7
Renal insufficiency	4
Cancer	5
Lupus erythematosus	1
Colonic diverticulosis	1

insufficiency resulted from the involvement of the leaflet tissue by a cardiac tumour.

Associated pathology and contraindications to heart transplantation

Associated non-cardiac diseases were present in the majority of these patients and precluded heart transplantation (Table 32.3). The five patients with a malignancy (Hodgkin's disease, lymphoma, thyroid carcinoma and two renal carcinomas) had been treated in the years preceding cardiomyoplasty and were considered cured or in remission.

Forty-two patients (64%) had one or several contraindications to cardiac transplantation: medical in 24, tumours in five, age over 65 in four, socioeconomical or geographical in 10. Among the 23 patients who had no contraindication to cardiac transplantation, 11 refused transplantation and five were judged to have a lower risk associated with a cardiomyoplasty than with cardiac transplantation (EF > 20% in four patients and isolated right ventricular failure in one). None of these five patients died.

Survival

Our experience demonstrates that cardiomyoplasty improves long-term survival. The 68.3% actuarial survival at 4 years contrasts with the survival of medically treated patients.[12] Improved survival in patients with cardiomyoplasty was demonstrated by Jatene and Moreira who compared medically treated patients with cardiomyoplasty patients.[24] The 2-year survival was 80% in the cardiomyoplasty group and 30% in the medically treated group. Survival can further be improved by taking into consideration the risk factors of the pre-assist and the post-assist periods (Table 32.4).

Table 32.2 Clinical status of the 65 patients prior to cardiomyoplasty.

Functional class IV	21
III	44
Left heart failure	41
Right heart failure	6
Biventricular failure	17
Cardiothoracic ratio	54 ± 5%
Indexed LV end-diastolic volume	178 ± 31 ml/m^2
Maximal oxygen consumption	12.8 ± 3.5 ml/min/kg
Left ventricular ejection fraction (at rest)	17 ± 6%

Table 32.4 Preoperative risk factors influencing hospital and late mortality (multivariate analysis).

Factors increasing hospital mortality
Clinical factors
Age >65 years
Filing pressures >45 mmHg
Patients on preoperative inotropic drug support
Biventricular heart failure
Pulmonary vascular hypertension

Surgical factors
'Cardiac suture' technique
Cardiopulmonary bypass
Associated valve procedures

Factors increasing late mortality
Permanent NYHA functional class IV
Cardiothoracic ratio >0.60
LV ejection fraction <15%
Biventricular heart failure
Pulmonary vascular hypertension
Atrial fibrillation

Functional benefit

A significant functional improvement was found in the great majority of the patients (Tables 32.5 and 32.6). Functional class decreased from an average 3.3 preoperatively to 1.5 postoperatively. Exercise capacity was generally improved, the number of episodes of hospitalizations per patient/year was reduced from 2.5 to 0.4 and in 64% of patients the need of drugs was significantly reduced. Similar improvements have been described by others.[11,24,25] Also of interest is the fact that functional improvement was progressive over a period of up to one year, which shows the capacity of the muscle to adapt to its new function. Functional improvement varied, however, from patient to patient, the least improvement being seen in patients with preoperative biventricular failure, excessive cardiac enlargement and ejection fraction below 15%.

Haemodynamics

Most disappointing was the fact that functional improvement did not always imply haemody-

namic improvement (Figs 32.3 and 32.4). Ejection fraction (radioisotopic) did increase in the majority of the patients (17% preoperatively versus 25% postoperatively), but no significant changes in filling pressures could be documented in the majority of the patients in this series (Table 32.7). In a recent report, however, Jatene and Moreira reported a significant reduction of the mean pulmonary artery pressure (from 37.4 mmHg to 26.6 mmHg) and of the mean pulmonary wedge pressure (from 24.8 mmHg to 16.6 mmHg) 12 months after the operation.[13] Patients with greater LV dimensions presented lesser LV ejection fraction improvements. More precisely, significant improvement in left ventricular function was found in patients whose left ventricular diastolic diameter was below 70 mm whereas no change was found in patients with a ventricular diastolic diameter greater than 75 mm. Both in Jatene's experience and in our experience, LV dimensions throughout the years showed a *stabilization in the process of ventricular dilatation in the majority of the patients.*

Mechanism of enhanced heart function

The improved ejection fraction observed in most cases, although limited, demonstrates that the functional improvement results from enhanced heart function. A placebo effect can therefore be ruled out. This is confirmed by the functional impairment following battery depletion observed in two patients and its complete reversibility after a new battery was implanted. Enhanced heart function involves several mechanisms.

Active reinforcement

The heart and the wrapped skeletal muscle behave like a cybernetic system with two interactive components, the heart governing the muscle and the muscle reinforcing heart contraction. The efficiency of the system depends on the

Table 32.5 Functional improvement in 29 patients surviving cardiomyoplasty and not transplanted.

	Preoperative	Postoperative	
Functional class (mean)	3.3	1.5	$p < 0.05$
Exercise capacity (watts)	60 ± 24	96 ± 18	$p < 0.1$
Hospitalizations (number/pt/year)	2.5	0.4	$p < 0.05$
Oxygen consumption (ml/min/kg)	12.8 ± 3.5	18.6 ± 4	$p < 0.05$

Table 32.6 Haemodynamic evaluation by aortic flow Doppler study (cardiomyostimulator off/on comparison).

| | Follow-up | |
	2 years	3 years
Patient numbers	21	11
Patients with Doppler improvements	15 (71%)	7 (63%)
LV stroke volume (% increase)	+27±8%	+22±4%
Cardiac output (% increase)	+12±3%	+10±2%
	$p < 0.05$	$p < 0.05$

Table 32.7 Haemodynamic data ($n = 20$).

	Pre-operative	Post-operative (2 years)	
MPAP (mmHg)	24.4±6.2	26.2±4	NS
MPWP (mmHg)	15.8±2.8	17.6±3.1	NS
LEVDP (mmHg)	20.3±4.2	18.7±2.6	NS
CI (l/min/m²)	2.38±0.41	2.87±0.63	$p = 0.049$
LVEF (%)	24±6.2	30.6±5	$p = 0.043$
LVED vol (ml/m²) indexed	178±31	186±36	NS

mechanical characteristics of these two components and the synchronization of their action. According to Laplace's law, the larger the ventricles the greater the tension which must be generated to produce a given pressure. Indeed, greater left ventricular dimension presented lesser left ventricular ejection fraction improvement.[12] Active reinforcement depends also on the size of the muscle and the amount of wrapping. The power of the transformed muscle has been calculated to be 40 W/kg, identical to the power developed by cardiac muscle during systolic contraction.[26] It is unfortunate that only a portion of this force is used since only a part of the muscle can be wrapped around the heart so as to prevent excessive tension on the neurovascular pedicle. Even though the free portion of the graft may also participate to some extent in cardiac assistance by traction and elevation of the heart during contraction, more than 50% of the force of the muscle is lost. A technique to elongate the neurovascular pedicle needs to be developed.

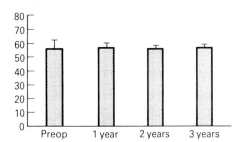

Fig. 32.3 Cardiothoracic ratios.

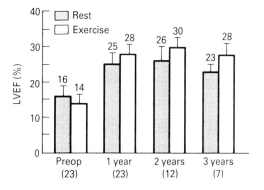

Fig. 32.4 Cardiomyoplasty LV ejection fraction (radioisotopic).

Passive reinforcement

By its intrinsic tension, the muscle prevents further dilatation of the ventricles and can restore more orderly cardiac contraction. In our experience, a stabilization of the process of ventricular dilatation could be documented as well as reduction in the paradoxical motion of the ventricular septum. Even in the case of passive reinforcement, stimulation of the muscle is important since it increases the tension of the muscle at the appropriate time.

Biological effect

By taking part of the workload of the heart without increasing the myocardial oxygen requirement, the muscle actually increases the oxygen supply to the heart so that some recovery of the cardiac function may result from this mechanism. This biological effect is suggested by two patients of our series who kept the full functional benefit of the operation for several days after the battery had been removed because of infection.

Enhanced coronary revascularization

Scattered coronary capillaries have been stained by dye injections into the latissimus dorsi artery in experimental animals after one year. However, this has not been documented in the human thus far.

Conclusions

Although some positive conclusions can be given at this stage, numerous points remain obscure and serious drawbacks must be underlined. The two most important are the variability of the results and the limited improvement observed after this operation. Numerous factors may explain these drawbacks, including heterogeneous patient population, heart size, suboptimal indications, variable muscle anatomy and vascularization. Some of these factors have been improved. They may be further improved upon in the future, especially patient selection. Table 32.8 summarizes the indications and contraindications as we consider them today.

In contrast, some positive points must be recognized which justify and stimulate our continuing effort to develop this operation. The fact that continuous fatigueless contraction of a skeletal muscle at the frequency of the heart has been obtained for periods of more than nine years in the human is in itself remarkable. The fact that patient survival was increased and that most patients were functionally improved with a significant increase in cardiac output and ejection fraction in many is most encouraging. Finally, the fact that similar results have been obtained by various groups throughout the world, provided that they had access to burst train generators, demonstrates that the operation is reproducible. All new operations face uncertainties and shortcomings in their developmental phases. As experience has accumulated, some of them have already been solved. Further progress is necessary, however, in order for this operation to face the challenge of the growing lack of donors for cardiac transplantation.

Table 32.8 Optimal indications and contraindications for cardiomyoplasty.

Optimal indications
Patients below 70 years of age
Dilated cardiomyopathy (idiopathic or ischaemic)
Functional class III or intermittent class IV
Sinus rhythm
Coronary arteries: good collateral circulation and no critical stenosis

Mitral valve regurgitation <++
LV ejection fraction >15%
LV end diastolic volume <250 ml

Contraindications
Hypertrophied cardiomyopathy
Permanent functional class IV
Severe, intractable ventricular arrhythmia
Pulmonary artery hypertension
Biventricular failure
Mitral valve incompetence >++ (temporary contraindication)

Neurovascular disease, or cachexia
Left pleura calcifications
Severe respiratory insufficiency (<55% predicted)

Ejection fraction <10%
Cardiac index <1.5 l/min/m^2
LV end diastolic volume >300 ml
LV end diastolic pressure >45 mmHg

References

1. Franciosa JA, Wilen M, Ziesche S, Cohn JN. Survival in men with severe chronic left ventricular failure due to either coronary heart disease or idiopathic dilated cardiomyopathy. *Am J Cardiol* 1983; **51**, 831–836.
2. Carpentier A, Chachques JC, Grandjean PA, Perier P, Mitz V, Bourgeois I. Transformation d'un muscle squelettique par stimulation séquentielle progressive en vue de son utilisation comme substitut myocardique. *CR Acad Sciences Paris* 1985; **301**, 581–586.
3. Chachques JC, Grandjean PA, Schwartz K, Mihaileanu S, Fardeau M, Swynghedauw B, Fontaliran F, Romero N, Wisnewsky C, Perier P, Chauvaud S, Bourgeois I, Carpentier A. Effect of latissimus dorsi dynamic cardiomyoplasty on ventricular function. *Circulation* 1988; **78**(suppl III), 203–216.
4. Termet H, Chalencon JL, Estour E, *et al.* Transplantation sur le myocarde d'un muscle strié excité par pace-maker. *Ann Chir Thorac Cardiovasc* 1966; **5**, 568–571.
5. Nakamura K, Glenn WI. Graft or diaphragm as a functioning substitute for myocardium. *J Surg Res* 1964; **4**, 435–439.
6. Macoviak J, Stephenson LW, Spielman S, *et al.* Replacement of ventricular myocardium with diaphragmatic skeletal muscle: short-term studies. *J Thorac Cardiovasc Surg* 1981; **81**, 519–527.

7. Dewar ML, Drinkwater DC, Chiu RC-J. Synchronously stimulated skeletal muscle graft for myocardial repair. *J Thorac Cardiovasc Surg* 1984; **87**, 325–331.

8. Carpentier A, Chachques JC. Myocardial substitution with a stimulated skeletal muscle: first successful clinical case. *Lancet* 1985; **i**, 1207.

9. Magovern GJ, Heckler FR, Park SB, Christlieb IY, Liebler GA, Burkholder JA, Maher TD, Benekart DH, Magovern GJ, Kao RL. Paced skeletal muscle for dynamic cardiomyoplasty. *Ann Thorac Surg* 1988; **45**, 614–619.

10. Carpentier A. The use of autologous pericardium for tissue patching. *Le Club Mitrale Newsletter* 1992; **2**, 7.

11. Magovern GJ, Park SB, Kao RL, Christlieb IY, Magovern GJ. Dynamic cardiomyoplasty in patients. *J Heart Transplant* 1990; **9**, 258–263.

12. Moreira LF, Stolf NA, Bocchi EA, Barretto AP, Meneghetti JC, Giorgi MC, Moraes AV, Leite JJ, da Luz PI, Jatene AD. Latissimus dorsi cardiomyoplasty in the treatment of patients with dilated cardiomyopathy. *Circulation* 1990; **82**(suppl IV), 257–263.

13. Jatene AD, Moreira LFP, Stolf NAG, Bocchi EA, Seferian P, Fernandes PMP, Abensur H. Left ventricular function changes after cardiomyoplasty in patients with dilated cardiomyopathy. *J Thorac Cardiovasc Surg* 1991; **102**, 132–139.

14. Moreira LFP, Chagas ACP, Camarano GP, Cardiomyoplasty benefits in experimental myocardial dysfunction. *J Cardiac Surg* 1989; **4**, 164–170.

15. Moreira LF, Seferian P, Bocchi EA, Pego-Fernandez PM, Stolf NA, Pereira-Barretto AC, Jatene AD. Survival improvement with dynamic cardiomyoplasty in patients with dilated cardiomyopathy. *Circulation* 1991; **84**(suppl III), 296–302.

16. Almada H, Molteni L, Ferreira R, Ortega D. Clinical experience with dynamic cardiomyoplasty. *J Cardiac Surg* 1990; **5** 193–198.

17. Carpentier A, Chachques JC. The use of stimulated skeletal muscle to replace diseased human heart muscle. In: Chiu RC-J (ed), *Biomechanical Cardiac Assit*. New York: Futura, 1986: 85–102.

18. Carpentier A, Chachques JC. Latissimus dorsi cardiomyoplasty to increase cardiac output. In: Rubago G, Cooley BA (eds), *Heart Valve Replacement and Future Trends in Cardiac Surgery*. New York: Futura, 1987: 473–486.

19 Carpentier A, Chachques JC. Surgical technique. In: Carpentier A, Chachques JC, Grandjean PA (eds), *Cardiomyoplasty*. New York: Futura, 1991: 105–122.

20. Carpentier A, Chachques JC, Acar C, Relland J, Mihaileanu S, Bensasson D, Kieffer JP, Guibourt P, Tournay D, Roussin I, Grandjean PA. Dynamic cardiomyoplasty at seven years. *J Thorac Cardiovasc Surg* 1993; **106**, 42–54.

21. Kao RL, Christlieb IY, Magovern GJ, Park SB, Magovern GJ. The importance of skeletal muscle fiber orientation for dynamic cardiomyoplasty. *J Thorac Cardiovasc Surg* 1990; **99**, 134–140.

22. Molteni L, Almada HE, Ferreira RP, Ortega D. Assessment of the optimal time interval between QRS and simple pulse stimulation in dynamic cardiomyoplasty. In: Chiu RC-J, Bourgeois I (eds), *Transformed Muscle for Cardiac Assist and Repair*. New York: Futura, 1990: 189–196.

23. Chachques JC, Acar C, Portoghese M, Bensasson D, Guibourt P, Grare P, Jebara VA, Grandjean PA, Carpentier A: Dynamic cardiomyoplasty for long-term cardiac assist. *Eur J Cardiothorac Surg* 1992; **6**, 642–648.

24. Moreira LFP, Bocchi EA, Stolf NAG, Pileggi F, Jatene AD: Current expectations in dynamic cardiomyoplasty. *Ann Thorac Surg* 1993; **55**, 299–303.

25. Jegaden O, Delahaye F, Finet G, Van Der Veen F, Montagna P, Eker A, Ossete J, Rossi R, Saint Pierre A, Mikaeloff Ph: Late hemodynamic results after cardiomyoplasty in congestive heart failure. *Ann Thorac Surg* 1994; **57**, 1151–1157.

26. Salmons S, Jarvis JC: Cardiomyoplasty: A look at the fundamentals. In: Carpentier A, Chachques JC, Grandjean PA (eds), *Cardiomyoplasty*. New York: Futura, 1991: 3–17.

Section VII _____

Problems

33

Valves in pulsatile devices

Scott Lick, Jack G Copeland, Richard G Smith, Christopher T Bowles,
Martyn Leat and John Fisher

Introduction

Mechanical, tissue, and polyurethane cardiac
valves are used in current Food and Drug Administration (FDA) approved pulsatile blood pumps.
Forces created by pulsatile pumps place greater
loads on valves than does the natural heart. This
was dramatically exemplified by the failure of the
mitral valve strut 13 days after the first total
artificial heart (TAH) implant in Dr Barney
Clark.[1]

This chapter reviews the current generation of
pulsatile devices (Table 33.1) and then discusses
the mechanics of valve failure and parameters
used by designers to reduce forces of blood on
valves.

Pulsatile devices in use today

The Thoratec ventricular assist device (VAD)
system uses Bjork–Shiley monostrut valves for
both inflow and outflow regulation. Instead of
pyrolytic carbon, as is used in standard Bjork–
Shiley valves, the discs are made of Delrin. Delrin
is a plastic that was used in first-generation valves.
It is relatively soft and prone to wear after five
years of use. However, it is less brittle than pyrolytic carbon, and less likely to crack when
opened and closed vigorously when solidly
mounted in an assist device. Wear has not been a
problem in clinical use. The Delrin valve has
higher regurgitation than the pyrolytic carbon
model. This reduces the 80 cm^3 stroke volume to

Table 33.1 Five pulsatile pumps currently being used in the United States.

Pulsatile devices	Heart valves	Inflow (mm)	Outflow (mm)
Thoratec ventricular assist device (VAD)	Bjork–Shiley Delrin	29	25
CardioWest total artificial heart (C-70 TAH)	Medtronic–Hall	27	25
Novacor left ventricular assist system (LVAS)	Carpentier–Edwards pericardial	21	21
Thermo Cardiosystems left ventricular assist device (TCI LVAD)	Medtronic–Hancock porcine	25	25
Abiomed biventricular assist device (BVAD)	Polyurethane tri-leaflet	18.5	18.5

an effective 65 cm^3, but in a device with an external power source this inefficiency is easily overcome.

The CardioWest C-70 (formerly Jarvik-70) total artificial heart uses pyrolytic disc Medtronic–Hall valves at all four positions. The predecessor to this heart, the 100 cm^3 Jarvik-7, was initially constructed using standard Bjork–Shiley valves. After the failure of the valve in the mitral position in Dr Barney Clark (and many failures in animal studies), a change was made to the Medtronic–Hall.[2] It was recognized that the tradeoff for a stronger valve might be haemolysis. Animal experiments conducted in Utah showed that in identical hearts with identical driving parameters, animals with the Medtronic–Hall valve hearts had a 23% decrease in haematocrit, a 75% increase in plasma free haemoglobin, and a 26% increase in lactate dehydrogenase (LDH) compared with Bjork–Shiley valve control hearts.[3,4] This increased blood trauma was believed to be caused in part by the central hole in the disc around the titanium strut. Lowering the driver dP/dT (which can be as high as four times that of a normal heart)[5] reduced haemolysis and valve trauma to acceptable levels. Further modifications of the system have included redesign of the junction between the polyurethane housing and titanium valve ring to eliminate the thrombus-forming gap. This reduced the incidence of thrombus formation at the titanium–polyurethane junction from 83% to 7% in calves and sheep.[6] A further refinement was made using a modified tubular ringed Medtronic–Hall valve custom-made to extremely close tolerances, which reduced the incidence of thrombus formation at this junction to zero. This tubular ringed valve was used in the Symbion acute ventricular assist device (AVAD),[7] but was not incorporated into the TAH for regulatory reasons. The incidence of strokes steadily declined as experience with the device grew and the design was modified.[3]

Notably missing from these devices is the St Jude valve. The haemodynamic properties of the valve are similar to the Medtronic–Hall valve in pulsatile VADs.[8] However, the outer pyrolytic carbon ring is brittle and non-uniform in shape which would require 'custom fitting'. The inner diameter is also non-uniform with flat pivot areas which would either result in turbulence or require custom stent ring adapters. One can compensate for these problems when making the VAD, but a custom fit is required, which is impractical.

The Novacor left ventricular assist system (LVAS) utilizes a relatively flat circular blood chamber with tangential blood flow. This system works best with a central opening valve that allows an inflowing stream of blood to be directed into a circular or vortex flow pattern, which creates better washout. Carpentier–Edwards pericardial 21 mm valves are used in both the inflow and outflow positions. Tissue valves have less regurgitation and hence are more efficient than mechanical valves, which is an advantage in this system that is designed to be mated to a portable transmitted power source. The use of tissue valves may decrease the need for anticoagulation. The valve incorporates a silicon elastomer flange, providing a compliant, energy-absorbing mount in the VAD housing. Also, the flexible wires form stents and the tissues themselves serve to disseminate forces. Implants in humans for up to one year have not resulted in valve failures. However, a peculiar form of red thrombus has been noted on the device side of the inflow valve on some of our implants at the University of Arizona (Fig. 33.1). This has not, however, compromised function of the device.

The Thermo Cardiosystems (TCI) left ventricular assist device (LVAD) utilizes 25 mm Medtronic–Hancock bioprostheses at both the inflow and outflow positions. These valves are not mounted directly to the device but are sewn into a Dacron conduit which is contained within a titanium support.[9] Mounting the valve away from the pump housing junction inside the flexible conduits allows for better dissipation of closing energy. The overall strategy of the device is to eliminate the need for anticoagulation. The interface between blood and pump is coated with textured surfaces with the hope of decreasing thrombogenecity by stimulating the growth of a cellular lining. The success of this idea remains unproven.[10] A tissue valve is the obvious choice for this pump. These valves are stentless modifications of the standard valve created to minimize dead space between leaflet and conduit. To date, 85 device explants have been performed for a total of 170 valves analysed. Thrombus and valve failure have not been a problem. As in the Novacor, a thin collagenous investment on the upstream side of the inflow valve has been noticed, but this has not compromised valve function (K Dasse, personal communication).

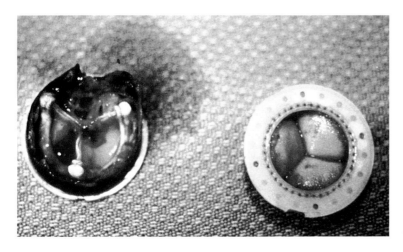

Fig. 33.1 Thrombus on the inflow valve of the Novacor LVAS (left). The outflow valve is shown on the right.

Polyurethane valves

The use of polyurethane valves in pulsatile assist devices has attracted considerable interest owing to their good hydrodynamic properties,[11–13] low manufacturing cost[11,14] and acceptable fatigue life in relation to the anticipated duration of support.[15] In common with many other types of assist device valves, characteristics should include: rapid synchronous leaflet opening, an open geometry which minimizes leaflet bending stresses, smooth closing with minimal regurgitation, a stable closed geometry with low membrane stresses, low back-flow when closed, a fatigue life typically in excess of 400 million cycles, good flow characteristics (especially behind the leaflets), a blood path free from surface discontinuities, and a biocompatible surface.

Polyurethanes are considered the most appropriate of the biocompatible elastomers for pulsatile assist device valve production, and each of the many biomedical grades which are available has different mechanical properties.[16] The correct choice of material is essential for a successful design. In contrast to the anisotropy of natural leaflet tissue,[17,18] which is believed to be of importance in native valve function,[19] polyurethanes are isotropic. The design of the geometry of a polyurethane valve must take into account the isotropic nature of the leaflet material. Polyurethanes are also linearly elastic over low strain ranges, in contrast to the highly nonlinear elasticity of native tissue. It has also been noted that the elastic modulus of polyurethanes at low strains is high in comparison with tissue valves,[20] and this is believed to be an important factor in the design of

valve leaflets with respect to leaflet opening.[21] In common with bioprostheses, polyurethane valves have been shown to calcify in long-term animal implants.[22] It has also been shown that the calcification of polyurethanes can be accelerated by pressure.[23] Calcification is undesirable because it is associated with a reduced life of the flexible valve leaflet owing to an increase in stiffness and local stress concentration, which may accelerate mechanical failure. The rate of calcification of polyurethane valves in clinical use may be sufficiently low for the problem not to be significant over the course of a relatively short period of support.

All polyurethane valves used in pulsatile assist devices are of the trileaflet design and similar in haemodynamic performance to pericardial valves.[11–13] During opening, the leaflets fold away to reveal a central flow orifice which presents a low resistance to flow. The central flow orifice of polyurethane valves is generally regarded as a desirable feature. When polyurethane valves are conduit mounted, there is usually a requirement for sinus-like cavities to encourage washing of the outer aspect of the valve leaflets. A recirculation may be established in the sinus cavity during forward flow which may continue after valve closure. However, it is more likely that the dominant mechanism of washing is retrograde blood flow when the valve is closed.

The Helmholtz Institute group have developed a pneumatic VAD incorporating polyurethane valves to the point of commercialization. These developments have been reported extensively[24–28] and considerable attention has been focused on valve leaflet stress analysis in relation to design.[26]

The early spherical leaflet valve had an optimum stress distribution when closed but was associated with flow separation, a high pressure drop and high strains due to kinking in the open position. Valve performance and durability were enhanced by selecting a conical leaflet geometry.[27] It has been shown that polyurethane valves compare favourably to tilting disks with respect to noise, VAD housing acceleration and thrombogenicity.[28]

Polyurethane trileaflet valves are incorporated into the Abiomed BVS 5000 biventricular device. This pneumatically driven twin-chamber system is gravity-filled and is thus non-ambulatory. Low cost is a key feature of this system and polyurethane is the logical choice of valve design. The valves are manufactured from a proprietary elastomer on a stainless steel mandrel. There is no seam between the cusps and the conduit walls. The neutral geometry of the leaflets corresponds to the fully closed configuration. This creates a spring action which resists opening but enhances leaflet closure and minimizes reverse flow. Sinuses similar to the Sinuses of Valsalva in the native aorta, downstream of the cusps, aid in closure and washout. The internal diameter of the valve is 18.5 mm and the maximum orifice area is 1.5 cm^2. *In vivo* experiments using these valves in ventricular apex-to-aorta conduits in calves showed no angiographic evidence of failure at 4.5 months.[15] Explantation after 29 days in a human showed no gross wear but deterioration of the closing edge of one of the leaflets was evident by scanning electron microscopy.[29]

Mechanisms of valve failure

One of the major design problems associated with pulsatile ventricular assist devices, particularly extracorporeal systems, is the requirement for long cannulae, stiff enough to withstand kinking and of low external diameter to allow sternal closure without cardiac compression. These requirements result in high blood velocities during pump ejection and filling, the rapid deceleration of blood at the end of pump systole and diastole, the reversal of flow through the valve, and the initiation of a pressure oscillation in the cannulae analogous to the water hammer effect.

There are two aspects of this pressure oscillation: the frequency, which increases as the cannula stiffness increases;[30] and the pressure amplitude, which increases with cannula length and is inversely related to its cross-sectional area. The resultant effect is to augment the pressure gradient across the valve, thereby reducing its fatigue life (Fig. 33.2). The key to reducing the water hammer effect is to use wide-bore, short, compliant cannulae and to minimize the reverse flow through the valve at the end of the ejection phase.

An alternative mechanism of valve failure is cavitation which occurs as a result of a transient reduction in local pressure and entails the rapid formation and collapse of vapour-filled bubbles. This phenomenon is well demonstrated in the Venturi tube which is a convergent/divergent flow channel. As the fluid velocity increases, the static pressure decreases and this may cause the liquid to rupture. Downstream of the narrow section, the tube cross-sectional area increases and there is pressure recovery. The cavitation bubbles that form in the constriction implode upon themselves into smaller bubbles, creating high-energy microjets (Fig. 33.2).[31,32]

In a non-occlusive mechanical valve, these phenomena may work together. The driving force is the water hammer pulse pressure on the outflow side of the valve and the vapour pressure created on the inflow side of the valve. The pressure drop across the valve may be 1550–1800 mmHg and exist for 600 milliseconds.[32]

The most important determinant of cavitation and water hammer is the rate of rise of transvalvular pressure prior to prosthetic valve closure (dP/dT). The initial rise in pressure of the outflow side causes fluid to flow retrograde through the prosthetic valve until the occluder seats in the housing. The faster the pressure rises, the higher the blood velocity will be and higher the water hammer pressure pulse. One can reduce the dP/dT in a pneumatically driven device by decreasing drive pressure or by using a gradually increasing dP/dT driver such as the Philadelphia system (Cardiac Systems Inc.).

Lowering the closure volume of the prosthetic valve will lower the water hammer pressure pulse. The blood is accelerated from zero to maximum velocity before coming to an abrupt stop when the valve seats. The lower the closing volume, the lower the velocity reached at valve occlusion.

An elastic mount for the valve lowers the instantaneous change in velocity and thus the water hammer pressure pulse. The Novacor device gains this benefit with its silicone valve mount.

The TCI LVAD achieves this goal by placing the valves within the Dacron conduits. A softer polyurethane valve mount has also been used in the Utah TAH, a device that is still in preclinical development.[33] The use of a soft ventricle as is being developed by the Utah group adds to the compliance of the system.[34]

Increasing the static valve leak of the valve will lower the water hammer. Given the same peak velocity at valve closure, a high-leak valve will change the velocity of the blood less than a low-leak valve. The Delrin disc Bjork–Shiley valve used

in the Thoratec is a high-leak valve. The tradeoff, however, is turbulence in the fluid.[35]

We thus see that numerous factors—such as valve mount, valve location, pattern of flow, duration of implant, anticipated need for anticoagulation, and ease of incorporation into production—are involved in choosing a particular valve for a device. Water hammer and cavitation are major determinants of valve failure, and several strategies are used to lower the mechanical load on valves.

Acknowledgement

The work upon which this chapter is based was supported by the University Medical Center, the Marshall Foundation and the University Heart Center, Arizona.

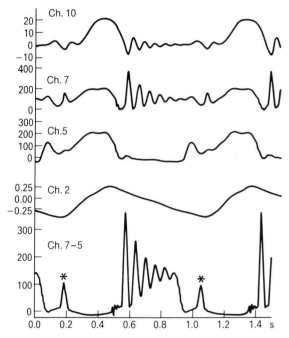

Fig. 33.2 Demonstration of the water hammer effect in the outflow cannula of a prototype adult paracorporeal ventricular assist device coupled to a mock circulation.

Operating conditions were: preload: 14 mmHg; Windkessel afterload: 100 mmHg: afterload compliance: 1000 cm³ air: test fluid: aqueous glycerol, density and dynamic viscosity at 37 °C, 1123 kg/m³ and 3.6 centipoise, respectively; outlet cannula length, compliance and mean internal diameter were 300 mm, 0.01 ml/mmHg and 12.5 mm, respectively.

Waveforms depicted are: Channel 10: instantaneous volumetric flow rate in the outflow cannula (l/min); Channel 7: outlet cannula pressure (mmHg); Channel 5: VAD blood chamber pressure (mmHg); Channel 2: the driver timing signal (positive and negative inflection: pump systole and diastole, respectively); Channel 7-5: the pressure gradient across the outflow valve.

Note that the pressure gradient across the closed outflow valve (pump diastole) is augmented by the pressure oscillation in the outflow cannula. The additional pressure peak across the outflow valve (indicated by *) is associated with inlet valve closure.

References

1. Joyce LD, DeVries WC, Hastings WL, Olsen DB, Jarvik RK, Kolff WJ. Response of the human body to the first permanent implant of the Jarvik-7 total artificial heart. *ASAIO Trans* 1983; **29**, 81–87.
2. Dew PA, Olsen DB, Kessler TR, Coleman DL, Kolff WJ. Mechanical failures in *in vivo* and *in vitro* studies of pneumatic total artificial hearts. *ASAIO Trans* 1984; **30**, 112–116.
3. Olsen DB. Current and future valves for blood pumps. *Artif Organs* 1988; **12**, 239–241.
4. Hughes SD, Butler MD, Holmberg DL, Chiang BY, Grevelink JM, Crump C, Burns GL, Deu PA, Olsen DB, Kolff WJ. Comparative hematological data from animals implanted with a total artificial heart containing different valves. *ASAIO Trans* 1985; **31**, 224–229.
5. Dew PA, Pantalos GM, Holfert JW, Murray KD, Olsen DB. Mechanical failures of the pneumatic Utah-100 and Jarvik total artificial hearts: a comparative study. *ASAIO Trans* 1989; **35**, 697–699.
6. Holfert JW, Riebman JB, Dew PA, DePaulis R, Burns GL, Olsen DB. A new connector system for the total artificial hearts: preliminary results. *ASAIO Trans* 1987; **33**, 151–156.
7. Icenogle TB, Smith RG, Cleavinger M, Vasu MA, Williams RJ, Sethi GK, Copeland JG. Thromboembolic complications of the Symbion AVAD system. *Artif Organs* 1989; **13**, 532–538.
8. Kovacs SG, McKeown PP. Prosthetic valve selection for a pulsatile LVAD. *J Clin Eng* 1991; **16**, 515–519.
9. Graham TR, Marrinan MT, Frazier OH, Macoviak J, Dasse K, Poirer V, Lewis CT. Current clinical experience with Medtronic porcine xenograft

valves in the Thermo Cardiosystems (TCI) implantable left ventricular assist device (LVAD). Presented at the International Seminar on Surgery for Valvular Diseases, London, 12 June 1989.

10. Dasse KA, Chipman SD, Sherman CN, Levine AH, Frazer OH. Clinical experience with textured blood contacting surfaces in ventricular assist devices. *ASAIO Trans* 1987; **33**, 418–425.

11. Chandran KB, Schoephoerster RT, Wurzel D, Hansen G, Yu LS, Pantalos G, Kolff WJ. Haemodynamic comparisons of polyurethane trileaflet and bioprosthetic heart valves. *ASAIO Trans* 1989; **35**, 132–138.

12. Chandran KB, Fatemi R, Schoephoerster R, Wurzel D, Hansen G, Pantalos G, Yu LS, Kolff WJ. *In vitro* comparison of velocity profiles and turbulent shear distal to polyurethane trileaflet and pericardial prosthetic valves. *Artif Organs* 1989; **13**, 148–154.

13. Stewart SFC, Burté F, Eidbo E, Kolff WJ, Yu LS, Clark RE. *In vitro* characterisation of a polyurethane trileaflet valve. *ASAIO Trans* 1990; **36**, M532–535.

14. Poirier V. The quest for the permanent LVAD. *ASAIO Trans* 1990; **36**, 787–788.

15. Russel FB, Lederman DM, Singh PI, Cumming RD, Morgan RA, Levine FH, Austen WG, Buckley MJ. Development of seamless trileaflet valves. *ASAIO Trans* 1980; **26**, 66–71.

16. McMillam CR. Physical testing of elastomers for cardiovascular applications. *Artif Organs* 1983; **7**, 78–91.

17. Mayne SD, Cristie GW, Smaill BH, Hunter PJ, Barret-Boyes BG. An assessment of the mechanical properties of leaflets from four second-generation porcine bioprostheses with biaxial testing techniques. *J Thorac Cardiovasc Surg* 1989; **98**, 170–180.

18. Clark RE. Stress–strain characteristics of fresh and frozen human aortic and mitral leaflets and chrodae tendineae. *J Thorac Cardiovasc Surg* 1973; **66**, 202–208.

19. Chong M, Missirlis YF. Aortic valve mechanics. II: Stress analysis of the porcine aortic valve leaflets in diastole. *Biomat Med Dev Art Org* 1978; **6**, 225–244.

20. Hayashi K. Fundamental and applied studies of mechanical properties of cardiovascular tissues. *Biorheology* 1982; **19**, 425–436.

21. Fisher J, Fisher AC, Evans VM, Wheatley DJ. Investigation of solvent cast polyurethane film as a material for flexible leaflet prosthetic heart valves. In: Paul *et al.* (eds), *Progress in Bioengineering*. London: Adam Hilger, 1988: 41–47.

22. Hoffman D, Sisto D, Yu LS, Dahm M, Kolff WJ. Evaluation of a stented polyurethane mitral prosthesis. *ASAIO Trans* 1991; **37**, M354–355

23. Shunmugakumar N, Jayabalan M. The pressure-induced calcium deposition on cross-linked polyurethanes. *Artif Organs* 1992; **16**, 256–262.

24. Knierbein B, Rosarius N, Reul H, Rau G. New methods for the development of pneumatic displacement pumps for cardiac assist. *Int J Artif Organs* 1990; **13**, 751–759.

25. Knierbein B, Mohr-Matuschek U, Rechlin M, Reul H, Rau G, Michaeli W. Evaluation of mechanical loading of a trileaflet polyurethane blood pump valve by finite element analysis. *Int J Artif Organs* 1990; **13**, 307–315.

26. Knierbein B, Rosarius N, Unger A, Reul H, Rau G. CAD-design, stress analysis and *in vitro* evaluation of three leaflet blood-pump valves. *J Biomed Eng* 1992; **14**, 275–286.

27. Eilers R, Harbott P, Reul H, Rakhorst G, Rau G. Design improvements of the HIA-VAD based on animal experiments. *Artif Organs* 1995. In press.

28. Reul H, Taguchi K, Herold M, Lo HB, Reck B, Mückter H, Messmer BT, Rau G. Comparative evaluation of disk- and trileaflet valves in left-ventricular assist devices (LVAD). *Int J Artif Org* 1988; **11**, 127–130.

29. Bohle AS, Sievers HH, Bernhard A. Scanning electron microscopy evaluation of the Abiomed 5000 ventricular support system after clinical biventricular assistance. *Eur J Cardiothorac Surg* 1990; **4**, 671–674.

30. Ogiro H, Klangsuk N, Jin W, Bowles CT, Yacoub MH. Influence of the compliance of the pump housing and cannulae of a paracorporeal pneumatic ventricular assist device on the transient pressure characteristics. *Artif Organs* 1995. In press.

31. Leuer L. *In vitro* evaluation of drive parameters and valve selection for the total artificial heart. *Trans Can Council Cardiovasc Perf*, Oct 1986. Reprints available through Medtronic Inc., Minneapolis, MN.

32. Lamson TC, Stinebring DR, Deutsch S, Rosenberg G, Tarbell JM. Real-time *in vitro* observation of cavitation in a prosthetic heart valve. *ASAIO Trans* 1991; **37**, M351–353.

33. Kolff WJ, DeVries WC, Joyce LD, Olsen DB, Jarvik RK, Nielsen S, Lastings L, Anderson J, Anderson F, Menlove R. Lessons learned from Dr Barney Clark, the first patient with an artificial heart. *Prog Artif Organs* 1983; **1**, 165–174.

34. Smulders YM, *et al.* The concept of a soft, compressible artificial ventricle under evaluation. *Artif Organs* 1991; **15**, 96–102.

35. Baldwin JT, Tarbell JM, Deutsch S, Geselowitz DB. Mean velocities and Reynolds stresses within regurgitant jets produced by tilting disc valves. *ASAIO Trans* 1991; **37**, M348–349.

34

Bleeding complications in patients requiring mechanical circulatory support

D Glenn Pennington and Marc T Swartz

Introduction

Bleeding is a complication often encountered in patients requiring mechanical circulatory support. The incidence of postoperative bleeding complications in post cardiopulmonary bypass (CPB) patients (recovery) receiving advanced mechanical circulatory support devices has ranged from 33% to 73%.[1-7] Between 29% and 53% of patients receiving ventricular assist devices or total artificial hearts as bridges to cardiac transplantation have required reoperation for bleeding.[8-14] During the past several years, the frequency and severity of bleeding has been reduced by improved insertion techniques, meticulous haemostasis, reversal of heparin used for CPB, the liberal use of platelets and fresh frozen plasma, and the use of thrombostatic agents, such as Surgicel, fibrin glue, and topical thrombin. In many cases bleeding seems to be related to a coagulopathy, but a specific pattern of haemostatic abnormalities has not been identified.

Blood–artificial surface interactions

When blood comes in contact with an artificial surface, a complex series of events is initiated that involves activation of platelets and white blood cells, the blood coagulation fibrinolytic system and the complement system.[15] Activation of platelets and the complement system may lead to local thrombus formation, thromboembolic complications, consumption coagulopathy, and excessive local or generalized bleeding. Systemic heparinization prevents the conversion of fibrinogen to fibrin. However, it does not initially affect platelet function, as evidenced by normal bleeding times shortly after heparinization.[16] During CPB there is a progressive prolongation in the bleeding time, which becomes greater than 30 minutes after two hours of bypass. Platelet activation occurs as a result of their contact with the artificial surface of the oxygenator, and this blood–artificial surface interaction renders the platelets refractory and dysfunctional. In routine cardiac surgical patients, normalization of the haemostatic function of platelets occurs shortly after CPB is discontinued, usually within 30 minutes.

However, the effects of continuous contact of platelets with an artificial surface are more complex. The duration of time during which the platelets are in contact with the artificial surface is important. When platelets come in contact with artificial surfaces at high sheer rates, von Willebrand factor is absorbed into the artificial surface. This leads to conformational changes of the von Willebrand factor molecule, which then interacts with its main platelet receptor. Platelets then undergo changes in shape associated with pseudopod formation. Resulting platelet adherence leads to a release of adenosine diphosphate, which attracts other platelets passing close to the adherent platelet. This results in platelet–platelet interaction or aggregation, an event governed primarily by fibrinogen and two other adhesive plasma glycoproteins. Theoretically, the artificial surfaces eventually undergo progressive passivation, presumably a result of protein absorption and desorption and protein–protein interaction. Patients with mechanical circulatory support devices have a continued activation of platelets until passivation of the artificial surfaces takes place. This activation of platelets may continue for several days and is often associated with low platelet counts. During this interval it is sometimes necessary to give platelet transfusions.

Factors affecting bleeding

Patients requiring mechanical circulatory support are at risk of developing postoperative bleeding complications due to a variety of factors, including preoperative use of the anticoagulants heparin or warfarin, low preoperative platelet counts as a result of cardiogenic shock or chronic congestive heart failure, long CPB times, and multiple sites of cannulation. Pulsatile devices also produce a large dP/dT, which may cause bleeding at the suture lines used to place the pump outflow graft or through the graft itself. These sites often require suture reinforcement to prevent postoperative bleeding.

Consequences of excessive bleeding

Bleeding is often a severe complication since it extends the period of haemodynamic instability. Hypovolaemia reduces native cardiac and support device output and lowers perfusion pressure, increasing the risk of ischaemic damage to already injured organs. Cardiac tamponade may also be quite harmful to vital organs. Tamponade is particularly difficult to diagnose in patients with ventricular assist devices since the mechanical device continues to function in spite of moderately severe tamponade. The usual pattern in patients with ventricular assist devices is an increase in right and left atrial pressures, which are associated with decreased pump filling that does not improve with volume loading. Unfortunately, by the time these signs are apparent, a significant degree of cardiac tamponade has already taken place and immediate exploration is necessary.

The need for blood or blood product transfusions increases the likelihood of the development of antibodies and may limit the ability to locate a donor organ in the bridge-to-transplant population. Massive blood transfusions may also contribute to the development of other complications, such as infection and renal failure. Depending on the amount of blood–prosthetic surface interface, haemostasis returns to near normal levels in 2–5 days. In most patients, severe bleeding complications are corrected within 24 hours. Bleeding is often complicated by the need for continuous systemic heparin, as required with less sophisticated systems such as centrifugal pumps and extracorporeal membrane oxygenation (ECMO). The detrimental effects of CPB and circulatory support devices on platelets are well known. In recipients of the Jarvik-7 total artificial heart, plasma levels of beta-thromboglobulin, fibrinopeptide-A and antithrombin-III were increased to levels higher than those seen after routine cardiac surgery.[17]

The type of volume to be replaced in bleeding patients is a critical consideration. Instead of reinfusing shed mediastinal blood, which may aggravate a coagulopathy, we infuse only washed red cells. Fresh frozen plasma restores decreased levels of antithrombin III and other coagulation factors and platelet transfusions are given for platelet counts <100 000/mm^3. Patients who are being bridged to cardiac transplantation receive pheresis platelet products which are human lymphocytic antigen type specific. Myocardial recovery patients receive random platelets. Red blood cells are given to maintain the haematocrit at 25–35%. We transfuse cardiac transplant candidates with red blood cells that are cytomegalovirus negative. In addition, red blood cells should be filtered to remove the leucocytes and reduce the exposure to antigens. In our experience, volume replacement with fresh frozen plasma, platelets and packed red blood cells is most effective.

In some patients, the impact of these risk factors can be reduced. For example, patients who are on warfarin preoperatively can receive fresh frozen plasma to normalize the prothrombin time prior to placement of the circulatory support device. It is often possible to insert the aortic graft of the assist device prior to establishing CPB. In some cases, it is even possible to place the entire VAD without the use of CPB, allowing for a lower dose of heparin.[18] In patients with postcardiotomy cardiogenic shock, the duration of CPB can be reduced if the decision to insert the assist device is made rapidly. Strict attention to haemostasis and wiring of the sternotomy often decreases the amount of sternal oozing.

Clinical experience at St Louis University

Since 1982, 86 patients have had investigational pulsatile mechanical circulatory support devices inserted, either to allow myocardial recovery ($n = 42$) or as a bridge to transplantation ($n = 44$). Patient characteristics for myocardial recovery and bridge groups are shown in Tables 34.1–34.3. Eleven patients died in the operating room (nine recovery and two bridge-to-transplant). Table 34.4 shows the total chest tube drainage, chest tube drainage per square metre of body surface area, as well as the amounts of blood products transfused in the first 48 hours in both myocardial recovery and bridge patients. Additionally, the mean number of times that each patient was re-explored for bleeding is shown. The myocardial recovery group had significantly more total chest tube drainage, and also received significantly more packed red blood cell transfusions. Table 34.5 shows the effect postoperative bleeding had on survival in the myocardial recov-

Table 34.1 Patient characteristics: myocardial recovery.

Gender: 34 male, 8 female
Age: 15–71 years (mean 52 years)
Duration of support: 0.2–17 days (mean 4.4 days)

Procedure	
CABG	21
MVR with/without CABG	6
AVR with/without CABG	4
Post cardiac transplant	4
AMI	3
ASD—hypoplastic LV	1
Aortic aneurysm	1
VSD, LVA and CABG	1
LVA and CABG	1

Type of device	
Thoratec	
LVAD	17
BVAD	16
RVAD	9

CABG = coronary artery bypass graft; MVR = mitral valve replacement; AVR = aortic valve replacement; AMI = acute myocardial infarction; ASD = atrial septal defect; VSD = ventricular septal defect; LVA = left ventricular aneurysm; LVAD = left ventricular assist device; BVAD = biventricular assist device; RVAD = right ventricular assist device.

Table 34.2 Patient characteristics: bridging.

Gender: 34 male, 10 female
Age: 12–65 years (mean 43 years)
Duration of support: 0.125–440 days (mean 45 days)

Type of cardiomyopathy	
Ischaemic	25
Idiopathic	11
Postpartal	4
Congenital	1
Valvular	1
Doxorubicin toxicity	1
Post-transplant rejection	1

Type of device	
Thoratec	32
LVAD	19
BVAD	13
Novacor LVAS	10
Symbion J-7 TAH	2

LVAD = left ventricular assist device; BVAD = biventricular assist device; LVAS = left ventricular assist system; TAH = total artificial heart.

ery group. There was no significant difference in any of the measured parameters between survivors and non-survivors, suggesting that bleeding is not a critical predictor of survival in patients who are supported with VADs until myocardial recovery occurs. This finding is consistent with data from the combined registry of the American Society of Artificial Internal Organs and the International Society for Heart and Lung Transplantation (CA Miller, personal communication).

Table 34.6 compares total chest tube drainage and blood products transfused for survivors and non-survivors in the bridge-to-transplant patient population. Unlike the myocardial recovery group, several of these parameters were statistically significant, showing that the development of post-device bleeding reduces the chances to receive a transplant and survive.

A review of the clinical data from 72 patients at St Louis University who received Thoratec ventricular assist devices over the last 10 years showed a marked decrease in blood product transfusions

Table 34.3 Results of recovery and bridge patients at St Louis University (SLU).

	Myocardial recovery	Bridging to transplantation
Patients	42	44
Number weaned	18	2
Transplanted	–	26
Survivors	11	27

Table 34.4 Postoperative bleeding with mechanical circulatory support.

	Recovery (n = 42)	Bridge (n = 44)	p value
Chest tube drainage (ml)	4683 ± 4155*	2733 ± 1912†	0.007
Chest drainage/m² (ml)	2454 ± 2194*	1481 ± 1052†	0.005
PRBCs (units)‡	16.5 ± 8.5	11.6 ± 8.9	0.23
Washed RBCs (ml)	681 ± 1124	401 ± 539	0.14
Autotransfused cells (ml)	776 ± 1925	233 ± 740	0.08
Fresh frozen plasma (units)	8.3 ± 6.4	8.5 ± 6.6	0.91
Platelets (units)§	29.1 ± 20.7	25.1 ± 22.8	0.40
Times re-explored (per patient)	0.38 ± 0.66	0.67 ± 1.11	0.18

*$n = 33$ (9 patients who died in operating theatre not included); †$n = 42$ (2 died in operating theatre); ‡PRBC = packed red blood cells; § one pheresis product equals 10 units of platelets.

in recent patients (1988–92) when compared with patients treated earlier (1982–87). Possible reasons for these improved results are shorter CPB times, earlier implantation of devices, and more vigorous, early transfusion of platelets and fresh frozen plasma. Despite these improvements, haemostatic studies have shown consistent evidence for the activation of platelets, impairment of platelet function and activation of blood coagulation with variably severe depletion of antithrombin-III.[15–17] Once the bleeding stops and the transfusion of blood produce ceases, haemostatic alterations return to normal. In some patients, mild thrombocytopenia persists with or without activation of platelets.

Discussion

Over the last decade, there have been some improvements in the understanding and treatment of postoperative bleeding complications associated with advanced mechanical circulatory support devices. The deleterious effects of pro-longed CPB are better understood and some of the specific haematologic alterations associated with blood–artificial surface interaction have been identified. However, most of the improvement in this area has been clinical. Clinicians now recognize that CPB times must be reduced as much as possible and that heparin should be reversed as soon as the device is in place and functioning. In all devices, a 24-hour period of heparin-free support may allow the haemostatic variables to correct themselves. At the same time, alterations in prothrombin time, partial thromboplastin time, platelet count and haematocrit need to be corrected using appropriate blood product transfusions. The platelet count should be maintained above 100 000/mm³ if possible. The prothrombin time should be normalized as much as possible with transfusions of fresh frozen plasma. Partial thromboplastin time should be corrected with protamine if necessary.

Much of the St Louis University data presented in this chapter is taken from patients who were supported prior to 1988. In many of these patients, especially those requiring postcardiot-

Table 34.5 Postoperative bleeding and survival in the myocardial recovery patients.

	Survivors (n = 11)	Non-survivors (n = 31)	p value
Chest tube drainage (ml)	4628 ± 3112	4709 ± 4658*	0.96
Chest drainage/m² (ml)	1609 ± 823	1738 ± 1431*	0.78
PRBCs (units)‡	19.2 ± 7.9	15.6 ± 8.6	0.23
Washed RBCs (ml)	760 ± 1077	654 ± 1156	0.79
Autotransfused cells (ml)	308 ± 240	942 ± 2222	0.35
Fresh frozen plasma (units)	7.9 ± 6.6	8.5 ± 6.4	0.80
Platelets (units)	26.4 ± 13.4	30 ± 22.8	0.61
Times re-explored (per patient)	0.33 ± 0.82	0.39 ± 0.65	0.57

*$n = 22$ (9 patients who died in operating theatre not included); ‡PRBC = packed red blood cells.

Table 34.6 Postoperative bleeding and survival in the bridge patients.

	Survivors (n = 27)	Non-survivors (n = 17)	p value
Chest tube drainage (ml)	2077 ± 1343	3883 ± 2240*	0.002
Chest drainage/m² (ml)	1104 ± 742	2143 ± 1204*	0.003
PRBCs (units)‡	9.1 ± 6.9	15.9 ± 10.3	0.011
Washed RBCs (ml)	350 ± 517	484 ± 581	0.43
Autotransfused cells (ml)	80 ± 173	484 ± 1162	0.076
Fresh frozen plasma (units)	6.8 ± 4.2	11.2 ± 8.9	0.29
Platelets (units)§	20 ± 18.1	33.5 ± 27.4	0.05
Times re-explored (per patient)	0.33 ± 0.68	1.25 ± 1.44	0.009

*n = 15 (2 patients who died in operating theatre not included); ‡PRBC = packed red blood cells; § one pheresis product equals 10 units of platelets.

omy support, the incidence and severity of post-operative bleeding complications was unacceptable. However, with better clinical management and understanding of the haematological alterations involved, as well as refined anticoagulation protocols, the morbidity associated with bleeding has decreased. As shown in Table 35.4, myocardial recovery patients had significantly more blood loss than bridge patients. They also required more packed red blood cell transfusion. Part of this disparity is due to the fact that bridge patients are often haematologically more stable than recovery patients, as the result of shorter CPB times. Most of the bridge-to-transplant patients were supported during the last five years.

In our experience, postoperative bleeding in recovery patients does not predict survival. However, there is little doubt that excessive bleeding is detrimental to the patient's postoperative course. Results in a larger group may yield different results. In the future, it is hoped that bleeding complications will continue to diminish. Earlier use of devices, new biomaterials, improved implantation techniques and better patient selection should diminish this common and often lethal complication.

References

1. Pennington DG, McBride LR, Swartz MT, Kanter KR, Kaiser GC, Barner HB, Miller LW, Naunheim KS, Fiore AC, Willman VL. Use of the Pierce Donachy ventricular assist device in patients with cardiogenic shock after cardiac operations. *Ann Thorac Surg* 1989; **47**, 130–135.
2. Golding LR, Jacobs G, Groves LK, Gill C, Nose Y, Loop FD. Clinical results of mechanical support of the failing left ventricle. *J Thorac Cardiovasc Surg* 1982; **83**, 597–601.
3. Killen DA, Piehler JM, Borkon AM, Reed WA. BioMedicus ventricular assist device for salvage of cardiac surgical patients. *Ann Thorac Surg* 1991; **52**, 230–235.
4. Wareing TH, Kouchoukos NT. Postcardiotomy mechanical circulatory support in the elderly. *Ann Thorac Surg* 1991; **51**, 443–447.
5. Pennington DG, Swartz MT. Temporary circulatory support in patients with postcardiotomy cardiogenic shock. In: Spence PA, Chitwood WR (eds), *Cardiac Surgery: State of the Art Reviews*, vol 5. Philadelphia: Hanley and Belfus, 1991: 373–392.
6. Curtis JJ, Walls JT, Schmaltz R, Boley T, Nawarawong W, Landreneau RJ. Experience with the Sarns centrifugal pump in postcardiotomy ventricular failure. *J Thorac Cardiovasc Surg* 1992; **104**, 554–560.
7. Pae WE, Miller CA, Matthews Y, Pierce WS. Ventricular assist devices for postcardiotomy cardiogenic shock. *J Thorac Cardiovasc Surg* 1992; **104**, 541–553.
8. Pifarre R, Sullivan HJ, Montoya A, Bakhos M, Grieco J, Foy BK, Blakeman B, Costanzo-Nordin M, Altergott R, Lonchyna V. The use of the Jarvik-7 total artificial heart and the Symbion ventricular assist device as a bridge to transplantation. *Surgery* 1990; **108**, 681–685.
9. Joyce LD, Emery RW, Eales F, Von Rueden TJ, Kiser JR, Hoffman FM, Johnson KE, Toninato CJ, Kersten TE, Nicoloff DM, Pritzker MR. Mechanical circulatory support as a bridge to transplantation. *J Thorac Cardiovasc Surg* 1989; **98**, 935–941.
10. Farrar DJ, Lawson JH, Litwak P, Cederwall G. Thoratec VAD system as a bridge to heart transplantation. *J Heart Lung Transplant* 1990; **9**, 415–423.
11. Portner PM, Oyer PE, Pennington DG, Baumgartner WA, Griffith BP, Frist WR, Magilligan DJ, Noon GP, Ramasamy N, Miller PJ, Jassawalla JS. Implantable electrical left ventricular assist system: bridge to transplantation and the future. *Ann Thorac Surg* 1989; **47**, 142–150.

12. Oaks TE, Pae WE, Miller CA, Pierce WS. Combined registry for the clinical use of mechanical ventricular assist pumps and the total artificial heart in conjunction with heart transplantation: fifth official report 1990. *J Heart Lung Transplant* 1991; **10**, 621–625.

13. Frazier OH, Rose EA, Macmanus Q, Burton NA, Lefrak EA, Poirier VL, Dasse KA. Multicenter clinical evaluation of the HeartMate 1000 IP left ventricular assist device. *Ann Thorac Surg* 1992; **53**, 1080–1090.

14. Johnson KE, Prieto M, Joyce LD, Pritzker M, Emery RW. Summary of the clinical use of the Symbion total artificial heart: a registry report. *J Heart Lung Transplant* 1992; **11**, 103–116.

15. Joist JH, Pennington DG. Platelet reactions with artificial surfaces. *ASAIO Trans* 1987; **33**, 341–344.

16. Copeland JL, Harker LA, Joist JH, DeVries WC. Bleeding and anticoagulation. *Ann Thorac Surg* 1989; **47**, 88–95.

17. Walenga JM, Hoppensteadt D, Fareed J, Pifarré R. Hemostatic abnormalities in total artificial heart patients as detected by specific blood markers. *Ann Thorac Surg* 1992; **53**, 844–850.

18. Brugger JP, Bonandi L, Meli M. SWAT team approach to ventricular assistance. *Ann Thorac Surg* 1989; **47**, 136–141.

35

Bleeding in extracorporeal membrane oxygenation (ECMO)

GA Pearson, MJ Underwood and RK Firmin

Introduction

In the animal laboratory, attempts to provide direct support for circulation and gas exchange started over 100 years ago. The notable contribution of Benjamin Ward Richardson[1] anticipated intermittent positive pressure ventilation, cardiac and respiratory pacemakers as well as variations upon the theme of extracorporeal oxygenation and circulatory assist devices. In 1865 he published a synthesis of his experiments in reanimation.[2] Richardson had attempted to reanimate animals (usually rabbits) which he had sacrificed using chloroform, carbonic acid or drowning. However, in his attempts to reanimate these animals (and indeed human patients) using extracorporeal circulation, he was confounded by the blood itself and the *'rapid coalescence of the blood corpuscles as the motion of the blood ceases'*. The issues of spontaneous coagulation aggravated by low blood flow or stasis within ECMO circuits remain pertinent today. The risks of thrombus formation are minimized as far as possible by modern circuit design,[3] but the 'coalescence of the corpuscles' and the manner in which current routines interfere with this process remain highly topical.

In 1916 McLean, a medical student of Johns Hopkins University, demonstrated anticoagulant activity in extracts of liver, and the active component (a glycosaminoglycan) was named 'heparin'. This extremely potent natural anticoagulant is discussed below. It acts by blocking or inhibiting multiple steps of the intrinsic and final common pathways of the coagulation cascade. The use of heparin allowed the further development of extracorporeal circulation, so enabling the birth of cardiac surgery.[4] However, recognition of the dangers of haemorrhagic complications during prolonged extracorporeal circulation has meant that, during ECMO, some attempt has to be made to monitor its effects and to titrate infusion regimens against them.[5] This process is made easier by the fact that it has a comparatively short half-life *in vivo*.

Predisposition of ECMO patients to haemorrhage

The institution of an extracorporeal circulation may predispose to both thrombosis within the circuit and bleeding from the patient. Anticoagulants such as heparin may be used to minimize the dangers from the former, but any tendency to haemorrhage not only remains but is potentiated. It is important to note, however, that bleeding in ECMO patients is related to several factors and not just the use of heparin (see below). For example, in many patients the severity of illness prior to ECMO may mean that the coagulation system is already abnormal. Additionally, as well as the more obvious haematological abnormalities, there are changes in the local tissues and microcirculation of sick patients which predispose to bleeding. Such changes may be induced by sepsis, hypoxia, hypovolaemia and reperfusion. Hypertension, which is a possible sequel to venoarterial ECMO, may also predispose to bleeding, particularly intracerebral haemorrhage. In addition there may be local factors in particular organs. For example, both the prior administration of tolazoline in neonates and the occurrence of 'stress ulcers' predispose to gastrointestinal bleeding. A patient ductus arteriosus may predispose to pulmonary haemorrhage. There are other examples.

The pattern and incidence of bleeding

The reported incidence of haemorrhage in ECMO patients in various sites is summarized in Table 35.1. This, being cumulative data,[6] does not accurately reflect any reduction in the incidence over time. It is more difficult to gather quantitative data on the significance of any reported haemorrhage. The severity of haemorrhage in those patients contributed to the registry by our own centre is often minimal. Catastrophic haemorrhage can occur but is mercifully rare.

Intracranial haemorrhage remains an important cause of neurological morbidity and mortality in neonatal ECMO patients. However, since original reports, its incidence has been greatly reduced.[7,8] This has been achieved, firstly, by the preference for accepting only infants of a predetermined maturity, and secondly by refinements in bedside protocol. This latter has probably been the major factor, since a recent review[9] and anecdotal reports suggest favourable experience in situations where the customary limits of neonatal size and gestation have been relaxed.

Patterns of intracranial haemorrhage seen in the ECMO population may differ from the classical intraventricular haemorrhage of the preterm neonate.[10] In our series, post mortem of patients who have died from catastrophic intracranial haemorrhage far more frequently confirms the ultrasound impression of haemorrhage into ischaemic lesions. We can presume that the origin of these lesions predates the referral for ECMO. The position of the 'watershed' for such ischaemic lesions changes with fetal maturity. Additionally the occurrence of posterior fossa haemorrhage has been observed[11] which may have been contributed to by cervical venous occlusion.

The other common sites of bleeding in all ECMO patients are cannulation sites, the gastrointestinal tract, surgical incisions and needle punctures. Care must be taken with chest drains, particularly those inserted prior to referral for ECMO. Haemothorax, intrapulmonary haemorrhage and cardiac tamponade may all occur, and drains present at referral should be left *in situ*, in order to avoid bleeding from the chest wall or to allow drainage of blood from the penetrating lung injuries incurred at their insertion. In most cases haemorrhage can be prevented by careful technique. Many centres, including our own, routinely conduct major surgery during ECMO. Generous use of fibrin glue and electrocautery are customary but postoperative haemorrhage is rare.

Management of bleeding

The incidence of bleeding complications may be reduced by maintaining the levels of routinely detectable soluble clotting factors as near normal as possible, thus minimizing unintentional changes in the coagulation profile. This is achieved by

Table 35.1 Sites of haemorrhage during ECMO (percentages).*

Patient category	Intracranial infarct or haemorrhage	Cannula site	Surgical site	Gastrointestinal	Other
Neonatal	16	7	6	3	7
Paediatric					
Respiratory	8	Not reported	28	6	12
Cardiac	5	Not reported	22	2	9
Adult	3	Not reported	39	1	17

*Cumulative data from the registry of the Extracorporeal Life Support Organization, October 1992; displayed as the percentage of all ECMO cases in that category reported to have displayed haemorrhage at the specified site.

the periodic infusion of fresh frozen plasma and cryoprecipitate as required and by maintaining a platelet count >100 000/mm³. Traditionally heparin infusions are titrated against a whole blood activated clotting time (ACT). There are many variables which can alter the level of the ACT other than the dose of heparin (not least active haemorrhage), and so a degree of lability of this somewhat coarse measure is to be expected. A general consensus for what constitutes an appropriate ACT level exists and has fallen over recent years. A value of 160–180 s (compared with a normal range of 100–120 s) is often considered acceptable, though many centres still run a little higher than this (ACT 180–200). Ideally under conditions of haemorrhage the ACT should be controlled as close to the limits of safety as is possible, but these limits are not well defined. Nonetheless it is possible to maintain patients without heparin for limited periods.[12] Under such circumstances, the use of high blood flow rates through the circuit reduces the likelihood of any areas of stasis which might promote thrombosis. The shear stresses induced by such flow have been shown *in vitro* to cause cultured epithelial cells to release tissue plasminogen activator (tPA) in quantities proportional to the shear stresses.[13] Endogenous tPA may contribute to anticoagulation during extracorporeal circulation (see below). ECMO patients are dependent on the circuits for their gas exchange, and so it is customary to have a preprimed replacement circuit at the bedside in anticipation of disaster when one is forced into such a situation.

When active bleeding occurs or a surgical procedure is necessary, it is customary to reset the targets of haematology and coagulation profiles. This is again achieved by transfusion of blood products and heparin titration. In our institution under such circumstances, the platelet count is maintained above 150 000/mm³ and the target for ACT is set close to 160 s. If the site of haemorrhage is a surgical one or there is bleeding into the pericardium or pleura, early consideration should be given to surgical exploration.

Effects of extracorporeal circulation on coagulation

Early extracorporeal circuits generated severe haemolysis within hours of their application. The principal site of red cell damage was the oxygenators which relied on an inherently destructive direct contact between blood and oxygen in order to achieve respiratory gas exchange. The development of the membrane oxygenator minimized this particular problem. Nevertheless there are many complex reactions initiated when blood interfaces with the artificial surfaces in the circuit—the tubing, oxygenator and heat exchanger.[14] In a modern circuit these surfaces include polyvinyl chloride (PVC), silastic, polycarbonate, polyurethane, other plastics and stainless steel.

The use of extracorporeal circulation is still associated with a 'whole-body inflammatory response'. Impaired haemostasis occurs as a part of this response, and abnormal bleeding may occur in up to 3% of patients receiving short-term CPB for cardiac surgery.[15,16] The mechanism of this haemostatic defect involves platelet dysfunction as well as activation of closely interrelated humoral systems such as the complement, coagulation, fibrinolytic and kallikrein/kinin systems. As discussed, these factors occur in addition to the deliberate inhibition of the intrinsic pathway, routinely achieved by heparin administration, which enhances the activity of the endogenous protease inhibitor, antithrombin-III.

There is considerable evidence that the major defect in haemostasis created by extracorporeal circulation is a reversible defect in platelet function. Under normal circumstances, platelets are involved in the formation of a 'haemostatic plug', which along with vasoconstriction (mediated by thromboxane A_2) is the mechanism by which bleeding from a 'damaged' capillary bed is stopped. The initial events which enable normal platelets to adhere to damaged tissue include the interaction of adhesive proteins (e.g. von Willebrand factor) and components of the subendothelium (e.g. collagen), with platelet receptors (e.g. glycoprotein-Ib and blycoprotein-IIb/IIIa). Platelet glycoprotein-Ib (GPIb) is essential for anchoring platelets to the sites of vascular injury, a function it performs through its binding to von Willebrand factor in the vessel wall. Platelet glycoprotein-IIb/IIIa (GPIIb/IIIa) is a member of a family of adhesion receptors collectively called 'integrins'. As well as binding von Willebrand factor, GPIIb/IIIa binds fibrinogen which forms the molecular link between aggregating platelets. The major role of GPIIb/IIIa, therefore, is to mediate the spread of platelets on to thrombogenic surfaces and recruit further platelets into the developing 'haemostatic plug'. Along with the well recognized thrombocytopenia associated with mechanical damage at the blood–gas interface and haemodilution (due to the priming fluids), a variety of complex mechanisms (involving the GPIb and GPIIb/IIIa receptors) may lead to platelet dysfunction following extracorporeal circulation, with a consequent reduction in their adhesive and aggregatory properties.

When blood first contacts the foreign materials of the bypass circuit, Hageman factor (factor XII) is activated and plays a central role in activating the fibrinolytic, coagulation, complement and kallekrein–kinin systems. Activation of the fibrinolytic system following extracorporeal circulation may be reflected by an increase in concentrations of tissue-type plasminogen activator.[17] tPA converts inactive circulating plasminogen into the enxymatically active plasmin, which in turn lyses fibrin. Thus enhanced fibrinolysis following extracorporeal circulation may contribute to the haemostatic deficit by prematurely destroying any haemostatic clot. It has also been suggested (based on *in vitro* data) that plasmin, generated during extracorporeal circulation, may adversely affect platelet function by hydrolysing and degrading the platelet GPIb receptor, thereby reducing its adhesive properties.[18] Certainly there have been clinical reports of a reduction in GPIb function following extracorporeal circulation,[19] but the underlying mechanism of this remains unclear. Fibrin-degradation products (generated following plasmin-mediated lysis of fibrin) are known to bind platelets (at the GPIIb/IIIa receptor site), and the occupancy of this receptor with an inert clotting fragment leads to defective clot formation.[20] Binding of GPIIb/IIIa receptor fragments to components of the extracorporeal circuit has been demonstrated,[21] and this may also be a contributory factor in post-extracorporeal circulation platelet dysfunction.

Conversion of plasminogen to plasmin may also be mediated by a kallikrein-dependent process[22] and lead to the secondary effects on platelet function and thence haemostasis described above. Activation of the kallekrein–kinin system following extracorporeal circulation has been demonstrated in clinical studies,[23] and importantly, the naturally occurring inhibitor of plasmin (alpha$_2$-antiplasmin) has been shown to be reduced.[24] The concentrations of other naturally occurring protease inhibitors such as C1-esterase (which inhibits the action of kallikrein, factor XIIa and urokinase), have also been shown to be

decreased following a period of extracorporeal circulation.[25] So it appears that not only are plasmin-generating enzymes stimulated by extracorporeal circulation, but the natural inhibitors of this process are diminished. Generation of kallikrein during extracorporeal circulation may also amplify the activation of factor XII to XIIa and further augment plasmin generation and subsequent fibrinolysis.

Complement activation and leucocyte elastase production (from activated polymorphonuclear leucocytes (PMN) are a well recognized component of the 'inflammatory response' to extracorporeal circulation.[26] Production of these factors may, however, indirectly affect haemostasis. PMN-derived elastase may have adverse effects on the platelet GPIb receptor,[27] potentiated by the PMN-chemotactic properties of complement.[28] Elastase is also able to convert plasminogen to mini-plasminogen[29] which is less susceptible to inhibition by alpha$_2$-antiplasmin, and readily converted to plasmin by tPA and urokinase-type plasminogen activator (uPA).[30] Kallikrein is also a potent stimulus for elastase release from neutrophils,[31] and hence may also contribute to this elastase-mediated platelet dysfunction and enhancement of fibrinolysis. Fibrinolysis following extracorporeal circulation may also be indirectly augmented by the proteolysis of alpha$_2$-antiplasmin and plasminogen activator inhibitor 1 (the naturally occurring inhibitor of tPA), by PMN-derived elastase.[32] The net result of the interaction between these various humoral and cellular systems is a reduction in platelet function, enhanced fibrinolysis and consequently impaired haemostasis.

All these influences contribute to generation of the observed clinical effects. The platelet count and the level of soluble clotting factors fall precipitately at the point of initiation of extracorporeal circulation. Subsequently the consumption of platelets and other factors continue as low-grade active processes. Ordinarily the essential elements of these can be compensated for by transfusion. However, on occasion during ECMO, there may be excessive consumption of clotting factors mirroring disseminated intravascular coagulopathy (DIC) with acutely raised levels of fibrin degradation products. Systemic sepsis and other medical causes need to be excluded, but this presentation can reflect runaway activation of the coagulation cascade within the oxygenator and the circuit. We have seen this effect on two occasions during prolonged paediatric ECMO cases. In each instance the problem presented before oxygenator function had deteriorated perceptively. Successful treatment necessitated changing the oxygenator (or circuit).

Despite improving understanding of the processes by which ECMO may aggravate a predisposition towards haemorrhage, the number of therapeutic options is limited. Every ECMO centre has a series of protocols to address thrombotic and coagulation issues of the type outlined above, but there is intense interest in possible therapeutic advances.

Modifying the effects of ECMO on haemostatic mechanisms

The use of albumin and blood in the prime, at least in theory, serves to coat and 'pacify' the artificial surfaces of the circuit to some extent.[33] However, during perfusion, platelet sequestration persists[8] and clotting factors and other blood proteins still tend to adhere to the circuit roughly in proportion to their concentration in plasma. Much research has been devoted to the possibility of reducing this problem by improving the biocompatability of artificial surfaces.

Currently the most topical advance in this field is the development of techniques of heparin bonding. The chemistry of these developments is complex and a variety of potential mechanisms have been explored. Of these, the widely preferred option is one of covalently bonding the heparin to the surface using a spacer molecule so that the active heparin molecules protrude into the lumen in the manner of a brush border. Alternatives include:

1. Binding the heparin ionically to a positively charged surface.
2. Using an ionically bound heparin polymer as a coating on a substrate polymer.
3. Applying heparin as a cross-linked surface.
4. Applying heparin as an immobilized layer at the luminal surface.
5. Heparin dispersed in a hydrophobic polymer layer on the luminal surface from which it leaches into the circulation.
6. Using a conjugate surface of heparin bound to an albumin coat.

Heparin-bonded tubing and hollow fibre oxygenators have been commercially available for some time.[34] Heparin-bonded membrane oxygenators have also been developed. The clinical impact of these devices remains to be assessed. Certainly the currently available apparatus can reduce the requirement, but does not yet negate the need, for the systemic administration of heparin, particularly at low blood flow rates.

Additionally a number of drugs are available which may modulate the effects that extracorporeal circulation may have upon haemostatic mechanisms. Four are worthy of mention here. A more comprehensive review is provided by Eberhart.[33]

Prostacyclin administration exerts a sustained but reversible inhibition upon platelet aggregation, which is antagonistic to that of thromboxane A_2. The mechanism of action is through alteration of the intracellular ratio of cyclic adenosine monophosphate to guanine monophosphate, and the effect has been demonstrated to improve platelet survival in extracorporeal circuits.[35] In pharmacological doses, prostacyclin is also a potent short-acting vasodilator which is in widespread use in the conventional treatment of pulmonary hypertension in neonates, and so may prove useful in the ECMO treatment of the same. Some caution is required in such an application since prostaglandins are ubiquitous compounds which extensively affect a diversity of biological systems. However, the application of prostacyclin to the ECMO population is worthy of further laboratory research and prospective clinical trials.

Epsilon amino caproic acid (EACA) is a synthetic amino acid which competes with plasminogen for plasmin activator and is hence a potent antifibrinolytic. It is capable of producing a hypercoagulable state by completely preventing fibrinolysis. Tranexamic acid is also a synthetic amino acid that is more potent than EACA but has a similar mode of action. Both compounds have been used in the context of extracorporeal circulation in attempts to reduce the likelihood of haemorrhage.

Aprotonin is an exogenous serine protease inhibitor. It is a basic, water-soluble polypeptide which is active against plasmin and possibly against plasminogen activator. It blocks the formation of thromboplastin and does not carry the risk of creating a hypercoagulable state. It is hence (amongst other things[25]) an antifibrinolytic. Accompanying such clinically beneficial effects there is evidence of platelet preservation.[19] Its use in ECMO patients with active haemorrhage has not been subject to controlled trial, but it is known to have dramatic effects on bleeding in patients after cardiac surgery). Paradoxically it elevates the ACT, so that when therapy is commenced the target ACT for heparin titration has to be reset. We have found an elevation of 40 s to be common after its administration to patients with stable heparin control at an ACT of 180 s. We have used this agent in the event of haemorrhage during ECMO (particularly in ECMO after cardiac surgery). Our subjective impression is favourable but our data insufficient to constitute proof of its efficacy.

Conclusions

Extracorporeal circulation leads to a systemic inflammatory reaction, resulting in activation of the kinin, coagulation, complement and fibrinolytic systems. Through a complex series of reactions, which are still not fully understood, platelet function and the formation of a protective 'haemostatic clot' are impaired. This may lead to a generalized impairment of normal haemostatic function and bleeding, with its associated morbidity and mortality. Meanwhile the prevention of thrombus formation within extracorporeal circuits still necessitates the administration of heparin.

The clinical response is to pay close attention to the management of anticoagulation and the detection and treatment of haemorrhage in the ECMO patient. The most productive approaches in this regard are those which emphasize *prevention*. Thrombotic and haemorrhagic complications remain potentially the most serious and certainly the most well known of the patient-related complications. Their decreasing incidence is largely the result of fastidious monitoring and meticulous ECMO technique and should not therefore give cause for complacency.

New agents, technological developments and basic scientific research currently promise rapid developments in this field. Despite his difficulties over 100 years ago, Benjamin Ward Richardson concluded his thesis with the assertion: *'Resuscitation by artificial means is a possible process and it only requires the elements of time, experiment and patience for its development'.*[2] Parts of his vision have been realized but the need for experiment and research continues, particularly in the same

aspects of extracorporeal circulation that confounded him even then.

References

1. Obituary of Benjamin Ward Richardson. *Lancet* 1896; **2**, 1575–1576.
2. Richardson BW. An enquiry into the possibility of restoring the life of warm blooded animals in certain cases where the respiration, the circulation and the ordinary manifestations of organic motion are exhausted or have ceased. *Proc Roy Soc Lond* 1865.
3. Fink SM, Bockman DE, Howell CG, Falls DG, Kanto WJ. Bypass circuits as the source of thromboemboli during extracorporeal membrane oxygenation. *J Pediat* 1989; **115**, 621–624.
4. Gibbon JH. Application of a mechanical heart and lung apparatus to cardiac surgery. *Minn Med* 1954; **37**, 171.
5. Bartlett RH, Isherwood J, Moss RA, Olszewski WL, Polet H, Drinker PA. A toroidal flow membrane oxygenator: four day partial bypass in dogs. *Surg Forum* 1969; **20**, 152–153.
6. Registry of the Extracorporeal Life Support Organisation, Ann Arbor, Michigan.
7. Bartlett RH, Gazzaniga AB, Toomasian J, Coran AG, Roloff D, Rucker R, Corwin AG. Extracorporeal membrane oxygenation (ECMO) in neonatal respiratory failure: 100 cases. *Ann Surg* 1986; **204**, 236–45. An erratum appears in *Ann Surg* 1987; **205**, 11A.
8. Bartlett RH. Extracorporeal life support for cardiopulmonary failure. *Curr Prob Surg* 1990; **27**, 621–705.
9. Bui KC, LaClair P, Vanderkerhove J, Bartlett RH. ECMO in premature infants: review of factors associated with mortality. *ASAIO Trans* 1991; **37**, 54–59.
10. Taylor GA, Fitz CR, Kapur S, Short BL. Cerebrovascular accidents in neonates treated with extracorporeal membrane oxygenation: sonographic–pathologic correlation. *Am J Roentgen* 1989; **153**, 355–361.
11. Bulas DI, Taylor GA, Fitz CR, Revenis ME, Glass P, Ingram JD. Posterior fossa intracranial hemorrhage in infants treated with extracorporeal membrane oxygenation: sonographic findings. *Am J Roentgen* 1991; **156**, 571–575.
12. Whittlesey GC, Drucker DE, Salley SO, Smith HG, Kundu SK, Palder SB, Klein MD. ECMO without heparin: laboratory and clinical experience. *J Pediat Surg* 1991; **26**, 320–324.
13. Diamond SL, Eskin SG, McIntire LV. Fluid flow stimulates tissue plasminogen activator secretion by

cultured human epithelial cells. *Science* 1989; **243**, 1483–1485.

14. Westaby S. Organ dysfunction after cardiopulmonary bypass: a systemic inflammatory reaction initiated by the extracorporeal circuit. *Intens Care Med* 1987; **13**, 89–95.

15. Mammen EF, Koets MH, Washington BC, *et al.* Hemostasis changes during cardiopulmonary bypass surgery. *Semin Thromb Hemostas* 1985; **11**, 281–292.

16. Saltzman EW, Weinstein MJ, Weintraub RM. Treatment with desmopressin acetate to reduce blood loss after cardiac surgery: a double blind randomised trial. *New Engl J Med* 1986; **314**, 1402–1406.

17. Stibbe J, Kluft C, Brommer EJ. Enhanced fibrinolytic activity after cardiopulmonary bypass surgery in man is caused by extrinsic (tissue type) plasminogen activator. *Eur J Clin Invest* 1984; **14**, 375.

18. Ademan B, Michelson AD, Loscalzo J. Plasmin effect on platelet glycoprotein Ib–von Willebrand interactions. *Blood* 1985; **65**, 32–40.

19. Van-Oeveren W, Eijsman L, Roozendaal KL, Wildevuur CRH. Platelet preservation by aprotonin during cardiopulmonary bypass. *Lancet* 1988; **i**, 644.

20. Kolawski E. Fibrinogen receptors and their biological significance. *Semin Haematol* 1968; **5**, 45–59.

21. Musial J, Niewiarowski S, Hershock D, Morinelli TA, Colman RW, Edmunds LH. Loss of fibrinogen receptors from the platelet surface during simulated extracorporeal circulation. *J Lab Clin Med* 1985; **105**, 514–522.

22. Kluft C, Dooijewaard G, Emeis JJ. Role of the contact system in fibrinolysis. *Thromb Haemostas* 1987; **13**, 50–68.

23. Fuhrer G, Gallimore MJ, Heller W. Studies on the components of the plasma kallikrein–kinin system in patients undergoing cardiopulmonary bypass. In: Greenbaum LW, Margolis HS (eds), *Kinins IV: Advances in Experimental Medicine and Biology.* New York: Plenum, 1984: 53–61.

24. Fuhrer G, Gallimore MJ, Heller W, Hoffmeister HE. Aprotonin in cardiopulmonary bypass: effects on the Hageman factor–kallikrein system and blood loss. *Blood Coag Fibrinol* 1992; **3**, 99–104.

25. Blauhut B, Gross C, Necek S. Effects of high-dose aprotonin on blood loss, platelet function, fibrinolysis, complement and renal function after cardiopulmonary bypass. *J Thorac Cardiovasc Surg* 1991; **101**, 958–967.

26. Chenoweth DE, Cooper SW, Hugli TE. Complement activation during cardiopulmonary bypass. *New Engl J Med* 1981; **304**, 497–503.

27. Korecki E, Erlich YH, Mars DD, Lennox RH. Exposure of fibrinogen receptors in human platelets by surface proteolysis with elastase. *J Clin Invest* 1986; **77**, 750–756.

28. Westaby S. Aspects of biocompatability in cardiopulmonary bypass. *CRC Crit Rev Biocompat* 1987; **3**, 193–234.

29. Machovich R, Owen WG, An elastase-dependent pathway of plasminogen activation. *Biochemistry* 1989; **28**, 4517–4522.

30. Takada A, Takada Y, Sugawata Y. Activation of val442-plasminogen (mini plasminogen) by urokinase, streptokinase and tissue plasminogen activator. *Thromb Res* 1988; **49**, 253–263.

31. Huisveld IA, Haspers H, van Heeswijk GM, *et al.* Contribution of contact activation factors to urokinase-related fibrinolytic activity in human whole plasma. *Thromb Haemostas* 1985; **54**, 102.

32. Brower MS, Harpel PC. Proteolytic cleavage and inactivation of alpha$_2$-antiplasmin inhibitor and C1 inhibitor by human polymorphonuclear leucocyte elastase. *J Biol Chem* 1982; **257**, 9849–9854.

33. Eberhart RC. Interactions of blood and artificial surfaces: in search of 'heparin free' cardiopulmonary bypass. In: Arensman RM, Cornish JD (eds), *Extracorporeal Life Support.* Boston: Blackwell Scientific, 1993: 105–125.

34. Toomasian JM, Hsu LC, Hirschl RB, Heiss KF, Hultquist KA, Bartlett RH. Evaluation of Duraflo II heparin coating in prolonged extracorporeal membrane oxygenation. *ASAIO Trans* 1988; **34**, 410–414.

35. Cottrell ED, Kappa JR, Stenach N, Fisher CA, Tuszynski GP, Switalska HI, Addonizio VP. Temporary inhibition of platelet function with iloprost (ZK36374) preserves canine platelets during extracorporeal membrane oxygenation. *J Thorac Cardiovasc Surg* 1988; **96**, 535–541.

36

Anticoagulants and the artificial heart

Jack G Copeland and Jacques Szefner

Thromboembolism following implantation of the total artificial heart (TAH) is well known. It may be that the strokes that occurred in two of the first four 'permanent' implants[1] which were so vividly described in the lay press have left us with a feeling that stroke is synonymous with the device itself. DeVries pointed out in his description of those patients: 'Animals have been proved to be inadequate to study the effects on the coagulation system.' The 'human model' which in those days so fascinated the media was from the start infinitely more sensitive to thromboembolism.

It is, therefore, not surprising that the device has lost favour. The former manufacturer, Symbion, which lost the support of its venture capital backer after failing to meet the standards set by the Food and Drug Administration for IDE (investigation device exemption) reporting is out of business. A new company (CardioWest, based out of the University of Arizona Medical Center and Med Forte of Utah) has been formed for the purposes of maintaining the technology which existed and initiating new studies.

No one can be certain of the extent to which 'bad publicity' may have influenced the attitudes of the medical profession, the general public, and many other sectors including the politicians and bureaucrats in our governments. Yet, it would appear that the most lasting impression upon all has resulted from the device and its interaction with the coagulation system. It seems reasonable for those who still believe there may be a place for

the TAH as a bridge-to-transplantation to review current practices with anticoagulation and the TAH and examine results that have been accumulated in over 170 patients.

Our first experiences with the TAH were filled with dread of massive clotting, embolism, and stroke. Our first successful bridge-to-transplant patient[2] was, therefore, followed closely with frequent monitoring of his platelet count, prothrombin time (PT), APTT, thrombin time, fibrinogen, antithrombin-III (AT-III), and factor X levels. He was treated with progressively increasing doses of heparin starting 24 hours postoperatively. Our goal was to maintain his thrombin time at twice normal, which was accomplished while we watched the PT and APTT remain normal and the fibrinogen, platelet count, factor X, and antithrombin-III rise to peak on the seventh day when the patient suffered a small (undetectable by CT scan) stroke with complete reversal of the two deficits, expressive aphasia and left upper extremity weakness. He was transplanted on the ninth day and went on to survive, return to work for several years, and finally die from an unsuspected small-bowel obstruction secondary to lymphoma 4.5 years after transplant.

Did we benefit from all the coagulation studies? Did the patient derive optimal results from our high-dose heparin up to 2000 IU per hour? Obviously the answer is 'no or not much'. When we explanted the device and examined the aortic outflow areas, the valve mount, and the quick connect, and found macron thrombi in the inner crevice of the quick connector, the junction of the quick connector and the aortic Dacron graft, and the inflow and outflow crevices of each valve, we quickly published this information together with the incriminating pictures.[3] We also mentioned in the report that better methods for anticoagulation and haematological monitoring were 'desperately needed', but clearly, the pictures left us with the impression that we had documented the weakness of the Jarvik total artificial heart (J-TAH).

We mention this case, not just to reminisce over the first successful TAH bridge-to-transplant, but to dramatize the current therapy which to our minds has improved some, but not enough from those early days. We at the University of Arizona were then, as we are now, quick to blame the device and point out new possibilities for design iterations, and perhaps too slow to examine more carefully the idea that the device might be adequate or better if we simply understood coagulation and anticoagulation.

Current results with the J-TAH summarizing the registry kept by the Minneapolis artificial heart group[4] include 171 bridge-to-transplant patients dating from our first patient in August 1985 up to January 1991. They observed: 'Anticoagulation regimens were variable and no correlation between neurologic complications and specific anticoagulation regimens could be detected'. Even though there was variation in regimens and undoubtedly some which were not optimal, there were only 16 neurologic events reported, among which nine (5.3%) patients had strokes and seven (4.1%) had transient ischaemic attacks. These data were received from 28 institutions and from patients with implantation times of from one to 603 days, with the great majority having an implantation time of 2 days to 2 weeks. Sixty-nine per cent of these patients were transplanted (31% died on the device) and 57% of those receiving a transplant (39% of the total) survived for at least one year.

From the most recent international conference summarizing the status of circulatory support devices (Circulatory Support 1991 sponsored by the Society for Thoracic Surgeons),[5] it would appear that many investigators are using an anticoagulation regimen that includes post-implant treatment (when significant haemorrhage has stopped) with low-molecular-weight dextran (dextran 40 at 25 ml/h) and dipyridamole in relatively small doses (75–100 mg three or four times a day, starting per nasogastric tube and continuing by mouth). Once the patient has demonstrated the ability to clot well as evidenced by the presence of serous, and minimally bloody, chest tube drainage, heparin is started by continuous infusion. When adequate heparinization is attained (APTT elevation to around twice the control values), dextran is stopped. When the patient reaches a post-implantation time of 1–2 weeks, warfarin is often instituted to replace the heparin (with a therapeutic target similar to that used for anticoagulation in mechanical valve patients of 1.5 to 2-fold prolongation of the PT). Thus, in the supported patient, after a period of one or two weeks, the consensus regimen seems to be warfarin and low-dose dipyridamole monitored by the prothrombin time. In patients with neurologic events of even the mildest variety, addition of aspirin (325–975 mg/day) appeared to be common. Such a protocol seemed to be most commonly used in the segmented polyurethane lined devices, and thus would most likely be used in J-TAH patients if there were a considerable number of implants today. Also, this treatment corresponds exactly to our own protocol in the most recent TAH recipients as well as recipients of pulsatile assist systems.

Standing apart from this consensus approach in both anticoagulation therapy[6] and results[7,8] is the team from La Pitié Hospital in Paris. Having a full-time physician in charge of coagulation dedicated to the cardiothoracic surgery service and having the largest experience (currently 63 J-TAH implants) has permitted study of the haemostatic mechanism. Therapies based upon these findings were proposed that not only seem to be reasonable but also have produced some incredibly good results. The approach includes extensive testing of the coagulation system and, thus, is applicable to a wide variety of coagulopathies encountered in cardiovascular surgery.

The La Pitié team views the TAH implant as a 'strong and permanent aggression' against the various pro- and anticoagulation systems (Fig. 36.1). Contact with a large foreign surface, the presence of shearing forces, non-laminar flow, and eddy currents provide a constant stimulus causing platelet degranulation, with the liberation of platelet factor 4 (PF4), beta-thromboglobulin (BTG), thrombin, thromboxane A_2, and other substances, resulting in some hypoactive platelets intermingled with some

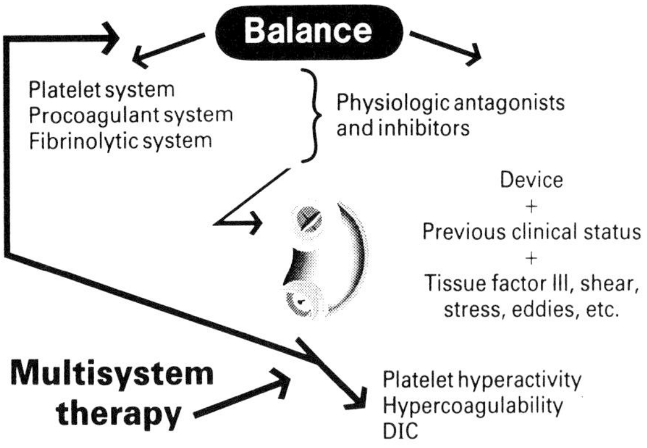

Fig. 36.1 Before administration of multisystem therapy the normal balance of the platelet, procoagulant and fibrinolytic systems is disturbed.

platelets that have normal function and may be stimulated by those factors that have been released. This activation spills over to the coagulation system that has already been stimulated by cardiopulmonary bypass, factor XII activation by foreign surface contact, the liberation of tissue factor III by the trauma of the operation. As more factor V and X become activated, there is a tendency to generate large amounts of thrombin over a short time, which in turn stimulates fibrin formation leading to thrombosis. This in turn leads to antithrombotic activity of antithrombin-III and activation of plasminogen and further instability of this extremely complex system. This sort of stimulation—particularly when associated with the surgical trauma of an already compromised patient with end-stage heart disease that may be associated with some organ dysfunction causing decreased production of clotting factors and/or platelet dysfunction—may lead rapidly to disseminated intravascular coagulation, and drastically reduce the implant patient's chance for survival.[9]

They have clearly demonstrated these pathological conditions to a greater or lesser extent in all the La Pitié TAH recipients. They have also demonstrated that in those patients developing DIC either in the immediate postoperative period or in association with sepsis developing later (or in the worst case when both are present) the chance of going on to transplantation is markedly reduced. Thus, they have adopted a vigorous approach to the stabilization of the coagulation systems from the time the potential implant recip-

ient is identified (see Tables 36.1 and 36.2).

Platelet stabilization is sought from the preoperative period onwards. Increasing doses of dipyridamole are given by either intravenous or oral routes in sufficient amounts to inhibit platelet phosphodiesterase, and thus increase platelet cyclic AMP which in turn makes platelets less susceptible to external forces that lead to degra-

Table 36.1 Coagulation monitoring checklist.

Platelet activation
Platelet count
Haematocrit
Platelet aggregation to ADP, adrenalin, collagen, arachidonic
  acid
Platelet factor 4 (PF4)
Beta-thromboglobulin (BTG)

Procoagulant system and its inhibitory regulation
Prothrombin time
Activated partial thromboplastin time (APTT)
Fibrinogen
Thromboelastography on recalcified whole blood (TEG)
Raby's transfer test on plasma
Antithrombin-III in plasma and in serum
Calculation of antithrombinic potential index (API)
Activated factor X in plasma and in serum

Fibrinolytic system
Reptilase time
Alpha$_2$-antiplasmin
Fibrinogen/fibrin degradation products (FDP)

Other tests
Ivy–Borchgrevink bleeding time
Wu–Hoak test
Platelet aggregation with other inductors
Raby's K test
Protein C, protein S and heparin cofactor II
D-dimer and/or fibrinopeptide A
Plasminogen
tPA, PAI, and venous occlusion test

Table 36.2 Multisystem therapy.

Heparin 1000–6000 IU/day
Dipyridamole 600–1500 mg/day
Aspirin 50–100 mg/day
Aprotinin 125 000 kIU IV injection followed by 500 kIU
  continuous IV infusion*
Pentoxifylline 400–1200 mg/day*
Ticlopidine 250 mg every 2 or 3 days*
Packed red blood cells*
Fresh frozen plasma*
Antithrombin-III concentrates*
Fibrinogen concentrates or cryoprecipitates*

*Only when indicated.

nulation. Doses necessary to accomplish this are in the range 600–1500 mg/day. Measurements used for assessment of the condition of the platelets and the effects of their therapy include PF4, BTG, and *in vitro* platelet aggregability in response to four different stimulators. Of course the platelet count is also of great importance, particularly decreasing serial measurements that may indicate consumption.

Aspirin in a low dose (50–100 mg/day by intravenous or oral route) is given to inhibit platelet cyclo-oxygenase, thus avoiding the liberation of thromboxane A_2 and inhibiting aggregation, but not enough to inhibit endothelial PGI_2 that has vasodilating and antiaggregant effects.

The coagulation system is stabilized primarily with low-dose heparin (1000–6000 IU/day by intravenous route). This agent acts in combination with antithrombin-III in its low-molecular-weight form against the low-grade continuous formation of small amounts (microdoses) of thrombin and in its high-molecular-weight form against rapid pathway formation of large amounts (macrodoses) of thrombin[6] (Fig. 36.2).

In order to judge the effectiveness of this therapy, in addition to the usual PT and APTT (10–20% APTT prolongation is usual), at La Pitié they examine factor Xa (plasma and serum), fibrinogen, antithrombin-III in the plasma and in the serum, and from that calculate the antithrombinic potential index (AT-III plasma – AT-III

serum). This activity allows one to know the amount of AT-III which is available to interact as well as its ability to be active against thrombin, which in turn reflects the relative amount of thrombin production.

The thrombodynamic potential index (TPI) taken from the whole blood thromboelastogram gives a measurement of the coagulability of the blood by looking at the rapid phase of clot formation. If this is very short (corresponding to a TPI >15), the test is said to demonstrate hypercoagulability; or if it is very long (corresponding to a TPI <6), the test indicates hypocoagulability. With this test, the ideal is a value of 6–15. Raby's transfer test (utilizing thromboelastography on plasma) is a measure of heparin therapy and is also used for the detection of circulating thromboplastinic material as in the assessment of DIC. The test is made using thromboelastography, this time looking at the first sign of clot formation (1 mm deflection) in two samples, one being a control and the other being a mixture of control and patient. If the ratio of mixture to control is less than one, this indicates unneutralized hypercoagulability and calls for increasing heparin. The goal is to maintain the patient in a stabilized condition that prevents stimulation by the TAH from leading to thrombosis or to DIC, yet leaves the patients free of the risk of bleeding.

To further stabilize these antagonistic systems if fibrinolytic activity is exaggerated, aprotinin is

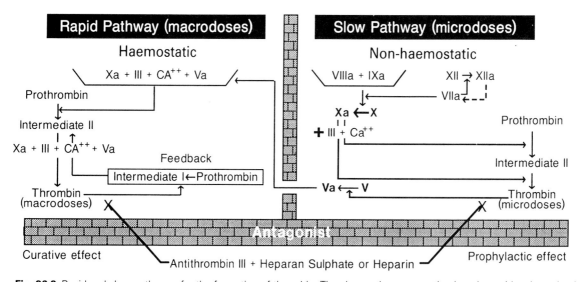

Fig. 36.2 Rapid and slow pathways for the formation of thrombin. The slow pathway may stimulate the rapid pathway by the activation of factor V.

used in a low dose (125 000 kIU IV injection followed by 500 kIU per minute continuous IV infusion). This inhibitor of plasmin makes possible the recovery of the natural plasmin inhibitor, $alpha_2$-antiplasmin, which in turn inhibits plasmin, thus 'protecting' the clot that has been produced in response to the trauma of the implantation. The aim is to allow the patient to remain free of abnormal bleeding. Measurements of $alpha_2$-antiplasmin and fibrin degradation products are used to follow these questions. Finally, pentoxifylline, an agent that improves red blood cell flexibility, is given to inhibit rouleaux formation and agglomeration. It also indirectly decreases fibrinogen concentration by acting through tumour necrosis factor. It is generally started on the third day and used empirically at a dose of 400–1200 mg/day (Fig. 36.3).

All of these concepts and treatments would have very little meaning if it were not for the nearly perfect track record for absence of cerebral and other embolism in 63 consecutive cases at La Pitié. Also they have noted extremely 'clean' devices at post-explanation examination. In a series of 15 autopsies of patients after J-TAH implantation, there were no cerebral emboli. They did find scattered haemorrhages in six cases with histories and findings compatible with DIC. There were two cerebral abscesses, and two cases of cerebral air embolism. In a series of 19 cases of device inspection for any evidence of macroscopic foci, a nearly perfect score was obtained, far from

what was reported from the University of Arizona in 1986. Finally, from the reports on the implantations by the French team there have been no cases of clinically detectable cerebral or other end-organ embolism.

In conclusion, we clearly have much to learn about how to use the artificial heart. Coagulation and anticoagulation problems have at first appeared to contraindicate further investigation, then later (as documented in the Minneapolis registry) to have been present but not nearly as severe as we had anticipated. We now, thanks to the work of the La Pitié group, have some evidence to support the concept that this device may not be so bad and that design changes may not be necessary. What needs improvement is our approach to coagulation. Heparin or coumarin therapy with the addition of low-dose dipyridamole is inadequate, as is dependence upon one test to determine the function of a coagulation system which has been continuously disturbed in many ways. A protocol which examines many of the features of the resulting coagulopathy seems indispensable. Examination of platelet function, coagulability, fibrinolysis and rheology should be available in artificial heart centres. Therapy tailored for treatment of abnormalities in each of these domains as outlined by the French team[6] is recommended.

Acknowledgement

The work upon which this chapter is based was supported by the University Medical Center, The Marshall Foundation and the University Heart Center, Arizona.

References

1. DeVries W. The permanent artificial heart. *JAMA* 1988; **259**, 849–859.
2. Copeland JG, Levinson MM, Smith RG, Icenogle TB, Vaughn C, Cheng K, Ott RA, Emery RW. The total artificial heart as a bridge to transplantation. *JAMA* 1986; **256**, 2991–2995.
3. Levinson MM, Smith RG, Cork RC, Gallo J, Emery RW, Icenogle TB, Ott RA, Burns GL, Copeland JG. Thrombolic complications of the Jarvik-7 total artificial heart: case report. *Artif Organs* 1986; **10**, 236–244.
4. Johnson KE, Prieto M, Joyce LD, Pritzker M, Emery RW. Summary of the clinical use of the Symbion total artificial heart: a registry report. *J Heart Lung Transplant* 1992; **11**, 103–116.

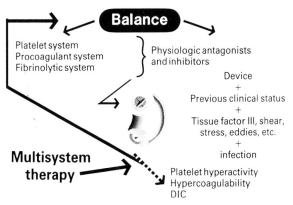

Fig. 36.3 After institution of multisystem therapy there is a return to equilibrium of the platelet, procoagulant and fibrinolytic systems. However, a constant tendency to disruption of the balance is caused by the device, the patient's condition, surgical trauma and infection. This 'strong and permanent aggression' must be meticulously documented with tests and corrected by modulation of therapy.

5. Copeland JG (ed). Circulatory Support 1991. *Ann Thorac Surg* 1991; **52**.

6. Bellon JL, Szefner J, Cabrol C. *Coagulation et Coeur Artificiel*. Paris: Masson, 1989.

7. Cabrol C, Gandjbakhch I, Pavie A, Bors V, Cabrol A, Leger P, Szefner J. Total artificial heart as a bridge to transplantation: La Pitié 1986 to 1987. *J Heart Transplant* 1986; **7**, 12–17.

8. Chomette G, Auriol M, Louahlia S, Leger P, Cabrol C. Artificial heart (Jarvik-7): anatomical consequences, apropos of 15 autopsies. *Arch Anat Cytol Pathol* 1987; **35**(5/6); 273–277.

9. Szefner J, Miralles A, Bors V, Gandjbakhch I, Cabrol A, Cabrol C. Disseminated intravascular coagulation: our experience with 40 patients with total artificial heart. *J Heart Transplant* 1990; **9**, 56.

37

Cannulation techniques in cardiac support systems

J Donald Hill and David J Farrar

Introduction

Providing sufficient blood flow to help or sustain a patient with compromised cardiac function is the most important specification of any prosthetic heart. Even though this has been recognized for several decades, it is surprising how little investigation and development into improved systems and cannulae have taken place. Cannulae and cannula technology do not represent a large enough market for industry to invest the money required for development. In most cardiac support systems, cannulae function adequately but can be considered a weak link in the system. This chapter describes the functions of a good cannula, some of the current shortcomings, and some clinical haemodynamic and thromboembolic aspects of different cannulation approaches.

Classification

Accessing blood via a cannulation system with the heart left in place (e.g. by a heterotopic system) can be by means of one of two techniques—direct cannulation of the heart, or peripheral vascular cannulation through medium-to-large vessels, usually in the groin. A complimentary system of classification is based on the length of time the cannula would be in place (e.g. temporary = 2–7 days; intermediate-term = 1 week to 6 months; long-term or permanent).

Specifications

The length of time a cannula is going to be in place increases the demands on the engineering specifications. Table 37.1 lists some of the characteristics a cannula should possess. Each of these will be important to a greater or lesser extent depending on the eventual specific application of the cannula.

A few of the specifications stand out when one reviews the current state of the art. Antithrombogenicity is an area in which great strides have been made but still falls short of the desired clinical performance. Antibacterial biomaterials are equally important for intermediate or permanent devices but are an area which is just beginning to be understood. There is a large body of data emerging that tie thrombosis and infection together.

The inability of the cannula to adapt to the patient's anatomical demands is a continuing frustration to the surgeon. This is particularly the case with desired features such as intraoperative custom shaping, cutting to length and forming a seamless connection, with proper length of reinforced areas and a non-kink, non-collapsible cannula that can be clamped. These are mechanical and chemical engineering challenges that must be addressed.

Table 37.1 Cannula ideal specifications.

Physical
Durable
Flexible
Non-kinking
Non-collapsible
Clampable
Thin-walled

Chemical
Durable
Non-toxic
Antithrombogenic surfaces
Antibacterial surfaces
Tissue in-growth to cannula surface

Surgical specifications
Different lengths
Different diameters
Different blood-accessing tips
Segmental reinforcement
Thin-walled
Modular

Custom adjustment
Bend to shape at tableside
Cut to length
Quick connections
Surgically 'friendly'

Cost
Inexpensive

Anatomical and physiological goals

As noted in the introduction, the one goal that cannot be compromised while improving other anatomical and physiological characteristics is adequate blood flow through the pump. Table 37.2 lists some of the important goals of cannulation systems.

The anatomical and physiological priorities sec-

Table 37.2 Anatomical and physiological goals of cannulation.

Good flow
Easy insertion
Easy late removal
Easy to de-air
No damage to the heart
No pressure points on adjacent tissues
Pulsatile flow
No haemolysis
No cannula–blood interface thrombosis
No intracardiac blood stasis
No ascending peri-cannula infection
No cannula–blood surface tissue overgrowth
No intra-atrial shunt

ond to obtaining good flow are dependent upon the type of clinical support that is necessary. For example, the important specifications in temporary support systems are ease of insertion, late removal and de-airing, and the absence of haemolysis. In systems for intermediate to long-term support, prevention of peri-cannula or device infection, or damage to the heart or adjacent organs, take on increased importance. Bridge-to-transplantation support systems usually require the specifications of an intermediate (1 week to 6 months) support system, although duration of support can be longer or shorter. Table 37.3 lists some of the specifications of an ideal bridge-to-transplant system.

Peripheral vascular cannulation

The use of peripheral vascular cannulation is almost entirely confined to temporary support systems. Access is usually via the femoral vessels in the groin. The traditional approach to the groin vessels is direct surgical exposure for insertion and removal. In recent years, percutaneous insertion systems using a needle, guidewire and dilator have become available and are popular with some physicians, especially cardiologists. Our experience with this technique resulted in many vascular problems in the groin that required surgical repair at the time of cannula removal. It is now our practice to use this technique only when speed of insertion is important. A potential problem with all peripheral vascular cannulation systems is the size and degree of disease in the access

Table 37.3 Goals of the ideal system for bridging to transplantation.

Uni- or bi-ventricular support
No patient size restrictions
Provides total oxygen requirements
Consistently good flow
Pulsatile flow
Durability
Minimal surgical procedure
Minimal anticoagulation required
No risk of infection *in situ*, peri-cannula or blood-borne
No damage to the blood formed elements or immunosupportive components)
No secondary organ physical or metabolic morbidity (lungs, liver, brain, renal)
Reasonable patient mobility
Low cost

vessel. Flexible, thin-walled, non-collapsible cannula features are mandatory in peripheral vascular access if successful cannulation is to be accomplished.

Another type of cardiac support system using peripheral vascular access is the Hemopump.[1] This device is covered thoroughly in Chapter 13 and will not be discussed in any detail here, except to note two issues that arise during its insertion. Firstly, the Hemopump cannula that is inserted in the femoral artery is 6 mm in diameter and may be too large for a small and/or atherosclerotic vessel. In this situation the surgeon must use the iliac vessels or occasionally the lower abdominal aorta to gain access. The second potential difficulty with the Hemopump system is in passing the cannula across the aortic valve, but improvements have been made in this system.

Direct cannulation for cardiac support

Direct cannulation of the heart is used in all three types of clinical cardiac support (short, intermediate and long-term) but with distinct differences in the sophistication of the cannulae.

These available cannulation systems range from standard open-heart surgical cannulae for temporary cardiac support, to long-term implant systems.

Standard open-heart surgery cannulae inserted into the atrial chambers of the heart, aorta or pulmonary arteries and brought out through the chest wall are surprisingly effective as cardiac support systems. They can only be used safely for 2–7 days. The overwhelming disadvantage is the requirement for heparin to prevent thrombosis from occurring in the system. Advances have been made to minimize or eliminate the need for anticoagulation with the development of covalently bonded heparin surfaces by Carmeda of Sweden and Bentley Laboratories.[2,3]

The Abiomed system is uniquely designed for temporary uni- or bilateral cardiac support. It has polymer trileaflet valves in the pole-mounted pumping chamber and is connected by cannulae and tubing to the heart.[4]

The cannulae and cannulation techniques of intermediate (1 week–6 months) and long-term or permanent systems require a maximum degree of sophistication and quality assurance of the system to minimize or eliminate any morbidity associated with their use.[5] These systems include the Thoratec and Berlin heart, Toyobo and Nippon Zeon for intermediate-term support (1–6 months) and the TCI and Novacor for implanted devices potentially for longer-term support.[6–11]

The pulmonary artery and aortic return cannulae in these systems are most commonly fabricated of woven Dacron that is sutured directly to the vessel. This minimizes the risk of thromboembolism and provides maximum cannula flexibility for the most favourable positioning in the mediastinum. The woven Dacron is usually preclotted by one of several standard methods. The preclotting method we prefer to use is cryoprecipitate followed by thrombin. This method avoids the necessity for autoclaving, which may damage the polymer portions of the cannula, and provides prevention against leakage through the graft. Some devices provide a cannula insertion system that, when in place, protrudes into the aorta or pulmonary artery. The advantages of this are speed and simplicity of insertion. However, because the cannula protrudes into the vessel the risk of thromboembolism is increased over a long period of support, and this method should only be used for short-term support.

Atrial and/or left ventricular chamber cannulation is the most important surgical aspect of these systems and one that continues to be the centre of a lot of controversy. After 10 years of clinical use and assessment of cardiac support systems, no one approach stands out clearly as the system of choice for all situations. Experience and surgical judgement are still important in selecting the best approach for an individual patient. Table 37.4 summarizes the advantages and disadvantages of the different approaches for accessing blood.

In cannulating the left atrium from either the right or the left side, it is imperative that the cannula enters the atrium on its free wall, well away from the pulmonary veins. The size of the cannula (32 to 51F) is large enough that any obstruction or stasis it might cause to the pulmonary veins could result in thrombosis and the risk of thromboembolism. This is especially true in patients who are on little or no anticoagulation. The left atrial appendage should also be avoided for two reasons: firstly, it is often too small for inserting a large cannula; and secondly, there is a site of stasis surrounding the cannula in the appendage that may result in thrombosis and embolization later when the cannula is removed. The preferred cannulation sites for the left atrium are shown in Figs 37.1 and 37.2. The Berlin heart cannulation system has unique cannulae with open-ended short tips that protrude only slightly into the atrium from the free wall. They are sometimes difficult to insert and remove. The Thoratec is a 51F curved cannula with a pointed caged tip that is inserted into the left atrial chamber. It is easy to insert and remove. Both approaches drain the atrium well.

It should be noted that, no matter how well atrial cannulae are designed or surgically implanted, they will never completely capture all the blood returning to the atrium. Some blood will always escape into the ventricular chamber. If there is profound ventricular dysfunction without any ejection, there will be significant stasis thrombosis in the ventricular chamber, making recovery of the heart impossible and presenting an increased risk of thromboembolism. This situation is particularly dangerous with recurring arrhythmias or frank ventricular fibrillation that persist over an extended period.

The left ventricular apex has many advantages over the other direct cannulation approaches. The LV apex approach provides the most consistent flow which is not affected by movement or the position of the patient, minimizes the risk of stasis in the heart, conserves space for chest closure in small patients, and allows easy postoperative patient management.[12] One disadvantage is that the patient must be on some means of extracorporeal support to make the insertion safely. Before utilizing the LV apex as a cannulation site one should be confident that the ventricle is not likely to recover. Some degree of muscle damage always occurs with this approach that can jeopardize ventricular recovery and weaning the patient from the cardiac support system. Despite this, several centres have reported using an LV apex cannulation approach in patients who were weaned from support with

Table 37.4 Cannulation sites.

Site	Advantages	Disadvantages
Base of the left atrial appendage or left atrial free wall	Easy cannulation	Poor LV decompression
	Good flow	Risk of blood stasis in the heart
	No damage to heart	Less postoperative mobility
	Easy to wean	Occupies anterior mediastinal space
	Easy to decannulate	Risk of vein graft damage
Trans mitral valve – left ventricle	Moderately easy cannulation	Hard to wean (e.g. mitral regurgitation)
	Good flow	Risk of mitral valve damage
	Easy to decannulate	Less postoperative mobility
	Good LV decompression	Occupies anterior mediastinal space
		Risk of vein graft damage
Left ventricle	Excellent flow	ECC for cannulation
	Excellent LV decompression	Bleeding difficult to fix
	No blood stasis	Difficult to decannulate
	Conserves space	Damages myocardium
	Stable patient mobility	
	Easy to wean	
Left atrium – intra-atrial groove (adjacent to right SPV)	Easiest cannulation (no ECC)	Poor LV decompression
	Good flow	Risk of blood stasis in the heart
	No myocardial damage	Less patient mobility
	Easy to wean	Occupies anterior mediastinal space
	Easy to decannulate	Risk of right superior pulmonary vein obstruction

successful removal of the apex cannula without significant residual damage to the LV muscle.

One important aspect about the decreased risk of thromboembolism with LV cannulation needs to be emphasized. In the Thoratec series of the first 166 patients supported for bridging to transplantation, 71 (43%) had LV apex cannulation, 38 (23%) had left atrial cannulation and 57 (34%) had intra-atrial groove cannulation on the right side of the left atrium in the free wall between the superior and inferior pulmonary veins. Of special interest is that the incidence of thromboembolism was significantly reduced with LV apex cannulation. Two patients out of 71 (2.8%) with LV cannulation had cerebral events, compared with five events (13.5%) in the left atrial cannulation group and six events (10%) in patients who were cannulated via the intra-atrial groove. Many of these events were transient and the patients made satisfactory recoveries; but the point that must be made is that LV apex cannula-

tion minimizes stasis of blood in the chambers of the heart, which is probably the explanation for the decrease in thromboembolic events. Despite the data on the incidence of thromboembolism, there were no differences in the long-term survival rates between patients who had atrial and those who had ventricular cannulation.

The continued interest and controversy over uni- versus biventricular support systems identifies another subtlety of left ventricular cannulation. The success of univentricular support of the left heart depends on the right ventricle functioning satisfactorily. The larger the LV apex cannula, the better the unloading of the left side, which can result in passive reduction of pulmonary artery pressures and therefore improved RV afterload. Good LV drainage is mandatory for univentricular systems, and this is aided by the size of the LV cannula.

Cannulation of the right atrium is a more standard procedure. Of primary importance is

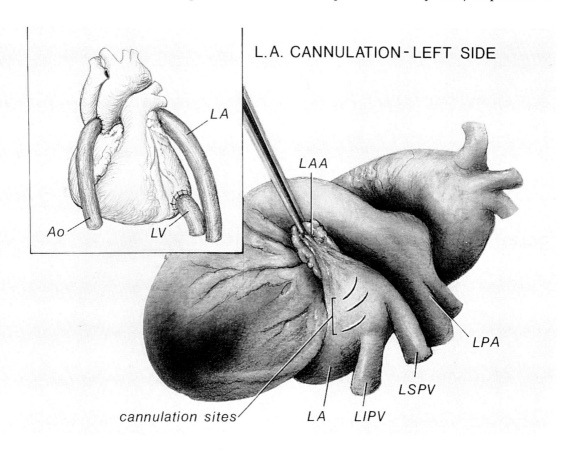

Fig. 37.1 Preferred left-side cannulation sites for the left atrium.

that the tip of the cannula should be well centred in the right atrium so that the maximum amount of blood can be captured before it escapes through the tricuspid valve into the right ventricle. Commonly, RV flow is less than LV bypass flow. In most instances the right ventricle tolerates this well and has a tendency to recover independently of the left ventricle. In bridge-to-transplant patients it is important to insert the cannula at a site that can be excised at the time of pump removal and transplant leaving an adequate remnant of right atrium to anastomose to the donor heart.

Conclusions

Cannulae and cannulation systems for cardiac support are an imperfect technology, and the clinical state of the art can be improved. The key is to have improved biomaterials and fabrication techniques to allow cannulae to be customized to the anatomic needs of the patient at the operating table. The most important thing every cannula and cannulation system must provide is adequate bypass flow. The second and third most important features of cannulae are antithrombogenic and antibacterial characteristics, which are still limiting factors in the long-term success of chronically implanted systems.

Despite these shortcomings, surgeons throughout the world have demonstrated great successes with a variety of different approaches. With more clinical experience, the state of the art will slowly develop to provide good results on a consistent basis.

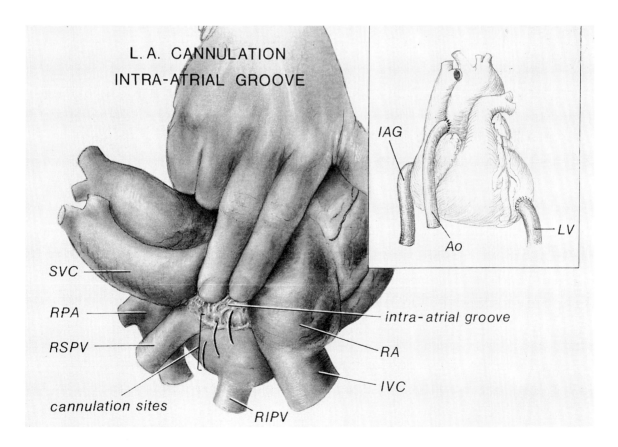

Fig. 37.2 Preferred cannulation sites for the left atrium via the intra-atrial groove (IAG).

References

1. Wampler RK, Frazier OH, Lansing AM, *et al.* Treatment of cardiogenic shock with the Hemopump left ventricular assist device. *Ann Thorac Surg* 1991; **52**, 506–513.
2. Magovern GA. The Biopump and postoperative circulatory support. *Ann Thorac Surg* 1993; **55**, 245–249.
3. Arnander C, Olsson P, Larm O. Influence of blood flow and the effect of protamine on the thromboresistant properties of a covalently bonded heparin suture. *J Biomed Mater Res* 1988; **22**, 859–868.
4. Dixon JF, Farris CD. The Abiomed BVS 5000 system. *Clin Iss Crit Care Nursing* 1991; **2**, 552–561.
5. Ganzel BL, Gray LA, Slater AD, *et al.* Surgical techniques for the implantation of heterotopic prosthetic ventricles. *Ann Thorac Surg* 1989; **47**, 113–120.
6. Farrar DJ, Hill JD, Gray LA, *et al.* Heterotopic prosthetic ventricles as a bridge to transplantation: a multicenter study in 29 patients. *New Engl J Med* 1988; **318**, 333–340.
7. Farrar DJ, Lawson JH, Litwak P, Cederwall. Thoratec VAD system as a bridge to heart transplantation. *J Heart Lung Transplant* 1990; **94**, 15–23.
8. McCarthy PM, Portner PM, Tobler HG, *et al.* Clinical experience with the Novacor ventricular assist system: bridge to transplantation and the transition to permanent application. *J Thorac Cardiovasc Surg* 1991; **102**, 578–586.
9. Portner PM, Oyer PE, Pennington DG, *et al.* Implantable electrical left ventricular assist system: bridge to transplantation and the future. *Ann Thorac Surg* 1989; **41**, 142–150.
10. Hetzer R, Hennig E, Schiessler, *et al.* Mechanical circulatory support and heart transplantation. *J Heart Lung Transplant* 1992; **11**(4,Pt 2), S175–181.
11. Takano H, Hakatani T, Taenaka Y. Clinical experience with ventricular assist systems in Japan. *Ann Thorac Surg* 1993; **55**, 250–256.
12. Reedy JE, Swartz MT, Lohmann DP, Moroney DA, Vaca KJ, McBride LR, Pennington DG. The importance of patient mobility with ventricular assist device support. *ASAIO J* 1992; **38**, M151–153.

38

Cannulation for ECMO

RK Firmin, J Waggoner and GA Pearson

Introduction

The correct placement of appropriately sized cannulae is essential for the satisfactory performance of any extracorporeal circuit. The cannula dimensions tend to be the rate-limiting step in terms of venous drainage, and resistance to return of blood to the patient. Correct selection is critical to avoid the dangers of high pressure gradients and suction within the circuit. Although many types of cannulae can be used for extracorporeal membrane oxygenation (ECMO), several are specifically designed for this purpose (Elecath, Biomedicus). Cannulae are designed to impart low resistance to flow at the rate anticipated to be required. They are therefore thin-walled, and relatively short, flexible yet kink-resistant. Venous cannulae have multiple side and end holes to afford the maximum blood drainage, whereas arterial cannulae have an end hole and few if any side holes. It should be remembered that the resistance to linear flow through a cannula is governed by Poiseuille's law and is therefore a function of its length and the fourth power of its internal radius.[1,2]

A limited number of double-lumen cannulae are available for venovenous ECMO (Kendall, Jostra). These cannulae with conjoined venous drainage and arterial return lumens avoid the need for carotid artery cannulation and ligation. All cannulae must be radio-opaque so that correct placement can be verified by radiography.

The operator performing cannulation must have a clear idea of what type of extracorporeal life support is required for a particular patient and what is the maximum anticipated flow. Cannulae and circuit design for neonatal ECMO have become relatively standardized. Cannulation for older children and adults, however, may be more difficult partly because of the heterogeneous nature of the clinical problems encountered and partly because a full range of high-quality cannulae and bladder reservoirs have yet to be marketed. A guide to cannula size, circuit tubing size, oxygenator size and priming volume is shown in Table 8.2 in Chapter 8.

Modes of cannulation

The two principal methods of cannulation for ECMO are venoarterial (VA) and venovenous (VV). Venoarterial perfusion is used when cardiac support is, at least in part, necessary. Venovenous perfusion is usually adequate for isolated pulmonary support and is the preferred option,[3] as lung perfusion seems to boost pulmonary healing and surfactant production.[4] Venovenous perfusion may be achieved by:

1. Two venous cannulae, one drainage and one return.
2. A double-lumen catheter.
3. Tidal drainage and return through a single lumen catheter.[5]

Cannulation procedures

Most patients are paralysed and on opiate sedation at the time of referral for ECMO. Further anaesthesia, therefore, takes the form of either local anaesthetic infiltration, an intravenous agent (e.g. ketamine 2 mg/kg) or an inhalational agent administered to the ventilator circuit (e.g. isoflurane). The patient is prepared and draped in the intensive care unit with all clinical staff taking operating room precautions. Care must be taken to avoid leaking oxygen under the drapes as explosions have occurred when 100% oxygen and spirit vapour from the skin preparation have been ignited by electrocautery.

For neonatal ECMO, the right supraclavicular region alone is prepared. A transverse supraclavicular incision is made through the skin and platysma using cautery for all except the skin edge. The deep fascia is opened at the anterior border of the sternomastoid muscle and the muscle retracted laterally. The omohyoid muscle usually requires division before opening the carotid sheath vertically. The right internal jugular vein and the right common carotid artery are exposed and cleared of fascia over a 2 cm length. Either thread ligatures or silastic slings are placed around the vessels. Silastic ligatures are preferable when it is intended to repair the vessel at decannulation. Absolute haemostasis is obtained. Heparin 40–100 units/kg is then given into the internal jugular vein. The sash is divided and the appropriate venous and arterial cannulae or double-lumen venous cannula selected. In general, the largest cannula that will fit is the correct one. For neonates it is usual to use a 10 or 12 French gauge arterial cannula and a 12 or 14 French venous catheter. Currently, 12 and 14 French gauge double-lumen catheters are available (Kendall, Jostra). It helps to moisten the cannula with saline before insertion. The arterial and venous cannulae are then inserted in turn to a distance dictated by the patient's size. The usual range for neonates is 2–4 cm for the arterial cannula and 5–8 cm for the venous catheter. In each case the vessel is ligated cranially and a clamp placed caudally. An arrowhead slit is made in the anterior part of each vessel and the opening gently dilated. During insertion there should be no resistance. If resistance is encountered, the cannula may be too large or the tip is catching the orifice of another vessel, usually the right subclavian branch. On occasions the arterial cannula may go into the subclavian artery instead of the aortic arch. This is easily recognizable as the cannula will not flush back as expected, and if connected to the circuit the line pressure does not reflect aortic pressure. If crossing the subclavian vessels poses difficulty, movement of either the neck, the arm or both will usually allow the cannula to pass. Some centres routinely place a cephalad venous cannula in addition to the atrial cannula. This boosts venous drainage and probably reduces intracranial venous pressure. It also provides an opportunity to get some indication of the adequacy of cerebral oxygen delivery. A one-size smaller cannula should be used and the cannula inserted only 2–2.5 cm. Having secured the ligatures around the cannulae, further stitches are placed to secure the cannulae to the skin. Fibrin glue and oxycel are placed around the cannulae and the incision closed. Cannula position is checked on X-ray and also on cardiac ultrasound. The most common error is to insert the arterial cannula too close to the aortic valve; such an error is readily identified by echocardiography.

In older children and adults, venoarterial ECMO may be used through a cervical incision as for neonates. Venovenous perfusion, however, usually requires the placement of two catheters as large double-lumen cannulae are not readily available. In such cases, the best venous drainage is achieved from right internal jugular cannulation and return is to a cannula placed into the femoral vein through the stump of the saphenous opening. This is often done at surgical cut-down. However, with the newer cannulae that are becoming available, percutaneous placement using a Seldinger technique may be possible.

A special consideration of cannulation is necessary relating to patients who have undergone cardiac surgery, which will usually have been for repair of congenital heart defects. In some cases cannulation will be performed in the operating theatre and, under these circumstances, cannulation of the aorta and right atrium may be direct through the median sternotomy or indirect through a standard cervical incision. Serious consideration should be given to a left-sided vent to prevent left ventricular distension. In cases in which the pulmonary or cardiopulmonary failure occurs later in intensive care, cannulation is preferable through a cervical incision. In cases in which one of the many variations of a total cavopulmonary anastomosis (Fontan) operation have been performed, obtaining adequate venous drainage may be difficult and require careful thought.

Decannulation

After a successful trial off ECMO, cannulae are removed under local or general anaesthesia. In the case of the internal jugular vein and carotid artery, it may be possible to reconstruct them, particularly the artery. This may be desirable theoretically and is practised routinely in some centres. However, any cerebrovascular compromise is likely to occur at cannulation and so by this time the merits of repair remain to be proven. In Leicester, we have also witnessed aneurysm formation at the site of previous vascular repair and thus use reconstruction selectively dependent on the state of the vessels at the time of decannulation. We do not believe that a difficult, prolonged operation is justified at this time and are conscious of the potential adverse embolic consequences of an inadequate result. The immediate and short-term results of simple ligation are surprisingly good,[6-11] though extreme long-term follow-up will be necessary to finally arbitrate differences in vessel repair strategy.

References

1. Montoya JP, Merz SI, Bartlett RH. A standardized system for describing flow/pressure relationships in vascular access devices. *ASAIO Trans* 1991; **37**, 4–8.
2. Sinard JM, Merz SI, Hatcher MD, Montoya JP, Bartlett RH. Evaluation of extracorporeal perfusion catheters using a standardized measurement technique: the M-number *ASAIO Trans* 1991; **37**, 60–64.
3. Ratliff JL, Hill JD, Fallat RJ. Complications associated with membrane lung support by veno-arterial perfusion. *Am Thorac Surg* 1975; **19**, 537–539.
4. Koul B, Wollmer P, Willen H, Kugelberg J, Steen S. Venoarterial extracorporeal membrane oxygenation—how safe is it? Evaluation with a new experimental model. *J Thorac Cardiovasc Surg* 1992; **104**, 579–584.
5. Durandy Y, Chevalier JY, LeCompte Y. Single-cannula venovenous bypass for respiratory membrane lung support. *J Thorac Cardiovasc Surg* 1990; **99**, 404–409.
6. Wiznitzer M, Masaryk TJ, Lewin J, Walsh M, Stork EK. Parenchymal and vascular magnetic resonance imaging of the brain after extracorporeal membrane oxygenation. *Am J Dis Child* 1990; **144**, 1323–1326.
7. Towne BH, Lott IT, Hicks DA, Healey T. Long-term follow-up of infants and children treated with extracorporeal membrane oxygenation (ECMO): a preliminary report. *J Pediat Surg* 1985; **20**, 410–414.
8. Perlman JM, Altman DI. Symmetric cerebral blood flow in newborns who have undergone successful extracorporeal membrane oxygenation. *Pediatrics* 1992; **89**, 235–239.
9. Glass P, Miller M, Short B. Morbidity for survivors of extracorporeal membrane oxygenation: neurodevelopmental outcome at 1 year of age. *Pediatrics* 1989; **83**, 72–78.
10. Campbell LR, Bunyapen C, Holmes GL, Howell CJ, Kanto WP. Right common carotid artery ligation in extracorporeal membrane oxygenation. *J Pediat* 1988; **113**, 110–113.
11. Campbell LR, Bunyapen C, Gangarosa ME, Cohen M, Kanto WP. Significance of seizures associated with extracorporeal membrane oxygenation. *J Pediat* 1991; **119**, 789–792.

39

Infectious complications associated with ventricular assist device support

D Glenn Pennington and Marc T Swartz

Introduction

The use of mechanical circulatory support devices in patients with refractory cardiogenic shock is gaining wider acceptance owing to technological advancements, as well as improvements in patient management and survival.[1] Currently, devices are inserted as either a bridge to cardiac transplantation or to provide circulatory support until myocardial recovery occurs. Despite increasing clinical experience and the maintenance of adequate haemodynamics in most patients, a significant number develop infectious complications, many of which are directly related to the mechanical device.[2] At present, all available mechanical circulatory support systems require transcutaneous cannulae, power cables or drive lines, and are associated with a risk of device-related infections. The development of a device-related infection is often dependent on the duration of support, whereas patient-related infections are more dependent on pre-device risk factors.[3–4] Factors such as the number of transcutaneous exit sites, anatomic position of the device, as well as the amount of host–device surface interaction are also believed to influence the incidence of infection.[2,5,6]

Pathophysiology

Implantation of any circulatory support device requires a moderate to large amount of host–device interaction between the artificial surfaces of the device and the body. These interactions can be divided into two categories: the interaction between the device and tissue cells, and the interaction between the device and the blood. The initial interactions between the artificial surfaces and tissue sets in motion a series of events which has been labelled 'the race to the surface'.[7] This theory describes the competition between healthy tissue and bacterial cells for implanted device surfaces in the early postoperative period. Bacteria may win out over the host/tissue cells in the race for the biomaterial surface, leading to infections that are extremely difficult to eradicate without removal of the device. If healthy tissue cells are the first to attach to the artificial surface, subsequent pathogens encounter living cells which are able to mount their own defence against the invading bacteria, and allow antibiotics to be delivered directly to the site of infection.

Circulatory support devices are constructed of materials that must be reasonably compatible with tissue as well as blood. Host–device interaction becomes an even more complex problem, considering that most devices contain several polymers, and often stainless steel or titanium. A wide range of organisms are attracted to these various materials in the early period after implantation. There are some data to support the concept that many bacteria are material-specific.[5] If bacteria arrive at the artificial surface composed of materials for which they have an affinity before the ingrowth of healthy tissue, they have an excellent opportunity for integration. The likelihood of eliminating such an infection without removal of the device is extremely low.

Blood components are also significantly affected by their initial interactions with an artificial surface. Several reports have described a profound T-cell lymphopenia which may be a contributory factor in the development of septic complications. Decreases in T-cell counts have been found in patients undergoing cardiopulmonary bypass (CPB) as well as in those supported with a total artificial heart.[8,9] The aetiology of the lymphopenia is unclear and may be due to multiple factors independent of the assist device, including pre-insertion cardiogenic shock, CPB and immunosuppression. A recent report showed that T-cell recovery is influenced more by the patient's clinical status than by the presence of a mechanical circulatory support device.[10] Complement activation occurs during CPB and haemodialysis.[11,12] This is believed to be a result of the interaction of blood with the artificial surfaces, as well as increased shear rates within some systems. Rapid complement activation results in consumption of serum complement components. Because the complement system contributes to the immunological defence mechanisms, a decrease in circulating complement levels may increase the risk of infection. In addition, there is evidence that complement activation results in the formation of several anaphylatoxins (C3a, C5a).[13] When complement activation occurs, the C3 molecule enzymatically attaches to the artificial material. The C3a segment is then released into the circulation, leaving most of the molecule (C3b) attached. A similar event occurs with the C5 molecule, producing a C5b portion attached to the surface and freeing the C5a segment to the circulation. While C5a is suspected of being a potent pulmonary vasoconstrictor, normally C5a acts as a moderator of the acute inflammatory response because it promotes granulocytic activation, adherence and chemotactic migration. Complement activation after CPB has been associated with a variety of clinical problems, including post-CPB pulmonary dysfunction, acute respiratory distress syndrome, increased infection, myocardial ischaemia, and hypotension induced by the heparin–protamine complex. Like most blood–surface interactions, activation of complement in patients with mechanical circulatory support devices is probably initially similar to those events which occur after routine CPB. After passivation of the artificial surface and/or clinical stabilization, complement activation probably ceases. Since complement activation has not been well documented in studies of patients with mechanical circulatory support devices, our current understanding is based upon data obtained from patients undergoing elective CPB.

Clinical results

The reported incidence of infectious complications in postcardiotomy ventricular assist device (VAD) patients ranges from 18% to 27% in larger series, and is 15% from the ASAIO/ISHLT registry.[14–17] It is unclear in many of these patients whether the infection was device-related or patient-related. It is often difficult and sometimes impossible to make this distinction, especially in cases of bacteraemia and mediastinitis. Since most postcardiotomy patients are supported for less than 7 days, many of the infections (such as pneumonia and line sepsis) are related to the patient or the procedure rather than the presence of the VAD. The development of infection is *not* a predictor of mortality in the postcardiotomy group.[17] Risk factors for infection in this group include long operative procedures, long CPB times, extensive transfusions, prolonged invasive monitoring, immobility, and bleeding that requires reoperation. These risks are compounded in patients who are operated upon under emergency conditions. The need for percutaneous cannulae may increase the risk of infection, but the development of device-related infections is related more to the amount of time the device is in place than to the number of cannulae.[3,4,18] Currently available devices all require at least one percutaneous power cable, pneumatic drive line or cannula that communicates with the mediastinum. Implantable VADs have the least number of transcutaneous exit sites (one) and are well suited for long durations of support. For shorter durations of support, the surgical complexity associated with inserting an implantable VAD outweighs the potential advantages of having only one percutaneous site as opposed to several.

Table 39.1 Clinical results at St Louis University.

	Recovery	Bridge
Number of patients	42	44
Mean duration of support (days)	4.4	43
Duration of antibiotics (days)	4.3	27.4
Infections (patients)*		
Pre-device	4	9
Post-implant (patient-related)	16	29
Post-implant (device-related)	1	15

*Clinically significant infection requiring antibiotics.

Reports from multicentre bridge-to-transplant clinical trials document a 24–40% incidence of infectious complications during support, and 20% of bridge patients are excluded from transplant as a result of infection.[19–23] Unlike in the postcardiotomy patient population, the presence of infection during the interval of assist device support in a bridge-to-transplant patient has a negative effect on survival. This negative effect is related to the clinician's hesitancy to transplant patients who are infected, since all these patients will require immunosuppression after transplantation. Clinical data relating to infection from the St Louis University experience are shown in Table 39.1. Our bridge-to-transplant population had considerably higher infection rates than the recovery group. This is most likely due to the longer durations of support. In the bridge group, 15 patients developed device-related infections, 9 of whom were transplanted. Eight of these 9 patients survived. None of the patients with active patient-related infections was transplanted. Predictors for the development of infection have yet to be identified.

Discussion

Infection is one of the more frequent contributors to death in patients undergoing mechanical circulatory support. Infection and thromboembolism, or infection and renal failure often occur simultaneously, and these combinations are almost uniformly lethal. Most of the patient-related infections are nosocomial bacterial infections similar to those occurring after routine cardiac surgery. Bacteraemia is usually the result of extensive and prolonged intravascular monitoring or the development of an abscess adjacent to one of the device components. Infections may originate at the exit sites of cannulae or transcuta-

neous power cables, and migrate up the prosthetic materials to invade the mediastinum. If such infections are detected early and treated aggressively with wound drainage and antibiotics, mediastinitis may be avoided. The shorter the duration of support, the less likely that device-related infections will occur. As clinical experience grows and less invasive monitoring is required in patients with mechanical devices, rates of infection should decrease. The development of mediastinal infections seems to be more prevalent in patients who undergo orthotopic total artificial heart replacement than in those who undergo heterotopic assist device placement. Griffith *et al.*[6] postulated that placement of a total artificial heart within the mediastinum creates a large dead-space with an abundant culture medium. Infection that develops within this dead-space cannot be treated effectively with systemic antibiotics. A recently published report suggests that mediastinal infection in patients with orthotopic total artificial hearts may not be as common as once thought.[24] However, the length of time the devices were in place was short.

Debate continues over how best to handle the threat of infections in patients who require prolonged support. Continuous antibiotics do not prevent infection and may allow superinfection. At present, the best rationale appears to be a short course of perioperative prophylactic antibiotics, followed by specific antibiotic treatment when clinically significant infections are detected. Infections are also less likely in patients who have few invasive monitoring lines, are haemodynamically stable, and have good nutritional status. Few patients develop opportunistic infections while on mechanical support. If an opportunistic infection does occur, it is usually in patients who have had prolonged multiple antibiotic therapy, or in patients who have poor nutritional status and were immunosuppressed as a result of the severity of their illness prior to device insertion. In most cases, device-related infections will respond well to treatment and clear once the device has been removed. For this reason, cardiac transplantation requiring immunosuppression can be safely undertaken in patients with controlled, non-mediastinal device-related infections. Patient-related infections (wound, pneumonia) should be eradicated and, if possible, an 'antibiotic free' period should be allowed prior to transplantation.

The role of percutaneous drive lines and cannulae in the initiation of infectious processes is not entirely clear. However, it has been generally presumed that the need for such lines will ultimately lead to local infections which are a constant risk for extending along the drive lines to the mediastinum. The early experience reported by DeVries and coworkers in long-term recipients of the Jarvik total artificial heart demonstrated this phenomenon in four patients.[25] However, the incidence of mediastinitis has been lower in VAD patients who retain their hearts, presumably because bacteria do not have the space and culture media in which to proliferate. Several other factors probably influence the development of ascending infections, including the degree of ingrowth of skin into the material at the skin entry site and the degree of mobility of the drive line, with minimal mobility being the goal. The establishment of a stable 'skin button' for prosthetic drive lines has been a laboratory goal for many years.[26,27] Although considerable progress has been made, there are no techniques which might ensure an infection-free site for long-term mechanical devices that require an external drive line. In our experience at St Louis University with the Novacor and Thoratec devices, some patients have had very well healed entry sites with excellent skin bonding to the prosthetic drive line, while others have had constant drainage, non-healing, and even purulent drainage. Since these drive line infections have led to mediastinitis or even prohibited transplantation, they undoubtedly would present a significant risk for a permanent system.

There is still much to be learned concerning host–device interactions as they relate to infection. Studies have shown that certain organisms have a special affinity for specific materials, including materials used in circulatory assist systems. Short-term antibiotic prophylaxis that is specific for the material involved may allow the natural protective factors to win the race to the surface and form protective barriers against subsequent invasion. Externally driven assist devices always carry the risk of bacterial infection. Future permanent systems are designed to be totally implantable, eliminating any need for lines or cables to transverse the body wall. It is hoped that elimination of these external routes of infection will greatly diminish the risk of infection, but the answers await the beginning of the clinical use of totally implantable LVAS systems.

References

1. Pennington DG, Swartz MT. Assisted circulation and the mechanical heart. In: Braunwald E (ed), *Heart Disease: A Textbook of Cardiovascular Medicine*. Philadelphia: WB Saunders, 1992: 535–550.
2. Didisheim P, Olsen DB, Farrar DJ, Portner PM, Griffith BP, Pennington DG, Joist JH, Schoen FJ, Gristina AG, Anderson JM. Infections and thromboembolism with implantable cardiovascular devices. *ASAIO Trans* 1989; **35**, 54–70.
3. McBride LR, Ruzevich SA, Pennington DG, Kennedy DJ, Kanter KR, Miller LW, Swartz MT, Termuhlen DF. Infectious complications associated with ventricular assist device support. *ASAIO Trans* 1987; **10**, 201–202.
4. McBride LR, Swartz MT, Reedy JE, Miller LW, Pennington DG. Device-related infections in patients supported with mechanical circulatory support devices for greater than 30 days. *ASAIO Trans* 1991; **37**, M258–259.
5. Gristina AG, Dobbins JJ, Giammara B, Lewis JC, DeVries WC. Biomaterial-centered sepsis and the total artificial heart: microbial adhesion *vs* tissue integration. *J Am Med Ass* 1988; **253**, 870–874.
6. Griffith BP, Kormos RL, Hardesty RL, Armitage JM, Dummer JS. The artificial heart: infection-related morbidity and its effect on transplantation. *Ann Thorac Surg* 1988; **45**, 409–414.
7. Gristina AG. Biomaterial-centered infection: microbial adhesion versus tissue integration. *Science* 1987; **237**, 1588–1595.
8. Ide H, Kakiuchi T, Furuta N, Matsumoto H, Sudo K, Furuse A, Asano K. The effect of cardiopulmonary bypass on T-cells and their subpopulations. *Ann Thorac Surg* 1987; **44**, 277–282.
9. Stelzer GT, Ward RA, Wellhausen SR, McLeish KR, Johnson GS, DeVries WC. Alterations in select immunologic parameters following total artificial heart implantation. *Artif Organs* 1987; **11**, 52–62.
10. Termuhlen DF, Pennington DG, Roodman ST, Ruzevich SA, Swartz MT, Reedy JE, McBride LR, Tsai CC, Kennedy DJ. T-cells in ventricular assist device patients. *Circulation* 1989; **80**(5) (suppl III), 174–182.
11. Chiu RC, Samson R. Complement (C3, C4) consumption in cardiopulmonary bypass, cardioplegia and protamine administration. *Ann Thorac Surg* 1984; **37**, 229–232.
12. Craddock PR, Fehr J, Brigham KL, Kreneberg RJ, Jacob HS. Complement and leukocyte-mediated pulmonary dysfunction in hemodialysis. *New Engl J Med* 1977; **296**, 769–774.
13. Chenoweth DE, Cooper SW, Hugli TE. Complement activation during cardiopulmonary bypass: evidence for generation of C3a and C5a anaphylatoxins. *New Engl J Med* 1981; **304**, 497–502.
14. Joyce LD, Kiser JC, Eales F, King M, Toninato CJ,

Hansen J. Experience with the Sarns centrifugal pump as a ventricular assist device. *ASAIO Trans* 1990; **36**, M619–623.

15. Killen DA, Piehler JM, Borkon AM, Reed WA. Biomedicus ventricular assist device for salvage of cardiac surgical patients. *Ann Thorac Surg* 1991; **52**, 230–235.

16. Pennington DG, McBride LR, Swartz MT, Kanter KR, Kaiser GC, Barner HB, Miller LW, Naunheim KS, Fiore AC, Willman VL. Use of the Pierce–Donachy ventricular assist device in patients with cardiogenic shock after cardiac operations. *Ann Thorac Surg* 1989; **47**, 130–136.

17. Miller CA, Pae WE, Pierce WS. Combined registry for the clinical use of mechanical ventricular assist devices: postcardiotomy cardiogenic shock. *ASAIO Trans* 1990; **36**, 43–46.

18. Pennington DG, Reedy JE, Swartz MT, McBride LR, Seacord LM, Naunheim KS, Miller LW. Univentricular *vs* biventricular assist device support. *J Heart Lung Transplant* 1991; **10**(2), 258–263.

19. Johnson KE, Prieto M, Joyce CD, Pritzker M, Emery RW. Summary of the use of the Symbion total artificial heart: a registry report. *J Heart Lung Transplant* 1992; **11**, 103–116.

20. Farrar DJ, Lawson JH, Litwak P, Cederwall G. Thoratec VAD system as a bridge to heart transplantation. *J Heart Lung Transplant* 1990; **9**, 415–423.

21. Frazier OH, Rose EA, Macmanus Q, Burton NA, Lefrak EA, Poirier VL, Dasse KA. Multicenter clinical evaluation of the HeartMate 1000 IP left ventricular assist device. *Ann Thorac Surg* 1992; **53**, 1080–1090.

22. Portner PM, Oyer PE, Pennington DG, Baumgartner WA, Griffith BP, Frist WR, Magilligan DJ, Noon GP, Ramasamy N, Miller PJ, Jassawalla JS. Implantable electrical left ventricular assist system: bridge to transplantation and the future. *Ann Thorac Surg* 1989; **47**, 142–150.

23. Oaks TE, Pae WE, Miller CA, Pierce WS. Combined registry for the clinical use of mechanical ventricular assist pumps and the total artificial heart in conjunction with heart transplantation: fifth official report, 1990. *J Heart Lung Transplant* 1991; **10**, 621–625.

24. Lonchyna VA, Pifarre R, Sullivan H, Montoyo A, Bakhos M, Grieco J, Foy B, Blakeman B, Altergott R, Calandra D, Hinkamp T, Istanbouli M, Sinno J, Bartlett L. Successful use of the total artificial heart as a bridge to transplantation with no mediastinitis. *J Heart Lung Transplant* 1992; **11**, 803–811.

25. Kunin CM, Dobbins JJ, Melo JR, Levinson MM, Love K, Joyce LD, DeVries W. Infectious complications in four long-term recipients of the Jarvik-7 artificial heart. *J Am Med Ass* 1988; **259**, 860–864.

26. Kantrowitz A. Development of a percutaneous access device. *ASAIO Trans* 1980; **26**, 444–449.

27. Topaz PA, Topaz SR, Kolff WJ. Molded double-lumen silicone skin button for drivelines to an artificial heart. *ASAIO Trans* 1991; **37**, 222–223.

40

Optimizing flow in centrifugal blood pumps

Leonard AR Golding

Introduction

In short-term support, the optimal flow from a ventricular assist device (VAD) is that amount necessary to maintain and/or aid the recovery of organ function. This can range from full replacement of cardiac output to lesser flows that together with partial ventricular function result in an adequate systemic flow. Thus the required flow varies with the clinical situation of various patients as well as with the time for an individual patient. Critical to the determination is the ability to quantitate the varying contributions from the injured ventricle by appropriate monitoring of flows, oxygenation and biochemical indices of organ function.

For short-term support, centrifugal blood pumps are the most frequently used and readily available ventricular replacement devices. Their role following cardiac surgical procedures is now well-established for patients who, in general, require 3–5 days of support.[1–8] More recently these pumps have been utilized as a component of emergency cardiopulmonary bypass (CPB) systems that can be instituted rapidly by the use of a percutaneous cannulation system.[4,9] This short-term technique has been used for resuscitation and/or support during diagnostic/therapeutic cardiology interventions. It can also permit resuscitation and allow a more studied decision as to the use of ECMO, a standard ventricular support device or corrective cardiac surgery. Centrifugal pumps have also found a role as a part of ECMO systems and, less frequently, as a bridge to cardiac transplantation.[1,3,10,11] For the latter, however, the durability and reliability of pulsatile devices pose significant advantages for their use instead.

Blood flow produced by centrifugal blood pumps is a function of the revolution speed produced as well as the pressure drop generated from the inlet to the outlet of the device. The basic premise in the use of centrifugal blood pumps is the concept that there is a reversible myocardial injury,[8] and their use will be to maintain systemic blood flow, to decrease the work of the failing ventricle and so decrease the myocardial oxygen consumption while improving the myocardial perfusion through the coronary arteries. The use of a centrifugal blood pump must be seen as a part of management of the whole patient, and this necessitates appropriate monitoring of haemodynamic and biochemical data. Thus the optimal flow for a particular clinical situation is that flow required to maintain systemic blood flow at $2.2-2.4 \, l/min/m^2$, normal atrial pressures, and adequate systemic perfusion pressure, while minimizing, as far as possible, any detrimental effects of the pump on blood elements by avoiding excessive motor speeds.

Simplistically, four major factors must be considered in attempts to optimize the flow produced by a centrifugal blood pump. These are: (a) patient factors; (b) inlet factors; (c) pump factors; and (d) outlet factors.

Patient factors

The use of centrifugal blood pumps for post-cardiotomy, short-term support is based upon the premise that the patient has a reversible myocardial injury that will recover with time. During the period of support, the goal is to minimize the workload on the failing ventricle; but equally important is the maintenance of systemic blood flow and perfusion pressure. With few exceptions, most patients will have undergone a trial period of support with intra-aortic balloon pumping, and this will be continued throughout the period of centrifugal support providing pulsatility. To optimize the flow necessitates adequate monitoring capability of haemodynamic function, and monitoring of atrial pressures, pulmonary artery pressures and thermodilution cardiac outputs is essential for providing information concerning haemodynamics as well as pump function. It is now accepted by most groups that pump flows of $2-2.4 \, l/min/m^2$ should be the goal during the initial 24-hour period of support and that the amount of pump flow thereafter is dependent upon recovery of the failing ventricle. In many cases, control of circulating blood volume is difficult and this should be by replacement of blood components, particularly in the initial 24 hours to control any bleeding tendency and maintain osmotic pressure.[12] Not infrequently, such patients become overloaded with fluid, but this can be controlled by the use of diuretics. In some cases, the early institution of slow, continuous ultrafiltration to remove excess water will expedite recovery of the patient.[12] Renal function must be maintained by providing good systemic flows and pressures, and instituting renal dose dopamine is routine. After the initial 24 hours of full support, pump flow can be decreased provided that systemic blood flow is maintained without significant increases in the atrial pressures, showing that the ventricle is recovering.

The centrifugal device can only pump volume that reaches it. The most frequent causes of inadequate centrifugal flow are the result of factors existing prior to blood entering the flow cannula. The most frequent of these causes are hypovolaemia, right ventricular failure, and tamponade (Table 40.1). Haemodynamic monitoring will show a lowered systemic flow, low left atrial pressure, with right atrial pressure helping to determine the cause (Table 40.2). Additionally, hypovolaemia and RV failure occur earlier than

Table 40.1 Patient factors in optimizing pump flow.

Bleeding
Right ventricle function
Patent foramen ovale
Pulsatility
Pulmonary vasoconstriction
Renal function
Delay to use
Circulating volume
Thrombosis/emboli
Infection (shunting)
Arrhythmias

does tamponade which tends to be a later event. Hypovolaemia is evidenced by low left and right atrial pressures, high systemic vascular resistance, and there is often associated bleeding. Right ventricular failure can also occur at an early stage, but in contrast, there is an elevated right atrial pressure and in the operating room the right ventricle is visibly distended. During the initial 24 hours, fluid replacement is preferably with blood, or blood components to maintain the haematocrit at near 30% while the use of blood components to control any bleeding diathesis is essential. The use of albumin for volume replacement when the haematocrit is at adequate levels has a useful effect by helping to maintain the osmotic pressure and retain fluid in circulation. Right ventricular failure is present in most cases, requiring left ventricular assist; treatment is by pharmacological means in most cases, particularly the use of isoproteranol (isoprenaline). In some cases, prostaglandin E_1 has proven effective,[13,14] but when there is an inadequate response to these measures, consideration of biventricular support is appropriate.[15-17] Cardiac tamponade tends to occur later in the course of the support and because of the frequency of bleeding many groups will now leave the sternum open for the initial 24 hours. Removal of any clot will produce a dramatic improvement in flow in such situations. Clinically, differentiation between RV fail-

Table 40.2 Causes of low pump flow in left ventricular assistance.

	Right atrial pressure	Left atrial pressure	Pulmonary atrial pressure
Hypovolaemia	↓	↓	↓
RV failure	↑	↑	↓
Tamponade	↑	↓	↑↓

ure and tamponade can be extremely difficult and is often solved only be exploration of the mediastinum.

Infrequently oxygenation can be difficult in spite of adequate flow and maximal ventilatory support, and it is essential to exclude the presence of a patent foramen ovale as the cause.[18] In some patients, not approximating the sternum during the initial 24–28 hours will improve the pulmonary function by limiting the compression of the oedematous lungs, and there is time to use diuresis or remove fluid by ultrafiltration.

Inflow factors

The inflow cannula and tubing can have an effect on flow. The pressure drop is a function of the flow generated, and to minimize this pressure drop and improve pump performance necessitates optimization of the tubing size and length (Tables 40.3 and 40.4). For clinical purposes, a venous inflow cannula of 32–36F size (wire reinforced) connected to slightly over a metre of $\frac{3}{8}$-inch (10 mm) tubing is now the standard (Table 40.5).

The cannulation site is usually into the atrial chamber rather than directly into the injured ventricle. This has become the preferred tech-

Table 40.3 Pressure drop along $\frac{3}{8}$-inch (10 mm) tubing (mmHg).

Flow	Tubing length		
	36 inches	60 inches	84 inches
1 l/min	4	5	9
2 l/min	5	14	20
3 l/min	10	25	35
4 l/min	20	35	52
5 l/min	30	50	75

Table 40.4 Effect of tubing size on pressure drop (mmHg) over 60 inches (1.5 m).

Flow	Tubing size	
	$\frac{3}{8}$ inch	$\frac{1}{4}$ inch
1 l/min	5	11
2 l/min	14	47
3 l/min	25	78
4 l/min	35	135

Table 40.5 Pressure drop (mmHg) across venous cannulae.

Flow	Cannula size		
	22F	28F	32F
1 l/min	40	25	17
2 l/min	88	60	33
3 l/min	175	109	63
4 l/min	300	175	102

nique because it avoids further myocardial injury and, in general, is an easier technical procedure. Some groups advance the atrial cannula across the mitral valve into the ventricle, but there appears to be no obvious advantage to this method for short-term support. Experimental studies tended to suggest that ventricular-to-aortic bypass produced better unloading of the ventricle in contrast to atrial-to-aortic pumping.[19] Such studies, however, were undertaken in animals with normal ventricles, and a study by Cohen *et al.*[20] compared the two methods in an animal model with induced infarction. This study compared the effects on the major factors determining myocardial oxygen consumption (e.g. contractility, wall tension and heart rate) and showed minimal differences between the two techniques for the decrease in the myocardial oxygen consumption achieved as well as for the maximal flow attainable by each of the versions.

Pump factors

All centrifugal pumps produce some degree of red cell injury. Flow produced by such pumps generally is in proportion to the revolution speed, but excessive speeds can cause haemolysis. In situations of low pump flow, it continues to be important to treat the cause rather than simply continuing to increase the pump speed in an attempt to improve blood flow. Clinical experience has shown that, in general, centrifugal pump-heads will function for the duration of short-term support of 3–5 days. The development of noise in the pump-head, or where increasing pump speed is necessary to maintain the same flow with no other change in haemodynamic parameters, suggests malfunction of the pump-head and the need for a replacement.

In general, for the biopump, speeds in excess of 2800 rev/min should be questioned as to their effectiveness. Sudden changes in pump flow can be a sign of dysfunction of the pump-head itself, or may simply be evidence that there is intermittently inadequate flow reaching the pump. Further evidence of this may be the occurrence of 'thudding' of the inflow tubing which disappears with decrease in pump speed.

After any bleeding tendency has been controlled, patients are given heparin to maintain the activated clotting time at approximately $1\frac{1}{2}$ times normal. More recently, the introduction of heparin-bonded systems has allowed the use of these devices without administering heparin and the associated risks of bleeding and/or thrombocytopenia.[21,22]

Outlet factors

Centrifugal pumps are somewhat sensitive to the afterload, and with increasing resistance to outflow, pump flow will decrease. The major causes of outflow problems are related to either the vascular resistance or to cannulae themselves. In most cases, $\frac{3}{8}$-inch tubing connected to a 22F or 24F arterial cannula will comprise the outflow system and prove more than adequate. The use of a narrow-bore arterial cannula or kinking can, however, result in significant haemolysis with some restriction of flow (Table 40.6). High vascular resistance can be controlled by the use of vasodilator therapy and tends to be a problem seen in the early phases soon after initiation of flow. Hypothermia will also cause peripheral vasoconstriction and limit the effectiveness of vasodilator therapy. Avoidance of cardiotonics which have a significant vasoconstrictive effect can also be helpful to maximize flow. Preferential cardiotonics are Isuprel, amrinone and dobutamine.

Table 40.6 Pressure drop (mmHg) across aortic cannulae.

Flow	Cannula size		
	22F	28F	32F
1 l/min	25	125	0
2 l/min	90	65	20
3 l/min	252	132	54
4 l/min	320	220	88

References

1. Golding LA, Crouch RD, Stewart RW, Novoa R, Lytle BW, McCarthy PM, Taylor PC, Loop FD, Cosgrove DM. Postcardiotomy centrifugal mechanical ventricular support. *Ann Thorac Surg* 1992; **54**, 1059–1063.
2. Noon GP, BioMedicus ventricular assistance. *Ann Thorac Surg* 1991; **52**, 180–181.
3. Zumbro GL, Kitchens WR, Shearer G, Harville G, Bailey L, Galloway RF. Mechanical assistance for cardiogenic shock following cardiac surgery, myocardial infarction, and cardiac transplantation. *Ann Thorac Surg* 1987; **44**, 11–13.
4. Moore CH, Dailey JW, Canon DS, Rubin JMO. Non-pulsatile circulatory support in 90 cases. *ASAIO J* 1992; **38**, M627–630.
5. Killen DA, Piehler JM, Borkon AM, Reed WA. BioMedicus ventricular assist device for salvage of cardiac surgical patients. *Ann Thorac Surg* 1991; **52**, 230–235.
6. Joyce LD, Kiser JC, Eales F, King RM, Toninato CJ, Hansen J. Experience with the Sarns centrifugal pump as a ventricular assist device. *ASAIO Trans* 1990; **36**, M619–623.
7. Drinkwater DC, Laks H. Clinical experience with centrifugal pump ventricular support at UCLA Medical Center. *ASAIO Trans* 1988; **34**, 505–508.
8. Braunwald E, Kloner RA. The stunned myocardium: prolonged, postischemic ventricular dysfunction. *Circulation* 1982; **66**, 1146–1149.
9. Dembitsky WP, Moreno-Cabral RJ, Adamson RM, Daily PO. Emergency resuscitation using portable extracorporeal membrane oxygenation. *Ann Thorac Surg* 1993; **55**, 304–309.
10. Bolman RM, Cox JL, Marshall W, *et al.* Circulatory support with a centrifugal pump as a bridge to cardiac transplantation. *Ann Thorac Surg* 1989; **47**, 108–112.
11. Pae WE, Pierce WS. Combined registry for the clinical use of mechanical ventricular assist pumps and the total artificial heart: second official report, 1987. *J Heart Transplant* 1989; **8**, 1–4.
12. Pierce WS, Hershon JJ, Kormos RL, Dembitsky WP, Noon GP. Circulatory Support 1991. The Second International Conference on Circulatory Support Devices for Severe Cardiac Failure. Panel IV: Management of secondary organ dysfunction. *Ann Thorac Surg* 1993; **55**, 222–226.
13. D'Ambra MN, LaRaia PJ, Philbin DM, *et al.* Prostaglandin E1: a new therapy for refractory right heart failure and pulmonary hypertension after mitral valve replacement. *J Thorac Cardiovasc Surg* 1985; **89**, 567–572.
14. Fonger JD, Borkon AM, Baumgartner WA, *et al.* Acute right ventricular failure following heart transplantation; improvement with prostaglandin

E1 and right ventricular assist. *Heart Transplant* 1986; **5**, 317–321.

15. Pennington DG, Merjavy JP, Swartz MT, Codd JE, Barner HB, Lagunoff D, Bashiti H, Kaiser GC, Willman VL. The importance of biventricular failure in patients with postoperative cardiogenic shock. *Ann Thorac Surg* 1985; **39**, 16–26.

16. Pennington DG, Farrar DJ, Loisance D, Pae WE, Emery RW. Circulatory Support 1991. The Second International Conference on Circulatory Support Devices for Severe Cardiac Failure. Panel I: Patient selection. *Ann Thorac Surg* 1993; **55**, 206–212.

17. Young JN, Iverson LI, Ennix CL, Ecker RR, May IA. Biventricular support is superior to univentricular support for mechanical circulatory assistance in patients after cardiotomy. *J Heart Transplant* 1987; **6**, 313–314.

18. Baldwin RT, Duncan JM, Frazier OH, Wilansky S. Patent foramen ovale: a cause of hypoxemia in patients on left ventricular support. *Ann Thorac Surg* 1991; **52**, 865–867.

19. Laks H, Ott RA, Standeven JW, Hahn JW, Blair OM, Willman VL. Servocontrolled cardiac assistance: effects of left ventricular to aortic and left atrial to aortic assistance on infarct size. *Am J Cardiol* 1978; **42**, 244–250.

20. Cohen DJ, Kress DC, Swanson DK, DeBoer LW, Berkoff HA. Effect of cannulation site on the primary determinants of myocardial oxygen consumption during left heart bypass. *J Surg Res* 1989; **47**, 159–165.

21. Bianchi JJ, Swartz MT, Raithel SC, Braun PR, Illes MZ, Barnett MG, Pennington DG. Initial clinical experience with centrifugal pumps coated with the Carmeda process. *ASAIO J* 1992; **38**, M143–146.

22. Magovern GJ. The biopump and postoperative circulatory support. *Ann Thorac Surg* 1993; **55**, 245–249.

41

Use of aprotinin in mechanical circulatory support

DY Loisance, PH Deleuze, JP Mazzucotelli and P Lebesnerais

Introduction

Implantation of mechanical circulatory assist systems has been shown to be associated with a high risk of intra- and postoperative bleeding.[1] This has led to an unacceptable rate of mediastinal re-entry in the first postoperative days, and to a need for massive transfusion of homologous blood derivatives with the risk of a complex immunological stimulation just before heart transplantation.

There has been considerable enthusiasm in Europe for the use of high-dose aprotinin in cardiac surgery, to prevent bleeding and to minimize blood requirements.[2-5] This led us to evaluate the beneficial effects of aprotinin during and after implantation of mechanical circulatory assist systems. Our study was performed in 1991 and 1992, and our data have been compared with those obtained earlier in patients not receiving aprotinin.

The aprotinin regimen used in our study included a 30-minute intravenous infusion at a dose of 2 million kallikrein inactivator units (kIU) at the time of the induction of anaesthesia. Furthermore, the extracorporeal circuit when used was primed with 2 million kIU of aprotinin in addition to routine fluids (crystalloids, bicarbonates, heparin). A continuous infusion of aprotinin was maintained throughout the surgical procedure, at a dose of 500 000 kIU per hour.[2] Heparin administration (300 IU/kg of bodyweight intravenously before cannulation and

5000 IU in the circuit), and post-bypass protamine infusion (1.5 × dose of heparin), were not different from the protocol used in routine cardiac surgery. The activated clotting time (ACT) was controlled during bypass and maintained above 500 s by heparin bolus top-up.

The anaesthesia did not differ from the protocol used in routine cardiac surgery. Emphasis was put on the level of arterial systemic pressure at the time of induction and intubation: the dosage was adjusted to avoid hypertensive episodes and/or hypotensive periods which would lead to the need for massive fluid infusion.

Extracorporeal perfusion was performed in a routine fashion. The circuit, equipped with membrane oxygenators and Sarns roller pumps, was primed with a minimal volume of fluid. Patient blood (500–1000 ml) was withdrawn at the start of perfusion, stored during the entire period of bypass and reinfused after discontinuation of perfusion. Details of the protocol have been published.[6]

Patient selection

The patients included in the study were in cardiogenic shock, despite optimal medical therapy including sympathomimetic agents and PDI inotropic agents.[7] The patients were grouped according to the type of mechanical assist system. In group A ($n = 4$), an electrical intracorporeal left ventricular assist system (Novacor) was implanted, with the use of an extracorporeal circulation. In group B (*n* = 4), external pneumatic ventricles (Nippon–Zeon) were implanted, without the need for bypass. Group C consisted of four patients, operated on before the start of the aprotinin protocol, who had received a Jarvik orthotopic total artificial heart with extracorporeal circulation. This group was used for comparison purposes. Anaesthetic management and surgeons were identical in all groups.

The small numbers in the three groups precluded formal statistical comparisons. Only tendencies were sought to draw out preliminary conclusions.

Results of the study

Demographic and major clinical characteristics of the patients are shown in Tables 41.1 and 41.2. The volume of postoperative bleeding and the amount of homologous blood material transfused during the first 24 hours are summarized in Table 41.3.

Pneumatic external biventricular assist devices (BVADs) were preferentially used in patients of low bodyweight because the Jarvik total artificial heart requires patients over 80 kg. Bypass duration was twice as long with Jarvik implantation, but the bleeding risk with Novacor implantation was greatly increased by the extended abdominal intraparietal dissection needed for device placement. Mediastinal bleeding in group A (with

Table 41.1 Patient characteristics (all male).

	Mean age (year)	Bodyweight (kg)	Aetiology	Previous surgery	CPB use
Group A (*n* = 4)	54.5 ± 9	72 ± 4	2 ischaemic 2 idiopathic	0	4
Group B (*n* = 4)	36.7 ± 8	70 ± 13	4 idiopathic	0	0
Group C (*n* = 4)	41.5 ± 5	87 ± 8	1 chronic graft rejection 3 ischaemic	2	4

Table 41.2 Perioperative data.

	Duration of CPB (min)	Haemoglobin (g/dl)		Platelets (×10³/ml)	
		Preop	Postop	Preop	Postop
Group A	107 ± 45	12.6 ± 2.3	9.4 ± 1.2	169 ± 90	60 ± 30
Group B	0	11.4 ± 2	9.3 ± 1.7	175 ± 90	122 ± 50
Group C	230 ± 50	10.4 ± 1.1	8 ± 0.8	236 ± 90	90 ± 40

Table 41.3 Postoperative bleeding after 24 hours, and the need for transfusion.

	Mediastinal bleeding (ml)	RBC (units)	Frozen plasma (units)	Platelets (units)
Group A	480 ± 90	4 ± 1.6	1.5 ± 2	0
Group B	2000 ± 2100 (median = 1000)	4 ± 5	4.2 ± 5	10*
Group C	1510 ± 600	4 ± 2	2.8 ± 2	10†

*One patient; †two patients.

aprotinin) was about half that in group C, but a similar decrease in postoperative haemoglobin was related to additional bleeding at the abdominal site of device implantation for group A. Platelet counts decreased similarly below the normal range, but platelet function seemed more preserved in group A with less bleeding, and less need for coagulation factors during the first postoperative day. In group B, without the use of bypass (CPB), the effect of aprotinin was less convincing because postoperative bleeding was more like in group C. Furthermore, in this group, bleeding in the first 24 hours was aggravated in one particular case where coagulation was dramatically disturbed preoperatively (by acute hepatic failure); this patient bled 5250 ml and needed 12 RBC units, 14 frozen plasma units and 10 platelet units. In group B, platelet counts remained within the normal range postoperatively.

Discussion

Surgery in patients in cardiogenic shock, submitted to the implantation of a mechanical circulatory support system, is associated with a high risk of bleeding and requires a large volume of fluids and homologous blood transfusion. This is a consequence of the frequently seen hepatic dysfunction leading to a drop in coagulation factors, together with the high-dose regimen of anticoagulant therapy given for days, and platelet dysfunction associated with poor haemodynamical function. Use of an extracorporeal circulation further alters the coagulation system: platelet numbers are decreased within a few minutes of bypass, platelets are activated during CPB, and there is substantial evidence that platelet granules are released during CPB.[9] In addition, the bleeding time, which is affected by platelet microvascular reactions, is prolonged by a few minutes after the onset of bypass. Finally, the fibrinolytic cascade is activated, as is complement. All these lead to an increased risk of bleeding, in addition to the risks directly related to the surgical technique involving suture of rigid materials to friable and fragile tissues. On this latter surgical cause of bleeding, surgical skill and a few technical details such as extensive use of mattressed sutures and gelatine resorcine formol glue are important.

Improvement in the haemostatic condition of patients by the use of aprotinin has been investigated extensively, both clinically and in the laboratory.[2-5] These studies have produced conflicting data, and so the precise mechanism of action of aprotinin remains to be clarified. Nevertheless, there seem to be beneficial effects on platelet activation during CPB,[3,9] reduction of plasmin activation, and a reduction of the increased bleeding time.

One of the major benefits of aprotinin therapy during implantation surgery is the immunological consequence of avoiding a major blood transfusion. Another benefit may be found in the prevention of a rise in pulmonary vascular resistance during and after CPB, a phenomenon which may compromise the functioning of the device. This problem is of crucial importance when implantation of a left ventricular assist system is considered, because maintaining the pulmonary vascular resistances at their low preoperative levels is a major requirement during the procedure.

It can be asked by the use of aprotinin was more efficacious when CPB was adopted for the surgical procedure. In our series, bleeding after BVAD implantation without the use of CPB was related more to preoperative liver failure than to platelet dysfunction. In all BVAD cases, bleeding was consistent with postoperative platelet count remaining in the normal range. However, the platelet count fell below the normal range in all procedures using CPB, but bleeding was much lower in the aprotinin group.

In conclusion, our experience with this small number of patients tends to suggest that the beneficial effects of a high-dose regimen of aprotinin, already demonstrated in cardiac surgery, may be observed in a population of high-risk patients submitting to major procedures such as the implantation of a mechanical assist device. The effect seems more marked in procedures requiring the use of extracorporeal circulation. The mechanism of action of aprotinin remains unclear and deserves more extensive investigation.

References

1. Oaks TE, Pae WE, Miller CA, Pierce WS. Combined registry for the clinical use of mechanical ventricular assist pumps and the total artificial heart in conjunction with heart transplantation: fifth official report, 1990. *J Heart Lung Transplant* 1991; **10**, 621–625.
2. Royston D, Bidstrup BP, Taylor KM, Sapsford

RN. Effect of aprotinin on need for blood transfusion after repeat open-heart surgery. *Lancet* 1987; **2**, 1289–1291.

3. Van Oeveren W, Harder MP, Roozendaal KJ, Eijsman L, Wildewuur CRH. Aprotinin protects platelets against the initial effect of cardiopulmonary bypass. *J Thorac Cardiovasc Surg* 1990; **99**, 788–797.

4. Bidstrup BP, Royston D, Sapsford RN, Taylor KM. Reduction in blood loss and blood use after cardiopulmonary bypass with high dose aprotinin. *J Thorac Cardiovasc Surg* 1989; **97**, 364–372.

5. Deleuze PH, Loisance DY, Feliz A, *et al.* Réduction des pertes sanguines per- et post-opératoires par l'aprotinine au cours de la circulation extra-corporelle. *Arch Mal Coeur* 1991; **84**, 1797–1802.

6. Tixier D, Loisance DY, Deleuze PH, *et al.* Blood saving in cardiac surgery: simple approach and tendencies. *Perfusion* 1991; **6**, 265–273.

7. Loisance DY, Dubois-Rande JL, Deleuze PH, *et al.* Pharmacological bridge to cardiac transplantation. *Eur J Cardiothorac Surg* 1989; **3**, 196–202.

8. Deleuze PH, Loisance DY, Shiiya N, *et al.* Irreversible drop of systemic vascular resistances in patients implanted with a Jarvik total artificial heart. *Int J Artif Organs* 1991; **14**, 286–289.

9. Lavee J, Savion N, Smolinsky A, Goor DA, Mohr R. Platelet protection by aprotinin in cardiopulmonary bypass: electron microscopic study. *Ann Thorac Surg* 1992; **53**, 477–481.

42

Device linings

Timothy R Graham and A Coumbe

Introduction

All mechanical circulatory support devices are required to be lined by biomaterials. These biomaterials need to be biocompatible. Biocompatibility, in this respect, is the ability of any biomaterial to perform or have an appropriate host response within a specific application.

In circulatory devices, biomaterials are required to be durable, flexing possibly over 40 million times per year, they should be non-toxic, maintain haematological homeostasis and remain non-thromboembolic (Table 42.1).[1]

It is important to consider the mechanical properties of biomaterials. Within different devices, different mechanical properties are required. In some device types the biomaterials need to be elastic and flexible, while in others they need to be plastic and stiff. These biomaterials may be fashioned in a smooth or textured manner and they need to be more durable in the longer term devices. Other properties are required in the shorter term devices. In most devices there are known areas of high flow and areas of stasis or low

Table 42.1 Ideal requirements for blood-contacting biomaterials within circulatory support devices.

Durable
Flexible
Non-toxic
Haematological homeostasis
Non-thromboembolic

flow, so that biomaterials with different mechanical properties and thrombo-resistance may be needed within the various parts of a device.[2]

Diaphragms

Table 42.2 lists diaphragm materials currently available. The choice of an acceptable biomaterial represents one of the more difficult issues in the development of an artificial ventricle.[3]

The material must be an elastomer, in order that it may be moved reproducibly back and forth

Table 42.2 Device diaphragm materials.

Silicone–polyurethane elastomers
  Cardiothane[a]

Polyurethane elastomers
  Biomer[b] (urea–urethane) MDI–PTMG
  Hemothane[c] (urea–urethane) (MDI–PTMG)
  Mitrathane[d] (urea–urethane) MDI–PTMG
  TLC-15 series[e] (urea–urethane) MDI–PTMG with additives
  Pellethane[f] 2363-80A (urethane) MDI–PTMG
  Tecoflex[g] hylene W–PTMG

Polyolefin elastomers
  Hexsyn[h] (polyhexene)
  Bion[i] (polyhexene)

[a]Kontron Instruments, Everett, MA; [b]Ethicon Corp., Sommerville, NJ; [c]3M Corp., St Paul, MN; [d]Mitral Medical Ltd, Wheat Ridge, CO; [e]Thoratec, Berkeley, CA; [f]Dow Chemical Co., Midland, MI; [g]Thermedics Inc., Woburn, MA; [h]Goodyear Tire and Rubber Co., Akron, OH; [i]Lord Corp., Erie, PA.

during the pump cycle. Second, the elastomer must not exhibit fatigue failure over the designated lifetime for the device. Third, the material surface must have low propensity for thrombus initiation. Finally, the elastomer must be capable of being formed into the shape dictated by the pump design in such a way that its mechanical and surface properties meet design specifications.

The criterion of fatigue resistance represents one which is particularly restricting because an average heart rate of 70 beats per minute amounts to approximately 40 million beats (cycles) per year. A fatigue life of 10^7 cycles is considered the maximum lifespan. The development of elastomers with improved fatigue resistance will play a significant part in realizing the objectives of a long-term artificial ventricle.

Design of the ventricle is an important factor in defining the 'degree' to which the material from which the diaphragm is made should be able to eliminate or retard the induction of thrombus.[3] A critical factor is the residence time of blood at the diaphragm surface, the ideal being that all blood which enters during diastole shall be expelled at the next systole.

Interactions

There are many possible interactions between biomaterials and tissues (Table 42.3). Of most importance within circulatory assist devices is the effect on the circulating blood.

Thrombosis on blood-contacting biomaterials relates to Virchow's triad—namely the haemodynamic conditions within the device, the thrombo-resistance of the underlying biomaterial surface, and the coagulability of the blood (Table 42.4). Good device design may alter these conditions. A good design is one which has adequate flow with

Table 42.3 Biomaterial – tissue interactions.

Blood surface
Potentiate infection
Foreign-body response mechanism
Cell activation/cytokine production by biomaterials
Vascular graft healing/intimal proliferation
Systemic effects
Calcification of biomaterials*
Enzymatic degradation (hydrolysis)*
Phagocytic effects*

*Effect of tissue on biomaterials.

Table 42.4 Thrombosis on blood-contacting biomaterials.

Triad of:
• Haemodynamic conditions
• Thrombo-resistance of biomaterial
• Coagulability of the blood

Pump design may alter:
• Haemodynamic conditions
  Good washing
  Eliminate seams
• Biomaterial
  Design thrombo-resistant material

good washing of all surfaces within the device. Seams should be eliminated wherever possible. Biomaterials which line these devices should be as thrombo-resistant as possible. Native haematological considerations have a great part to play in the thrombosis associated with artificial surfaces (see Chapter 3). Thrombosis has been noted, in particular, with several problem areas within devices.[4] These are the creases and flaws within the linings (Fig. 42.1), the diaphragm/housing junction, conduits and connectors, prosthetic valves (within the device or within the native heart) and areas of mineralization. Importantly the native myocardium and valves may be diseased and have a propensity to thromboembolic formation. The presence of systemic infection is also associated with thrombosis and subsequent embolism.

Materials currently available

Several types of biomaterial linings are available for use in circulatory support devices (Table 42.5).

Intra-aortic balloon pumps use smooth segmented polyurethanes on the surface of the intra-aortic balloon.

Centrifugal blood pumps use acrylic plastic for the inverted plastic cones (Biomedicus) or the impellars (Sarns, St Jude). These rigid vanes are responsible for moving blood on through the device.

Extracorporeal intermediate devices use smooth segmented polyurethanes and have copolymers added to them in order to try and make them increasingly thrombo-resistant (see Fig. 42.2).

The *Novocor implantable left ventricular assist device* uses a smooth-surfaced polyurethane Biomer for the blood sac within the pump. The *TCI device* uses an integrally textured polyurethane Biomer on the flexible pusher plate side, and sintered titanium microspheres on the static blood-contacting side of the rigid housing (Fig. 42.3).

The majority of *total artificial hearts* use smooth-surfaced polyurethanes as the blood-contacting biomaterial for the blood pump sac.

Smooth versus textured surfaces

The majority of circulatory support devices currently use smooth-surfaced polyurethanes.[5] However, microscopic imperfections may remain in them during the manufacturing process (Fig. 42.1) and the long-term durability may be affected by the cracking of the lining because it has to flex so many times. Platelets recognize imperfections of only a few nanometres and thus these areas have a propensity to become thrombogenic. Seams and junctions within smooth-surfaced sacs may also be a problem, as may be the variability of the adsorbed proteins upon the surface. It is currently recommended that devices using the smooth-surfaced polyurethanes require formal anticoagulation (warfarin/coumadin).

The alternative is to use a textured surface.[6] These include textured polyurethanes and textured metals. The textured-surface polyurethanes, when used within implantable circulatory support devices, mimic the textured vascular grafts (e.g. Dacron) which are commonly used in vascular surgery. There is, however, one important difference. The surfaces within circulatory support devices are impermeable compared with the peripheral vascular grafts (because of the metal pump housing).

Textured polyurethane surfaces encourage the development of an adherent coagulam and the subsequent development of a neo-intima.[7] Surface imperfections are covered by the development of this biological lining, and seams and junctions may be incorporated. It has been advo-

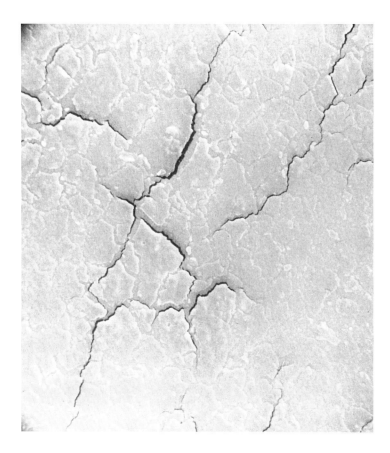

Fig. 42.1 Scanning electron microscopy (×950) of smooth surface polyurethane 'Biomer', showing 'microscopic' fissures.

Table 42.5 Biomaterial linings.

Short-term devices
IABP
- Datascope — Smooth segmented polyurethane
- Aries/St Jude — Smooth segmented polyurethane

Centrifugal heads
- Biomedicus — Acrylic plastic
- Aries/St Jude — Acrylic plastic
- Sarns/3M — Acrylic plastic

Intermediate-term devices
Extracorporeal/
paracorporeal devices
- Thoratec — Biomer®
- Zeon Nippen — Cardiothane®
- Toyobo — Cardiothane®
- Abiomed — Angioflex®

Long-term devices
TAH
- Utah/Jarvik/CardioWest — Biomer®
- Philadelphia Heart — Pellathane®
Implantable LVAS
- Novocor — Biomer®
- TCI — Textured Biomer® and Sintered titanium

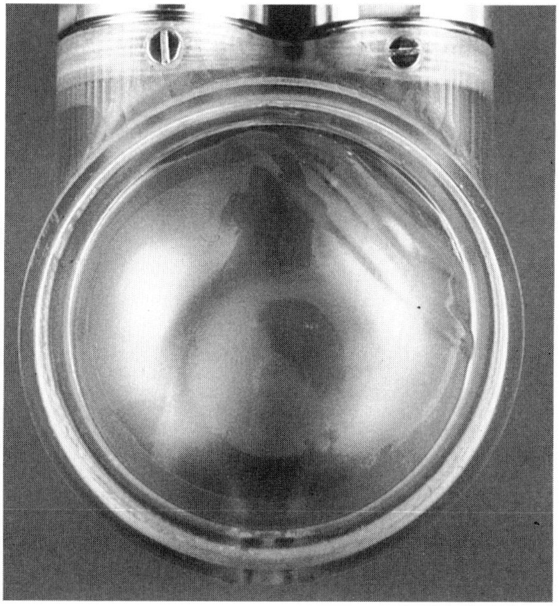

Fig. 42.2 Smooth surface polyurethane blood sac for the Thoratec device.

cated that antiplatelet therapy only is required for devices utilizing these linings. These linings may have the capacity to impart the properties of a biological lining to the surface of a man-made device.

Evaluation of the developing biological lining on textured surfaces within the TCI device

Linings that are still satisfactory have been observed following explantation of TCI devices at up to 223 days post-implantation (Fig. 42.4). There has been no evidence of thrombosis. The linings are thin and closely adherent. There are areas of apparent collagenous ingrowth on both the pusher plate and titanium surfaces. Histological examination has revealed on the ITP side a relatively thin lining with cellular components present upon the surface (Fig. 42.5). These cells appear to be multinucleated and contain inclusion bodies. Histological evaluation of the sintered titanium side reveals a thin compact fibrin lining without the same cellular surface appearances.[7] On scanning electron microscopy (Fig. 42.6), a compact fibrin lining can be seen developing upon the sintered titanium. On the polyurethane fibrils, closely adherent cellular elements are seen developing (Fig. 42.7).[7] On transmission electron microscopy, large multinucleated cells with many inclusion bodies are observed populating the surface of the lining on the polyurethane fibrils (Fig. 42.8). Deeper within the lining, similar cellular elements appear closely adherent to the underlying polyurethane fibrils (Fig. 42.9).[7] These cells contain large amounts of rough endoplemic reticulum and appear metabolically active.

Immunocytochemical techniques have identified several different cell types—activated macrophages, fibroblasts and smooth muscle cells (as encountered in areas of healing and in areas of granulation).[8] Endothelial cells have been grown out of this tissue in cell culture. It has also been possible to identify several different collagen types.

There are potentially four options for the possible origin of these developing cellular elements. These are: locomotion along the surface of the conduits and the device surface, transmural migration through the biomaterial, cellular seeding before implantation, or circulating native cells which have settled upon these biomaterial surfaces.

These cellular elements have not been observed on examination of the Dacron conduit; the device is impermeable and the devices have not been pre-seeded. Therefore the only option is that these cellular elements are circulating cells which are within the blood and have settled upon these developing biological surfaces, transforming into the various observed cellular elements.[8]

This has obvious potential implications for the ability of the body to 'self-seed' implanted cardiovascular prostheses.

Summary

Obtaining a successful interface between blood and biomaterials within these devices remains a complex issue. Controlled deformation of the biomaterials is important to prevent areas of stasis and thus the design of devices and the choice of biomaterial remains interrelated. Surface modifications are possible and are being investigated currently (Table 42.6). Flow conditions within the devices remain as vital as the component interfaces and the inherent thrombogenicity of the blood.

Unfortunately thromboembolism does still occur following implantation of mechanical circu-

Table 42.6 Ways to modify biomaterial surfaces.

Immobilize biomolecules
Alter electrical charge
Self-assembly of ordered synthetic structures
Cellular adhesion/seeding

Table 42.7 Device linings.

Current alternatives
* Acrylic plastics
* Smooth polyurethanes (copolymers)
* Textured surface (polyurethane, powdered metals)

Future alternatives
* Biolized polyurethanes
* Heparin bonding
* Protein-specific absorbing surface

latory support devices, and it is in part related to lining/blood interactions. The biomaterials currently available remain limited (Table 42.7). This area warrants further research and development as devices are being used in increasing numbers for 'short-term' support, prolonged bridging to transplantation and eventually for permanent implantation.

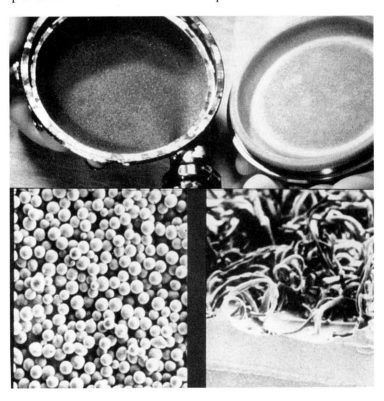

Fig. 42.3 A TCI device opened to reveal the sintered titanium surface on the static housing (left) and a textured polyurethane 'Biomer' on the diaphragm surface. Below are respective scanning electron microscopy appearances (approximately ×50 and ×100).

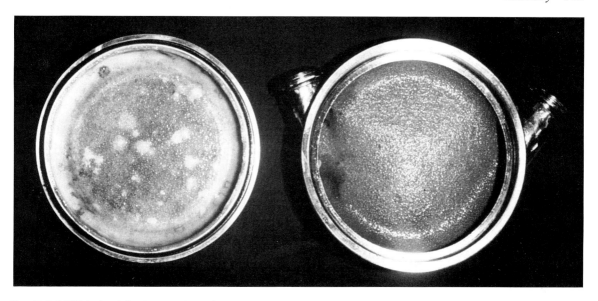

Fig. 42.4 A TCI device following 223 days of implantation (textured polyurethane on left, sintered titanium on right).

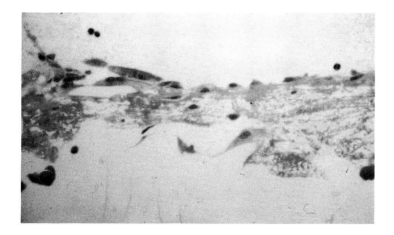

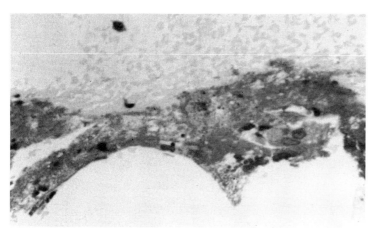

Fig. 42.5 Light microscopy appearances of linings in TCI device following 13 days' implantation (×90): textured polyurethane surface (top) and sintered titanium surface (bottom).

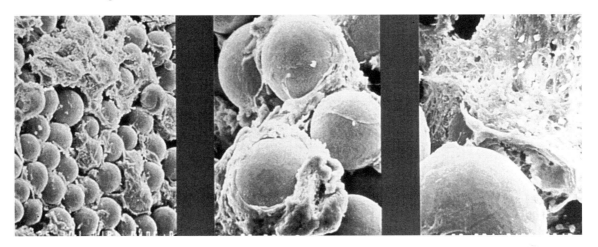

Fig. 42.6 Scanning electron microscopy appearances of a sintered titanium surface at 37 days. Left to right: (×100, ×300, ×500).

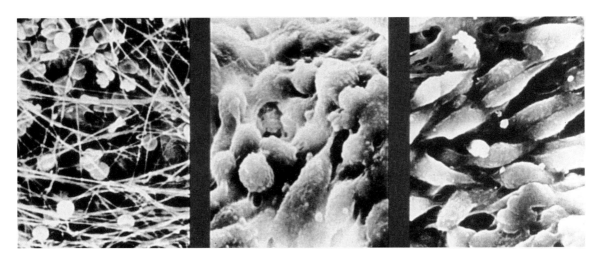

Fig. 42.7 Scanning electron microscopy appearances of a textured polyurethane surface (×1000). Left to right: (5 days, 19 days, 41 days).

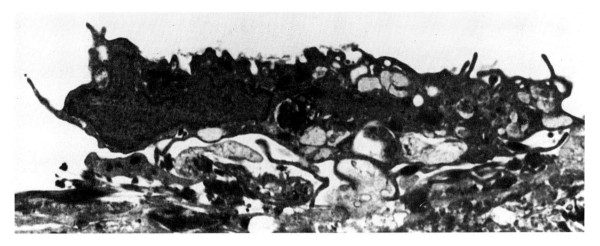

Fig. 42.8 Transmission electron microscopy of cellular elements on a textured polyurethane lining surface at day 13 (×10 000).

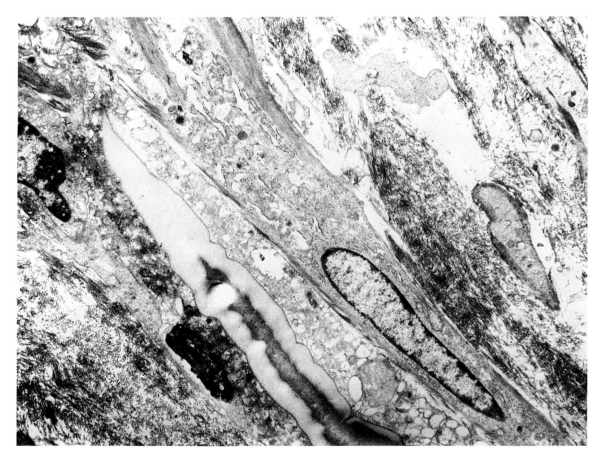

Fig. 42.9 Transmission electron microscopy of cellular elements within a textured polyurethane lining adjacent to Biomer fibril (×10 000).

References

1. Graham TR, Lewis CT. Lining artificial ventricles—status 1990. In: Salmons S, Jarvis JC (eds), *Heart Harnessing Skeletal Muscle Power for Cardiac Assistance.* Commission of the European Communities, secretariat: CCBMT, University of Twente, Box 217, 7500 AE Enschede, Netherlands.
2. Hill JD. Polymer surfaces for prosthetic ventricles. In: Chiu RC-J, Bourgeois I (eds), *Transformed Muscle for Cardiac Assist and Repair.* Mount Kisco, NY, Futura Publishing 1990.
3. Gibbons DF. Cardiac assist devices. In: Hastings G (ed), *Cardiovascular Biomaterials.* New York: Springer Verlag, 184–194.
4. Olsen DB, Unger F, Oster H, Lawson J, Kessler T, Kolff J, Kolff WJ. Thrombus generation within the artificial heart. *J Thorac Cardiovasc Surg* 1975; **70**, 248–255.
5. Portner PM, Green GF, Ramasamy N. The blood interface at artificial surfaces within a left ventricular assist system. *Ann NY Acad Sci* 1983: 471–503.
6. Dasse KA, Chipman SD, Sherman CN, Levine, Frazier OH. Clinical experience with textured blood contacting surfaces in ventricular assist devices. *ASAIO Trans* 1987; **33**, 418–425.
7. Graham TR, Dasse K, Coumbe A, Salih V, Marrinan MT, Frazier OH, Lewis CT. Neo-intimal development on textured biomaterial surfaces during clinical use of an implantable left ventricular assist device. *Eur J Cardiothorac Surg* 1990; **4**, 182–190.
8. Salih V, Graham TR, Berry CL, Coumbe A, Smith SC, Dasse K, Frazier OH. The lining of textured surfaces in implantable left ventricular assist devices. *Am J Cardiovasc Pathol* 1992; **4**, 317–325.

Section VIII _____

General Issues

43

Regulatory and informed consent issues in circulatory support

J Donald Hill and S Jill Ley

Editors' note

The following extremely important chapter has been contributed by Donald Hill and Jill Ley of the California Pacific Medical Centre, San Francisco, and as such is principally a discussion of the situation as it occurs in North America. This is not inappropriate, as a large share of the research and clinical work on most of the devices discussed in this book have been undertaken in the USA.

In addition, the USA has a society where a written constitution defines very clearly the responsibilities of the individual and the state. Historically the situation has been very different elsewhere. Certainly in the past, medical practitioners in many countries in Europe have been answerable principally to God and only secondarily to the state. This situation is rapidly changing as European Community Directives control increasingly all forms of professional behaviour. It is likely that questions of informed consent and regulatory mechanisms controlling the use of experimental devices will become more like the system seen in the USA, inheriting both its manifest advantages and its disadvantages.

The responsibilities of, and relationships between, manufacturers, clinicians and patients pertaining in any one country must be fully appreciated as the world, particularly the medical world, gets smaller.

*As an **appendix** to this chapter we show a consent form used at the Pacific Presbyterian Hospital, San Francisco, entitled 'Ventricular assist device for bridge to cardiac transplantation' and a further similar form from St Luke's Episcopal Hospital, Texas, entitled*

'Informed consent for use of an intermediate-term ventricular assist device for non-reversible ventricular dysfunction'. These two examples may be of considerable help to workers and institutions new to this field contemplating the clinical use of such devices.

Introduction

Guidelines for the protection of patient rights have been established by both United States case law and biomedical ethics. Federal regulations specific to the protection of human research subjects were first issued in 1974 by the US Department of Health, Education and Welfare. One of the fundamental principles of this and future documents is a respect for persons as autonomous individuals who must be given an opportunity to 'choose what shall or shall not happen to them'.[1] This principle is applied to human research subjects via the process of informed consent.

Issues of informed consent fall within the purview of three distinct but interrelated regulatory bodies in the USA. Federal regulations are delineated by the Department of Health and Human Services (DHHS), with implementation and supervision provided by hospital-based institutional review boards (IRBs) and the Joint Council for Accreditation of Hospital Organizations (ICAHO). This chapter will review the complementary roles of these groups in ensuring protection of human research subjects, and will discuss issues of informed consent for patients requiring mechanical circulatory support.

The role of the federal government

The *Code of Federal Regulations Regarding Protection of Human Subjects, Title 45 CFR Part 46*, delineates DHHS regulations on this subject, which are administered by the Food and Drug Administration (FDA). This policy defines its scope as applicable to all research involving human subjects with a few specific exceptions (i.e. educational testing, study of public records, food quality evaluations, etc.).

In defining federal rules regarding informed consent, it states that a person may not be involved as a research subject unless the investigator first obtains 'the legally effective informed consent of the subject or the subject's legally authorized representative'.[2] Furthermore, 'coercion or undue influence' are forbidden, information must be provided in a 'language understandable to the subject', and the subject's legal rights cannot be waived in any manner.[2] A provision for protection of children, defined as persons who have not attained the legal age for consent in the jurisdiction where the research will be conducted, is also included. Criteria for obtaining permission from parents or legal guardians are defined, with reference to state or local law in identifying these individuals.

Also included are critical elements of the consent process and documentation guidelines, as defined by the DHHS, for all research studies conducted in the USA. In addition, regulations pertaining to the functions and operations of an IRB in implementing these policies are provided. *Under the current system, the federal government defines policy and regulations regarding issues of informed consent, with implementation and enforcement carried out at a local level by the IRB.* This board is accountable to federal regulations and is subject to periodic FDA reviews to ensure compliance with federal standards.

Role of the Institutional Review Board

The mandate of a local IRB, which is a committee of the medical staff in a hospital with research

funded by the National Institutes of Health, is to ensure that all research conducted under its jurisdiction is of scientific merit and complies with federal regulations regarding protection of human subjects. A signed agreement for 'Assurance of Compliance' is maintained between all IRBs and the DHHS. The IRB's responsibility lies in 'protection of subjects from undue risk and from deprivation of personal rights and dignity'.[3] This mandate is carried out by ensuring that subjects participate on a voluntary basis and indicate their informed consent, and that an appropriate balance between risks and benefits to the subject exists.

All research proposals must be submitted to an IRB for evaluation of these elements *prior* to study implementation. Once a study is approved the IRB requires annual status reports by the investigator, as well as reporting of adverse events (either serious clinical events or problems with patient recruitment or participation). Adverse events may warrant a modification in consent procedures, study procedures, or halting of the study altogether.

Investigational devices

In the case of research involving investigational devices, protection of human subjects is a shared responsibility of the IRB, FDA and device manufacturer. Following submission of a device protocol by a site investigator, the IRB classifies the relative risk the device poses to subjects as either significant (SR) or non-significant (NSR). Device studies are considered SR if they involve the diagnosis, cure or treatment of a disease while posing a potential for serious risk to the health, safety or welfare of the subject.[4] If the IRB deems the study to be NSR and approves the research protocol, investigation may begin immediately without requiring FDA notification or approval.

All device studies classified as SR must be submitted to the FDA for approval under an investigational device exemption (IDE) protocol. The FDA evaluates data from European or worldwide centres. The FDA will accept these data provided by the device manufacturer regarding bench and animal testing, as well as produce biomaterials, for safety and durability. If preclinical results are favourable, clinicians are granted an IDE to begin human trials. Once granted, investigators report clinical data to the manufacturer for compilation of multi-site findings, which are then reported to the FDA. In granting an IDE the FDA establishes limits on the number of sites and participants. Ongoing monitoring of IDE studies for safety and efficacy occur primarily via the FDA, with annual updates provided by the investigator to the IRB as well. In large double-blind clinical studies, government agency oversight committees follow the accruing patient data and can stop the study at any time when the data indicate the outcome even though the study is not concluded. When the FDA has sufficient evidence of product performance, pre-market approval (PMA) is granted allowing for wide distribution but with ongoing follow-up. The transition of a cardiac device from an IDE to a PMA is a painstaking process that takes years to complete. To support US experience with a device, manufacturers may submit data provided there is documentation that the centres outside the US followed the protocol and informed consent was obtained from every patient.

The FDA recognizes a one-time emergency exception to IDE approval in life-threatening situations, if no other acceptable alternatives to the investigational device exist. The investigating physician is expected to obtain an independent assessment of the emergency by an uninvolved physician, obtain informed consent from the patient or legal representative, and confer with the IRB chairperson prior to proceeding with use of the device. A written report of the circumstances must then be submitted to the FDA and IRB within five working days. Should an IDE application be denied by the FDA, the device cannot be used under any circumstances, including emergencies.

Excluding intra-aortic balloons, all mechanical circulatory support devices currently being used in the US are under an IDE with two exceptions. The Medtronic–Biomedicus centrifugal ventricular assist device (Eden Prarie, MN) was already in use for cardiopulmonary bypass prior to institution of the Rodgers Act of 1976 and IDE regulation, and was therefore exempt from its jurisdiction. Other centrifugal pump manufacturers have enjoyed this exception based on the Biomedicus precedent. The FDA is currently re-evaluating the status of centrifugal pumps and will almost certainly bring them under closer FDA scrutiny and control. The Abiomed BVS 5000 biventricular support system (Danvers, MA) recently completed the IDE process and received

pre-market approval in 1992.

There is another category the FDA has for a device in addition to an IDE and PMA. A device that is presented by a manufacturer to be *substantially equivalent* to existing approved devices, upon review by the FDA, can be granted a 510K status. A 510K is equivalent to a PMA and once obtained the device can be distributed widely. No cardiac support devices have or are likely to ever qualify for a 510K category.

The Joint Commission for Accreditation of Hospital Organizations (JCAHO)

The JCAHO is the accreditation body for all hospitals. It sets guidelines for medical staff organization and committee structure (including the IRB), and enforces government regulations and professional standards for medicine. The overriding focus of the JCAHO is quality assessment and improvement. Through a review and audit process, the JCAHO evaluates each hospital's ability to carry out quality medical care in compliance with government (state and federal) regulations. Recommendations made by the JCAHO on hospital performance are binding to maintain accreditation.

Ethical issues in the IDE process for cardiac devices

Paramount in the FDA's decision to grant an IDE and later in reviewing the data to grant a PMA is the protocol. Two themes have evolved that are the subject of continued debate between the FDA, industry and investigators/physicians. They are the principal reasons for the long delay time in PMAs being granted to cardiac support devices in the USA. First is the FDA's insistence on strict adherence to every aspect of the approved protocol, and the detailed record-keeping by the clinical investigators and industry sponsor. This involves improved discipline on the part of the investigators and manufacturers. If the protocol is not followed precisely, data that could be used in assessing efficacy for the PMA from a study patient can be excluded from review by the FDA. If the protocol is followed but there is missing data, a patient may also be excluded from review. If deviations from the protocol occur often, the FDA can withdraw an IDE. Strict adherence to a protocol raises particular problems for physicians in emergency and life-threatening situations.

The second point of contention between the FDA, industry and investigators is the study design. The FDA has a responsibility to verify that a device is equal to or better than the standard of care. In their eyes, to demonstrate efficacy and safety adequately requires an uncompromised (randomized, blinded) control group. The FDA will accept historical controls but consider this a weak aspect to a protocol. The FDA does not dictate the choice of control group for a study but the merit of the protocol will be judged by the strength of its ability to statistically demonstrate efficacy and safety.

In choosing a control group there is a clash between the FDA and the physician. The physician is held to a standard to represent the patient's best opportunity to survive, and as Shakespeare's Hamlet declared: '...ay, there's the rub'. In a life-threatening situation a physician is loathe to randomize a patient to a control group whose end-point is death, when the condition in his or her judgement carries a 100% mortality on standard care over a short time span. The FDA's position is that the physician cannot be certain of the outcome of the control group and resist the idea of compromising the study by relaxing its definition of a control group. This states the issue in its simplest form. There are many current variations on this theme. Both groups are seeking a satisfactory compromise that will meet the biostatistical needs of the FDA and the conscience of the physician.

Consent requirements

The DHHS considers the following elements as general requirements for informed consent:[2]

1. A statement that the study involves research, an explanation of its purpose and the procedures required (identifying those that are experimental), and the duration of participation.
2. Foreseeable risks or discomforts to the subject.
3. Expected benefits to the subject or others.
4. Disclosure of appropriate alternative treatments.

5. A description of confidentiality offered to the subject.
6. If more than minimal risk is involved, an explanation of any compensation or treatment available in the event of injury.
7. An explanation of whom to contact for questions about the study, subjects' rights, or research-related injury.
8. A statement that participation is voluntary, a refusal to participate is without penalty, and the subject has the right to discontinue at any time.

Additional elements (i.e. costs to the subject, consequences of withdrawal, etc.) may also be required by the FDA or IRB, in certain circumstances. The IRB may approve a consent form that does not include all of these elements provided the subjects' rights and welfare are maintained. Generally, written consent forms documenting these elements are signed by the subject or representative, although the IRB can waive written consent in special circumstances. Once a consent form has been approved by the IRB, it cannot be altered in any way without resubmission for approval.

Informed consent with mechanical circulatory support devices

Mechanical circulatory support by its very nature is used for critically ill patients, with informed consent often provided by extremely anxious spouses or guardians. As stated by Schiedermayer and Shapiro: 'Given the inevitable vulnerability of the patient and the necessary enthusiasm of the clinician, the process of obtaining informed consent for bridge implantation must be safeguarded'.[5] When support devices are used as a bridge-to-transplant, federal regulations require that risks and benefits of both the specific device as well as cardiac transplantation be discussed. If patient risk increases with the duration of circulatory support, this should also be presented to the patient prior to implant.

The process of informed consent includes disclosure of 'the consequences of a subject's decision to withdraw from the research and procedures for orderly termination of participation by the subject', when deemed appropriate.[2] A legal precedent is clearly established regarding a patient's right to terminate even life-sustaining treatment.[6] Barney Clark, the first recipient of the total artificial heart, reportedly was given a key to turn off the device at any time he wished to withdraw from treatment.[7] Both case law and biomedical ethics would dictate that respect for patient autonomy be paramount to the clinician, and the symbolic key 'must remain in the hands of the patient'.[5]

For patients requiring mechanical circulatory support, the right to stop treatment must be discussed in the consent document and remain as an option for the patient and family, despite the inevitable fate that will befall a patient wishing to withdraw from such treatment. The National Heart, Lung and Blood Institute Working Group states that these situations 'call for careful and searching discussions involving the patient, health professionals and, as appropriate, members of the patient's family'.[8]

It is clear that informed consent is an ongoing process that cannot be satisfied by merely signing a written document. The critical nature of the patient requiring circulatory support coupled with the experimental nature of our current technology creates a unique challenge to the physician in ensuring that patient rights and dignity are maintained. Clinicians should ask: 'How can a fuller, shared understanding by patient and professional of their common enterprise by promoted, so that patients can participate, on an informed basis and to the extent they care to do so, in making decisions about their health care?'[9] The dialogue that ensues from answering this question will do much to promote both human rights and our knowledge of circulatory support technology.

References

1. US Department of Health, Education and Welfare. *Belmont Report: Ethical Principles and Guidelines for the Protection of Human Subjects of Research.* Report of the National Commission for the Protection of Human Subjects of Biomedical and Behavioral Research, 1979.
2. Department of Health and Human Services, National Institutes of Health. *Code of Federal Regulations: Title 45, Part 46, 18 June 1991*: 1–17.
3. Institutional Review Board at California Pacific Medical Center. *Guidelines for Research Involving Human Subjects*, 1992, section 1.
4. Department of Health and Human Services. *FDA IRB Information Sheets*, 15 February 1989: 1–94.
5. Schiedermayer DL, Shapiro RS. The artificial heart as a bridge to transplant: ethical and legal issues at the bedside. *J Heart Transplant* 1989; **8**, 471–473.
6. Schloendorff *v* Society of New York Hospital, 211 NY 125, 105 NE 92, 95 (1914).
7. Rachels J. *Hastings Center Report* 1983; **13**, 17–19.
8. Levine RJ. Mechanical circulatory support systems: ethical considerations. *Transplant Proc* 1990; **22**, 969–970.
9. President's Commission for the Study of Ethical Problems in Medicine and Biomedical and Behavioral Research. *Making Health Care Decisions: Vol 1—A Report on the Ethical and Legal Implications of Informed Consent in the Patient–Practitioner Relationship.* US Government Printing Office, 1983: 31.

Editors' appendix: Research consent forms

I—The essential text of a form used at Pacific Presbyterian Hospital, San Francisco

'Ventricular assist device for bridge to cardiac transplantation'

Patient _____ Hospital # _____

1. I understand that I have a heart condition from which I cannot recover using conventional medical and surgical therapy. I further understand that I am in imminent danger of dying within the next few hours or several days. I further understand that should a human donor heart become available, cardiac transplantation would increase my opportunity for survival to approximately 50% at 5 years.

2. I understand that during this waiting period for a donor heart, the pumping function of my heart can be supported by a **Thoratec Ventricular Assist Device** (VAD) on the left side alone or in association with one on the right side as well. I understand that the VAD will be connected to my heart during an open chest surgical procedure and it will assist and bypass the heart for a number of days while waiting for a donor heart (this is known as a bridge to transplantation). The VAD will be placed outside the chest and it will be connected to the heart with two tubes

(cannulae) going through the chest wall. The VAD is controlled and powered by an external drive console to which the VAD must be connected at all times.

3. I understand that there is no guarantee that a donor heart will be found. I am aware that I am categorized as a 'most urgent need' patient for donor heart procurement. Donor hearts for 'most urgent need' patients can often be located within 5 days, and usually within 10 days. Situations that could lengthen the procurement time include body size and difficulty in tissue matching.

4. I further understand that at this moment the medical and surgical opinion is that 'bridge to transplantation' is my only opportunity to substantially extend my life by years.

5. I understand that the temporary ventricular assist device is an investigational device under regulation by the US Food and Drug Administration, and that it has been developed under sponsorship of the National Heart, Lung and Blood Institute. I further understand that it has been extensively tested in the laboratory and has provided effective circulatory support in animals for an average duration of 84 days and a maximum duration of 141 days. To date it has been used in over 100 humans as part of a study that will involve over 200 patients. During the last 12 months, half of the transplanted VAD patients have received donor hearts within 21 days, and half between 21 and 91 days. The average length of VAD support has been between 21 and 91 days. The average length of VAD support has been 27 days, and the longest duration, 91 days.* I understand the temporary nature of the device (expected duration of the pumping, 1–10 days) and agree to the second surgical procedure under general anesthesia necessary to remove it and implant a human donor heart.

6. I understand that potential alternative procedures or courses of treatment such as intra-aortic balloon pump counter-pulsation and drug therapy will be considered. The experimental temporary ventricular assist device will be utilized only after all other treatment alternatives have been exhausted, at which point it will be the only other alter-

* The data refers to June 1991.

native which affords any possibility of preserving my life.

7. The potential complications associated with use of the device have been explained to me, and I understand that beyond the risks normally associated with any cardiovascular surgical procedure under general anesthesia, the most significant risks associated with use of the device are:

• Thromboembolism—The production of small clots which become lodged in blood vessels and impair blood circulation to vital organs.
• Mechanical failure—the pump or one of its components might break down and fail to operate. Although mechanical failure is a life-threatening risk associated with use of this device, backup systems are on hand to decrease the event of such an emergency.
• Bleeding—There may be unusual and excessive bleeding from both surgical cases (cut vessels) and coagulation disorders (the blood does not clot normally).
• Infection—The pump with its attached tubing could present an opportunity for infection that would not normally exist.

8. I understand that if the device is used, I can anticipate essentially the same postoperative discomfort experienced by any patient following cardiovascular surgery. I do understand, however, that use of the device would necessitate additional instrumentation and studies in order that adequate information can be obtained about the mechanical function of the device. Such instrumentation and studies would consist of, or be similar to, those experienced in cardiac catheterization and the attendant discomfort would be essentially the same.

9. I understand that at the time of implantation and afterward an evaluation of how well my heart is functioning is important in order to properly manage my care. To add considerably to this information an esophageal (food tube to my stomach) ECHO probe may be inserted into my esophagus which will be able to accurately assess the function of my heart. The main potential risk of this could be perforation (tear) of the esophagus; however there has never been a perforation recorded in association with the use of the ECHO probe in evaluation of the heart. The tube is not painful but can cause discomfort if I am

awake. I understand I will either be asleep (during surgery) or sedated (postoperatively) if this procedure is performed. A second potential risk is a burn on the esophagus from the ECHO sound transmission. There has never been any patient who complained of this and current power levels used are so low it is very unlikely.

10. I acknowledge that no guarantees have been made to me concerning the results of my surgery or the performance of the temporary ventricular assist device.

11. I hereby give my permission for California Pacific Medical Center and the physician providing my care, to release any or all of the information contained in my medical records as in the judgment of Dr _____ may be necessary for the proper scientific evaluation of the temporary ventricular assist pump. This includes any review necessary for the Food and Drug Administration to conduct an evaluation of the device.

12. I understand that Dr _____ (telephone _____) is available and willing to answer any questions concerning my rights as a research subject. I understand that I may contact Dr _____ in the event of a research-related injury.

13. I understand that I (and/or my insurance carrier) am responsible for the cost of the VAD and for the costs of surgery and my hospitalization during the use of the VAD that are in addition to the costs for cardiac transplantation.

14. I understand that at this moment I am a suitable candidate for heart transplantation, but the development of a contraindication during the period of VAD support could make me no longer a candidate for transplantation. Such complications include infection and thromboembolism, as discussed above.

15. I understand that it is possible that I could become a permanent VAD recipient. In this case I understand that the hospital will provide continuous care, as it would for any patient. I understand that I am responsible for the cost of this care.

16. I understand that participation is voluntary and I am free at any time to withdraw my consent for use of the assist device, without penalty or loss of benefits to which I am otherwise entitled. I recognize that the exercise of such an option after the pump is in use would likely result in my death.

17. I understand that California Pacific Medical Center and the Medical Research Institute have no special program by which they can provide compensation or medical treatment if physical injury occurs during the biomedical or behavioral research.

18. Should I have any questions about my rights as a subject, I may call the Joint Council on Human Research (telephone _____).

19. I have been given a copy of the experimental subject's 'Bill of Rights'.

20. I have read the above and, by signing below, agree to be a subject in this investigation.

Patient's signature and date
(or legal representative)† _____

Witness' signature and date _____

II—The essential text of a form used at St Luke's Episcopal Hospital, Texas*

'Intermediate-term ventricular assist device for non-reversible ventricular dysfunction'

PURPOSE:

We would like to enroll you as a participant in a research study. The purpose of the study is to use a mechanical heart assist device to assist your heart which is failing. The device is designed to keep you alive until a heart transplant is available. The device is investigational and we are studying its safety and ability to pump blood to provide your body with flow which is necessary to live. Although this device may improve your chances for survival, the nature and the severity of your heart disease may override any benefits from the device and death is still a possible outcome.

* This form has been used in addition to a regular treatment consent form at St Luke's Hospital.

PROCEDURE:

- The surgical approach in your body will be done using standard surgical procedures and care. The placement of the device in the abdomen and the connection of the device to the heart and aorta are investigational.
- The device may be implanted in your abdomen until a heart transplant is available, and you are in good enough condition to receive such a transplant. Generally, this will be for 2 to 4 weeks to allow your organs to recover before a transplant is done. It may be longer if you are too sick or if a donor heart is not available.
- The actual procedure entails opening the chest and abdominal cavities in surgery and connecting the devices described below. There will be a tube passing through the skin of the abdomen to the power console which drives the device. This in turn is plugged into an electrical outlet. There is a battery that allows the patient to be unplugged for about 30 minutes at a time.

RISKS AND DISCOMFORTS:

Potential complications
The potential complications associated with the use of the TCI HeartMate LVAD have been explained to me, and I understand that beyond the risks normally associated with any cardiovascular surgical procedure under general anesthesia, the most significant risks associated with its use are believed to be:

- excessive bleeding
- thromboembolism (blood clots that form and can travel to other parts of the body—this could result in a stroke or loss of a limb or other organs and could require surgery)
- infection (due to the pneumatic drive tube penetrating the skin)
- hemolysis (the destruction of red blood cells), and
- mechanical failure (the assist device or one of its components might break down and fail to operate).

Any of these complications may cause loss of limb, stroke, or death. I understand that I can anticipate postoperative discomfort similar to that experienced by a patient following cardiovascular surgery and specifically related commonly to the device. I will hear and feel the pump working in my body and I will experience some pain in the skin area around the drive line.

Pump dependence
I understand that if after 40 days I am still being supported by the TCI HeartMate LVAD and I am not a transplant candidate, Dr _ _____ or whomever he may designate from the hospital will consult with me, if possible, or with my family or legal representative if I am unconscious or incapacitated, and reach a decision whether to remove the TCI HeartMate LVAD and support my heart with conventional measures, such as the intra-aortic balloon and pharmacologic therapy, or to continue supporting my heart with the TCI HeartMate LVAD. Also, the facilities, emergency treatment and professional services of the hospital will be available as long as necessary (at cost to me) if I become permanently dependent upon the device.

I understand that while the device is in place I must remain hospitalized. I also realize that I will possibly feel very well on the device but still have end-stage heart disease which can only be treated by a transplant. This device cannot be permanent; it could fail suddenly and therefore must be removed as soon as possible when a donor heart becomes available.

Quality of life
Physical limitations can range from totally bedridden and ventilator dependent to fully ambulatory. If full ambulation is possible, it will be encouraged. All normal physical activities within the hospital confines may then be feasible. The degree to which this can result is unpredictable.

BENEFITS:

Expected benefit to patient
I, _____, understand that due to the nature of my end-stage heart disease, I am an accepted candidate for cardiac transplantation. I also understand that a donor organ for transplantation is not available at this time, but that my natural heart is unable to maintain adequate blood flow to sustain my life.

I also understand that implantations of a temporary ventricular assist device in such cases may provide sufficient circulatory support until such time as an appropriate donor heart is available for transplantation. The average waiting time for a heart varies with size, blood type and quality of heart that is acceptable as well as a good crossmatch.

Potential benefit to others
I understand that my participation in this research study may benefit future patients with ventricular dysfunction for whom mechanical support with a temporary ventricular assist device could be an accepted therapy.

NATURE AND USE OF DEVICE:

I understand that the TCI HeartMate LVAD is intended for temporary support of the failing heart for a period of up to 40 days.

I understand that the device will be implanted in the abdomen and connected between the heart and the aorta. The assist device will be powered by compressed air from a portable, external drive console via a tube passing through the skin.

Research program on this experimental device
I understand that the TCI HeartMate LVAD has been developed over the last 10 years, has been extensively tested in the laboratory and in animals, and has been used in humans in several clinical investigations. In animal tests, the device was evaluated for as long as 393 days, with the average duration of all implants being 92 days. In human studies as of October 1990, the device was evaluated for as long as 233 days, with the average duration of implants being 59 days. I understand that the results of prior research with this device will be explained to me, if I so desire and request an explanation. I understand that the TCI HeartMate LVAD is an investigational device that will be evaluated in additional patients over the next year at this hospital. During the research program, clinical data will be collected and analyzed objectively to determine the safety and efficacy of the TCI HeartMate LVAD.

Decision to use device
I request and authorize Dr _____ and whomever he/she may designate from the hospital to proceed with the implantation of a TCI HeartMate LVAD because my natural heart is unable to sufficiently support my circulation, and Dr _____ of the hospital has determined in his/her judgment that the TCI HeartMate LVAD may help to augment and support my failing heart and circulation.

I understand that the device will be utilized only after other conventional treatment alternatives (e.g. medication and/or the intra-aortic balloon pump) have been utilized or clinically excluded.

Patient participation
I understand that implantation of the TCI HeartMate LVAD requires surgery to my chest and abdomen, and because it is temporary, a second operation under appropriate anesthesia will be necessary for removal of the device. I hereby consent to this second operation for such removal.

MEDICAL RECORDS/CONFIDENTIALITY:

I hereby give permission to the hospital and the physicians providing my care to release any or all of the information contained in my medical records that, in the judgment of Dr _ _____ or whomever he/she may designate from the hospital may be necessary for the proper scientific evaluation of the TCI HeartMate LVAD. I understand that my identity will remain confidential. I also understand that the Food and Drug Administration may inspect records of this research project at any time.

COST TO PATIENT:

I understand that I will be responsible for the costs associated with implantation of the TCI HeartMate LVAD and that these costs will be similar to those of open-heart surgical procedures. I understand that I will not be responsible for the cost of the TCI HeartMate LVAD and drive console. In the event that I become permanently dependent upon the TCI HeartMate LVAD, I understand that I will be responsible for the costs associated with pump dependence.

I understand that in the event of injury resulting from the research procedures described to me, financial compensation will not be available from the hospital, TCI, or Dr _ _____ nor will any of them be able to offer to absorb the costs of medical treatment. However, necessary facilities, emergency treatment, and professional services will be available to me just as they are to the community generally. In this event, I understand that I can contact Dr _____ to discuss my rights and options.

RESULTS AND LIABILITY:

I acknowledge that no guarantees have been made to me concerning the results of my surgery or the performance of the TCI Heart-Mate LVAD and that the possibility exists that complications arising from its use, such as:

• severe infection
• kidney dysfunction
• liver dysfunction
• stroke

may preclude cardiac transplantation. I also understand that any of these complications or others that have been explained to me may cause the waiting period for a donor heart to be extended. I understand that, under situations where a patient is being supported by a circulatory support system, the longest wait and the average wait for a donor heart at this institution has been _____ and _____ respectively.

It is understood that nothing in this informed consent shall act to waive any of my legal rights or to release the hospital, TCI, or Dr _____ or any of their agents from liability for negligence.

QUESTIONS ABOUT PARTICIPATION:

I understand that a copy of this form will be given to me as a subject in this study if I agree to participate, and that a Patient Care Representative is available to talk with me about my participation in or concerns regarding the study, if I so desire.

I understand that participation is voluntary and that I am free to refuse to participate, to withdraw consent, or to discontinue participation in the study at any time without penalty or prejudice to my care.

I understand that any significant new findings that may affect my willingness to participate will be provided to me as they become available. I also understand that, if during my treatment, it is found that the TCI HeartMate LVAD is ineffective or harmful, Dr _____ or whomever he/she may designate from the hospital may elect to cease treatment with the TCI HeartMate LVAD and remove it at his/her discretion.

I understand that Dr _____ and the hospital are available at (telephone _____) and are willing to answer any questions I or my family or authorized representative may have during the study. I also understand that I may contact the secretary of the hospital's Investigational Review Board if I require any additional information about my rights as a research subject.

PHYSICIAN'S STATEMENT:

I have fully explained the procedures, identifying those which are investigational, and have explained their purpose. I have asked whether or not any questions have arisen regarding the procedures and have answered these questions to the best of my ability.

Signature and date _____

PATIENT'S ACKNOWLEDGEMENT:

I have been fully informed as to the procedures to be followed including those which are investigational, and have been given a description of the attendant discomforts, risks and benefits to be expected and the appropriate alternative procedures. In signing this consent form, I agree to this method of treatment and I understand that I am free to withdraw my consent and have this study discontinued at any time. I understand also that if I have any questions at any time, they will be answered.

Patient's signature and date
(or legal representative)† _____

Witness' signature and date _____

† If the patient, due to his/her grave medical condition, is unable to give full consent, it is to the best knowledge of the patient's representative (next-of-kin, guardian, legal representative, physician) that the patient has not expressed the desire to refuse extraordinary means to prolong his/her life.

44

Economic evaluation of therapies for end-stage heart failure

Martin Buxton

Introduction

Any realistic consideration of the service relevance of a new health care technology, however technically exciting it may be, must recognize the situation in which all health care systems find themselves: health care resources are scarce relative to what is already technically possible. It is not just a problem in the relatively impoverished UK. Even in the USA, which spends the largest proportion of the highest gross domestic product on health expenditure of all OECD countries, there is a recognition that not all that is technically feasible is economically or socially desirable. There must be choices and this necessarily involves rationing of one sort or anther.[1] If rationing decisions are not to be merely arbitrary, good information is needed to permit a comparison of the net health benefits of an intervention with its net costs. In that way, resources can be directed towards interventions that achieve most with the available scarce resources. Costs are important because they provide the linkage to benefits that will have to be foregone elsewhere in the health care system if resources are used in a particular way. The emerging technologies for end-stage heart failure are no exception: they need to be subjected to rigorous evaluation, not simply out of scientific curiosity, but as part of an evaluative ethic.[2]

Evaluation of heart transplantation: a model for the future

It is notable that heart transplantation has been more thoroughly, comprehensively and internationally subjected to economic evaluation at a reasonable early stage in its development than perhaps any other health care technology. Major prospective studies were undertaken contemporaneously in the USA[3] and the UK[4] and subsequently in the Netherlands.[5] Each was a publicly funded prospective study commissioned by national health-care funding and regulatory authorities. All three major studies looked at survival and quality of life of patients, and costs of the programmes. Each emphasized the good, and improving, post-transplant survival, the remarkable improvements in quality of life to near normal levels and the high costs, of which a major element was the on-going costs of immunosuppression. Each suggested (implicitly or explicitly) that heart transplantation, in those centres and at that time, generated additional life years of sufficient quality at a reasonable cost relative to other accepted procedures within the particular health-care systems.

The greatest weakness in all three studies was the absence of a formal control group to provide firm evidence of survival, quality of life and costs for equivalent patients in the absence of transplantation. Both the British and Dutch studies used survival experience on the waiting list to statistically estimate survival without transplantation.[5,6]

Each appeared to contribute to decisions about the transition from an experimental to a routinely funded service; about the appropriate scale of provision and the necessary funding to support it; and the rate of diffusion of the technology to additional centres. It is, of course, debatable how much difference the evaluations made to national policies, given that we do not know what would have been policy in the absence of evaluation. It is certainly the case that in the UK, the Department of Health's funding policy appeared to follow rather than precede local decisions,[7] although the evaluation provided a firm evidential basis to lend support to a policy that heart transplantation should be accepted for specific earmarked funding in designated centres. In the USA, the Medicare decision to cover heart transplantation was consistent with the findings of Evans[8] and was similarly selective, not in terms of named centres but in approving Medicare reimbursement only in centres that performed a minimum of 24 heart transplants over two years with a minimum 65% 2-year survival rate. The Dutch study most directly affected future policy in a system that now requires formal technology assessment including economic evaluation of all such new medical technologies.[9] But perhaps Lord Balniel was right in 1969 in suggesting in a House of Lords debate that there was 'an inevitability about the development of heart transplant surgery'.[10]

Obviously estimates of cost-effectiveness are dependent on available data, and this is limited by the extent of extant experience. The original UK evaluation of the heart transplant programmes resisted attempting to integrate cost and effectiveness data because of the sensitivity of the result to assumptions about long-term survival.[6] Subsequently, estimates were made in 1989 on the basis of updated cost information and rather longer survival experience. These are summarized in Table 44.1. These figures were intended to be conservative and reflected the then observed medium-term survival results of the programme (rather than an extrapolation of the most recent short-term survival). A mean survival with transplant of 5.9 years is estimated, which adjusted for imperfect quality of life and discounted at 5% would be in the order of 4.7 quality-adjusted life years (QALYs). Transplantation and all follow-up costs, including immunosuppression, for a mean survival of 5.9 years are estimated at a (dis-

Table 44.1 Estimates of cost per QALY for heart transplantation (1989).

	With transplant	Without transplant	Net gain
Life years	5.9	0.7	5.2
QALYs*	4.7	0.3	4.4
Costs (£000)*	36.9	7.6	29.3

*Discounted at 5% per annum.
Source: Author's own estimates based on reference 4 and unpublished Papworth data.

counted) cost of £36 000. By comparison, it is estimated that survival without transplant would have been 0.7 years (or 0.3 discounted QALYs) and this survival without transplantation would be associated with a cost of £7600. This gives a net cost per QALY gained from transplantation of £6700; or realistically, given the uncertainties, a figure somewhere within the range £6000–8000.

More important than the specifics of this calculation is the framework and the logic that this approach offers: it involves estimates of survival, quality of life and the full costs of the intervention, and of what would happen in the absence of intervention. The net gain in health outcomes needs to be related to the net increase in costs. Additionally, the logic of this analysis emphasizes that the lower limit to the cost per QALY is the on-going annual maintenance cost of post-transplant care, monitoring and immunosuppression. However long the post-transplant survival, however good the quality of life, and however low-cost the operative stay, the cost per QALY cannot fall below the floor set by these on-going costs per year of post-transplant life, and the same logic will apply to any future long-term therapy.

The total artificial heart

The long-term research programme in the USA to develop a satisfactory total artificial heart (TAH) has been the subject of much debate and dispute, and a number of studies have attempted to estimate the likely future cost-effectiveness of the technology once available. Many studies have been undertaken as part of an assessment of the potential value of continuing to invest public money in the research and development programme.

In a background paper for the Office of Technology Assessment of the US Congress in 1982, Lubeck and Bunker[11] made some initial estimates of the cost of treatment using an artificial heart. These estimates included the costs of the device and implantation, and the continuing costs of medical and technological care. The authors drew on the limited extant experience with left ventricular assist devices and with heart transplantation, as well as data on the more commonly used coronary artery bypass grafting and the artificial cardiac pacemaker. The study stressed that the opportunity cost of using resources in this way needed to be considered carefully, but emphasized that a prior consideration was whether, and how, the federal government could assure equitable access to such a high-cost technology.

In 1985, a report published by the US Department of Health and Human Services[12] suggested that the cost-effectiveness of a TAH, which it optimistically estimated as $28 000 per year of life gained, 'will likely fall within the broad range for currently accepted, expensive medical technologies'. It added:

> Furthermore, because the artificial heart does offer the promise of significantly improved survival and quality of life for some patients with end-stage cardiac disease, it will certainly be more efficient and a better use of resources than some "standard" treatments (p. 20).

In 1986, Lubeck[13] estimated the future size and costs of a programme of artificial heart transplantation and the likely resultant increase in life expectancy in the USA under a number of different assumptions. This study serves particularly to emphasize the potential magnitude of the programme costs. Assuming a 51% 5-year survival and an initial implantation cost of $100 000, Lubeck projected the total programme costs in the fifth year to $1.3 billion for a pool of 12 000 patients and $3.8 billion for 32 500 patients. The author concluded:

> ... it is imperative that such a potentially expensive innovation as the artificial heart be compared carefully with other social and medical programs designed to extend life and improve its quality (p. 380).

More recently, Garrison[14] presented, as part of a study by the Institute of Medicine of the artificial heart programme of the US National Heart, Lung and Blood Institute, a detailed analysis of the eventual cost-effectiveness of the use of the

TAH. Given the lack of clinical experience with the TAH, the study was intended:

> ... to explore some of the likely outcomes and trade-offs under alternative sets of plausible assumptions and scenarios that were developed through discussions with ... experts (p. 262).

The analysis used a 20-year Markov simulation model beginning in the year 2010—the earliest date at which, it was thought, a TAH might be in routine use. The model took a societal perspective of costs (as distinct from that of any particular individual or organization) and related these to estimates of life-years gained, adjusted for assumptions about their quality. The TAH was compared with both conventional medical therapy and heart transplantation. The results of the base case analysis are summarized in Tables 44.2 and 44.3. In this base case, conventional management is estimated as providing just 0.5 life years mean survival, transplantation (at that time) 11.3 life years, and the TAH 4.42 years. The analysis shows TAH as

Table 44.2 Predicted costs and outcomes for the total artificial heart.

Therapy	Cost* (US$ 000)	Life years	QALYs*
Total artificial heart	327.6	4.42	2.88
Heart transplantation	298.2	11.30	8.45
Conventional management	28.5	0.50	0.03

*Discounted at 3% per annum, 20-year time horizon.
Source: Reference 14, Table E6A.

Table 44.3 Incremental cost-effectiveness of the total artificial heart.

Comparison	Cost per life-year gained* (US$ 000)	Cost per QALY gained* (US$ 000)
Total artificial heart *versus* conventional management	76	105
Heart transplantation *versus* conventional management	25	32

*Discounted at 3% per annum, 20-year time horizon.
Source: Reference 14, Table E6B.

dominated by (that is, both more costly and less effective than) heart transplantation. When the survival figures are quality-adjusted and related to the expected costs, the cost per QALY gained by TAH is $105 000, compared with $32 000 for heart transplantation when each is compared with conventional management.

Clearly these figures are highly speculative, involving as they do numerous assumptions for which there is currently no firm evidential basis. Extensive sensitivity analysis is used to explore the implications of these assumptions, but this suggests that only on the most favourable combination of assumptions would the cost per QALY for TAH fall to $73 000. Garrison concluded that the cost per QALY for TAH would be 'considerably beyond the upper bound of what many would consider as generally acceptable for medical treatments and procedures.'

Cardiac assist devices

Garrison also noted that the cost per QALY of the ventricular assist device is likely to be somewhat more favourable than that for the TAH. In considering the future costs of cardiac assist devices (CADs) it is helpful to consider separately three major elements of cost: centre set-up costs, device and implantation costs, and patient maintenance costs.

The first of these, the costs necessary to enable a centre to undertake CAD implantation, are in a sense a fixed minimum overhead cost that is not directly variable with the centre's patient numbers. This element of cost can therefore be minimized by restricting the number of centres offering the technology. An additional argument for ensuring that a minimum number of large centres are involved is provided by the evidence, relating to the results from a variety of procedures including coronary artery bypass surgery, that suggests that centre and surgeon experience of a particular procedure, measured in terms of total or annual numbers of cases, are inversely related to negative patient outcomes.[15,16] Initially for CAD, even with a restricted number of centres this specific programme 'overhead' cost will be a relatively high proportion of the average cost per patient.

The device and implementation costs are the elements most likely to fall quickly in the early years of experience. For example, the length of

inpatient stay from transplant to discharge for cardiac transplantation fell at Harefield Hospital from 30.3 days in 1982 to 20.0 days in 1986, and at Papworth Hospital from 51.9 to 27.1 days.[17] Experience with pacemakers and implantable CADs similarly suggests that the initial device costs may well fall in real terms. But it is important not to forget that patents cover aspects of these devices and the firms involved will expect and aim to recoup their major financial R&D investment. To what extent they may try to increase market size by reducing costs considerably, depends much on the economics of the production of the devices and the manufacturers' expectations about their price-elasticity.

The maintenance costs (the on-going costs of supporting a patient on CAD therapy, including monitoring, treatment of problems, etc.) are likely ultimately, as with heart transplantation, to be the key factor. The Garrison estimate for TAHs was a monthly maintenance cost of $800 for a well-functioning device, but with considerable additional costs relating to the expected probabilities of various complications.[14] The comparable monthly 'maintenance' cost for a well-functioning transplant was $1500. The magnitude of these maintenance costs is likely to be crucial in the overall analysis, for it is these costs that are the limiting factor on cost per QALY.

Conventional therapy for end-stage heart failure

It is perhaps surprising that one of the weakest elements in these calculations of the additional benefits of transplantation or mechanical support devices is the poor information available on the costs and effectiveness of conventional (medical) therapy. An Institute of Medicine report[18] notes that there are important deficiencies in our knowledge of the epidemiology and natural history of end-stage heart failure, particularly as regards co-morbidities and the longitudinal tracking of clinical events and costs. The situation is no better in the UK.

Moreover, it is not clear to what extent existing medical therapies are used to their best. A study, using epidemiological and cost data from the Netherlands[19] but drawing on the clinical results of the CONSENSUS[20] and SOLVD trials,[21] suggests that:

... using ACE inhibitors as first-line therapeutic agents is highly cost-effective compared with standard therapy in the Netherlands in 1988, in which ACE inhibitors were prescribed only rarely and only for patients with very severe heart failure (p. 396).

In essence the authors argue that greater use of ACE inhibitors would offer overall cost savings, by reducing hospitalization whilst at the same time both improving quality of life and extending survival by slowing the rate of disease progression. Whilst their modelling involves a number of arguable assumptions, it lends strong weight to the view that current use of therapies may not be optimal.

Additionally it is possible that in the future new developments in medical therapy may provide more effective care for end-stage heart failure patients and offer an alternative to more dramatic surgical interventions. However, the recently announced withdrawal of flosequinan, an arteriolar and venous dilator for the treatment of heart failure,[22] and the early cessation of trials of epoprostenol sodium[23] as a treatment for congestive heart failure, suggest that major medical advances in the treatment of end-stage heart failure may be more elusive than was hoped.

Strategy for CADs in the UK

It is evident that implantable cardiac assist devices may potentially provide an important and cost-effective new therapy for end-stage heart failure, particularly as the shortage of donor organs becomes a more and more limiting factor on the use of heart transplantation.

Given the potential importance of CADs but the very great clinical uncertainties, the known high costs and, not least, the political visibility of the procedure, it would be inappropriate for any of these devices to be used as a last-ditch effort to save the life of a single patient. They must not be allowed to slip into routine patient care as a dramatic step of the sort that Cochrane[24] characterized with the following quote from TS Eliot:

Not for the good that it will do
But that nothing may be left undone
On the margin of the impossible.

Such one-off uses will merely maximize the costs of use, whilst minimizing the useful experience and evaluative data gained from that cost. Rather,

each and every use of a CAD in the UK should be part of a nationally planned research programme that is undertaken at a minimum number of centres and is competitively funded from research funds. It should be conducted according to a well-defined and peer-reviewed protocol and involve a formal randomized controlled trial. It should also be unconstrained by the commercial interests of the manufacturers, with all results publicly available and open to scrutiny. Whilst this takes place, a voluntary moratorium on all other uses of the device should be in place, backed up by the willingness of purchasers to exert financial sanctions on any NHS centre that does not 'toe-the-line'.

In this context, every application of a CAD would contribute to a better understanding of its appropriate use and its benefits and costs. Such controlled use of the devices could be justified in terms of the expected research gain for future patients, achieved in the most cost-effective manner. But *ad hoc* use of the devices would be unethical, because it would offer no such research gain but would simply be depriving other patients of scarce health-care resources for some of the interventions for which there is already plentiful research evidence to show benefits commensurate with the resources involved.

References

1. Buxton MJ. Scarce resources and informed choices. In: Ashton D (ed), *Future Trends in Medicine* (International Congress and Symposium Series 202). London: Royal Society of Medicine, 1993.
2. Fineberg HV. Reflections on medical innovation and health care reform. In: Gelijns AC (ed), *Medical Innovation at the Crossroads. Vol III: Technology and Health Care in an Era of Limits*. Washington, DC: National Academy Press, 1992.
3. Evans RW, Manninen DL, Overcast TD, *et al. The National Heart Transplantation Study: Final Report*. Seattle, Washington: Battelle Human Affairs Research Centres, 1984.
4. Buxton MJ, Acheson R, Caine N, *et al. Costs and Benefits of the Heart Transplant Programmes at Harefield and Papworth Hospitals* (DHSS Research Report 12). London: HMSO, 1985.
5. van Hout B, Bonsel B, Habbema D, *et al.* Heart transplantation in the Netherlands: costs, effects and scenarios. *J Health Econ* 1993; **12**, 73–93.
6. O'Brien BJ, Buxton MJ, Ferguson BA. Measuring the effectiveness of heart transplant programmes: quality of life data and their relationship to survival

analysis. *J Chron Dis* 1987; **40**, 137–153S.

7. Buxton MJ. Heart transplantation in the UK: the decision making context of an economic evaluation. In: Stocking B (ed), *Expensive Health Technologies: Regulatory and Administrative Mechanisms in Europe* (Commission of the European Communities, Health Services Research Series 5). Oxford: Oxford University Press, 1988.

8. Evans RW. Coverage and reimbursement for heart transplantation. *Int J Tech Assess Health Care* 1986; **2**, 425–449.

9. Borst-Eilers E. Assessing hospital technology in the Netherlands. *Br Med J* 1993; **306**, 226.

10. *Hansard*, 20 June 1969.

11. Lubeck DP, Bunker JP. *The Implications of Cost-Effectiveness Analysis of Medical Technology. Case Study 9: The Artificial Heart—Costs, Risks and Benefits.* Washington, DC: Office of Technology Assessment, 1982.

12. Working Group on Mechanical Circulatory Support (NHLBI). *Artificial Heart and Assist Devices: Directions, Needs, Costs and Societal Ethical Issues.* Washington, DC: National Institutes of Health, 1985.

13. Lubeck DP. The artificial heart: cost risks and benefits—an update. *Int J Tech Assess Health Care* 1986; **2**, 369–386.

14. Garrison P. Assessing the cost-effectiveness of development and use of the total artificial heart. Appendix E of *The Artificial Heart: Prototypes, Policies and Patients*, Washington, DC: Institute of Medicine, 1991.

15. Black N, Johnston A. Volume and outcome in hospital care: evidence, explanations and implications. *Health Serv Mgmt Res* 1990; **3**, 108–114.

16. Hannan E, *et al.* The relationship between in-hospital mortality rate and surgical volume after controlling for clinical risk factors. *Med Care* 1991; **29**, 1094–1107.

17. Buxton MJ. Resource implications of heart transplantation. In: Wallwork J (ed), *Heart and Lung Transplantation.* Philadelphia: WB Saunders, 1989.

18. Institute of Medicine. *The Artificial Heart: Prototypes, Policies and Patients.* Washington, DC: Institute of Medicine, 1991.

19. van Hout BA, Wielink G, Bonsel GJ, Rutten FFH. Effects of ACE inhibitors on heart failure in the Netherlands: a pharmacoeconomic model. *Pharmacoeconomics* 1993; **3**, 387–397.

20. CONSENSUS (Cooperative North Scandinavia Enalapril Survival Study). Effects of enalapril on mortality in severe congestive heart failure. *New Engl J Med* 1987; **316**, 1429–1435.

21. SOLVD Investigators. Effect of enalapril on survival in patients with reduced left ventricular ejection fractions and congestive heart failure. *New Engl J Med* 1991; **325**, 293–302.

22. Flosequinan withdrawn. *Lancet* 1993; **342**, 235.

23. Wellcome shares dip after heart drug study is halted. *The Times* 1993; 22 June: 24.

24. Cochrane AL. *Effectiveness and Efficiency: Random Reflections on Health Services* (The 1971 Rock Carling Fellowship Lecture). London: Nuffield Provincial Hospitals Trust, 1972.

45

The ethical considerations of circulatory support

Sir Terence English

The ethical issues faced by doctors involved with support systems are no different in kind from those we meet in our routine practice. However, there are some factors which make these ethical issues more acute at the present stage of development of this new technology. First, the devices are still largely at an experimental stage. Second, there are enormous resource implications. Third, the patients with whom we deal in these situations are often in a critical condition. These factors all tend to focus the ethical issues more sharply than in more established branches of medicine.

Before examining some of these issues in more detail, let us first be clear about some definitions. Originally, as I understand it, 'ethics' and 'morals' were two terms that were used by the Greeks and the Romans to describe something very similar conceptually, and that was the code of conduct which was acceptable and normal within a particular society. In the modern world this is no longer so. Medical *ethics* represents an accepted code of behaviour within a particular group, namely the medical profession, whereas *morality* implies acceptance of standards wider than that group, and usually based on either a philosophy or a religion. Both of these in turn need to be distinguished from *legality*, which is relatively easily determined by reference to statute law in individual countries. So it is possible, in the judgement of a particular group, for something to be legal but unethical, and conversely, in the judgement of a particular individual, for some-thing to be ethical but immoral.

As doctors we use technical skills and expertise which give us great power over patients, who by the nature of things are usually dependent and vulnerable. Patients, therefore, have the right to expect that the series of judgements and decisions which contribute to their overall management are made fairly in the light of our knowledge and our experience and which should be brought to bear wholly for the benefit of the individual patient. This concept is embodied in that part of the Hippocratic tradition which obliges the doctor to 'Follow that system and regimen, which according to my ability and judgement, I consider for the benefit of my patients and abstain from whatever is deleterious and mischievous'.

Let us now examine some of the more important ethical issues that are generated by the application of mechanical circulatory support systems. These can perhaps best be considered under the following headings:

1. The evaluation of the devices at our disposal.
2. The whole area of informed consent. Related to this is often the question of timing of insertion and removal of devices, and in that category I will touch on the question of bridging to transplantation.
3. The conflict over the use of resources both at an individual or local level and at a national level.

As far as the testing and evaluation of devices is

concerned, I think we can look at this with regard to the obligations of the manufacturers and the obligations of the clinicians. I believe that manufacturers have a clear ethical obligation to undertake the development and testing of devices in a responsible way and to pay careful attention to quality-control issues. I think also that clinicians and researchers who become involved in the assessment of devices should make sure that they have a solid background knowledge of the subject, should get properly trained in any of the specific techniques that are required, and should follow rigorous research protocols. Very importantly, I believe that honest and accurate reporting of the results of the work as it develops needs to be accomplished, both by manufacturers and by researchers.

Informed consent can obviously be difficult to obtain in this particular area. We get some solace from the fact that protocols are now scrutinized very carefully by local ethics committees who usually pay careful attention to how informed consent is to be achieved. However, many of the issues are complex and have implications which patients may find very difficult to follow; hence, the 17-page document which Barney Clark had to sign before he received the first permanent artificial heart. Problems may also arise with the intellectual function of the patient, if this is clouded by the consequences of low cardiac output and metabolic dysfunction. When we first started heart transplantation in 1979, I was reluctant to take on young children, largely because of problems with informed consent. Parents would inevitably make decisions that were determined by a desire to see their child alive whatever the consequences, and we were unable to explain to the patient, namely the child, what some of the consequences might be. Occasionally we are faced with the problem of it not being possible to obtain consent at all, and then we can only act on the basis of what we believe to be in the best interest of the patient at that particular time and be prepared to defend the decision later if necessary.

Important ethical issues are involved, too, in the debate on bridging to transplantation. There is no denying that we should use all donor organs to their best possible effect. There is, however, a fundamental contract that the doctor enters into when he or she accepts a particular patient for treatment. This is something which weighs heavily on most of us. There can be a very real conflict between the clinician's responsibility to the individual patient and the responsibility to all the other potential patients needing transplantation. This can create a difficult dilemma, but my own ethical inclination has always tended towards the patient who I had already accepted to treat to the best of my ability.

In addition, the question of bridging to transplantation and what impact this might or might not have on waiting lists is a very important one. The issue appears to be surfacing in the USA with liver transplantations, where on a number of occasions pig livers have been used as a bridge to transplantation, with these patients then moving to the top of the waiting list for human liver transplantation. I have grave doubts as to whether this is an ethical way of proceeding. The priority on our own waiting list is based primarily on when the patient is accepted into the programme, and we tell patients this at the time they go on the list. However, we also explain that when a donor organ becomes available we look first at blood group compatibility, and then at other matching requirements such as size and pulmonary vascular resistance; and then the first patient who fits these criteria would normally get the organ. This is something that most patients find easy to understand, but at the same time it is made clear that there may be occasions when we give preference to a patient who is going downhill fast and in whom we know that a particular organ could be life-saving. I suspect that British patients, being used to the National Health Service and to the concept of being on waiting lists for treatment, accept this as a way of dealing with a difficult problem. However, the whole question of how best to distribute donor organs raises ethical issues which need to be reviewed periodically, as we have been doing recently in Britain.

The conflicts over resource use can, as already indicated, be broken down into local and national dimensions. The impact of a large transplant programme on colleagues and other activities in a hospital are not inconsiderable, and it seems proper to obtain their cooperation and support where possible in order to ensure that other services in the hospital do not suffer. Similar considerations apply to mechanical circulatory support, which can be very resource hungry at a local level. On the wider social level, it should be emphasized that health care inevitably is rationed in every country in one way or another, and somehow as professionals we have to get involved with the setting of priorities. I have no doubt that over the next 5–10 years the priorities for mechanical circulatory assist devices in the overall context of provision of health care will receive a lot of ethical consideration, in those countries in which it is applied.

Finally, returning to the question of the need to look at costs and benefits, I believe that it is important to go beyond individual technologies and to embark on a comparative cost–benefit analysis in which attempts are made to compare other developing technologies using similar methodologies. This is something that several economists are currently addressing. At present their measurements are rather crude, but as decisions on priorities start to be made on the basis of the results of their analyses, so the techniques will become more refined. I think we are now at a stage when we can do useful comparative cost–benefit studies between mechanical assist devices and standard treatment for heart failure, and I hope very much that this will be accomplished.

Appendix: Technical review of circulatory support devices

Dereck Wheeldon and Terry McCarthy

The following review of mechanical circulatory support (MCS) devices is designed to provide the reader with an overview of the technical specifications of devices currently available and those which have reached a significant stage of development.

The information is categorized according to the placement of the pump: extracorporeal (E), paracorporeal (P) or implantable (I). There is a cross-reference to the manufacturer for each device.

The information was collected by questionnaire to all known manufacturers and developers, from whom we had an excellent response, in most cases. There were a few who declined to provide any information. These have been asterisked and whatever information is in the published literature has been collated. In other cases, the information requested was incomplete and, following further requests, still not provided. In these cases missing information is indicated by (–).

Whilst this review is not entirely comprehensive, we believe that it includes all the 'main players' and should serve to provide the reader with a good representation of the scope and variety of endeavours in this exciting and challenging field.

Extracorporeal devices

E1, E2	Metronic, Minnesota, USA
E3	Abiomed, Massachusetts, USA
E4	Sarns/3M Health Care, Michigan, USA
E5	St Jude Medical, Massachusetts, USA
E6	Helmholtz Institute, Aachen, Germany
E7	University Hospital Zurich, Switzerland

Paracorporeal devices

P1, P2	Pennsylvania State University, USA
P3	Thoratec Laboratories Corporation, California, USA
P4	Biomed SA, Madrid, Spain
P5	Helmholtz Institute for Biomedical Engineering, Aachen, Germany
P6	Fehling Medical/Free University of Berlin, Germany
P7	Vacord Bioengineering Res Co Ltd, Czech Republic
P8	KX Qian/Medical College of University of Taiwan, Taipei, Taiwan
P9, P10,	Baylor College of Medicine, Texas, USA
P11	
P12	Vacord Bioengineering Research Co Ltd, Czech Republic
*P13	Toyobo, Osaka, Japan
*P14	Nippon Zeon Co Ltd, Tokyo, Japan

Implantable devices

I1	Terracor SARL, La Vallette, France
I2	Johnson & Johnson Interventional Systems, California, USA
I3	SUN Medical Technology Research Corporation, Nagano-Ken, Japan
I4	Helmholtz Institute for Biomedical Engineering, Aachen, Germany
I5	Kyoto University Faculty of Medicine, Kyoto, Japan
I6	University of Utah, Utah, USA
I7, I8	Thermo Cardiosystems Inc, Mass., USA
I9	University of Vienna, Vienna, Austria
I10	Allegheny-Singer Research Institute, Pennsylvania, USA
I11	Pennsylvania State University, USA
I12, I13	Baxter Healthcare Corporation, Novacor Division, California, USA
I14	Thoratec Laboratories Corporation, California, USA
I15	University of Ottawa Heart Institute and University of Utah, Ottawa, Canada
I16, I17	Pennsylvania State University, USA
I18	Cleveland Clinic – Nimbus, Ohio, USA
I19	Helmholtz Institute, Aachen, Germany
I20	Bioengineering Laboratory, University of Vienna, Vienna, Austria
I21	Vacord Engineering Research Co Ltd, Czech Republic
I22	Centre for Cardiac Surgery, Salzburg, Austria
I23	CardioWest, Arizona, USA
I24, I25,	Baylor College of Medicine, Texas, USA
I26	

Addresses and contacts

Abiomed Inc, 33 Cherry Hill Drive, Danvers, MA
01923, USA
Tel: +1 508 777 5410
Fax: +1 508 777 1561
Contact: Bruce J Shook
R&D supported by Abiomed
DEVICE: E3

Allegheny-Singer Research Institute, 320 East North
Avenue, Pittsburgh, PA 15212, USA
Tel: +1 412 359 4912
Fax: +1 412 359 5071
Contact: Andrew H Goldstein
Investor-funded research
DEVICE: I10

Baxter Healthcare Corporation, Novacor Division,
7799 Pardee Lane, Oakland, CA 94621, USA
Tel: +1 510 568 8338
Fax: +1 510 633 1057
Contact: Phillip J Miller
Funded by Baxter
DEVICE: I12, I13

Baylor College of Medicine, Department of Surgery,
One Baylor Plaza, Houston, TX 77030, USA
Tel: +1 713 798 4434
Fax: +1 713 798 3985
Contacts: Yukihiko Nose/Michael E De Bakey (I24)
Funded by university/hospital
DEVICES: P9, P10, P11, I24, I25, I26

Biomed SA, Parque Tecnologico de Madrid,
C/Einstein 3, Tres Cantos, 28760 Madrid, Spain
Tel: +34 1 8039 193
Fax: +34 1 8036 668
Contact: Antonio Arribas
R&D supported by Biomed
Research funded by university/hospital
DEVICE: P4

CardioWest Technologies Inc, 1501 N. Campbell
Avenue, Suite 5505, Tucson, AZ 85724, USA
Tel: +1 602 694 6200
Fax: +1 602 694 2630
Contact: Richard G Smith
University/hospital funded research
DEVICE: I23

Centre for Cardiac Surgery, Salzburg, Austria
Tel: +43 662 4482 ext 3351
Fax: +43 662 433 840
Contact: Prof Felix Unger
Government funded research
DEVICE: I22

Cleveland Clinic Foundation – Nimbus Corporation,
9500 Euclid Avenue, Cleveland, OH 44195, USA
Tel: +1 216 445 7082
Fax: +1 216 444 9198
Contact: Raymond J Kiraly
85% of funding by government grants
15% by hospital/university
DEVICE: I18

Fehling Medical/Free University of Berlin, Usedomer
Strasse 4, D-13355 Berlin, Germany
Tel: +49 30 463 5008
Fax: +49 30 463 4059
Contact: Andreas Goullon
R&D supported by Fehling Medical
Funded by government, university and investors
DEVICE: P6

Helmholtz Institute for Biomedical Engineering,
Pauwelstrasse 30, D-5100 Aachen, Germany
Tel: +49 241 8088 766
Fax: +49 241 8089 416
Contacts: T Siep/H Reul
Government sponsored institution
DEVICES: E6, P5, I4, I19

Johnson & Johnson Interventional Systems, 2890
Kilgore Road, Rancho Cordova, CA 95656, USA
Tel: +1 916 631 1800
Fax: +1 916 638 4587
Contact: Mike Wright
Funded by parent company
DEVICE: I2

KX Qian/Medical College of University of Taiwan, 7
Chung Shan Road, Taipei, Taiwan
Tel: +886 2 3123456 ext 8728
Fax: +886 2 3224793
Contact: KX Qian
Government funded research
DEVICE: P8

Kyoto University Faculty of Medicine, Department of
Cardiovascular Surgery, 54 Shougoin-Kawaramachi,
Sakyo-ku, Kyoto 606, Japan
Tel: +61 75 751 3780
Fax: +61 75 753 2906
Contact: Teiji Oda
Research funded by university
DEVICE: I5

Medtronic Biomedicus, 9600 West 76th Street, Eden
Prairie, MN 55344, USA
Tel: +1 612 943 7733
Fax: +1 612 943 7714
Contact: Donald Georgi
R&D supported by Medtronic
DEVICES: E1, E2

Nippon Zeon Co Ltd, 2-6-1 Marunouchi Chiyoda-ku, Tokyo, Japan
Tel: +81 3 216 1771
Fax: –
Contact: –
Research: –
DEVICE: P14

Pennsylvania State University, College of Medicine, The Milton S Hershey Medical Center, 500 University Drive, Hershey, PA 17033, USA
Tel: +1 717 531 8328/7068/6301
Fax: +1 717 531 5011/4464/4464
Contact: William S Pierce/Alan J Snyder/Gerson Rosenberg
Research funded by the government, university and charity
DEVICES: P1, P2, I11, I16, I17

St Jude Medical, Cardiac Assist Division, 12 Elizabeth Drive, Chelmsford, MA 01824, USA
Tel: +1 508 250 8020
Fax: +1 508 250 1727
Contact: William Edelman
R&D for this device supported by St Jude
DEVICE: E5

Sarns/3M Health Care, 6200 Jackson Road, Ann Arbor, MI 48103, USA
Tel: 0101 492 861 803 739
Fax: 0101 492 861 803 444
Contact: Klaus Kiwitz
Funding unavailable owing to company constraints
DEVICE: E4

SUN Medical Technology Research Corporation, 1-3-11 Suwa, Suwa-shi, Nagano-ken, 392 Japan
Tel: +81 266 53 9630
Fax: +81 266 58 6443
Contact: Toshio Mori
Research funded by government grants and SUN Medical
DEVICE: I3

Terracor SARL, Parc Sainte Claire, Avenue des Freres Lumiere, F 83160 La Valette, France
Tel: +33 94 20 43 55
Fax: +33 94 27 35 57
Contact: Jean-Luc Tourres
Funded by government grants, charity, university or hospital funds
DEVICE: I1

Thermo Cardiosystems Inc (TCI), 470 Wildwood Street, PO Box 2697, Woburn, MA 01888-2697, USA
Tel: +1 617 932 8668
Fax: +1 617 933 4476
Contact: Betty Silverstein
R&D funded by Thermo Cardiosystems
DEVICES: I7, I8

Thoratec Laboratories Corporation, 2023 Eighth Street, Berkeley, CA 94710, USA
Tel: +1 510 841 1213
Fax: +1 510 845 3935
Contact: David J Farrar
DEVICES: P3, I14

Toyobo Co Ltd, 2–8 Dojima Harna 2-chome, Kita-ku, Osaka 530, Japan
Tel: +81 6 348 4209
Fax: +81 6 348 4492
Contact: –
Research: –
DEVICE: P13

University of Ottawa Heart Institute and University of UT, Cardiovascular Devices Division, 1053 Carling Avenue – Rm H560, Ottawa, Ontario K1Y 4E9, Canada
Tel: +1 613 761 4323
Fax: +1 613 724 7921
Contact: Dr Tofy Mussivand
Research funding by the university, charity, government, investor and parent company
DEVICE: I15

University of Utah, Artificial Heart Research Laboratory, 803 North 300 West, Salt Lake City, UT 84103, USA
Tel: +1 801 595 7256
Fax: +1 801 581 4044
Contact: Dr Donald Olsen
Research funded by university, government and charity
DEVICE: I6

University of Vienna, Bioengineering Laboratory, 2nd Dept of Surgery, Van Swietengasse 1, A-1090 Vienna, Austria
Tel: +43 1 40400 2424
Fax: +43 1 40400 2353
Contact: Dr H Schima/DiplIng A Prodinger
Funded by government, university and investors
DEVICES: I9, I20

University Hospital Zurich, Clinic for Cardiovascular Surgery, CH-8091 Zurich, Switzerland
Tel: +41 1 255 11 11
Fax: +41 1 255 44 49
Contact: Dr LK von Segesser
Research supported by University Hospital Zurich
DEVICE: E7

Vacord Bioengineering Research Co Ltd, 61400 BRNO-Husovicz, Cascovicka 53, Czech Republic
Tel: +42 5 577211
Fax: –
Contact: Prof Yaromir Vasku
Research: –
DEVICES: P7, P12, I21

Extracorporeal devices

Ao	aorta	LV	left ventricle	PV	peripheral vein
C	centrifugal	O	optional	RA	right atrium
D	diaphragm	P	preferred	SV	stroke volume
E	electrical	Pa	peripheral artery	TL	trileaflet
EM	electromagnetic	PA	pulmonary artery	VR	variable rate
FSV	fixed stroke volume	PC	power consumption	VSV	variable stroke volume
HEP	heparin	PN	pneumatic	WT	weight ± blood
LA	left atrial	Pu	polyurethane		

Code	Name	Position	Comments	Control	
				Ext	Type
E1	Biopump$_{50}$	Bedside	Concentric cone Biopump	✗	E
E2	Biopump$_{80}$	Bedside	Concentric cone Biopump	✗	E
E3	BVS-5000	Bedside	Pulsatile VAD	✗	E
E4	Delphin	Bedside	Vaned pump with pulsatile option	✗	E
E5	Isoflow	Bedside	Inclined vane pump	✗	E
E6	Helmholtz	Bedside	Seal-less vaned impeller	✗	E
E7	VFP	Bedside	Vane-less friction pump	✗	E

Code	Actuator		Pumping chamber	Category		Routine bypass
	On controller	Remote		C	D	
E1	✗	✗	EM	✗		✗
E2	✗	✗	EM	✗		✗
E3		✗	PN		✗	–
E4	✗		EM	✗		✗
E5	✗	✗	EM	✗		✗
E6	✗	✗	EM	✗		✗
E7	✗		EM	✗		✗

Code	Inflow						Outflow				Valves		
	LA	LV	Pa	RA	RV	Pv	Ao	Pa	PA	Pv	Type	In (mm)	Out (mm)
E1	✗	✗	✗	✗	✗	✗	✗	✗	✗	✗	None	None	None
E2	✗	✗	✗	✗	✗	✗	✗	✗	✗	✗	None	None	None
E3	✗			✗			✗			✗	PuTL	25	25
E4	✗	✗	✗	✗	✗	✗	✗	✗	✗	✗	None	None	None
E5	✗	✗	✗	✗	✗	✗	✗	✗	✗	✗	None	None	None
E6	✗	✗	✗	✗	✗	✗	✗	✗	✗	✗	None	None	None
E7	✗	✗	✗	✗	✗		✗		✗		None	None	None

Code	Pump characteristics					Control algorithms			
	Output max (l/m)	Pump vol (ml)	SV max (ml)	PC (watts)	Size L×W×D (mm)	Non-pulse	Pulse	FSV VR	VSV VR
E1	5.0	50	–	15	70×70×50	✗			
E2	10.0	80	–	30	70×70×70	✗			
E3	5.0	660	90	280	400×60×60		✗	✗	
E4	10.0	48	–	–	85×85×70	P	O		✗
E5	10.0	65	–	–	90×90×70	✗			
E6	15.0	25	–	25	70×70×60	✗			
E7	30.0	22	–	–	100×100×15	✗			

Code	Blood pump design characteristics					Stage of development
	WT + blood (g)	WT − blood (g)	Max duration (h)	Surface	Modification	
E1	40	20	4	Acryl	HEP bond	Clinical 17 years
E2	50	25	4	Acryl	HEP bond	Clinical 17 years
E3	2300	1600	None	Pu-multi		Clinical 6 years
E4	179	128	4	PU	–	Clinical 6 years
E5	350	290	6	Acryl	–	Clinical 5 years
E6	115	90	48	Acryl	–	Laboratory
E7	–	–	–	Acryl	HEP bond	Laboratory

Paracorporeal devices

Ao	aorta	O	optional	SMA	surface modifications agent (silicon polymers)
C	centrifugal	P	preferred	SV	stroke volume
D	diaphragm	Pa	peripheral artery	TL	trileaflet
FSV	fixed stroke volume	PA	pulmonary artery	VR	variable rate
HEP	heparin	PC	power consumption	VSV	variable stroke volume
LA	left atrial	Pu	polyurethane	WT	weight + blood
LV	left ventricle	RA	right atrium		
Mdisc	mechanical disc				

Code	Name	Application		Actuator				Category	
		Uni	Bi	Cable	Electric motor	Pneumatic	E/H motor	C	D
P1	Pierce–Donachy		✗			✗			✗
P2	Penn State (Paed)		✗			✗			✗
P3	Thoratec		✗			✗			✗
P4	BCM		✗			✗			✗
P5	HIA-VAD		✗			✗			✗
P6	Berlin Heart		✗			✗			✗
P7	BRNO-VAD	✗							✗
P8	KX QIAM		✗		✗			✗	
P9	Baylor-Nikkiso		✗	✗				✗	
P10	Baylor Gyro M		✗		✗			✗	
P11	Baylor Gyro C		✗		✗	✗		✗	
P12	TNS-BRNO LVAD	✗				✗			✗
*P13	Toyobo		✗			✗			✗
*P14	Xmex 60		✗			✗			✗

Code	Inflow				Outflow		Valves			
	LA	LV	RA	RV	Ao	PA	No.	Type	In (mm)	Out (mm)
P1	✗	✗	✗	✗	✗	✗		Mdisc	27	25
P2	✗		✗		✗	✗		Mdisc	–	–
P3	✗	✗	✗	✗	✗	✗		Mdisc	29	21
P4	✗		✗		✗	✗		MBL	29	21
P5	✗		✗		✗	✗		PuTL	21	21
P6	✗	✗	✗	✗	✗	✗		Mdisc or PuTL	22	22
P7	✗	✗			✗			PuBL	34	24
P8	✗		✗		✗	✗	✗			
P9	✗	✗	✗	✗	✗	✗	✗			
P10	✗	✗	✗	✗	✗	✗	✗			
P11	✗	✗	✗	✗	✗	✗	✗			
P12	✗	✗	–	–	✗	–		PuML	34	34
*P13	✗	–	✗	–	✗	✗		Mdisc	–	–
*P14	✗	–	✗	–	✗	✗		Mdisc	18	18

Code	Pump characteristics					Control algorithms					
	Output max (l/m)	Pump vol (ml)	Sv max (ml)	PC (watts)	Size L × W × D (mm)	Non-pulse	Pulse	Sync/async	FSV VR	VSV VR	VSV FR
P1	8.0	–	70	–	140 × 90 × 50		✗	O/P	P		
P2	1.0	25	14		47 × 54 × 33		✗	O/P			O
P3	6.5		65		140 × 90 × 50		✗	O/P	P	O	O
P4	7.0	125	75		100 × 100 × 95		✗	O/P	O	P	
P5a	9.8		70		190 × 90 × 50		✗	O/P	P	O	
b	8.4		60		180 × 85 × 47		✗	O/P	P	O	
c	1.4		10		100 × 50 × 30		✗	O/P	P	O	
P6a	8.5		80		185 × 70 × 80		✗	O/P	O	P	
b	6.5		50		160 × 60 × 75		✗	O/P	O	P	
c	1.6		8		160 × 60 × 75		✗	O/P	O	P	
P7	9.6		80	5	–		✗	P/O	P		
P8	10.0	20	–	–	38 × 38 × 65	O	P	P/O		P	
P9	10.0	25	–	15	66 × 66 × 58	✗		As	–	–	–
P10	5.0	30	–	15	75 × 75 × 100	✗		As	–	–	–
P11	10.0	38	–	–	84 × 84 × 10	✗		As	–	–	–
P12	7.2	–	80	–	85 × 55 × 75	✗		P/O	–	P	O
*P13	6.2	–	80	–	–	✗		–	–	–	–
*P14	7.5	–	100	–	–	✗		P/O	–	P	O

Code	Blood pump design characteristics					Stage of development
	WT + blood (g)	WT − blood (g)	Max duration (h)	Surface	Modification	
P1	460	390	–	Pu	–	Limited clinical
P2	86	58	–	Pu	–	Laboratory
P3	448	383	–	Pu-multi	SMA	63 centres worldwide
P4	244	112	–	Pu		Early clinical, single centre
P5a	370	180	3/12	Pu	HEP	Laboratory
b	320	155	3/12	Pu	HEP	Laboratory
c	60	30	3/12	Pu	HEP	Laboratory
P6a	290	160	6/12	Pu	HEP	Laboratory
b	220	160	6/12	Pu	HEP	Laboratory
c	210	160	6/12	Pu	HEP	Laboratory
P7	300	220		Pu-multi	–	Clinical 3 centres
P8	130	100	–	Pu	–	Laboratory
P9	170	145	2/7	Pu-multi	–	Clinical 3 centres
P10	430	400	2/7	Pu	–	Laboratory
P11	638	600	2/7	Pu	–	Laboratory
P12	280	–	–	Steel/Pu	–	Laboratory
*P13	–	–	–	Pu	–	Clinical
*P14	–	–	–	Pu	Cardiothane	Clinical 21 centres

Implantable devices

A	axial	EM	electromechanical	Pi piston
Abdom	abdominal cavity	IntraVasc	intravascular	PP push plate
C	centrifugal	Mdisc	mechanical disc	Pu polyurethane
D	diaphragm	O	optional	S skeletal
EH	electrohydraulic	P	preferred	Thorac thoracic cavity

Code	Name	Application			Category						Anatomical position		
		Uni	Bi	TAH	C	A	D	Pi	PP	S	Intra Vasc	Thorac	Abdom
I1	VAGSI	✗						✗					L wall
I2	Hemopump	Left				✗						LV-Ao		
I3	IVAX	Left				✗						LV-Ao		
I4	HIA-Microaxial	Left				✗						Ao-LV		
I5	Dual Skeletal	Left								✗		L pleura	
I6	EHTAH			✗			✗						Ortho	
I7	HeartMate IP	Left							✗				L wall
I8	HeartMate VE	Left							✗				L wall
I9	Vienna Centrifugal	L/R			✗								Int rib	
I10	Hemadyne AB180	L/R			✗								Int rib	
I11	Penn State RSVAD	L/R							✗				L or R
I12	Novacor N100P	Left							✗				L wall
I13	Novacor N100W	Left							✗				L wall
I14	Thoratec MVAD	L/R							✗				Pleural	
I15	Unified EVAD	L/R				✗							Pleural	
I16	Penn State Heart			✗			✗						Ortho	
I17	Penn State RS TAH			✗					✗				Ortho	
I18	Cleveland Nimbus E4T			✗					✗				Ortho	
I19	HIA-TAH			✗					✗				Ortho	
I20	New Vienna TAH			✗			✗						Ortho	
I21	TNS-BRNO TAH			✗			✗						Ortho	
I22	Unger TAH			✗			✗						Ortho	
I23	CardioWest C-70 TAH			✗			✗						Ortho	
I24	Baylor-NASA VAD		✗			✗							L pleura	
I25	Baylor Permanent LVAD	✗							✗				L wall
I26	Baylor Permanent TAH			✗					✗				Ortho	

Code	Inflow valves Type	Size (mm)	Outflow valves Type	Size (mm)	Cable	Pneumatic	EM	Max output (l/m)	Pump vol (ml)	Max SV (ml)	PC (watts)	Size H×W×D (mm)
I1	None		None			✗		9.0	75	60	20	50×9.5×9
I2	None		None		✗			5.0	5.02	–	70	8.0 dia
I3	None		None			✗		8.5	–	–	14	14.0 dia
I4	None		None		✗			3.0	–	–	2.5	6.5 dia
I5	Bio	–	Bio	–		✗		8.8	29.7	10.7	–	15×6 dia
I6	Disc	27	Disc	27			EH	12.8	700	92.0	40	90×117×114
I7	Bio	25	Bio	25		✗		10.0	–	83	–	40×112 dia
I8	Bio	25	Bio	25		✗		10.0	–	83	–	42×112 dia
I9	None		None					8.0	45	–	15	85×85×45
I10	None		None					7.0	5	–	4	50×60×60
I11								9.0	150	62	6.5	93×78×75
I12	Bio	21	Bio	21		✗		10.5	120	70	14.0	170×134×62
I13	Bio	21	Bio	21		✗		10.5	120	70	10.0	170×134×62
I14	Disc	–	Disc	–		✗		5.2	–	65	–	–
I15	Bio/Disc	–	Bio/Disc	–			EH	11.0	–	73	35	40×118×183
I16	Disc	27	Disc	25		✗		10.0	–	70	–	110×115×83
I17	Disc	27	Disc	25		✗		9.0	120	62	7.5	100×92×78
I18	Bio	29	Bio	25			EH	9.6	620	60	10.0	120×80×100
I19	PU	27	PU	23			EM	9.5	650	73	27	94×94×120
I20	Mdisc	23	Mdisc	23		✗		10.0	–	72	200	72×72×56
I21	PU	34	PU	24		✗		14.0	120	80	–	60×85×35
I22	Mdisc	29	Mdisc	27		✗		16.0	110	100	–	80×40×70
I23	Mdisc	27	Mdisc	25		✗		10	380	70	–	140×80×75
I24	None	None	None	None	✗			9.5	5.0	–	10	85×25 dia
I25	Bio	21	Bio	21			EM	9.6	–	63	11	115×97×32
I26	Bio	27	Bio	23			EM	9.6	–	63	14.6	83×97 dia

Code	Non-pulse	Pulse	Sync AS	FSV VR	VSR VR	VSV FR	Wt+ blood	Wt- blood	Max duration	Surface	Mod	Stage of development
I1		✗	AS	P	–	–	1500	1400	3 mths	Titanium	Diamond	Laboratory
I2	✗		AS	–	–	–	10	5.9	7 days	S. steel		Clinical 7 centres
I3	✗		AS	–	–	–	–	261	–	S. steel		Laboratory
I4	✗		AS	–	–	–	–	9.5	7 days	S. steel		Laboratory
I5		✗	S	P	–	–	–	–	Perm	Muscle		Laboratory
I6		✗	N/A	P	–	O	–	790	5 yrs	Pu		Laboratory
I7		✗	S	P	–	O	–	570	–	Tit/Pu	Rough	Clinical 72 centres
I8		✗	S	P	–	O	–	–	–	Tit/Pu	Rough	Clinical 9 centres
I9	✗		AS	–	–	–	400	355	7 days	Tit/epoxy		Laboratory
I10	✗		–	–	–	–	245	240	6 mths	Pu/C	Biomer	Laboratory
I11		✗	AS	P	–	O	865	700	–	Pu		Laboratory
I12		✗	S	–	P	O	900	850	>2 yrs	Pu	Biomer	Clinical 38 centres
I13		✗	S	–	P	O	900	850	>1 yr	Pu	Biomer	Clinical 38 centres
I14		✗	S	P	–	–	–	–	–	–		Laboratory
I15	X		S	P	O	O	810	750	>2 yrs	Pu		Laboratory
I16		✗	n/a	PL	–	PR	704	440	–	Pu		Clinical 1 centre
I17		✗	n/a	PL	–	PR	975	710	–	Pu		Laboratory
I18		✗	S	–	P	–	795	735	Perm	Pu	Gelatin	Laboratory
I19		✗	S	P	–	–	–	–	>2 yrs	Pu		Laboratory
I20		✗	AS	O	–	P	150	75	Weeks	Pu		Clinical 1 centre
I21		✗	S	P	–	–	300	–	–	Pu		Clinical 3 centres
I22		✗	S	P	–	O	–	–	–	Pu		Clinical 3 centres
I23		✗	n/a	–	–	P	–	1.95	–	Pu	Biomer	Clinical 9 centres
I24	✗		AS	–	–	–	70	65	3 mths	S. steel	Pu	Laboratory
I25		✗		–	P	O	635	570	5 yrs	Pu	Gelatin	Laboratory
I26		✗	n/a	–	O	P	685	620	5 yrs	Pu	Gelatin	Laboratory

Index